Nutrition and Meta

Edited on behalf of The Nutrition Society by

Michael J. Gibney, Ian A. Macdonald
and Helen M. Roche

Blackwell
Science

Published by Blackwell Science
a Blackwell Publishing company
Editorial offices:
Blackwell Science Ltd, 9600 Garsington Road,
Oxford OX4 2DQ, UK
  Tel: +44 (0) 1865 776868
Iowa State Press, a Blackwell Publishing Company,
2121 State Avenue, Ames, Iowa 50014-8300, USA
  Tel: +1 515 292 0140
Blackwell Science Asia Pty, 550 Swanston Street, Carlton, Victoria 3053, Australia
  Tel: +61 (0)3 8359 1011

First published 2003

SMC

Library of Congress
Cataloging-in-Publication Data
Nutrition and metabolism / edited on behalf of the
Nutrition Society by Michael J. Gibney, Ian MacDonald, and Helen M. Roche. – 1st ed.
    p. cm.
    ISBN 0-632-05625-8 (pbk. : alk. paper)
1. Nutrition. 2. Metabolism. I. Gibney, Michael J. II. Macdonald, Ian, 1921–
III. Roche, Helen M. IV. Nutrition Society (Great Britain)

    QP141.N7768 2003
    612.3–dc22

                                                    2003015190

ISBN 0-632-05625-8

A catalogue record for this title is available from the British Library

Set in Minion by Gray Publishing, Tunbridge Wells, Kent
Printed and bound in Great Britain using acid-free paper
by Ashford Colour Press, Gosport

For further information on Blackwell Publishing, visit our website:

www.blackwellpublishing.com

The Human Nutrition Textbook Series

The International Scientific Committee

Editor-in-Chief
Professor Michael J Gibney
Trinity College, Dublin, Ireland

Assistant Editor
Julie Dowsett
Trinity College, Dublin, Ireland

Professor Lenore Arab
University of North Carolina, USA

Professor Yvon Carpentier
Université Libre de Bruxelles, Belgium

Professor Marinos Elia
University of Southampton, UK

Professor Frans J Kok
Wageningen University, Netherlands

Professor Olle Ljungqvist
Ersta Hospital & Huddinge University Hospital, Sweden

Professor Ian Macdonald
University of Nottingham, UK

Professor Barrie Margetts
University of Southampton, UK

Professor Kerin O'Dea
Menzies School of Health Research, Darwin, Australia

Dr Helen Roche
Trinity College, Dublin, Ireland

Professor Hester H Vorster
Potchefstroom, South Africa

Textbook Editors

Introduction to Human Nutrition
Editor-in-Chief
Professor Michael J Gibney
Trinity College, Dublin, Ireland

Professor Hester H Vorster
Potchefstroom, South Africa

Professor Frans J Kok
Wageningen University, Netherlands

Nutrition and Metabolism
Editor-in-Chief
Professor Michael J Gibney
Trinity College, Dublin, Ireland

Professor Ian Macdonald
University of Nottingham, UK

Dr Helen Roche,
Trinity College, Dublin, Ireland

Public Health Nutrition
Editor-in-Chief
Professor Michael J Gibney
Trinity College, Dublin, Ireland

Professor Barrie Margetts
University of Southampton, UK

Professor Lenore Arab
University of North Carolina, USA

Dr John Kearney
Dublin Institute of Technology, Ireland

Clinical Nutrition
Editor-in-Chief
Professor Michael J Gibney
Trinity College, Dublin, Ireland

Professor Marinos Elia
University of Southampton, UK

Professor Olle Ljungqvist
Ersta Hospital & Huddinge University Hospital, Sweden

www.nutritiontexts.com

A unique feature of the Nutrition Society Textbook Series is that each chapter will have its own web pages, accessible at www.nutritiontexts.com. In the course of time, each will have downloadable teaching aids, suggestions for projects, updates on the content of each chapter and sample multiple choice questions. With input from teachers and students we will have a vibrant, informative and social website.

The Human Nutrition Textbook series comprises:

Introduction to Human Nutrition

Introduction to Human Nutrition: a global perspective on food and nutrition
Body composition
Energy metabolism
Nutrition and metabolism of proteins and amino acids
Digestion and metabolism of carbohydrates
Nutrition and metabolism of lipids
Dietary reference standards
The vitamins
Minerals and trace elements
Measuring food intake
Food composition
Food policy and regulatory issues
Nutrition research methodology
Food safety: a public health issue of growing importance
Food and nutrition: the global challenge

Nutrition and Metabolism

Core concepts of nutrition
Molecular nutrition
Integration of metabolism 1: Energy
Integration of metabolism 2: Protein and amino acids
Integration of metabolism 3: Macronutrients
Pregnancy and lactation
Growth and aging
Nutrition and the brain
The sensory systems: taste, smell, chemesthesis and vision
The gastrointestinal tract
The cardiovascular system
The skeletal system
The immune and inflammatory systems
Phytochemicals
The control of food intake
Overnutrition
Undernutrition
Exercise performance

Public Health Nutrition

An overview of public health nutrition
Nutrition epidemiology
Food choice
Assessment of nutritional status at individual and population level
Assessment of physical activity
Overnutrition
Undernutrition
Eating disorders, dieting and food fads
PHN strategies for nutrition: intervention at the level of individuals
PHN strategies for nutrition: intervention at the ecological level
Food and nutrition guidelines
Fetal programming
Cardiovascular disease
Cancer
Osteoporosis
Diabetes
Vitamin A deficiency
Iodine deficiency
Iron deficiency
Maternal and child health
Breast feeding
Adverse outcomes in pregnancy

Clinical Nutrition

General principles of clinical nutrition
Metabolic and nutritional assessment
Overnutrition
Undernutrition
Metabolic disorders
Eating disorders
Adverse reactions to foods
Nutritional support
Ethical and legal issues
Gastrointestinal tract
The liver
The pancreas
The kidney
Blood and bone marrow
The lung
Immune and inflammatory systems
Heart and blood vessels
The skeleton
Traumatic diseases
Infectious diseases
Malignant diseases
Pediatric nutrition
Cystic fibrosis
Clinical cases
Water and electrolytes

Contents

Series Foreword

The early decades of the twentieth century were a period of intense research on constituents of food essential for normal growth and development and saw the discovery of most of the vitamins, minerals, amino acids and essential fatty acids. In 1941, a group of leading physiologists, biochemists and medical scientists recognized that the emerging discipline of nutrition needed its own learned society and the Nutrition Society was established. Our mission was, and remains, *'to advance the scientific study of nutrition and its application to the maintenance of human and animal health'.* The Nutrition Society is the largest learned society for nutrition in Europe and we have over 2000 members worldwide. You can find out more about the Society and how to become a member by visiting our website at *www.nutsoc.org.uk*

The ongoing revolution in biology initiated by large-scale genome mapping and facilitated by the development of reliable, simple-to-use molecular biological tools makes this a very exciting time to be working in nutrition. We now have the opportunity to get a much better understanding of how specific genes interact with nutritional intake and other lifestyle factors to influence gene expression in individual cells and tissues and, ultimately, effects on health. Knowledge of the polymorphisms in key genes carried by a patient will allow the prescription of more effective, and safe, dietary treatments. At the population level, molecular epidemiology is opening up much more incisive approaches to understanding the role of particular dietary patterns in disease causation. This excitement is reflected in the several scientific meetings which the Nutrition Society, often in collaboration with sister learned societies in Europe, organizes each year. We provide travel grants and other assistance to encourage students and young researchers to attend and to participate in these meetings.

Throughout its history a primary objective of the Society has been to encourage nutrition research and to disseminate the results of such research. Our first journal, *The Proceedings of the Nutrition Society,* recorded, as it still does, the scientific presentations made to the Society. Shortly afterwards, *The British Journal of Nutrition* was established to provide a medium for the publication of primary research on all aspects of human and animal nutrition by scientists from around the world. Recognizing the needs of students and their teachers for authoritative reviews on topical issues in nutrition, the Society began publishing *Nutrition Research Reviews* in 1988. More recently, we launched *Public Health Nutrition,* the first international journal dedicated to this important and growing area. All of these journals are available in electronic as well as in the conventional paper form, and we are exploring new opportunities to exploit the web to make the outcomes of nutritional research more quickly and more readily accessible.

As protection for the public and to enhance the career prospects of nutritionists, the Nutrition Society is committed to ensuring that those who practice as nutritionists are properly trained and qualified. This is recognized by placing the names of suitably qualified individuals on our professional registers and by the award of the qualifications *Registered Public Health Nutritionist (RPHNutr)* and *Registered Nutritionist (RNutr).* Graduates with appropriate degrees but who do not yet have sufficient postgraduate experience can join our Associate Nutritionist registers. We undertake accreditation of university degree programs in public health nutrition and are developing accreditation processes for other nutrition degree programs.

Just as in research, having the best possible tools is an enormous advantage in teaching and learning. This is the reasoning behind the initiative to launch this series of human nutrition textbooks designed for use worldwide. The Society is deeply indebted to our former President, Professor Mike Gibney for his foresight, and to him and his team of editors for their innovative approaches and hard work, in bringing this major publishing exercise to successful fruition. Read, learn and enjoy.

John Mathers
President of the Nutrition Society

Preface

This is the second of a series of four textbooks which the Nutrition Society is preparing in association with Blackwell Publishing. Whereas the *Introduction to Human Nutrition* textbook was designed to be used not just by nutrition students, but also by students who might take nutrition as a minor option such as in food science, pharmacy, nursing, agriculture, etc., the present textbook is firmly aimed at the student opting to pursue nutrition as a main academic subject. The textbook, as the title implies, has as its focus the physiological and biochemical basis for the role of nutrients in metabolism. The first seven chapters cover some core areas, some traditional such as the integration of metabolic nutrition or those related to stages of growth, and one focussing on molecular nutrition, an area of great growth and one that will undoubtedly greatly shape the next edition of this textbook.

Thereafter, the chapters are organized somewhat differently to the usual format of nutrition textbooks. The editorial committee took the view that the role of individual nutrients needed to be integrated into chapters on 'systems' rather than nutrients. Issues of public health nutrition are by and large avoided, so that the forthcoming textbook of *Public Health Nutrition* can tackle these. However, the *Clinical Nutrition Textbook* will also tackle diet–disease links on a systems-by-systems basis.

As with the introductory textbook, the issue of within- and between-textbook overlap arose. As best we could, we tried to minimize within-textbook overlap and have tried to cross-reference chapters where possible. However, some level of overlap across texts will occur, but from a different perspective. Thus, the present text introduces an analysis of how nutrient influence risk factors for coronary heart disease with a perspective on the metabolic dimension. Much of this will again arise in both the Public Health and the Clinical Nutrition textbooks, from a population and preventive approach and from a patient and therapeutic approach, respectively.

I am, as ever, very grateful to all of the authors who suffered my regular electronic prompts of deadlines and details, and I am especially grateful to several authors who stepped in at the last minute to help out with the project. To the volume editors Helen and Ian, I am very grateful for their diligence, attention to detail and to timetables, and great teamwork. Again, Julie Dowsett was the catalyst that kept the project going and I am very grateful to Julie and her constant bonny humor. Finally, to the officers of the Nutrition Society, thank you for your confidence in supporting this project, which continues to be a labor of love.

Michael J Gibney
Editor-in-Chief

Sadly, we must remember three authors within this series of four textbooks who have passed away: Britt Marie Sandstrom, Peter Reeds and Vichai Tanphaichitr.

Contributors

Professor Abayomi O Akanji
Professor of Clinical Pathology
Department of Pathology
Kuwait University Faculty of Medicine
Safat, Kuwait

Dr Linda Bandini
Assistant Professor
Department of Health Sciences
Boston University
Boston, MA USA

Dr France Bellisle
Institut National de la Recherche Agronomique
Paris, France

Professor John Brosnan
Professor of Biochemistry
Department of Biochemistry
Memorial University of Newfoundland
St John's
Newfoundland, Canada

Dr Louise Burke
Department of Sports Nutrition
Australian Institute of Sport
Australia

Professor Philip C Calder
Professor of Nutritional Immunology
Institute of Human Nutrition
University of Southampton
Bassett Crescent East
Southampton, UK

Dr Aedin Cassidy
Head of Molecular Nutrition
Unilever Research
Colworth House,
Sharnbrook, Bedfordshire, UK

Professor Peter Cleaton-Jones
Professor of Experimental Odontology
and Director
MRC/Wits Dental Research Institute
Wits, South Africa

Dr Fabien Dalais
Senior Research Officer
Department of Epidemiology
and Preventive Medicine
Monash University, The Alfred Hospital
Prahan, Victoria, Australia

Dr Conor Delahunty
Department of Food and Nutritional Sciences
University College
Cork, Ireland

Dr Adam Drewnowski
Director, Center for Public Health Nutrition
School of Public Health and
Community Medicine
University of Washington
Seattle, WA, USA

Professor John D Fernstrom
Professor of Psychiatry, Pharmacology & Neuroscience
Research Director, UPMC Health System
Weight Management Center
University of Pittsburgh School of Medicine
Pittsburgh, PA, USA

Dr Madelyn H Fernstrom
Associate Professor of Psychiatry, Epidemiology & Surgery
Director, UPMC Health System Weight Management Center
University of Pittsburgh School of Medicine
Pittsburgh, PA, USA

Professor Albert Flynn
Department of Food and Nutritional Sciences
University College
Cork, Ireland

Professor Keith Frayn
Oxford Centre for Diabetes, Endocrinology and Metabolism
University of Oxford
Churchill Hospital
Oxford, UK

Professor Michael Gibney
Department of Clinical Medicine
Trinity College Medical School
St James' Hospital
Dublin, Ireland

Professor Ángel Gil
Department of Biochemistry and Molecular Biology
Faculty of Pharmacology
University of Granada
Granada, Spain

Dr Lisette de Groot
Division of Human Nutrition and Epidemiology
Wageningen University
Wageningen, The Netherlands

Dr Asker Jeukendrup
Senior Lecturer and Academic Director
School of Sport and Exercise Sciences
University of Birmingham
Birmingham, UK

Dr Antigone Kouris-Blazos
Research Fellow
Asia Pacific Health & Nutrition Centre
Monash Asia Institute, Monash University
Clayton, Victoria, Australia

Dr Xavier Leverve
Bioénergetique Fondamentale et Appliquée
Université Joseph Fourier
Grenoble, France

Professor Ian A Macdonald
Professor of Metabolic Physiology
School of Biomedical Sciences
University of Nottingham
Nottingham, UK

Professor Mariano Mañas Almendros
Catedrático de Fisiología
Departamento de Fisiología
Instituto de Nutricion y Tecnología de Alimentos
Universidad de Granada
Granada, Spain

Professor Emilio Martínez-Victoria
Institute of Nutrition and Food Technology
University of Granada
Granada, Spain

Professor John Mathers
Professor of Human Nutrition
Human Nutrition Research Centre
School of Clinical and Medical Sciences
University of Newcastle
Newcastle upon Tyne, UK

Professor Ronald P Mensink
Professor of Molecular Nutrition
Department of Human Biology
University of Maastricht
Maastricht, The Netherlands

Professor John M Pettifor
Professor of Paediatrics and Child Health
Chris Hani Baragwanath Hospital and the
University of the Witwatersrand
Johannesburg, South Africa

Dr Ann Prentice
MRC Human Nutrition Research
Elsie Widdowson Laboratory
Cambridge, UK

Dr Joop van Raaij
Division of Human Nutrition and Epidemiology
Wageningen University
Wageningen, The Netherlands

Professor Gabriele Riccardi
Department of Clinical and
Experimental Medicine
University of Naples Federico II
Naples, Italy

Dr Angela A Rivellese
Department of Clinical and
Experimental Medicine
University of Naples Federico II
Naples, Italy

Dr Helen Roche
Department of Clinical Medicine
Trinity College Medical School
St James' Hospital
Dublin, Ireland

Ms Katherine A Ross
Research Officer
Asia Pacific Health & Nutrition Centre
Monash Asia Institute, Monash University
Clayton, Victoria, Australia

Professor Tom Sanders
Director of the Nutrition, Food and Health Research Centre
Department of Nutrition and Dietetics
King's College London
London, UK

Ms Tracey L Setter
Research Officer, Asia Pacific Health & Nutrition Centre
Monash Asia Institute, Monash University
Clayton, Victoria, Australia

Dr Prasong Tienboon
Associate Professor of Pediatrics
Honorary Professor in Clinical Nutrition
Division of Nutrition, Department of Pediatrics
Faculty of Medicine,
Chiang Mai University
Chiang Mai, Thailand

Dr Mario Vaz
Associate Professor
Department of Physiology
St John's Medical College
Bangalore, India

Professor Mark L Wahlqvist
Director, Asia Pacific Health & Nutrition Centre
Monash Asia Institute, Monash University
Victoria, Australia

Professor Christine M Williams
Hugh Sinclair Unit of Human Nutrition
School of Food Biosciences
University of Reading
Reading, UK

Dr Maria D Yago
Institute of Nutrition and Food Technology
University of Granada
Granada, Spain

Dr Parveen Yaqoob
Reader in Cellular & Molecular Nutrition
School of Food Biosciences
The University of Reading
Reading, UK

Professor Vernon Young
Laboratory of Human Nutrition
Massachusetts Institute of Technology
Cambridge, MA, USA

1
Core Concepts of Nutrition

IA Macdonald and MJ Gibney

Key messages

- The change in body stores of a nutrient is the difference between the intake of that nutrient and the body's utilization of that nutrient. The time-frame necessary to assess the body's balance of a particular nutrient varies from one nutrient to another.
- The concept of turnover can be applied at various levels within the body (molecular, cellular, tissue/organs, whole body).
- The flux of a nutrient through a metabolic pathway is a measure of the rate of activity of the pathway. Flux is not necessarily related to the size of the pool or pathway through which the nutrient or metabolite flows.

- Nutrients and metabolites are present in several pools in the body. The size of these metabolic pools varies substantially for different nutrients/metabolites, and a knowledge of how these pools are interconnected greatly helps us to understand nutrition and metabolism.
- Darwinian theory of evolution implies a capacity to adapt to adverse conditions, including adverse dietary conditions. Many such examples can be cited. Some allow for long-term adaptation and others buy time until better conditions arrive.

1.1 Introduction

This textbook on *Nutrition and Metabolism* covers macronutrient aspects of nutrition in an integrated fashion. Thus, rather than considering the macronutrients separately, this book brings together information on macronutrients and energy in relation to specific states or topics (e.g. undernutrition, overnutrition, cardiovascular disease). Before considering these topics in detail it is necessary to outline the core concepts that underlie nutritional metabolism. The core concepts to be covered in this chapter are nutrient balance, turnover and flux, metabolic pools, and adaptation to altered nutrient supply.

1.2 Balance

As discussed in Chapter 3, nutrient balance must be considered separately from the concepts of metabolic equilibrium or steady state. In this present chapter, the concept of balance is considered in the context of the classical meaning of that term, the long-term sum of all the forces of metabolic equilibrium for a given nutrient.

The concept of nutrient balance essentially restates the law of conservation of mass in terms of nutrient exchange in the body. Thus, the idea of nutrient balance is summarized by the equation:

$$\begin{bmatrix} \text{Nutrient} \\ \text{intake} \end{bmatrix} - \begin{bmatrix} \text{Nutrient} \\ \text{utilization} \end{bmatrix} = \begin{bmatrix} \text{Change in body} \\ \text{nutrient stores} \end{bmatrix}$$

The above equation can have three outcomes:

- **zero balance** (or nutrient balance): intake matches utilization and stores remain constant
- **positive balance** (or positive imbalance): intake exceeds utilization and stores expand
- **negative balance** (or negative imbalance): utilization exceeds intake and stores become depleted.

In relation to macronutrient metabolism, the concept of balance is most often applied to protein (nitrogen) and to energy. However, many research studies now subdivide energy into the three macronutrients and consider fat, carbohydrate and protein balance separately. This separation of the macronutrients is valuable in conditions of altered dietary composition (e.g. low-carbohydrate diets) where a state of energy balance might exist over a few days but be the result of negative carbohydrate balance (using the body's glycogen store to satisfy the brain's requirement for glucose) matched in energy terms by positive fat balance.

Balance is a function not only of nutrient intake but also of metabolically induced losses. Fat balance is generally driven by periods where energy intake exceeds energy expenditure (positive energy balance) and by periods when intakes are deliberately maintained below energy expenditure such as in dieting (negative energy balance). However, nutrient balance can also be driven by metabolic regulators through hormones or cytokines. For example, the dominance of growth hormone during childhood ensures positive energy and nutrient balance. In pregnancy, a wide range of hormones lead to a positive balance of all nutrients through placental, fetal and maternal stores (Chapter 6). By contrast, severe trauma or illness will dramatically increase energy and protein losses, an event unrelated to eating patterns.

Balance is not something to be thought of in the short term. Following each meal, there is either a storage of absorbed nutrients [triacylglycerol (TAG) in adipose tissue or glucose in glycogen] or a cessation of nutrient losses (breakdown of stored TAG to non-esterified fatty acids or amino acid conversion to glucose via gluconeogenesis). As the period of postprandial metabolism is extended, the recently stored nutrients are drawn upon and the catabolic state commences again. This is best reflected in the high glucagon to insulin ratio in the fasted state before the meal and the opposite high insulin to glucagon ratio during the meal and immediate post-prandial period. However, when balance is measured over a sufficient period, and that varies from nutrient to nutrient, a stable pattern can be seen: zero, positive or negative (Figure 1.1). It is critically important with respect to obesity that the concept of balance is correctly considered. While at some stage energy balance must have been positive to reach an overweight or obese stage, once attained, most people sustain a stable weight over quite long periods.

In the context of the present chapter, it is worth reflecting on the reasons why the period to assess energy balance correctly varies for different nutrients.

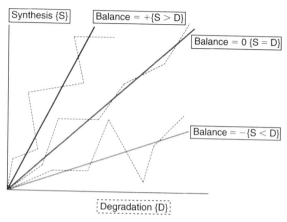

Figure 1.1 Positive, zero and negative nutrient balance over time with fluctuations upwards and downwards within that time.

Fat and adipose tissue (Chapter 5)

- There is a very large capacity to vary the body's pool of adipose tissue. One can double or halve the level of fat stored in the body.
- The capacity to vary the level of TAG in blood *en route* to and from adipose tissue can vary considerably.
- Almost all of the TAG stores in adipose tissue are exchangeable.

Calcium and bone (Chapter 12)

- The human being must maintain a large skeleton as the scaffold on which the musculature and organs are held.
- There is a very strict limit to the level of calcium that can be transported in blood. Excess or insufficient plasma calcium levels influence neural function and muscle function, since calcium is also centrally associated with both.
- Only a small fraction (the miscible pool) of bone is available for movement into plasma.

Because of these differences, calcium balance will require months of equilibrium while fat balance could be equilibrated in days or at most a few weeks.

1.3 Turnover

Although the composition of the body and of the constituents of the blood may appear constant, this does not mean that the component parts are static. In fact, most metabolic substrates are continually being utilized and replaced (i.e. they turn over). This process of turnover is well illustrated by considering protein metabolism in the body. Daily adult dietary protein intakes are in the region of 50–100 g, and the rates of urinary excretion of nitrogen match the protein intake. However, isotopically derived rates of protein degradation indicate that approximately 350 g is broken down per day. This is matched by an equivalent amount of protein synthesis per day, with most of this synthesis representing turnover of material (i.e. degradation and resynthesis) rather than being derived *de novo* from dietary protein (Chapter 4).

Similar metabolic turnover occurs with other nutrients; glucose is a good example, with a relatively constant blood glucose concentration arising from a matching between production by the liver and utilization by the tissues (Chapter 3).

The concept of turnover can be applied at various levels within the body (molecular, cellular, tissue/ organs, whole body). Thus, within a cell the concentration of adenosine triphosphate (ATP) remains relatively constant, with utilization being matched by synthesis. Within most tissues and organs there is a continuous turnover of cells, with death and degradation of some cells matched by the production of new ones. Some cells, such as red blood cells, have a long lifespan (c. 120 days), while others, such as platelets, turn over in a matter of 1–2 days. In the case of proteins, those with very short half-lives have amino acid sequences that favor rapid proteolysis by the range of enzymes designed to hydrolyze proteins. Equally, those with longer half-lives have a more proteolytic-resistant structure.

A major advantage of this process of turnover is that the body is able to respond rapidly to a change in metabolic state by altering both synthesis and degradation to achieve the necessary response. One consequence of this turnover is the high energy cost of continuing synthesis. There is also the potential for dysfunction if the rates of synthesis and degradation do not match.

The consequences of a reduction in substrate synthesis will vary between the nutrients, depending on the half-life of the nutrient. The half-life is the time taken for half of the material to be used up, and is dependent on the rate of utilization of the nutrient. Thus, if synthesis of a nutrient with a short half-life is stopped, the level of that nutrient will fall quickly. By contrast, a nutrient with a long half-life will disappear

more slowly. Since proteins have the most complex of structures undergoing very significant turnover, it is worth dwelling on the mechanism of this turnover. Synthesis is fairly straightforward. Each protein has its own gene and the extent to which that gene is expressed will vary according to metabolic needs. In contrast to synthesis, a reasonably small array of lysosomal enzymes is responsible for protein degradation.

1.4 Flux

The flux of a nutrient through a metabolic pathway is a measure of the role of activity of the pathway. If one considers the flux of glucose from the blood to the tissues, the rate of utilization is approximately 2 mg/kg body weight per minute. However, this does not normally lead to a fall in blood glucose because it is balanced by an equivalent rate of glucose production by the liver, so the net flux is zero. This concept of flux can be applied at the cellular, tissue/organ or whole body level, and can also relate to the conversion of one substrate/nutrient to another (i.e. the movement between metabolic pathways). Flux is not necessarily related to the size of the pool or pathway through which the nutrient or metabolite flows. For example, the membrane of a cell will have several phospholipids present and each will have some level of arachidonic acid. The rate at which arachidonic acid enters one of the phospholipid pools and exits from that phospholipid pool is often higher in the smaller pools.

1.5 Metabolic pools

An important aspect of metabolism is that the nutrients and metabolites are present in several pools in the body (Figure 1.2). At the simplest level, for a given metabolite there are three pools, which will be illustrated using

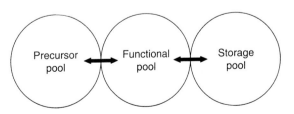

Figure 1.2 The pools in the body in which nutrients and metabolites may exist.

the role of dietary essential fatty acids in eicosanoid synthesis.

In *the functional pool*, the nutrient/metabolite has a direct involvement in one or more bodily functions. In the chosen example, intracellular free arachidonic acid, released from membrane-bound stores on stimulation with some extracellular signal, is the functional pool. It will be acted on by the key enzyme in eicosanoid synthesis, cyclo-oxygenase.

The storage pool provides a buffer of material that can be made available for the functional pool when required. Membrane phospholipids store arachidonic acid in the sn-2 position at quite high concentrations, simply to release this fatty acid when prostaglandin synthesis is needed. In the case of platelets, the eicosanoid thromboxane A_2 is synthesized from arachidonic acid released into the cytoplasm by stimuli such as collagen.

The precursor pool provides the substrate from which the nutrient/metabolite can be synthesized. Linoleic acid represents a good example of a precursor pool. It is elongated and desaturated in the liver to yield arachidonic acid. Thus, the hepatic pool of linoleic acid is the precursor pool in this regard. Not all nutrient pools should be thought of in the concept of precursor, storage and functional pool model outlined above. The essential nutrients and the minerals and trace elements do not have a precursor pool. Nevertheless, no nutrient exists in a single homogeneous pool and an awareness of the existence of metabolic pools is essential to an understanding of human metabolism. For example, one might expect that a fasted individual would show a fall in all essential nutrient levels in the plasma pool. In many instances this is not the case initially because of the existence of storage pools, such as liver stores of iron or vitamin A. In the case of folic acid, fasting causes a rise in blood folic acid levels and this is explained by the concept of metabolic pools. A considerable amount of folic acid enters the gut via the bile duct and is reabsorbed further down the digestive tract. Thus there is an equilibrium between the blood folate pool and the gut folate pool. Fasting stops gallbladder contraction and thus the flow of folate to the gut and hence folate is redistributed from one pool to another.

Another example of how an awareness of metabolic pools helps us to understand nutrition and metabolism is the intracellular free amino acid pool. This is the functional pool from which protein is synthesized. As this pool is depleted in the process of protein

synthesis, it must be repleted, otherwise protein synthesis stops. Moreover, its not just the intracellular pool of amino acids that matters but the intracellular pool of essential amino acids or, more precisely, the intracellular pool of the most limiting essential amino acid. Calculations show that if the pool of the most limiting amino acid in mammalian cells were not replenished, protein synthesis would cease in under 1 h. This highlights the need to transfer the limiting amino acid across the cell membrane, which raises the question of how that pool is repleted. Effectively, it can only be repleted if there is a comparable rate of protein degradation to provide the key amino acid, assuming the balance is zero. Thus there are links between the protein pool of amino acids and the extra and intracellular pools of amino acids.

The size of these various pools varies substantially for different nutrients and metabolites. When studying the activities of metabolic processes within the body, it is often necessary to measure or estimate the size of the various pools in order to derive quantitative information about the overall rates of the processes. In addition, the actual situation may be more complex than the simple three-pool model described above. Nutritional assessment often involves some biochemical assessment of nutritional status. Blood is frequently the pool that is sampled and even there, blood can be separated into:

- erythrocytes, which have a long half-life and are frequently used to assess folic acid status
- cells of the immune system, which can be used to measure zinc or ascorbic acid status
- plasma, which is used to ascertain the levels of many biomarkers
- fractions of plasma, such as cholesteryl esters used to ascertain long-term intake of polyunsaturated fatty acids.

In addition to sampling blood, nutritionists may take muscle or adipose tissue biopsies, samples of saliva, buccal cells, hair and even toenails. A knowledge of how a nutrient behaves in different metabolic pools is critically important in assessing nutritional status. For example, the level of folic acid in plasma is determined by the most recent intake pattern and thus is subject to considerable fluctuation. However, since erythrocytes remain in the circulation for about 120 days, a sample of erythrocytes will represent very recently synthesized cells right through to erythrocytes ready for recycling through the turnover mechanism previously described. As erythrocytes do not have a nucleus, they cannot switch on genes that might influence folate levels, and so the cell retains the level of folate that prevailed at the time of synthesis. Thus, erythrocyte folate is a good marker of long-term intake. The free form of many minerals and trace elements is potentially toxic, and for this reason their level in the serum is strictly regulated. Hence, blood levels are not used to assess long-term intake of selenium, but toenail clippings can be used.

1.6 Adaptation to altered nutrient supply

In many circumstances, the body is able to respond to altered metabolic and nutritional states in order to minimize the consequences of such alterations. For example, the brain has an obligatory requirement for glucose as a substrate for energy and it accounts for a significant part of resting energy expenditure. During undernutrition, where glucose input does not match glucose needs, the first adaptation to their altered metabolic environment is to increase the process of gluconeogenesis, which involves the diversion of amino acids into glucose synthesis. That means less amino acid entering the protein synthesis cycle of protein turnover. Inevitably, protein reserves begin to fall. Thus, two further adaptations are made. The first is that the brain concedes to the crisis and begins to use less glucose for energy (replacing it by ketones as an alternative metabolic fuel). The second is that overall, resting energy expenditure falls to help sustain a new balance if possible (Chapter 8). Stunting in infants and children, reflected in a low height for age, can be regarded as an example of successful adaptation to chronic low energy intake. If the period of energy deprivation is not too long, the child will subsequently exhibit a period of accelerated or catch-up growth (Chapter 7). If it is protracted, the stunting will lead to a permanent reprogramming of genetic balance. In many instances, the rate of absorption of nutrients may be enhanced as an adaptive mechanism to low

intakes. Some adaptations appear to be unsuccessful but work for a period, effectively buying time in the hope that normal intakes will be resumed. In essential fatty acid deficiency the normal processes of elongation and desaturation of fatty acids take place but the emphasis is on the wrong fatty acid, that is, the non-essential 18 carbon monounsaturated fatty acid (oleic acid, C18:1 n-9) rather than the deficient dietary essential 18 carbon polyunsaturated fatty acid (linoleic acid, C18:2 n-6). The resultant 20 carbon fatty acid does not produce a functional eicosanoid. However, the body has significant stores of linoleic acid and so the machinery of eicosanoid synthesis operates at a lower efficiency than normal in the hope that things will get better. Eventually, pathological consequences ensue. In effect, adaptation to adverse metabolic and nutritional circumstances is a feature of survival until the crisis abates. The greater the capacity to mount adaptations to adverse nutritional circumstances the greater the capacity to survive.

1.7 Perspectives on the future

These basic concepts of nutrition will remain forever but they will be refined in detail by the emerging subject of nutrigenomics (Chapter 2). We will develop a greater understanding of how changes in the nutrient content of one pool will alter gene expression to influence events in another pool and how this influences the flux of nutrients between pools. We will better understand how common single nucleotide polymorphisms will determine the level of nutrient intake to achieve nutrient balance in different individuals.

Further reading

Frayn KN. Metabolic Regulation: A Human Perspective, 2nd edn. Oxford: Blackwell Publishing, 2003.

Websites

www.nlm.nih.gov/medlineplus/foodnutritionandmetabolism.html
health.nih.gov/search.asp?category_id=29
www.indstate.edu/thcme/mwking/

2
Molecular Aspects of Nutrition

HM Roche and RP Mensink

Key messages

- The genome is the full complement of genes (genotype) that when expressed determines the phenotype. The genome determines nutritional requirements and metabolic responses. Nutrients can modulate gene expression. These interactions between nutrition and the genome are referred to as molecular nutrition or nutrigenomics.
- DNA is the most basic unit of genetic information. It is organized into chromosomes and every cell contains the full complement of chromosomes.
- Genetic variation can be the result of DNA damage and genetic mutations. Genetic polymorphisms are common forms of genetic heterogeneity whereby there are several different forms of the sample allele in a population.
- Gene expression refers to the process whereby information encoded in the genes is converted into an observable phenotype.

- There are several tools to investigate molecular aspects of nutrition: animal models, cell/tissue-culture models, molecular cloning, gene expression analysis [polymerase chain reaction (PCR) and DNA microarrays], protein analysis and stable isotopes.
- Genetic background or common polymorphisms can determine nutrient requirements, the metabolic response to nutrients and/or susceptibility to diet-related diseases.
- Nutrients can interact with the genome and modulate gene expression. Hence, it is possible that nutrients could be used to manipulate an individual's metabolic response or to reduce their predisposition to diet-related diseases.

2.1 Introduction

Our genes determine every characteristic of life: gender, physical characteristics, metabolic functions, life stage and responses to external or environmental factors, which include nutrition. Nutrients have the ability to interact with the genome and to alter gene expression, which in turn can affect normal growth, health and disease. It is true that we are only beginning to understand how nutrients interact with the genome. This aspect of nutritional science is known as **molecular nutrition** or **nutrigenomics**. Within the context of molecular nutrition this chapter will review the core concepts in molecular biology, introduce the genome and the process of gene expression, identify some important research tools to investigate molecular aspects of nutrition, examine how the genome influences the response to nutrients and

discuss some examples of how nutrients regulate gene expression. The human genome project has provided an enormous amount of genetic information and thus a greater understanding of our genetic background. Molecular nutrition looks at the relationship between the human genome and nutrition from two perspectives. First, the genome determines every individual's genotype (or genetic background), which in turn can determine their nutrient state, metabolic response and/or genetic predisposition to disease. Secondly, nutrients have the ability to interact with the genome and alter gene expression. But gene expression is only the first stage of the whole-body or metabolic response to a nutrient and a number of post-translational events (e.g. enzyme activity, protein half-life, co-activators, co-repressors) can also modify the ability of nutrients to alter an individual's phenotype. The principal aim of molecular nutrition is to understand how the genome interacts with nutrition and nutrition-related diseases; it attempts to determine nutrients that enhance the expression of the genes, proteins and metabolic pathways that are associated with health and suppress those that predispose to disease. While it is unrealistic to assume that nutrition can overcome our genetic fate, good nutrition can improve health and quality of life. Therefore, it is essential that we extend our understanding of the molecular interactions between the genome and nutrition and therefore have a greater understanding of the molecular relationship between diet, health and disease.

2.2 Core concepts in molecular biology

The genome, DNA and the genetic code

The **genome** refers to the total genetic information carried by a cell or an organism. In very simple terms the genome (or DNA sequence) is the full complement of genes. The expression of each gene leads to the formation of a protein, which together with many other proteins that are coded by other genes form tissues, organs and systems, which together constitute the whole organism. In complex multicellular organisms the information carried within the genome gives rise to multiple tissues (muscle, bone, adipose tissue, etc.). The characteristics of each cell type and tissue are dependent on differential gene expression by the genome, whereby only those genes are expressed that code for specific proteins to confer the individual characteristics of the cells that constitute each organ. For example, gene expression in muscle cells may result in the formation of muscle specific proteins that are critical for the differentiation, development and maintenance of muscle tissue, and these genes are completely different from those expressed in osteoblasts, osteoclasts and osteocytes, which form bone. These differentially expressed proteins can have a wide variety of functions: as structural components of the cell, or as regulatory proteins including enzymes, hormones, receptors and intracellular signalling proteins that confer tissue specificity.

It is very important to understand the molecular basis of cellular metabolism because incorrect expression of genes at the cellular level can disrupt whole-body metabolism and lead to disease. Aberrant gene expression can lead to cellular disease when proteins are produced in the wrong place, at the wrong time, at abnormal levels or as a malfunctioning isoform that can compromise whole-body health. Furthermore, different nutritional states and intervention therapies can modulate the expression of cellular genes and thereby the formation of proteins. Therefore, the ultimate goal of molecular nutrition is to understand how nutrients interact with the genome, and alter the expression of genes, and the formation and function of proteins that play a role in health and disease.

DNA (deoxyribonucleic acid) is the most basic unit of genetic information, as the DNA sequence codes for the amino acids that form cellular proteins. Individual DNA molecules are packaged as the chromosomes of the nucleus of animal and plant cells. The structure and composition of DNA is illustrated in Figure 2.1. DNA is composed of large polymers, with a linear backbone composed of residues of the five-carbon sugar residue deoxyribose, which are successively linked by covalent phosphodiester bonds. A nitrogenous base, either a **purine** [**adenine** (A) or **guanine** (G)] or a **pyrimidine** [**cytosine** (C) or **thymine** (T)], is attached to each deoxyribose. DNA forms **a double-stranded helical structure**, in which the two separate DNA polymers wind around each other. The two strands of DNA run **antiparallel**, such that the deoxyribose linkages of one strand runs in the 5′–3′ direction and the other strand in the opposite 3′–5′ direction. The double helix is mainly maintained by hydrogen bonds between nucleotide pairs. According to the **base-pair rules**, adenine always binds to thymine via two hydrogen bonds and guanine binds to cytosine via three hydrogen bonds. This complementary base-pair rule ensures that the sequence of one DNA strand specifies the sequence of the other.

The **nucleotide** is the basic repeat unit of the DNA strand and is composed of deoxyribose, a phosphate group and a base. The 5′–3′ sequential arrangement of the nucleotides in the polymeric chain of DNA is the **genetic code** for the arrangement of amino acids in proteins. The genetic code is the universal language that translates the information stored within the DNA of genes into proteins. It is universal between species. The genetic code is read in groups of three nucleotides. These three nucleotides, called a **codon**, are specific for one particular amino acid. Table 2.1 shows the 64 possible codons, of which 61 specify for 22 different amino acids, while three sequences (TAA, TAG, TGA) are stop codons. Some amino acids are coded for by more than one codon; this is referred to as **redundancy**. For example, the amino acid isoleucine may be coded by the DNA sequence ATT, ATC or ATA. Each amino acid

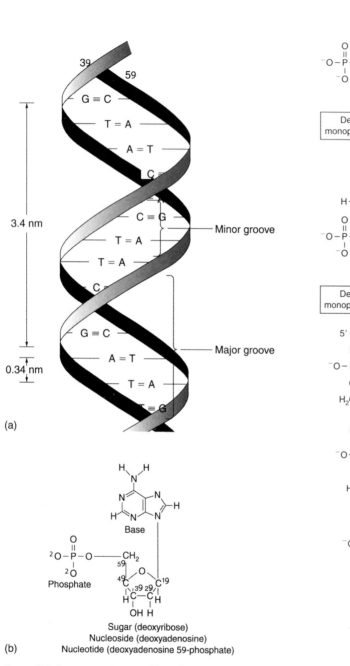

Figure 2.1 Structure and composition of DNA. DNA contains deoxynucleotides consisting of a specific heterocyclic nitrogenous base (adenine, guanine, cytosine or thymine) joined to a deoxyribose phosphate moiety. Adjacent deoxynucleotides are linked through their phosphate groups to form long polynucleotide chains. (a) The DNA double helix; (b) a nucleotide; (c) the purine and pyrimidine bases. (Reproduced from Cox and Sinclair, 1997.)

Table 2.1 The genetic code

First base	Second base				Third base
	T	C	A	G	
T	TTT (Phe)	TCT (Ser)	TAT (Tyr)	TGT (Cys)	T
	TTC (Phe)	TCC (Ser)	TAC (Tyr)	TGC (Cys)	C
	TTA (Leu)	TCA (Ser)	TAA (Stop)	TGA (Stop)	A
	TTG (Leu)	TCG (Ser)	TAG (Stop)	TGG (Trp)	G
C	CTT (Leu)	CCT (Pro)	CAT (His)	CGT (Arg)	T
	CTC (Leu)	CCC (Pro)	CAC (His)	CGC (Arg)	C
	CTA (Leu)	CCA (Pro)	CAA (Gln)	CGA (Arg)	A
	CTG (Leu)	CCG (Pro)	CAG (Gln)	CGG (Arg)	G
A	ATT (Ile)	ACT (Thr)	AAT (Asn)	AGT (Ser)	T
	ATC (Ile)	ACC (Thr)	AAC (Asn)	AGC (Ser)	C
	ATA (Ile)	ACA (Thr)	AAA (Lys)	AGA (Arg)	A
	ATG (Met)	ACG (Thr)	AAG (Lys)	AGG (Arg)	G
G	GUU (Val)	GCT (Ala)	GAT (Asp)	GGT (Gly)	T
	GTC (Val)	GCC (Ala)	GAC (Asp)	GGC (Gly)	C
	GTA (Val)	GCA (Ala)	GAA (Glu)	GGA (Gly)	A
	GTG (Val)	GCG (Ala)	GAG (Glu)	GGG (Gly)	G

Ala: alanine; Arg: arginine; Asn: asparagine; Asp: aspartic acid; Cys: cysteine; Gln: glutamine; Glu: glutamic acid; Gly: glycine; His: histidine; Ile: isoleucine; Leu: leucine; Lys: lysine; Met: methionine; Phe: phenylalanine; Pro: proline; Ser: serine; Thr: threonine; Trp: tryptophan; Tyr: tyrosine; Val: valine.

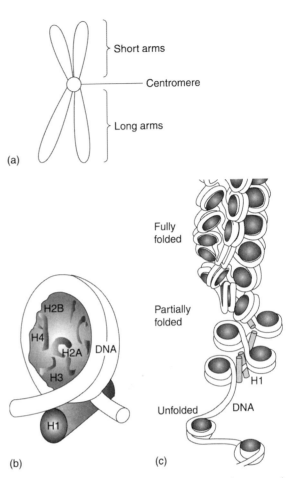

Figure 2.2 Structure of (a) a chromosome, (b) the nucleosome and (c) chromatin. (Reproduced from Cox and Sinclair, 1997.)

sequence of a protein always begins with a methionine residue because the start codon (ATG) codes for methionine. The three stop codons signal the end of the coding region of a gene and the resultant polypeptide sequence.

Chromosome (karyotype)

In eukaryotic cells, DNA is packaged as **chromosomes** and every cell contains a set of chromosomes (Figure 2.2). Each chromosome has a narrow waist known as the centromere, which divides each chromosome into a short and a long arm, labeled p and q, respectively. The tip of each chromosomal arm is known as the telomere. DNA is packaged in a very compact structure within the nucleus. Condensing of DNA is essential because the human cell contains approximately 4×10^9 nucleotide pairs, termed **base pairs (bp)** of DNA, whose extended length would approach more than 1 m. The most basic unit of the chromosome is the **nucleosome**, which is composed of a 145 bp linear strand of double-stranded DNA wound around a complex of **histone proteins** (H2a, H2b, H3 and H4). Nucleosomes are linked together by the histone protein H1 to form **chromatin**. This is then further compacted

with the aid of non-histone chromosomal proteins to generate a chromosome. The structure of DNA in chromatin is important, because it has profound effects on the ability of DNA to be transcribed.

The chromosomal complement or karyotype refers to the number, size and shape of the chromosomes. The human karyotype is composed of 22 pairs of autosomes and a pair of sex chromosomes: XX in the female and XY in the male. Most human cells contain 46 chromosomes, the **diploid** number. Chromosomal disorders are characterized by abnormalities of chromosomal number or structure. They may involve the autosomes or the sex chromosomes and may be the result of a **germ-cell mutation** in the parent (or a more distant ancestor) or a **somatic mutation** in which only a proportion of cells will be affected (mosaicism). The normal chromosome number is an exact multiple of the **haploid** number (23) and is referred to as the diploid number. A chromosomal number that exceeds the diploid number (46) is called **polyploidy**, and one that is not an exact multiple number is **aneuploidy**. Aneuploidy usually occurs when the pair of chromosomes fails to segregate (non-disjunction) during meiosis, which results in an extra copy of a chromosome (**trisomy**) or a missing copy of a chromosome (**monosomy**). Down's syndrome is a common example of trisomy, which is due to the presence of three copies of chromosome 21 (trisomy 21).

Structural abnormalities of chromosomes also occur. A **translocation** is the transfer of chromosomal material between chromosomes. Chronic myeloid leukemia results from the translocation of genetic material between chromosome 8 and chromosome 22. This results in an abnormal chromosome, known as the Philadelphia chromosome, the expression of which results in leukemia. **Chromosomal deletions** arise from the loss of a portion of the chromosome between two break points. **Inversions** arise from two chromosomal breaks with inversion through 180° of the chromosomal segment between the breaks.

Genotype, phenotype and allelic expression

The **genotype** of an organism is the total number of genes that make up a cell or organism. The term, however, is also used to refer to alleles present at one locus. Each diploid cell contains two copies of each gene; the individual copies of the gene are called **alleles**. The definition of an allele is one of two (or more) alternative forms of a gene located at the corresponding site (**locus**) on homologous chromosomes. One allele is inherited from the maternal gamete and the other from the paternal gamete. Therefore, the cell can contain the same or different alleles of every gene. **Homozygous** individuals carry two identical alleles of a particular gene. **Heterozygotes** have two different alleles of a particular gene. The term **haplotype** describes a cluster of alleles that occur together on a DNA segment and/or are inherited together. **Genetic linkage** is the tendency for alleles close together to be transmitted together through meiosis and hence be inherited together.

Genetic polymorphisms are different forms of the same allele in the population. The 'normal' allele is known as the **wild-type allele**, whereas the variant is known as the polymorphic or mutant allele. A polymorphism differs from a mutation because it occurs in a population at a frequency greater than a recurrent mutation. By convention, a polymorphic locus is one at which there are at least two alleles, each of which occurs with frequencies greater than 1%. Alleles with frequencies less than 1% are considered as a recurrent mutation. The alleles of the ABO blood group system are examples of genetic polymorphisms. The acronym **SNP** (single nucleotide polymorphism) is a common pattern of inherited mutation that involves a single base change in the DNA. A **RFLP** (restriction fragment length polymorphism) is another genetic marker that identifies genetic polymorphisms. RFLPs result in different lengths of DNA fragments when restriction enzymes cleave DNA at specific target sites because of nucleotide changes in the DNA sequence at the site where the restriction enzyme would usually cleave DNA. There is a considerable amount of research investigating the relationships between common genetic polymorphisms and disease because certain genetic polymorphisms may predispose an individual to a greater risk of developing a disease. The effect of genetic variation in response to dietary change is also of great interest because some polymorphisms may determine an individual's response to dietary change. Hence, genetic polymorphisms can determine the therapeutic efficacy of nutritional therapy, which may in turn determine the outcome of certain disease states. The interrelationship between diet, disease and genetic polymorphisms will be discussed in greater detail in Section 2.5.

The **phenotype** is the observable biochemical, physiological or morphological characteristics of a cell or individual resulting from the expression of the cell's genotype, within the environment in which it is expressed. Allelic expression can affect the phenotype of an organism. A **dominant allele** is the allele of a gene that contributes to the phenotype of a heterozygote. The non-expressing allele that makes no contribution to the phenotype is known as the **recessive allele**. The phenotype of the recessive allele is only demonstrated in homozygotes who carry both recessive alleles. **Codominant alleles** contribute equally to the phenotype. The ABO blood groups are an example of codominant alleles, where both alleles are expressed in an individual. In the case of **partial dominance** a combination of alleles is expressed simultaneously and the phenotype of the heterozygote is intermediate between that of the two homozygotes. For example, in the case of the snapdragon, a cross between red and white alleles will generate heterozygotes with pink flowers. **Genetic heterogeneity** refers to the phenomenon whereby a single phenotype can be caused by different allelic variants.

DNA damage, genetic mutations and heritability (monogenic and polygenic disorders)

Many agents can cause DNA damage, including ionizing radiation, ultraviolet light, chemical mutagens and viruses. DNA can also change spontaneously under normal physiological conditions. For example, adenine and cytosine can spontaneously undergo deamination to produce hypoxanthine and uracil residues. A change in the nucleotide sequence is known as a **mutation**. A mutation may be defined as a permanent transmissible change in the nucleotide sequence of a chromosome, usually in a singe gene, which may lead to loss or change of the normal function of the gene. A mutation can have a significant effect on protein production or function, because it can alter the amino acid sequence of the protein that is coded by the DNA sequence in a gene. **Point mutations** include i**nsertions**, **deletions**, **transitions** and **transversions**. Two types of events can cause a point mutation: chemical modification of DNA that directly changes one base into another, or a mistake during DNA replication that causes the insertion of the wrong base into the polynucleotide during DNA synthesis. Transitions are the most common type of point mutations, and result in the substitution of one pyrimidine (C–G) or one purine (A–T) by the other. Transversions are less common, where a purine is replaced by a pyrimidine or vice versa.

The functional outcome of mutations can vary very significantly. For example, a single point mutation can change the third nucleotide in a codon and not change the amino acid that is translated; or it may cause the incorporation of another amino acid into the protein – this is known as a **missense mutation**. The functional effect of a missense mutation varies greatly depending on the site of the mutation and the importance of the protein in relation to health. A missense mutation can have no apparent effect on health or it can result in a serious medical condition. For example, sickle cell anemia is due to a missense mutation of the β-globin gene; a glutamine is changed to valine in the amino acid sequence of the protein. This has drastic effects on structure and function of the β-globin protein which causes aggregation of deoxygenated hemoglobin and deformation of the red blood cell. A nucleotide change can also result in the generation of a stop codon

(**nonsense mutation**) and no functional protein will be produced. **Frameshift mutations** refer to small deletions or insertions of bases that alter the reading frame of the nucleotide sequence; hence, the different codon sequence will affect the expression of amino acids in the peptide sequence.

Heritability refers to how much a disease can be ascribed to genetic rather than environmental factors. It is expressed as a percentage, a high value indicating that the genetic component is important in the etiology of the disease. Genetic disorders can simply be classified as **monogenic** (or single gene disorders) or **polygenic diseases** (multifactorial diseases). In general, we have a far greater understanding of the **single gene disorders** because they are due to one or more mutant alleles at a single locus and most follow simple **Mendelian inheritance**. Examples of such disorders are:

- **autosomal dominant:** familial hypercholesterolemia, von Willebrand's disease, achondroplasia
- **autosomal recessive:** cystic fibrosis, phenylktonuria, hemochromatosis, α-thalassemia, β-thalassemia
- **X-linked dominant:** vitamin D-resistant rickets
- **X-linked recessive:** Duchenne muscular dystrophy, hemophilia A, hemophilia B, glucose-6-phosphate dehydrogenase deficiency.

Some single gene disorders show non-Mendelian patterns of inheritance, which are explained by different degrees of penetrance and variable gene expression. **Penetrance** means that a genetic lesion is expressed in some individuals but not in others. For example, people carrying a gene with high penetrance have a high probability of developing any associated disease. A low-penetrance gene will result in only a slight increase in disease risk. **Variable expression** occurs when a genetic mutation produces a range of phenotypes. **Anticipation** refers to the situation when a Mendelian trait manifests as a phenotype with decreasing age of onset and often with greater severity as it is inherited through subsequent generations (e.g. Huntington's chorea, myotonic dystrophy). **Imprinting** refers to the differential expression of a chromosome or allele depending on whether the allele has been inherited from the male or female gamete. This is due to selective inactivation of genes according to the paternal or maternal origin of the chromosomes. Although there are only a few examples of diseases that arise as a result of imprinting (e.g. Prader–Willi and Angelman's syndromes), it is thought that this form of gene inactivation may be more important than previously realized.

Polygenic (or multifactorial) diseases are those due to a number of genes (e.g. cancer, coronary heart disease, diabetes and obesity). Even though polygenic disorders are more common than monogenic disorders, we still do not understand the full genetic basis of any of these conditions. This reflects the fact that there is interaction between many candidate genes, that is, those genes that are thought to play an etiological role in multifactorial conditions. Furthermore, in polygenic inheritance, a trait is in general determined by a combination of both the gene and the environment.

The Human Genome Project

The Human Genome Project (HGP) is an important source of genetic information that will be a resource to molecular nutrition, especially in terms of understanding the interaction between nutrition and the human genome. The working draft sequence of the human genome was published in February 2001. The project showed that the size of the human genome is 30 times greater than that of the fruit fly and 250 times larger than yeast. Only 3% of the DNA in the human genome constitutes coding regions. Compared with the fruit fly, the human genome has much more non-coding or intronic regions. Although these intronic regions do not code for genes they may have a functional role, and these functional effects could, for example, include important promoter and/or repressor regions. The number of genes coded by the human genome was much less than expected. The human genome codes for only 30 000–40 000 genes. Indeed, a man has only two to three times as many genes as a fruit fly. The two- to three-fold difference between humans and fruit flies may largely be accounted for by the greater number of control genes (e.g. transcription factors) in the human genome.

In the future, we will have a greater understanding of the human genome and how it interacts with the environment. The HGP showed that humans are very alike: it estimated that humans are 99.8% genetically similar. Nevertheless, the implications of the HGP in relation to molecular nutrition are immense. The challenge is to identify the proportion of that genetic variation that is relevant to nutrition. The term 'gene mining' refers to the process that will identify the new genes involved in nutrition, health and disease. At the most basic level we already know that the human

genome determines nutrient requirements, for example gender determines iron requirements – the iron requirement of menstruating women is greater than that of men of the same age. In the case of folate, research would suggest that the methylenetetrahydrofolate reductase (MTHFR) polymorphism could determine an individual's folate requirements. Since there are fewer genes than anticipated, it has been proposed that different isoforms of the same gene with different functionality are important. Already there are examples of this (e.g. the three isoforms of the apolipoprotein E (Apo E) gene determine the magnitude of postprandial triacylglycerol metabolism). Furthermore, it has been proposed that the interaction between the human genome and the environment is an important determinant of within- and between-individual variation. Within the context of molecular nutrition we will have to determine how nutrients alter gene expression and determine the functional consequences of genetic polymorphisms. With the information generated from the HGP we will have a more complete understanding and information in relation to the relevance of genetic variation, and how alterations in nutrient intake or nutritional status affect gene expression in a way that is relevant to human health and disease processes. In essence, the challenge is to bridge the gap between the genome sequence and whole-organism biology, nutritional status and intervention.

2.3 Gene expression: transcription and translation

Gene expression

Gene expression refers to the process whereby the information encoded in the DNA of a gene is converted into a protein, which confers the observable phenotype upon the cell. A **gene** may be defined as the nucleic acid sequence that is necessary for the synthesis of a functional peptide or protein in a temporal and tissue-specific manner. However, a gene is not directly translated into a protein; it is expressed via a nucleic acid intermediary called **messenger RNA** (**mRNA**). The transcriptional unit of every gene is the sequence of DNA transcribed into a single mRNA molecule, starting at the promoter and ending at the terminator regions. The essential features of a gene and mRNA are presented in Figure 2.3. The DNA sequence of a gene comprises of two non-coding (or untranslated) regions at the

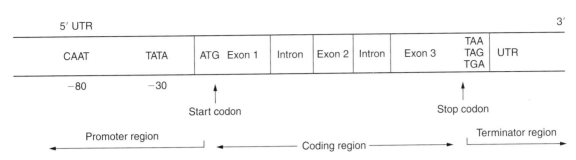

Figure 2.3 Essential features of the gene.

beginning and end of the gene coding region. The non-coding promoter and terminator regions of the DNA give rise to the 5′ and 3′ **untranslated regions** (**UTR**) of mRNA. Although the non-coding regions of a gene are not components of the protein product of the gene, they represent critical parts of the gene that regulate gene expression and the functional characteristics of the protein product. The **promoter region** is located immediately upstream of the gene coding region; it contains DNA sequences, known as the TATA and CAAT boxes, which define the site at which transcription starts and regulate the rate of gene expression. The **TATA box** is an AT-rich sequence that occurs about 30 basepairs (−30 bp) upstream from the transcriptional start site. The **CAAT box** contains this short DNA sequence about 80 bp upstream (−80 bp) of the start site. These sequences, together with binding sites for other **transcription factors**, regulate the rate of tissue-specific gene expression. Transcription starts at **the CAP site**, so called because following transcription the 5′ end of the mRNA molecule is capped at this site by the attachment of a specialized nucleotide (7-methyl guanosine). The CAP site is followed by the **initiation, or start codon** (ATG), which specifies the start of translation; hence, according to the genetic code every polypeptide begins with methionine. The DNA coding sequence for a gene is not contiguous or uninterrupted. Each gene contains DNA sequences that code for the amino acid sequence of the protein, which are called **exons**. The exons are interrupted by non-coding DNA sequences, which are called **introns**. The last exon ends with a **stop codon** (TAA, TAG or TGA), which represents the end of the gene-coding region and it is followed by the terminator sequence in the DNA sequence that defines the end of the gene-coding region. The **3 UTR** of the mRNA molecule includes a **poly(A) signal** (**AATAAA**) that is added to the mRNA molecule following transcription.

Ribonucleic acid (RNA)

RNA is like DNA because it carries genetic information. The composition of RNA is very similar to DNA, and it plays a key role in all stages of gene expression. RNA is also a linear polynucleotide, but it differs from DNA in that it is single stranded and composed of polymers of ribose rather than deoxyribose, and the pyrimidine base **uracil** (**U**) replaces thymine (T). There are three different types of RNA in eukaryotic cells and all are involved in gene expression.

- **Messenger RNA** (**mRNA**) molecules are long, linear, single-stranded polynucleotides that are direct copies of DNA. mRNA is formed by transcription of DNA.
- **Ribosomal RNA** (**rRNA**) is a structural and functional component of ribosomes. Ribosomes, the cytoplasmic machines that synthesize mRNA into amino acid polypeptides, are present in the cytoplasm of the cell and are composed of rRNA and ribosomal proteins.
- **Transfer RNA** (**tRNA**) is a small RNA molecule that donates amino acids during translation or protein synthesis.

RNA is about 10 times more abundant than DNA in eukaryotic cells; 80% is rRNA, 15% is tRNA and 5% is mRNA. In the cell mRNA is normally found associated with protein complexes called **messenger ribonucleoprotein** (**mRNP**), which package mRNA and aid its transport into the cytoplasm, where it is decoded into a protein.

Transcription

RNA transcription, which is the process whereby the genetic information encoded in DNA is transferred into mRNA, is the first step in the process of gene expression

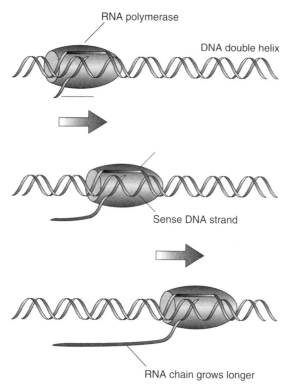

RNA polymerase

DNA double helix

Sense DNA strand

RNA chain grows longer

Figure 2.4 RNA polymerase II transcribes the information in DNA into RNA.

and occurs in the nucleus of the cell. It can be divided into four stages: template recognition, initiation, elongation and termination. Transcription is catalyzed by DNA-dependent **RNA polymerase (RNA pol)** enzymes (Figure 2.4). In eukaryotic cells RNA pol II synthesizes mRNA, while RNA pol I and RNA pol III synthesize tRNA and rRNA. RNA polymerase II is a complex 12-subunit enzyme, associated with several transcription factors, including TFIIA, TFIIB, TFIIC, TFIID, TFIIE, TFIIF, TFIIH and TFIIJ. The strand of DNA that directs synthesis of mRNA via complementary base pairing is called the template or **antisense strand**. The other DNA strand that bears the same nucleotide sequence is called the coding or **sense strand**. Therefore, RNA represents a copy of DNA. Transcription is a multistep process. An initiation complex (TFIID, TFIIA, TFIIB, TFIIF, TFIIE, TFIIH) assembles at the promoter, to which RNA pol II binds. TFIID recognizes the promoter and binds to the TATA box at the start of the gene. TFIIH unwinds double-stranded DNA to expose the unpaired DNA nucleotide and the DNA sequence is used as a template from which RNA is

synthesized. TFIIE and TFIIH are required for promoter clearance, allowing RNA pol II to commence movement away from the promoter. Initiation describes the synthesis of the first nine nucleotides of the RNA transcript. Elongation describes the phase during which RNA polymerase moves along the DNA and extends the growing RNA molecule. RNA is synthesized by adding nucleotides to the 3′ end of the growing RNA chain. Termination involves recognition of the **terminator sequence**, which signals the end of the gene, and the synthesis of the RNA polynucleotide ends. RNA synthesis is always in a 5′–3′ direction.

Post-transcriptional processing of RNA

After transcription of DNA into RNA, the newly synthesized RNA is modified. This process is called post-transcriptional processing of RNA (Figure 2.5). The **primary RNA transcript** synthesized by RNA pol II from genomic DNA is often called **heterogeneous nuclear RNA (hnRNA)** because of its considerable variation in size. The primary transcript consists of an RNA molecule that represents a full copy of the gene extending from the promoter to the terminator region of the gene, and includes introns and exons. While still in the nucleus, the newly synthesized RNA is capped, polyadenylated and spliced. **Capping** refers to the addition of a nucleotide cap on to the 5′ end of the mRNA. The 7-methylguanosine cap has three functions: it protects the mRNA from enzymic attack, it aids mRNA splicing and it enhances translation of the mRNA. **Polyadenylation** involves the addition of a string of adenosine residues, a **poly(A) tail**, to the 3′ end of the mRNA. Then the mRNA is spliced, which is performed by the splicosome. This RNA–protein complex recognizes the consensus sequences at each end of the intron (5′-GU and AG-3′) and excises the introns so that the remaining exons are spliced together. After capping, polyadenylation and splicing, the mRNA moves from the nucleus to the cytoplasm for translation.

Alternative splicing describes the process through which not all exons are included in the mature mRNA molecule. As illustrated in Figure 2.6, one primary RNA transcript can be spliced in three different ways, leading to three mRNA isoforms, one with five exons or two with four exons. Upon translation the different mRNA isoforms will give rise to different isoforms of the protein product of the gene. This is a relatively common phenomenon and although the physiological or metabolic relevance of the different isoforms of many

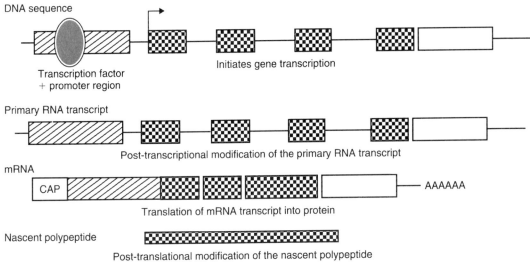

Figure 2.5 Transcription and processing of mRNA.

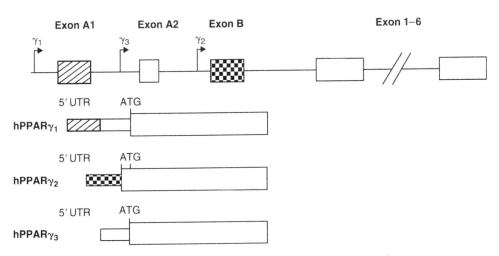

Figure 2.6 Alternative RNA splice variants of the peroxisome proliferator activator receptor-gamma (PPARγ) gene.

proteins is not fully understood it may be relevant to molecular nutrition. For example, the peroxisome proliferator activator receptor-gamma (PPARγ) gene can produce three different isoforms of mRNA (PPARγ$_1$, PPARγ$_2$, PPARγ$_3$) as a result of different promoters and alternative splicing. It would seem that the PPARγ$_2$ mRNA isoform is responsive to nutritional states. PPARγ$_2$ mRNA expression is increased in the fed state; its expression is positively related to adiposity and is reduced upon weight loss. Therefore, PPARγ$_2$ mRNA

may be the isoform that mediates nutrient regulation of gene expression.

RNA editing is another way in which the primary RNA transcript can be modified. Editing involves the binding of proteins or short RNA templates to specific regions of the primary transcript and subsequent alteration or editing of the sequence, either insertion of one or more different nucleotides or base changes. This mechanism allows the production of different proteins from a single gene under different physiological conditions. The two isoforms of apo B are examples of this. In this case, RNA editing allows for tissue specific expression of the apo B gene, such that the full protein apo B100 is produced in the liver and secreted on VLDL. By contrast, in the intestine the apo B48 isoform is produced because a premature stop codon is inserted so that transcription of the protein is halted and the resultant apoprotein is 48% of that of the apo B100 isoform.

Control of gene expression and transcription

All cells contain a complete set of genes. Therefore, it is of critical importance that genes are expressed in the correct tissue and at the correct time. Temporal and tissue-specific gene expression in eukaryotic cells is mostly controlled at the level of transcription initiation. Two types of factors regulate gene expression: *cis*-**acting control elements** and *trans*-**acting** factors. *Cis*-acting elements do not encode proteins; they influence gene transcription by acting as binding sites for proteins that regulate transcription. These DNA sequences are usually organized in clusters, which are located in the promoter region of the gene, that influence the transcription of genes. The TATA and CAAT boxes are examples of *cis*-acting elements.

The *trans*-acting factors are known as **transcription factors** or DNA binding proteins. Transcription factors are proteins that are produced by other genes, and include steroid hormone receptor complexes, vitamin-receptor proteins and mineral–protein complexes. These transcription factors bind to specific DNA sequences in the promoter region of the target gene and promote gene transcription. The precise mechanism(s) of how transcription factors influence gene transcription is not fully understood. It is possible that unfolding or folding of DNA to expose or hide sections of DNA may be important. Structures that favor the binding of proteins to DNA have been identified in some DNA binding proteins (zinc fingers, leucine zippers, etc.). Transcription factors play a key role in temporal and tissue-specific gene expression. For example, the genes for the enzymes of gluconeogenesis can be turned on in the hepatocyte, but not in the adipocyte. This is because the hepatocyte expresses the transcription factors that are required to initiate the expression of the gluconeogenic enzymes.

Master regulatory proteins regulate the expression of many genes of a single metabolic pathway. For example, in the lipogenic pathway the fatty acid

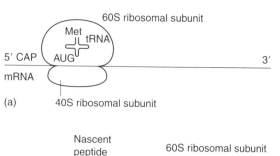

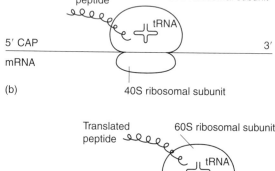

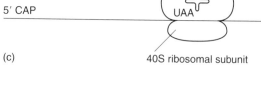

Figure 2.7 Three phases of translation. (a) Initiation: first codon methionine; (b) elongation: translation continues elongating the nascent peptide; (c) termination: translation ends upon recognition of the stop codon.

synthase complex codes for seven distinct genes that have to be coordinately expressed to form the enzymes required for fatty acid synthesis. This ensures that sufficient levels of all of the enzymes of this metabolic pathway are available simultaneously.

RNA translation: protein synthesis

Translation is the process by which the genetic information coded in mRNA is converted into an amino acid sequence (polypeptide) according to the trinucleotide or codon sequence (Figure 2.7). The three forms of RNA play an inherent role in this process. mRNA represents the template from which the protein is synthesized, rRNA is the cytoplasmic machine that synthesizes the protein product of the gene and tRNA donates the amino acids that are incorporated into the polypeptide during protein synthesis. The tRNA molecule has a very distinct structure that is used to deliver the amino acids of the nascent polypeptide. Protein synthesis occurs on the **ribosome** in the cytoplasm.

Ribosomes consist of two subunits, a 40S (small) and 60S (large), which combine to form the 80S particle. Protein synthesis begins by the formation of a complex involving a 40S ribosomal subunit carrying a methionine tRNA, which base pairs with the initiation codon AUG on the mRNA molecule. Translation is largely regulated by controlling the formation of the initiation complex, which is the 40S ribosomal subunit, the mRNA and specific regulatory proteins. The structure of the 5′ UTR is critical for determining whether mRNA is translated or sequestered in the untranslated ribonucleoprotein complex. Initiation of translation is also dependent on the presence of the 5′ cap structure and secondary structure of the mRNA next to the initiation codon. Secondary structures such as stem loops in the 5′ end of the mRNA inhibit the initiation of translation. Some of the translation regulatory proteins are cell specific and mRNA specific, allowing precise post-transcriptional control over the synthesis of specific proteins. The poly(A) tail also modulates translation. Although it is not essential for translation to occur, mRNA lacking the poly(A) tail is less efficiently translated.

Once the initiation complex has formed, synthesis of the polypeptide chain is driven by the interaction between **elongation factors** (elFs), the ribosome and tRNA along the length of the mRNA molecule. At each codon the ribosome and elFs promote the interaction between mRNA and tRNA. tRNA donates an amino acid that is added to the newly synthesized polypeptide which corresponds to the codon in the mRNA. The tRNA achieves this because it bears a triplet of bases (**anticodon**) which are complementary to the mRNA codon, and there is an amino acid attached to the acceptor arm of the tRNA that corresponds to the codon in the mRNA. When the anticodon of the tRNA matches the codon or trinucleotide sequence in the mRNA, the tRNA donates the amino acid to the newly synthesized polypeptide. For example, the first tRNA that carries methionine has the anticodon UAC; it recognizes the methionine codon AUG on mRNA. Similarly, the anticodon AAC recognizes the leucine codon TTG on the mRNA. This process continues until the ribosome reaches a termination codon (UAA, UAG, UGA) and then the completed polypeptide is released from the ribosomal units.

Post-translational modification

Post-translational modification refers to the process that converts the nascent polypeptide into the mature protein product of the gene. The nascent polypeptide may start to form the complex structure of the protein as it is being synthesized; otherwise, it will pass through the rough endoplasmic reticulum and move to the Golgi body for processing. The polypeptide may be modified further, by hydroxylation, phosphorylation or glycosylation, which will confer functional characteristics to the protein. For example, the phosphorylation status of a protein can determine whether it is active or inactive.

2.4 Research tools to investigate molecular aspects of nutrition

For many reasons, it is not always possible to examine the molecular aspects of nutrition in humans. Such studies may be very expensive, while in many cases it is simply not possible to obtain the tissues or cells of interest. Another pragmatic problem is that responses to dietary interventions may vary widely between individuals owing to differences in genetic background and in exposures to environmental factors. Therefore, various approaches such as animal and cell studies are used to gain a better understanding of the effects of diet or specific dietary constituents at the cellular and molecular level. Although such approaches are valuable, it should always be kept in mind that each one has its strengths and limitations. Extrapolation to the human situation will always be a problem and questions that can be addressed in humans should therefore ultimately be addressed in humans.

Animal models

Dietary studies with animals have been carried out for many decades. One advantage is that such studies can be done in a highly controlled way. Food intake can easily be monitored and manipulated, while factors such as temperature, humidity and the stage of the disease can be controlled for. In addition, tissues and cells can be obtained that cannot be readily sampled in humans. It should be appreciated that each animal model has specific advantages and disadvantages. Therefore, many factors need to be considered before a model is chosen, including animal size, the time needed for breeding, litter size, costs of animal housing, and the feasibility of performing blood sampling and vivisection. Then, as with human studies, it is possible to use techniques from the fields of genetics and molecular biology.

An important advantage of animal studies is that the effect of a nutrient can be investigated in animals with a similar genetic background. In this way, variation in responses between animals due to genetic heterogeneity is excluded. Genetic homogeneity can be obtained by inbreeding. For this, genetically related animals, such as brothers and sisters, are mated for many generations. The overall result will be that heterozygosity between animals will reduce and that in the end an inbred strain is obtained with a similar genetic, homozygous background. Genetic homogeneity, however, is not always an advantage. If, for example, the mode of action of a food component is not known or if the main purpose is to test the safety of nutrients or drugs, genetic heterogeneity may be preferable, because it increases the extrapolation of results. In addition, differences in responses between various strains can be helpful for elucidating the responses at the molecular level. Thus, it is evident that a clear research question is needed before the choice of an animal model can be made.

It is possible to insert an isolated (foreign) gene sequence into an animal's genomic material. The resultant animals that carry such a foreign gene are called transgenic animals and have traits coded by these genes. Another approach is to knock out a certain endogenous gene. With this technique, a specific gene is modified, which results in a loss of function. With such an approach it is possible to test candidate genes for their effects on the parameters of interest. Transgenic and knockout animals are valuable models for nutrition research. For example, mice have been generated that express human Apo AI. In this way, it was possible to examine in detail the role of this apolipoprotein in atherogenesis. By inserting or knocking out genes, the importance of specific genes on the genesis of disease and on complex biological pathways in various tissues can be addressed. Finally, by interbreeding mouse strains with different genetic backgrounds, the interaction between genes and the relative contribution of genes and diet on phenotype can be unraveled.

Another tool involves the generation of transgenic mice with tissue specific overexpression of a particular gene. This can be accomplished in several ways. It is, for example, possible to insert a tissue-specific promoter before the foreign gene of interest. This DNA construct can then be used to construct a transgenic animal. It is possible to make genes whose expression is dependent on the presence or absence of dietary components such as tetracycline. In this way, it is even possible to switch on the expression of a gene in a specific tissue at any stage of the disease just by taking away tetracycline from (or adding it to) the diet. Gene expression in the intact animal can also be manipulated by DNA electroporation or with adenovirus-mediated gene delivery. With these methods, DNA can be inserted into a specific tissue. This results in increased levels of mRNA and protein expression of the gene of interest. The effects of gene expression of macrophages, which are made by bone marrow, can be studied *in vivo* by bone-marrow transplantation. For these experiments two strains of inbred mice with similar genetic background are used. For example one strain has no functional apoE gene locus (apoE knockout mice) but the other strain has. After lethal irradiation of the bone marrow of the apoE knockout mice, a bone-marrow cell suspension from the wild-type animal is injected. Within about 4 weeks, the knockout animals are completely reconstituted with the bone marrow from the wild-type animals. As a consequence, their macrophages do not contain apoE and the specific effects of macrophage apoE production can be studied.

Tissue cultures

In vitro studies with intact tissues or isolated cells are an alternative to *in vivo* human and animal studies. If conditions are optimal, cells survive, multiply and may even differentiate after isolation. Tissue cultures can be divided into two categories: organ cultures and cell cultures. An organ culture is composed of a complete or a small part of an intact organ or tissue that is brought into the culture medium. The advantage is that, at least to some extent, the normal biochemical and morphological differentiation and communication routes between the various cell types of a tissue are still maintained. Further, it is possible to mimic closely the physiological environment. The survival time of organ cultures, however, is limited and generally not more than 24 h. In addition, it is not possible to culture the cells further and fresh material is needed for each set of experiments.

Cell suspensions are different to tissue cultures in that the extracellular matrix and intercellular junctions between cells are disrupted. For this, tissues are first treated with proteolytic enzymes and with components that bind calcium. Then, the tissue is mechanically dispersed into single cells. By doing so, a suspension is obtained that is composed of various cell types. If necessary, it is possible to isolate further one specific cell type that can be used for experiments or serve as starting material for a cell culture.

Cell cultures prepared directly from the organs or tissues of an organism are referred to as primary cultures. These cells may still have the potential to divide and in this way secondary and tertiary cell cultures are obtained. Depending on the type of cell and technique used, these cells can be cultured in a suspension or as a monolayer. As for tissue cultures, survival time is limited. However, cell lines can be used that do not lose their capability for indefinite replication. Such cells are frequently derived from cancerous tissue and are all derived from the same stem cell. Therefore, they have a similar genetic make-up. It should be emphasized, however, that after each cell passage these cells lose some of their biochemical and morphological characteristics: the older they are, the more differences can exist from the original stem cell. However, it is feasible to freeze cells after each passage. After thawing properly, these cells can be cultured again, which makes it possible to go back to a previous passage.

Studies with isolated tissue or cell models are very useful for mechanistic studies. Table 2.2 details common tissue-culture models. The effects of adding nutrients or combinations of nutrients can be studied in detail. The responses of cells to these stimuli can be examined under the microscope. It is also possible to examine the effects on mRNA or protein expression, and interactions between two or more different cell types. Finally, it is possible to insert isolated (foreign) gene sequences into the cells. However, extrapolation of the results to the intact animal or to the human situation is always a problem.

Molecular cloning

Molecular cloning refers to the process of making copies of a DNA segment, which is not necessarily the entire gene. This segment can be a piece of genomic DNA, but also complementary DNA (cDNA) derived from mRNA. The DNA fragment is isolated, then the segment is inserted into a vector. The vector with its piece of foreign DNA is subsequently inserted into bacterial cells. As a vector has the capability to replicate autonomously in its host and the host itself can also be grown indefinitely in the laboratory, huge amounts of the DNA segment of interest can be obtained. Many vectors are available and the selection of the vector depends, among other things, on the size of the DNA fragment, whether it is genomic DNA or cDNA, and

Table 2.2 Common tissue-culture models

Cell line	Organism	Tissue	Morphology
HUVEC	Human	Umbilical vein, vascular endothelium	Epithelial
HepG2	Human	Liver, hepatocellular carcinoma	Epithelial
Caco-2	Human	Colon, colorectal adenocarcinoma	Epithelial
CV-1	African green monkey	Kidney	Fibroblast
293	Human	Kidney	Epithelial
HeLa	Human	Cervical adenocarcinoma	Epithelial
THP-1	Human	Monocyte, acute monocytic leukemia	Suspension culture

on the host to be used. The purpose of cloning is to isolate a particular DNA sequence for further study.

Molecular cloning has important applications in a number of areas of molecular nutrition. For example, this method could be used to test the functionality of an SNP and determine whether the SNP is differentially affected by a nutrient. In this case, two DNA constructs could be made, one with and the other without the SNP. Each construct can be inserted into a vector that can be used to transfect a cell line of interest. After exposure of these cells to different nutritional interventions, it is possible to determine whether dietary effects on mRNA or protein expression are affected by this particular SNP.

Libraries are collections of clones, which are widely available nowadays. To construct a genomic library, DNA is first partially digested with restriction enzymes. The DNA fragments so formed are then cloned. An efficient way to limit the total number of clones is first to isolate the chromosomes and then to construct a library for that particular chromosome. Similarly, cDNA libraries have been constructed. Such libraries are constructed from the mRNA population present within a particular cell. A potential advantage of a cDNA library over a genomic library is that the cloned material does not contain the non-coding regions and the introns as present in the genomic DNA. Further, it is possible to make cDNA libraries from specific tissues or cells. In this way, cDNA libraries can be constructed that are enriched with clones for genes known to be expressed preferentially in a certain tissue, or during a specific disease or state of development.

Quantification of gene expression: single gene mRNA expression

Single gene expression is measured by quantification of the mRNA transcripts of a specific gene. It mainly gives information on the effects of, for example, nutrients at the transcriptional level. mRNA quantification can also provide a good estimate of the level of protein present in a sample, at least when production of the protein is transcriptionally regulated. Since only very small amounts of mRNA are present, mRNA samples are first translated into cDNA with the reverse transcriptase (RT) enzyme. To make detection possible, cDNA needs to be amplified by the polymerase chain reaction (PCR). To control for experimental variation in the RT and the PCR step, an internal control RNA can be used in the entire RT-PCR or a DNA competitor in the PCR only. The total procedure is then called competitive-RT-PCR or, when a DNA competitor is used, RT-competitive-PCR. For mRNA analyses, several procedures are available to extract RNA from lysed cells. With most methods, total RNA is isolated that consists of rRNA, mRNA and tRNA. Only approximately 5% of total RNA is mRNA. As eukaryotic cells contain natural RNAses, which are liberated during cell lysis, it is important to ensure that activity of these RNAses is minimized in order to avoid digestion of the isolated RNA. Therefore, it is essential to use RNAse inhibitors during RNA extraction and the following analytical steps. Glassware and plasticware should be RNAse free or be treated with RNAse inhibitors. After isolation, concentrations of RNA can be determined by measuring the optical density at 260 nm.

After RNA isolation, cDNA is synthesized from mRNA with the RT step. cDNA differs from genomic DNA in that it only contains the exons from DNA. RT or first strand synthesis can be done by several protocols. One possibility is to use random hexamers. These hexamers bind at many places to the RNA, while the gaps in between are filled with nucleotides by the enzyme reverse transcriptase. It is also possible to make use of the poly(A) tail, which is present on the 3′ UTR of all mRNA molecules. With both procedures, all mRNA present in the sample is copied into cDNA. It is also possible to make only cDNA for one gene in particular during the RT reaction. In this case, the first strand synthesis can be performed by a primer, which is specific for this gene.

The RT step has variable reproducibility and quality control for this step is crucial. Each difference in RT efficiency is augmented in the following exponential PCR. To overcome these problems, a known amount of a competitive RNA template can be added to the RNA sample as an internal control. The size of the internal standard is in general 20–30 bp longer or shorter than the gene of interest. This RNA standard is also copied into cDNA during the RT step with the same efficiency as the normal RNA transcripts present in the RNA sample. Both the competitor cDNA and the genomic cDNA are amplified in the following PCR. Isolation is always possible, as the two RT-PCR products have a different size.

After the RT step, cDNA is amplified by Taq DNA polymerase. For this reaction two primers are used, which are complementary to both ends of the targeted product. The primers are the starting points for the Taq DNA polymerase enzyme. The Taq polymerase reads the cDNA strand from the 3′ side to 5′, thus forming a complementary strand from 5′ to 3′ by incorporating the four available nucleotides A, T, G and C. This process of amplification requires a specific-temperature program, which is referred to as a PCR cycle. First, the double-stranded cDNA is denatured at 95°C. The temperature is then decreased to the annealing temperature, which is the temperature at which the primers bind to the individual strands, normally at about 60°C. Next, the temperature is increased to 72°C, the optimum temperature for Taq polymerase to incorporate nucleotides into the complementary strand. This is called extension. Thus, during one PCR cycle the number of the targeted product is doubled. This means that after n cycles the number of copies of only one cDNA molecule is 2^n. Thus, after 25 cycles 2^{25} (33×10^6) copies are formed from each cDNA molecule. Such a quantity can be visualized using a detection system.

If an internal control is used during the RT-PCR, the original number of mRNA molecules can be calculated by comparing the intensity of the PCR product of the mRNA of interest versus the intensity of the PCR product from the internal control. Since the initial amount of the internal standard is known, the unknown amount of mRNA can be calculated.

If no internal control is used, expression of a gene is related to the expression of a constitutive gene such as β-actin or GAPDH. These housekeeping genes are always expressed to the same extent and can therefore be used as a measure for the amount of RNA used in the reaction as well as for cDNA synthesis. The PCR for the housekeeping genes needs to be performed from the same cDNA as that for the gene of interest.

Detection of the PCR products formed is carried out by different methods. A frequently used method is by separation of the fragments by gel electrophoresis, followed by visualizing the fragments with ethidium bromide staining using ultraviolet (UV) light. Several other stains can be used, such as cybr green or gelstar. The intensities of the bands on the gels are analyzed by densitometry, which is proportional to the concentration.

Another method makes use of fluorescent labeled primers during the PCR. A laser beam, which visualized the signal, can detect the fluorescently labeled PCR products formed, by densitometry. The areas of the peaks on the densitogram are a measure for the amount of product formed in the RT-PCR. It is also possible to use a labeled (radioactive) probe, which is complementary to the amplified gene of interest. These probes bind the PCR product and this hybrid can be blotted, visualized and quantified.

PCR techniques are particularly useful for the quantification of mRNAs that are present at low concentrations. At higher concentrations, mRNA can also be identified by a technique called Northern blotting. For this, RNA or purified mRNA is first separated according to size by electrophoresis and transferred to a filter. This filter is then incubated with a labeled probe, which specifically binds to the mRNAs of interest. After washing to remove the non-hybridized probe, the specific RNA transcript can be detected. When the probe hybridizes with more than one transcript, more bands will appear on the filter.

Quantification of gene expression: multiple gene mRNA expression

In general, the expression of large numbers of genes changes when environmental conditions, such as nutrient exposure or nutritional status, are altered. For example, dietary interventions known to up-regulate the expression of the low-density lipoprotein (LDL) receptor may also change the expression of genes coding for cholesterol-synthesizing enzymes. Further, expression profiles may vary between tissues, and it is known that not all individuals respond similarly to changing conditions. This may be due to differences in genetic background, but also to conditions such as differences in gender, age, physical activity or state of the disease. DNA microarrays are useful to understand better the interactions between a large number of genes and to examine events at a transcriptional level.

DNA microarrays or chips are a tool to detect with a single assay differences between two or more samples in the expression of a large number of genes. The concept behind this technique is comparable to that underlying Northern blotting. First, gene-specific polynucleotides are individually spotted on a flat solid support at designated places by a robot. These polynucleotides, which may be from known and unknown genes, are then probed with cDNA from both the test and reference material. These two sources of cDNA, which each has its own specific label, compete for binding on the array. The intensity of the signal from the label can now be measured and gives a global indication of the amount of cDNA present in the test sample relative to that in the reference sample. For example, the test material can be fluorescence labeled with a red tag and the control material with a green tag. If expression of a certain gene is similar in the test and reference samples, a yellow signal will appear. The final step is to interpret the expression profiles for which computer software is available. Likewise, arrays exist that measure gene expression levels of one sample at a time.

In principle, it is possible to obtain with DNA microarrays information on the expression profiles of numerous known and unknown genes at the same time in different tissues at various stages of a disease. Such studies will give an enormous amount of data that need to be analyzed in a meaningful way. For this, use is made of bioinformatics tools, such as clustering analysis and principal component analysis.

Quantification of protein synthesis

Proteins fulfill a very diverse role, which varies from being structural and contractile components to being essential regulatory elements in many cellular processes in the form of enzymes or hormones. Although mRNA serves as a template for protein, it is important to realize that the amount of mRNA is not necessarily correlated with the amount of protein. For example, mRNA can be degraded without being translated. In addition, proteins can be modified after translation in such a way that it alters their half-life, functions or activities. Finally, genetic variation may also result in different molecular forms of the protein. Therefore, it is important to obtain information not only on gene expression, but also on protein synthesis, modification and activity.

Various techniques are used for protein analysis. The most sensitive techniques are a combination of one or two methods that make use of differences in molecular weight, electric charge, size, shape or interactions with specific antibodies. A frequently used technique is Western blotting. Proteins are first isolated from a tissue or cell extract and then separated according to size by electrophoresis. Proteins are then transferred and permanently bound to a filter, which is subsequently incubated with one or two antibodies. At least one antibody is raised against this protein. This or a second antibody that recognizes the first antibody is tagged with a detectable component, which makes it possible to quantify the amount of protein present in the sample. It is also possible to quantify amounts of protein using enzyme-linked immunosorbent assays (ELISAs) or radioimmunoassays (RIAs). These techniques are mainly based on immunoreactivity and can detect many proteins at physiological concentrations. However, they do not make use of differences in molecular weight as with Western blotting, and may therefore be less specific for determining post-translational modification of proteins. The most direct approach to detect differences in proteins is to determine the amino acid sequence. Typically, a purified protein is first cleaved into a number of large peptide fragments, which are isolated. The next step is to determine the amino acid sequence of each fragment. If a part or the total amino sequence is known, the mRNA and exon sequence of the corresponding gene can be generated as information of the amino acid sequence provides information on the nucleotide sequence. This can then be used to synthesize probes to build libraries or to synthesize these proteins on a large scale for further studies or for the production of drugs such as insulin.

Cleavage of the protein into fragments and then into amino acids is also helpful to determine those parts of the protein that are transformed after translation. In this way, for example, it is possible to identify sides and the degree of phosphorylation or glycosylation. Comparable to DNA microarrays, arrays have also been developed for protein profiling. Instead of gene-specific polynucleotides, antibodies raised against proteins are spotted on a flat solid support. However, there is still a long way to go before these techniques can be used on a routine basis.

Stable isotopes: a tool to integrate cellular metabolism and whole-body physiology

With DNA arrays and protein arrays it is possible to obtain information on the expression and formation of many genes and proteins, respectively. This provides valuable information for delineating how patterns are influenced by internal and external stimuli. It does not, however, provide information on enzyme activity or quantify metabolic events *in vivo*. For example, an increase in the synthesis of a certain protein for gluconeogenesis does not necessarily mean that glucose production is also increased. Glucose production is very complex and controlled at many levels. To address such issues, stable isotope technology is helpful, with which quantitative information can be obtained in humans on *in vivo* rates of synthesis, degradation, turnover, fluxes between cells and tissues, and so on.

Stable isotopes are molecules that differ slightly in weight owing to differences in the number of neutrons of one or more atoms. For example, ^{12}C and ^{13}C refer to carbon atoms with atomic masses of 12 and 13, respectively, which behave similarly metabolically. In nature, about 99% of the carbon atoms are ^{12}C and only 1% ^{13}C. As they are non-radioactive, they can be used safely in human experiments. In contrast, radioactive isotopes are frequently used in animal or cell studies.

With the appropriate analytical techniques, it is possible to separate atoms and molecules based on differences in weight. All of these characteristics make stable isotopes useful tools to integrate cellular metabolism and whole-body physiology. Experiments are based on the low natural abundance of one of the isotopes. To use a very simplistic example, if one is interested in the rate of appearance in breath $^3CO_2$ from the oxidation of an oral dose of glucose, ^{13}C-labeled glucose (which is prepared on a commercial scale) can be given. The expired air will become enriched with $^{13}CO_2$, which can be measured. One now has the certainty that this $^{13}CO_2$ is derived from ^{13}C-labeled glucose. Ultimately, this gives information on the rate, proportion and amount of glucose oxidized. Such an approach is instrumental to increase our understanding on the metabolic consequences of the effects found at the cellular and molecular level.

2.5 Effects of the genetic code on the response to nutrients

Genetic polymorphisms may affect metabolic responses to diet by influencing the production, composition and/or activity of proteins. A considerable amount of research has therefore been conducted on the effects of common genetic polymorphisms on the response to nutrients. This is of great interest for at least two reasons. First, such studies provide information on specific molecular process underlying dietary responsiveness. Secondly, if a common genetic polymorphism determines the dietary response, then people can be identified who will, or will not, benefit from specific dietary recommendations. This would allow targeted dietary treatment for specific metabolic aberrations and ultimately the outcome of certain disease states.

Several general criteria can be formulated to assess the impact of the results on studies between polymorphisms and dietary responses. First of all, the polymorphism should affect the metabolic response by influencing the production, composition and/or activity of the proteins. Mutations in the promoter region will not affect the composition of the protein, but may affect its production. In contrast, mutations in an exon may not affect the production, but can change the composition and consequently the structure or activity of a protein. However, it is also possible that mutations in introns are associated with dietary responses. In such cases, it is very likely that this mutation is associated with another mutation in the genetic code that is responsible for the effects found. For the practical applicability of the results, it is relevant that the number of subjects in the population with that mutation is sufficient. Further, there should be pronounced, biologically relevant, effects of the polymorphism on dietary responses. However, even if the number of subjects is limited or the effects are marginal, such studies may still provide important information at the molecular level. Finally, there should be a plausible mechanism to explain the results.

Common polymorphisms and disease: the cholesteryl ester transfer protein Taq IB polymorphism

Cholesteryl ester transfer protein (CETP) is an important protein that regulates cholesterol metabolism; therefore, genetic and nutritional factors that affect this protein are important with respect to coronary heart disease. In human plasma CETP facilitates the transfer of cholesteryl ester from high-density lipoprotein (HDL) to apo B-containing lipoproteins such as LDL and very low-density lipoproteins (VLDL). As high LDL and VLDL cholesterol concentration and low HDL cholesterol concentrations are related to increased cardiovascular risk, CETP could be regarded as a potentially atherogenic factor. Worldwide, a few people have been identified with no CETP activity. From *in vitro* studies it appeared that these subjects have a defect in the transfer of cholesteryl ester from HDL to LDL or VLDL. These patients also have increased HDL cholesterol and lowered HDL triacylglycerol levels. Animals with no plasma CETP activity are relatively resistant to atherosclerosis, while CETP transgenic mice have decreased HDL cholesterol levels. Specific CETP inhibitors increase HDL cholesterol and slow down the progression of atherosclerosis in rabbits. All of these findings are in agreement with the predicted metabolic and functional effects of CETP *in vivo*.

The primary structure of human plasma CETP is known. The initial studies used a human liver library, in which CETP cDNA was identified, isolated and cloned using a partial amino acid sequence from purified CETP. Further studies demonstrated that the gene is located on chromosome 16. Several DNA polymorphisms for the CETP gene have been described. One of these polymorphisms, the *Taq* IB, has been identified in intron 1 by the restriction enzyme *Taq* I. The presence of this DNA variation is frequently referred to as B1 and its absence as B2. The B1 allele frequency varies between populations, but is in general somewhere between 0.4 and 0.6. This means that 16–36% of the population has the CETP *Taq* IB-1/1 genotype. Cross-sectional epidemiological studies in various population groups have shown that the presence of the B2 allele is associated with decreased CETP activity and increased HDL cholesterol levels. Further, it has been reported that subjects with the B2 allele have a lower cardiovascular risk.

Although this CETP polymorphism determines HDL cholesterol levels, effects on dietary responses are less evident. Several studies did not see any effect at all, but other studies have suggested that this polymorphism modulates the HDL or LDL cholesterol response to alcohol and fat intake. Effects, however, are small and not found in all studies. Further, it should be realized that the CETP *Taq* IB mutation is situated in intron 1 and it is not very likely that this mutation is functional. This suggests that this mutation in the CETP gene is a marker for a mutation in another part of the same gene or in another gene involved in lipid metabolism. Indeed, it has been found that the *Taq* IB mutation is in linkage disequilibrium with a functional mutation in the CETP promoter region.

Gly972Arg polymorphism in insulin receptor substrate-1

Insulin is well known for its role in glucose and lipid metabolism. After binding of insulin to the insulin receptor, insulin receptor substrate-1 (IRS-1) is activated by phosphorylation. In this way, the signal from plasma insulin is mediated in a variety of insulin-responsive cells and tissues, through the insulin receptor at the cell surface, towards intracellular enzymes. Because of this central role in the signal transduction pathway, IRS-1 may be involved in the decreased insulin sensitivity observed in patients with non-insulin-dependent diabetes mellitus.

The IRS-1 gene was cloned from a human male placenta library and found to be located on chromosome 2. Mice with no functional IRS-1 gene have been bred. These animals have a clustering of metabolic abnormalities characteristic for diabetic subjects. The sensitivity of IRS-1-deficient cells for insulin could be partially restored by transfecting these cells with IRS-1. Such studies clearly demonstrate the importance of IRS-1 in the insulin signaling cascade and insulin secretion pathways. However, disruption of the IRS-1 gene is not lethal in mice, which suggests that other pathways exist that can pass the signal of plasma insulin.

There are several amino acid polymorphisms in IRS-1, one of which, a glycine to arginine substitution at amino acid 972 (Gly972Arg mutation), is quite common. In the heterozygous form, the codon-972 variant of IRS-1 is present in about 10% of the population, but may be more prevalent in subjects with non-insulin-dependent diabetes mellitus or dyslipidemia. Carriers of the Gly972Arg allele have lower fasting insulin concentrations and a less favorable plasma lipoprotein profile than non-carriers. Further, cultured cells transfected with either wild-type human IRS-1 or the Gly972Arg variant showed that this mutation impaired insulin-stimulated signaling. From these studies, it appears that this polymorphism may contribute to insulin resistance.

More interestingly from a nutritional point of view, an interaction between this Gly972Arg mutation of IRS-1 and body mass has been suggested. The already increased frequency of the Gly972Arg mutation in patients with coronary heart disease was even further increased in obese subjects. The results of the intravenous glucose tolerance test were less favorable in moderately overweight heterozygous carriers of this polymorphism than in wild-type subjects. These findings suggests that only overweight subjects with this Gly972Arg variant would benefit from weight loss with respect to improved insulin sensitivity. It should

be noted that this interaction with obesity has not been observed in all studies.

677C–T polymorphism of methylene-tetrahydrofolate reductase

Increased levels of plasma homocysteine, a sulfur-containing amino acid, are associated with an increased risk of various disorders such as neural tube defects, thrombotic disease and vascular disease. These associations do not prove a causal role for homocysteine in these diseases, but they do indicate that homocysteine plays an important role in many physiological processes. In homocysteine metabolism, a crucial role is fulfilled by the enzyme methylene-tetrahydrofolate reductase (MTHFR). The MTHFR gene is located on chromosome 1. Some subjects with MTHFR deficiency have been identified and they all have increased homocysteine levels. To study the *in vivo* pathogenetic and metabolic consequences of MTHFR deficiency, an MTHFR knockout mouse model has been generated. Homocysteine levels are slightly elevated in heterozygous animals and are increased 10-fold in homozygous knockout mice. The homozygous animals show similar diseases to human MTHFR patients, supporting a causal role of hyperhomocysteinemia in these diseases. Nevertheless, extrapolation from animal studies to the human situation remains a problem.

A common DNA polymorphism in the MTHFR gene is a C-to-T substitution at nucleotide 677, which results in the replacement of alanine for valine. The allelic frequency of the 677C–T genotype, which can be identified with the restriction enzyme *Hin*fI, is as high as 35% in some populations, but the allelic frequency of the 677C–T polymorphism varies widely between populations. Substitution of the alanine for valine results in a reduced enzyme activity and individuals homozygous for this polymorphism have significantly increased plasma homocysteine concentrations. Thus, the 677C–T mutation may have functional consequences. An increased frequency of the 677T allele in patients with pre-eclampsia, neural tube defects and cardio-vascular disease has been claimed by some studies, but refuted by others.

It has been hypothesized that the lack of association between MTHFR polymorphisms and disease in certain populations may be due to differences in dietary status. Homocysteine metabolism requires the participation of folate and vitamin B_{12}. In the plasma, a negative relationship exists between homocysteine levels and those of folate and vitamin B_{12}. Moreover, supplementation with folate in particular, but also with vitamin B_{12}, reduced fasting homocysteine levels. In this respect, subjects carrying the 677C–T mutation were more responsive. Thus, a daily low-dose supplement of folic acid will reduce and in many cases normalize slightly increased homocysteine levels, which is explained by a possible effect on the stability of folate on MTHFR. Whether this will result in a reduced disease risk or whether certain population groups are more responsive to folate intervention needs to be established.

Conclusions

Results of studies on the effects of genetic polymorphisms on the response to dietary interventions are often inconsistent. Several explanations can be offered for this. First of all, many of the earlier, pioneering studies were carried out in retrospect. This means that genotyping was performed after the study had ended and that groups were not well balanced. For example, if a study is carried out with 150 subjects and the allele frequency of a certain mutation is 10%, then the expected number of subjects homozygous or even heterozygous for that mutation will be low. As a consequence, groups will be small and it will be difficult to find any differences between the groups with respect to differences in responses to the diets, simply because of a lack of statistical power. Another explanation is that the effects of the polymorphism of interest depend on the make-up of other genes (gene–gene interaction). Human studies on gene–gene interaction are even more difficult to design. Suppose that the frequency of a certain polymorphism is 10% and that of another is 20%. Such values are not uncommon, but it means that only 2% of the subjects may have the combination of the two mutations of interest. Thus, one needs to screen many subjects to find appropriate numbers. Similarly, effects may depend on gender, age or other factors, such as body mass index, smoking or state of the disease. Without doubt, studies on gene–gene or environment–gene interaction will expand our knowledge on the effects of the genetic code on the response to nutrients. Finally, it is possible that in a certain population the polymorphism is a marker for another, unknown, genetic defect. Ideally, results should therefore always be confirmed in different, independent populations with different genetic backgrounds.

As already mentioned, one of the rationales for studies on genetic polymorphisms in relation to dietary responses is that people can be identified who will, or will not, benefit from specific dietary recommendations. It has become clear, however, that dietary responses are a complex combination of genetic and environmental factors. In general, the known relationships between responses to diet with genetic polymorphisms are not very strong and different combinations of genetic and environmental factors may ultimately lead to a similar response. To address such issues, cell and animal studies are also relevant. Another approach is to make a complete inventory of differences in gene expression or protein synthesis in a particular organ or cell type after changing dietary intake. For this, microarray analyses can be useful. It is clear that there is still a long way to go, but studies on specific molecular processes underlying dietary responsiveness remain a major challenge.

2.6 Nutrient regulation of gene expression

While nutritional recommendations strive to promote good health through good nutrition, it is clear that such population-based strategies do not account for variations in an individual's nutritional requirements. These variations are due to our genetic background and environmental factors, including nutrition. The previous section showed how different genetic variations or polymorphisms can alter an individual's nutritional responses to diet. This section will examine how nutrients affect gene expression. The expression of a gene that results in an active protein can be regulated at any number of points between transcription and the synthesis of the final protein product. While the process of gene expression is well understood, as detailed in Section 2.3, relatively little is known about how nutrients affect gene expression, at the level of either mRNA or protein. Nevertheless, there are a few examples of nutrients that affect gene expression to alter mRNA and/or active protein levels by interacting with transcriptional, post-transcriptional and post-translational events. The effect of nutrients on gene expression is a very intensive area of research. In light of the technological advances in molecular biology, as detailed in Section 2.4, the number of examples of nutrient regulation of gene expression will expand rapidly over the next few years. Ultimately, it is important not only to understand the concept of nutrient regulation of gene expression (at both the mRNA and protein level), but also to know how changes at the level of the gene relate to whole-body metabolism and health.

Nutrient regulation of gene transcription

Theoretically, gene expression can be regulated at many points between the conversion of a gene sequence in to mRNA and into protein. For most genes, the control of transcription is stronger than that of translation. As reviewed in Section 2.3, this is achieved by specific regulatory sequences, known as *cis*-acting control elements, in the promoter region of the gene, and *trans*-acting factors, known as transcription factors or DNA-binding proteins, that interact with the promoter region of genes and modulate gene expression. Nutrients can alter the transcription of target genes; some examples of this are detailed in Table 2.3.

Direct and indirect nutrient regulation of gene transcription

Certain dietary constituents can influence gene expression by direct interaction with regulatory elements in the genome, altering the transcription of a given gene. Examples include retinoic acid, vitamin D, fatty acids and zinc. However, nutrients can also have an indirect effect on gene transcription. It is often difficult to discern whether a gene–nutrient interaction is a direct effect of a particular nutrient, or an indirect effect of a metabolite or a secondary mediator such as a hormone, eicosanoid or a secondary cell message that alters transcription. For example, many genes involved in fat and carbohydrate metabolism have genes that have an insulin response element in their promoter region. Hence, a particular fatty acid or carbohydrate could mediate its effect via insulin. The indirect

route may be particularly important for the more complex dietary components because they have a number of bioactive constituents. For example, part of dietary fiber is metabolized by the colonic flora to produce butyric acid. Butyric acid, in turn, may affect gene expression by selective effects on G-proteins (which are intracellular messengers) or by direct interactions with DNA regulatory sequences.

Nutrient regulation of transcription factors

Nutrients can also regulate the expression of transcription factors and thereby alter gene expression. The peroxisome proliferator activated receptors (PPARs) are a good example of *trans*-acting transcription factors that can be modulated by nutritional factors. PPARs are members of the nuclear hormone receptor superfamily and these regulate the expression of many genes involved in cellular differentiation, proliferation, apoptosis, fatty acid metabolism, lipoprotein metabolism and inflammation. PPARs are ligand-dependent transcription factors, which are activated by a number of compounds, including fatty acids. There are several members of the PPAR family, PPARα, PPARγ and PPARδ (β) each with multiple isoforms. PPARα is primarily expressed in the liver, PPARγ in adipose tissue and PPARδ (β) is ubiquitously expressed. When activated by fatty acids (or eicosanoids and pharmacological PPAR agonists) the PPARs combine with the retinoid X receptor (RXR). This PPAR–RXR heterodimer binds to a PPAR response element (PPRE) in the promoter region of the target gene and induces transcription of the target gene. Many genes involved in lipid and glucose metabolism have PPRE, some of which are listed in Table 2.4. Therefore, the PPARs represent an example of how nutrients can regulate gene expression through transcription factors. Sterol regulatory

Table 2.3 Effect of nutrients on gene transcription

Nutrient	Gene	Transcriptional effect
Glucose	Glucokinase	Increase
Retinoic acid	Retinoic acid receptor	Increase
Vitamin B_6	Steroid hormone receptor	Decrease
Zinc	Zinc-dependent enzymes	Increase
Vitamin C	Procollagen	Increase
Cholesterol	HMG CoA reductase	Decrease
Fatty acids	SREBP	Increase

HMG CoA: 3-hydroxy-3-methylglutaryl-coenzyme A; SREBP: sterol regulatory response element binding protein.

Table 2.4 PPAR-responsive genes and their metabolic effect

PPAR target genes	Target cell	Metabolic effect
aP2	Adipocyte	Adipogenesis
FABP, ACS	Adipocyte	Fatty acid synthesis
Apo CIII, LPL	Hepatocyte	VLDL metabolism
Apo AI, Apo AII	Hepatocyte	HDL metabolism

PPAR: peroxisome proliferator activator receptor; VLDL: very low-density lipoprotein; HDL: high-density lipoprotein; FABP: fatty acid binding protein; ACS: acyl-CoA synthetase; LPL: lipoprotein lipase.

response element binding proteins (SREBPs) are another group of transcription factors that mediate the effects of dietary fatty acids on gene expression. There are two forms of SREBP: SREBP-1 regulates fatty acid and triacylglycerol synthesis, whereas SREBP-2 regulates the genes involved in cholesterol metabolism. Therefore, the SREBPs modulate the expression of the genes involved in cholesterol and fatty acid metabolism, in response to different fatty acid treatments.

Nutrients and post-transcriptional control of gene expression

It is generally accepted that the initiation of transcription is the primary mode of regulating gene expression, and there are good examples of different nutrients increasing and decreasing mRNA expression. However, there is increasing evidence that the response of gene expression to nutrients involves control of post-transcriptional events. Much of the evidence for post-transcriptional control comes from observed discrepancies between mRNA abundance and transcriptional rates (altered mRNA abundance associated with unchanged gene transcription implies altered mRNA stability). In addition, mRNA abundance is not necessarily correlated to protein concentration (altered protein concentration in the absence of any changes in mRNA abundance implies either altered translation of the mRNA or changes in the proteolytic breakdown of the protein). Since nutrients can regulate mRNA translation and stability, mRNA abundance may not reflect amounts of protein or rates of synthesis. Therefore, it is incorrect to assume that if a nutrient alters the level of mRNA then there is a concomitant change in protein levels. To assess with confidence the effect of a nutrient on gene expression, mRNA analysis should be accompanied by measurements of the protein product.

Table 2.5 Nutrient regulation of gene expression: post-transcriptional control

Gene	Nutritional factor	Control point	Regulatory element
Ferritin	Iron	Translation	5′ UTR
Transferrin receptor	Iron	Stability	3′ UTR
Glutathione peroxidase	Selenium	Translation	3′ UTR
Glucose transporter-1	Fed/fasted state	Translation	5′ UTR
Lipoprotein lipase	Fatty acid supply	Translation	3′ UTR
Apolipoprotein CIII	Hyperlipidemia	Unknown	3′ UTR

Some examples of post-transcriptional control of gene–nutrient interactions are presented in Table 2.5. It is important to note that often the non-coding region of the gene may play a key role in the regulation of gene expression whereby nutrients interact with regulatory elements located in the 5′ and the 3′ UTRs of a range of target genes, mediating the effect of nutrients on gene expression.

Iron is a classical example of how a nutrient regulates the expression of the genes involved in its metabolism (Figure 2.8). Transferrin and ferritin are key proteins involved in iron metabolism, and the expression of each is determined by the non-coding region of transferrin and ferritin mRNA. The transferrin receptor is required for the uptake of iron in cells. Transferrin receptor has five regulatory sequences, known as the iron response elements (IREs) in the 3′ UTR. In the absence of iron, trans-acting transcription repressor proteins, the iron regulatory proteins (IRPs), bind to the IRE and protect the mRNA from degradation. In the presence of iron, the IRPs are removed from the transferrin receptor mRNA, leading to mRNA destabilization, decreased translation of mRNA and decreased transferrin receptor synthesis. This mechanism therefore prevents excessive amounts of iron being taken up by a cell.

Ferritin is required for the storage of iron. It sequesters cellular iron which would otherwise be toxic. The expression of ferritin is also regulated post-transcriptionally. This controls the supply of free iron within the cell according to cellular iron levels. Ferritin has an IRE in the 5′ UTR that regulates transcription. When cellular iron levels are low the IRP binds the IRE and represses translation of ferritin, thus supplying free iron as required for cell metabolism. In the presence of iron the IRP does not bind the IRE and ferritin translation is increased to allow storage of iron. The presence of similar IREs in the transferrin receptor and ferritin mRNA is important because it allows coordinated regulation of the synthesis of the two proteins according to different cellular levels and requirements for protein.

Nutrient regulation of translation and post-translational protein modification

Hypothetically, a nutrient could regulate the translation of mRNA into protein. However, to date there are no examples of a direct effect of a nutrient on protein translation that is independent of alterations in mRNA. Similarly, there is little information on the effects of nutrients on post-translational protein

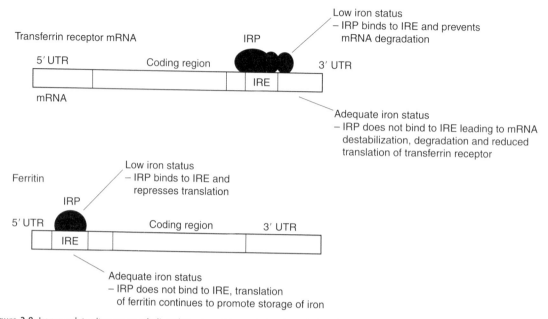

Figure 2.8 Iron regulates its own metabolism through post-transcriptional regulation of transferrin and ferritin.

modification. Vitamin K is one of the very few examples of nutrient regulation of post-translational protein modification, and it has this effect by regulating the activation of prothrombin. Prothrombin is an essential protein involved in the coagulation system. It is the proenzyme for thrombin, which is an inherent component of the clot. Prothrombin cannot function correctly unless its glutamic acid residues are carboxylated. Carboxylation of prothrombin allows it to bind to calcium, and prothrombin can only participate in the clotting process if it can bind to calcium. This post-translational modification means that the nascent prothrombin protein is dependent on the supply of vitamin K. Apart from the effect of overt vitamin K deficiency on coagulation, the extent to which an individual's vitamin K status affects clotting is unknown. Further research that specifically addresses whether and/or how nutrients modulate protein expression is required to gain a greater understanding of this aspect of molecular nutrition.

2.7 Perspectives on the future

Molecular nutrition represents a new phase of nutrition research that will provide a much greater understanding of the interactions between nutrients and the human genome. This chapter explored the technological opportunities in molecular biology that can be applied to nutrition research. These rapidly advancing technologies present tremendous opportunities for improving our understanding of nutritional science. The Human Genome Project will undoubtedly improve our understanding of genetic background and diversity. From the perspective of nutrition, we should be able to develop a greater understanding of how nutrients interact with genetic destiny, alter disease processes and promote health. Within the context of human nutrition probably the greatest challenge is to develop experimental models that mimic the *in vivo* response and whole-body metabolism. Such models need to be developed to maximize the potential of the novel molecular technologies to investigate the molecular and cellular effects of nutrients in experimental models that can be extrapolated and applied to human health. No doubt the next decade will be very exciting in terms of grasping the novel molecular technologies and applying them in an intelligent manner to nutrition research. It is hoped that the next phase of molecular nutrition research will generate a more comprehensive understanding of the cellular and molecular effects of nutrients and improve our understanding of whether and how nutrients modulate disease processes. The ultimate goal will be the ability to define scientifically sound, evidence-based nutritional strategies to promote health.

Further reading

Anon. Nutrition in the post-genomic era. Proc Nutr Soc 2002 ; 61(4): 401–463.

Berdanier CD, ed. Nutrient Regulation of Gene Expression: Clinical Aspects. Boca Raton, FL: CRC Press, 1996.

Cox TM, Sinclair J. Molecular Biology in Medicine. Oxford: Blackwell, 1997.

Hanash SM. Operomics: molecular analysis of tissues from DNA to RNA to protein. Clin Chem Lab Med 2000; 38: 805–813.

Hirschi KD, Kreps JA, Hirschi KK. Molecular approaches to studying nutrient metabolism and function: an array of possibilities. J Nutr 2001; 131: 1605S–1609S.

Luscombe NM, Greenbaum D, Gerstein M. What is bioinformatics? A proposed definition and overview of the field. Meth Inf Med 2001; 40: 346–358.

3
Integration of Metabolism 1: Energy

XM Leverve

Key messages

- Energy metabolism refers to the ways in which the body obtains and spends energy from food. In terms of energy transduction, part of nutrient energy is converted into chemical, mechanical, electrical or osmotic forms of energy.
- The steady state refers to when the production of final metabolites equals the consumption of the initial precursors: exactly the same amount of matter enters and leaves the system.
- The mitochondrion is the key cellular organelle involved in energy metabolism. The mitochondrion is also involved in other key cellular processes, including apoptosis, calcium signaling and reactive oxygen species production.
- The chemical energy in nutrients (redox energy) is converted into adenosine triphosphate (ATP). ATP is the universal currency of cellular energy metabolism; it is formed from adenosine diphosphate (ADP) by oxidative phosphorylation.
- At a given cellular level, ATP can be synthesized aerobically or anaerobically, that is in the presence or absence of oxygen. But when considering the whole organism, interorgan aerobic and anaerobic energy metabolism must be complementary and steady-state energy metabolism must be completely aerobic.
- Energy metabolism for the whole body is primarily due to resting energy expenditure. The thermic effects of food and physical activity are also important components of energy expenditure.

3.1 Introduction

From an energy point of view, life is a succession of transfers that obey the second law of thermodynamics stating that the entropy of the universe is steadily increasing. But, when considering living organisms as isolated systems, they appear to be a kind of exception to this principle since, by definition, a biosynthetic pathway would decrease the entropy of the newly synthesized biomolecules, at the expense of the universe free energy, through catabolism of nutrients. Unlike plants, animals, including humans, are unable to use the light directly as a source of energy. Hence, these living organisms must use another source of energy, provided from the catabolism of nutrients, the synthesis of which is directly or indirectly permitted via plant photosynthesis. Therefore, our life is indirectly but totally dependent on sunlight, as the unique energy source for plants, and on the complex, but highly regulated pathways that link nutrient degradation to adenosine triphosphate (ATP) synthesis.

All kinds of biochemical reactions are linked to energy transfer, therefore each physiological function, as well as each pathological disorder or therapy, must have a consequence for biological energy. It is probable that further investigation of energy disorders in pathological states will lead to a better understanding of the underlying pathophysiological mechanisms and to new therapeutic tools. Living systems must be efficient in situations of both abundance and penury; therefore, two distinct classes of diseases can be proposed. On the one hand are diseases of excess nutrients. For example, excess energy intake is associated with obesity, diabetes, hyperlipidemia and atherosclerosis.

On the other hand, diseases related to a deficit of nutrients can occur at the level of the whole body, individual organs or discrete cells. Diseases of scarcity include anorexia, cachexia, shock, hypoxia and ischemia, which can lead to acute or chronic nutrient imbalance.

The last introductory remark concerning energy metabolism is related to the fact that there is a peril to life related to respiratory chain activity. Indeed, energy metabolism is mainly based on redox reactions involving molecular oxygen as the final electron acceptor, and reactive oxygen species (ROS) represent a major danger to many biomolecules and therefore to life. ROS are probably one of the major determinants of the process of aging. In this view, understanding the mechanisms for sensing and transducing the surrounding oxygen concentrations, based on the flux of ROS production, represents a major field of research for possible applications oriented towards new therapies for several diseases such as anoxia, ischemia, diabetes, atherosclerosis, cancer and degenerative pathologies.

3.2 Energy metabolism at the cellular level

Thermodynamics

Energy is a property of the matter permitting it to be transformed, either as the result of a work or as achieving work. The common use of terms such as 'energy consumption' or 'energy production' is not proper. Indeed, in accordance with the first law of thermodynamics the amount of energy in the universe remains constant, so it is only possible to convert energy from one form to another, but not to produce or to consume it. This is known as energy transduction. Hence, humans transform the nutrient-contained energy into chemical, mechanical, electrical or osmotic forms of energy. The second law of thermodynamic indicates that the transformation of energy is always in the direction of a continuous increased universe entropy which is the ultimate form of energy that cannot be used for any further work. In simple terms entropy can be viewed as the degree of disorder of matter; it is a kind of waste after a work achievement. Whatever biochemical reactions are, fast or not, probable or not, reversible or not, they must always follow energy transfers and the general direction of metabolism always obeys the laws of thermodynamics.

Our world is the location of permanent energy exchanges between systems, which have different potentials. These energy exchanges are performed in strict accordance with two principles called thermodynamic laws. This statement, proposed by the French scientist Carnot more than a century ago, was never really demonstrated but so far it has never failed! The first law states that total energy of the universe is constant: 'Rien ne se perd, rien ne se crée, tout se transforme', while the second gives the direction of the exchanges: universe entropy must always increase.

The consequences of the second law may be illustrated by a simple example. According to this second law, entropy can never decrease. However, when a liter of water freezes, the degree of organization of its constitutive molecules increases and therefore entropy decreases. To achieve this result, the freezer produces heat on its back in such a way that the overall result (water in and freezer out) is increased entropy according to the second law. Life can be compared to this: although it leads to the organization of molecules, thus decreasing their own entropy, the degradation of nutrients initially produced from the energy of the light of the sun results in an increased entropy of the universe.

Equilibrium, steady state, metabolic control and metabolic regulation

One of the main features of any living system is represented by the achievement of real steady states. Metabolic reactions are completed close to or far from the equilibrium, leading to definition of two different fields of thermodynamics: equilibrium thermodynamics and non-equilibrium thermodynamics. Therefore, it is important to realize that the actual meaning of equilibrium is often misused. Equilibrium means that both forward and reverse reactions are strictly equal in such a way that the net flux is equal to zero and that reactant concentrations are constant. Such a state is incompatible with life and might be viewed as a definition of death: no change, no past, no future, but only an endless stable state. In the state of equilibrium, every event is completely reversible, leading to a total lack of evolution. In living organisms many of the biochemical reactions are not really at equilibrium but occur close to it. In terms of energy metabolism, this near state of equilibrium is often referred to as energy balance. However, it is important to realize that energy balance is not a state of equilibrium but is a steady state. Indeed, maintaining the energy content of the body depends on energy intake (in) and energy dissipation (out), so strictly speaking body composition (or its energy content) is maintained constant but at the expense of substrate supply and product removal, which is the definition of a steady state. In these near-equilibrium reactions both forward and reverse reactions are of large magnitude, but one of them is slightly greater than the other. This permits a real net flux to be achieved, while reactant concentrations are quickly equilibrated after any change in the concentration of the others. Thermodynamic strengths impose the direction of the reactions according to the second law of thermodynamics.

- Equilibrium equals death: no net flux, no work and definitive immobility.
- Steady state: constant renewal, characteristics of life, but exogenous systems are required for sustaining it with both input (nutrients and oxygen entering the system) and exit (wastage).

In any living system, the maintenance of a single metabolic parameter (blood glucose, cellular ATP, oxygen concentration, etc.) at a constant level can be referred to as substrate balance. It is important to appreciate that this is a limited part of a metabolic pathway, within the context of whole-body metabolism, which in turn has its metabolic steady state. The metabolic 'steady

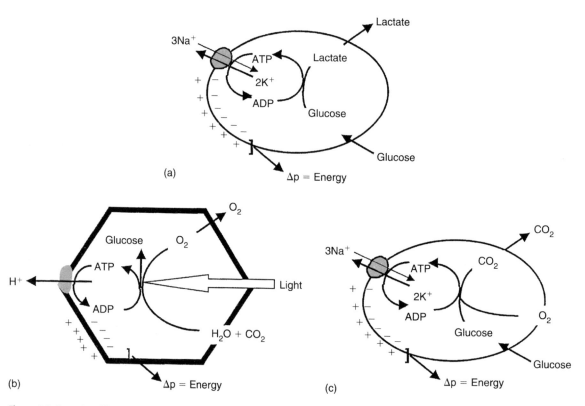

Figure 3.1 Examples of living energy transducing systems. (a) Anaerobic system: the energy source is provided by organic nutrients (i.e. made by a living system) converted through a pathway (fermentation) resulting in ATP generation (phosphate potential or ATP/ADP · Pi ratio). The plasma membrane ATPase (Na^+/K^+-ATPase) allows the conversion of to this phosphate potential into a membrane potential (Δp) because of the electrogenic exchange of $3Na^+$ with $2K^+$ and permits to the cell to generate some work. The erythrocyte represents a good example of a completely anaerobic cell, where the unique source of energy is glucose and the unique energy wastage is lactate, with a stoichiometry of 2 moles of ATP for 1 mole of glucose. (b) Phototrophic system: the energy source is light, which enables the extraction of hydrogen from water. The transduction of energy into ATP and then into membrane potential is similar to the anaerobic system except that Na^+/K^+-ATPase is replaced by a proton ATPase. (c) Aerobic system: the source of energy is the redox power contained in the nutrients (carbohydrates or lipids), electrons from hydrogen finally being transferred to oxygen, permitting the formation of water. The successive energy transduction processes are similar to those of the anaerobic system (a), but the production of ATP is much higher. The stoichiometry of ATP synthesis depends on the substrates used, and the waste products are water and carbon dioxide.

state' is also often referred to as 'metabolic balance'. For examples of this relating to fat and carbohydrate metabolism, refer to Chapter 5. Such a metabolic state can be defined as a peculiar condition where both net resulting flux and related intermediates are constant, meaning that production of final metabolite(s) equals consumption of initial precursor(s) (Figure 3.1). In this view, the 'milieu intérieur', as denominated by Bernard more than a century ago, is the result of the metabolism of every cell from every organ in a whole organism. Its steady-state composition can be viewed as the best compromise between cell priorities and needs for cellular or interorgan cooperation. Hence, each cell can theoretically interfere with the metabolism of every cell. The transition between different steady states is initiated by changes in intermediates and/or fluxes (pre-steady states) allowing the new steady state to be reached, as a consequence of the new physiological (i.e. fed versus fasted, sleep, physical activity, pregnancy, growth, etc.) or pathological states. The metabolic fluxes (e.g. ATP synthesis, oxygen consumption, gluconeogenesis, glycolysis, β-oxidation) are dependent on two different kinds of parameter:

- one pertaining to the thermodynamic strengths, which is the energetic result of reactant concentrations (i.e. substrates versus products) *pushing* the conversion of a precursor into a product
- the second pertaining to kinetic constraints, which might be viewed as the ability of a metabolic machinery (e.g. enzyme, carrier) to achieve the conversion (transport) of a substrate into a product.

When a system is in a steady state, any change in a given kinetic parameter (e.g. increase in enzymic activity or supply of a nutrient) will affect the entire network, causing it to achieve a new steady state. The information as to the 'new' rules of the system resulting from the change in one parameter can be relayed in two separate, but not mutually exclusive ways.

First, any change in one of the kinetic constraints of the system will affect in turn the different intermediates, upstream and/or downstream of the modified step (Figure 3.2). The magnitude of the transmitted effect on the different intermediates depends on the characteristics of each step. This parameter is called elasticity. This form of information transmitted by the changes in intermediate concentrations is called *metabolic control*.

Secondly, a given change in one of the intermediates can trigger a signal (e.g. hormonal or cellular signaling), which in turn affects the kinetics of one or more step(s) of the pathway. Such a mechanism is referred to as *metabolic regulation*.

- Metabolic control: a modification occurring on a step of a given pathway can be transmitted by adjacent modifications of all reactants involved in the pathway in order to affect the whole pathway.
- Metabolic regulation: a modification occurring on a step of a pathway can be transmitted to an effector, external to the system (any kind of signaling), which in turn can affect one or more step(s) of the pathway or of other pathways.

Cellular and mitochondrial aerobic energy metabolism

The transformation of a part of the energy contained in nutrients into a form that can be used by the cells for different types of work can be divided into two successive steps. First, the chemical energy contained in the nutrient must be converted into a redox form and then this redox potential must be transduced as a phosphate potential [ATP/(ADP · Pi, where ADP is adeno-

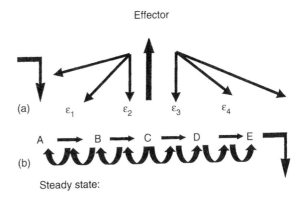

Effector

(a)

ε_1 ε_2 ε_3 ε_4

A → B → C → D → E

(b)

Steady state:

$$[A] = [B] = [C] = [D] = [E] = \text{constant}$$

(c) $\quad J_{A \to E} = J\varepsilon_1 = J\varepsilon_2 = J\varepsilon_3 = J\varepsilon_4$

Figure 3.2 Metabolic regulation, metabolic control and steady state: a schematic view. Capital letters (A, B, C, D, E) represent intermediates, ε_1, ε_2, ε_3, ε_4 are enzymes and J means flux. (a, b) Schematic representations of metabolic regulation and metabolic control, respectively; (c) metabolic characteristics of a steady state. In this view any metabolic intermediate (glucose, lactate, ATP, etc.) could be viewed as the intermediate B and ε_2 is a part of the downstream pathway (glycolysis, gluconeogenesis, ATPase, etc.).

sine diphosphate and Pi is inorganic phosphate)] by ATP synthesis.

From macronutrient to redox potential

The macronutrients, carbohydrates (glucose), amino acids and fatty acids, are catabolized by different pathways, including glycolysis, β-oxidation and amino acid pathways. However, all of them converge towards a common intermediate: acetyl-coenzyme A (acetyl-CoA). Glycolysis is the only energy-yielding pathway capable of producing ATP independently of the mitochondrion and without oxygen. This process is referred to as anaerobic metabolism (see later section). In the mitochondrial matrix, the tricarboxylic acid cycle, also known as the Krebs cycle, leads to a complete oxidation of acetyl-CoA, resulting in the formation of reducing equivalents (three NADH, H^+ and one $FADH_2$) and carbon dioxide (CO_2). The main result of the Krebs cycle activity is to provide reducing power to the respiratory chain in the form of $NADH/NAD^+$ or $FADH_2/FAD$, rather than ATP formation. (NAD^+ is nicotinamide adenine dinucleotide, NADH its reduced form and NAD^+ its oxidized form; FAD is flavin adenine dinucleotide.) Only one ATP, or guanosine triphosphate (GTP), is formed per mole of oxidized acetyl-CoA, compared with 14 ATP molecules that can result from reducing equivalent reoxidation.[1] Oxygen is not directly involved in this part of the pathway. However, the dehydrogenases that oxidize acetyl-CoA work at near-equilibrium and the accumulation of NADH, due to lack of oxygen, inhibits the net flux of acetyl-CoA through the Krebs cycle. Hence, although not directly involved, oxygen plays a crucial role in the Krebs cycle activity by maintaining adequate reducing potential.

A potential is the amount of a given form of energy that can be *potentially* used for a work. On top of a mountain, a liter of water represents a given amount of energy. If this water falls from the top of the mountain through a waterfall, a part of this energy is progressively converted into kinetic potential during the fall. At the bottom of the waterfall, when the water crashes on a rock, the kinetic potential is then converted to heat, i.e. to entropy. In this case some of the initial potential is directly converted to heat. If the waterfall is equipped with a turbine, some of the kinetic energy can be converted to electrical energy: this is an example of coupling machinery. But when the electrical energy is converted to light, it will result in an increase in entropy. In this case the potential energy is also finally converted to heat, but on the way it also provides light.

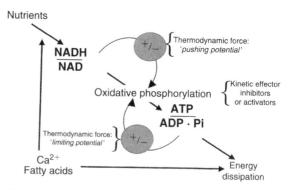

Figure 3.3 Regulation of oxidative phosphorylation flux. The control of oxidative phosphorylation is exerted by two different factors: kinetic parameters (i.e. kinetic properties of the different enzymes) and thermodynamic factors (i.e. forces exerted on the system). A dramatic change in the flux without a large change in either redox potential or phosphate potential implies subtle co-ordinated mechanisms, as is done for instance by calcium or fatty acids, which affect the oxidative phosphorylation pathway simultaneously upstream and downstream.

- Redox potential [$(NADH^+ \times H^+)/NAD^+$]: the amount of energy that can be released when one (or often two) electron(s) jump(s) from one compound (which will be oxidized) to another (which will be reduced).
- Phosphate potential [$ATP/(ADP \cdot Pi)$]: the amount of energy that can be released when ATP is converted to ADP and Pi.

From redox potential to ATP synthesis

Mitochondrial energy is supplied by proton oxidation, oxygen being the final electron acceptor:

$$4H^+ + 4e^- + O_2 \rightarrow 2H_2O + \text{energy}$$

This reaction leads to a large release of energy, which is normally dissipated as heat, pressure or an increase in volume. The unique property of the mitochondrial respiratory chain is to convert, with high efficiency, energy towards ADP phosphorylation. As first proposed by Mitchell, and now generally accepted, energy release during oxidation in the respiratory chain results in active proton transport outside the mitochondrial matrix. Hence, owing to the sequence of the respiratory chain complexes, the redox energy is converted into another form of potential: the mitochondrial inner membrane potential or proton-motive force. The next step in the oxidative phosphorylation pathway is to use this proton-motive force for ATP synthesis. The enzymic complex of mitochondrial ATP synthase (Figure 3.3) achieves this. It is important to note that oxidation (also known as respiration) and phosphorylation (or ATP synthesis) are connected through a common intermediate, the proton-motive force.

This proton-motive force depends on:

- the activity of the respiratory chain by pumping protons out of the matrix
- the ATPase by transferring protons back in the matrix when ATP is synthesized
- the properties of the inner membrane, creating a barrier that is impermeable to protons.

Practical assessment of oxidative phosphorylation

Although it is relatively simple to investigate the oxidative phosphorylation pathway in isolated mitochondria, this is much more difficult in an intact system or *in vivo*. The whole pathway of oxidative phosphorylation can be divided schematically in several steps:

1. cytosolic pathways that result in cytosolic redox potential.
2. mitochondrial oxidation of acetyl-CoA (Krebs cycle) that results in mitochondrial redox potential.
3. respiratory chain activity and its resultant proton-motive force.
4. ATP synthesis and resultant mitochondrial phosphate potential.
5. electrogenic ATP–ADP exchanges across the mitochondrial inner membrane (adenine nucleotide translocator) and resultant cytosolic phosphate potential.

The electrochemical potential across the inner mitochondrial membrane is of crucial importance for each of these steps. Therefore, any phenomenon that could affect it (e.g. proton leak, see below) would affect the complete pathway of ATP synthesis. Cytosolic lactate dehydrogenase and mitochondrial 3-hydroxybutyrate dehydrogenase work at near equilibrium state. Therefore, the cytosolic and mitochondrial redox state can be evaluated by measuring lactate-to-pyruvate and 3-hydroxybutyrate-to-acetoacetate ratios.[2] These measurements are useful tools that can be used to evaluate any defects in the oxidative pathway *in vivo*. The activity of the respiratory chain can be assessed by measuring the rate of oxygen consumption either at the level of the whole body or in an isolated organ, cell(s) or mitochondrion. The most difficult parameters of oxidative phosphorylation to assess are phosphate potential, ATP synthesis (or turnover rate) and the

yield of ATP synthesis, i.e. of oxidative pathway. Indeed, if ATP concentration could be calculated *in vivo* by nuclear magnetic resonance (NMR), then phosphate potential could be determined if the concentration of ADP was known. However, ADP concentration cannot be obtained directly. Moreover, since adenine nucleotides are highly compartmentalized in the cell (see below), average values for intracellular or tissue ATP levels are of limited interest.

Regulation of the flux through oxidative phosphorylation

Although much is known concerning the regulation of the different enzymes of the oxidative phosphorylation pathway, the actual regulation of mitochondrial respiration and the rate of ATP synthesis is not fully understood. The sophisticated machinery of this pathway can be simplified as a single step catalyzing the following reaction:

$$2NADH + 2H^+ + O_2 + 6ADP + 6Pi$$
$$\rightarrow 2NAD^+ + 2H_2O + 6ATP$$

As for any biochemical reaction, its rate is dependent on kinetic and thermodynamic parameters: the activity and affinity of enzymes and resulting thermodynamic strength applied to the system (i.e. the difference between upstream and downstream potentials). In the case of oxidative phosphorylation, redox potential (NADH/NAD) represents upstream potential and *pushes* the flux; while downstream, opposed to the redox potential and *limiting* the flux, is the phosphate potential (ATP/ADP · Pi) (Figure 3.3). Thus, an increased NADH/NAD ratio and/or a decreased ATP/ADP · Pi ratio will increase the flux. Conversely, a decrease in NADH/NAD and/or an increased ATP/ADP · Pi ratio will reduce oxidative phosphorylation flux. The mitochondrial redox potential depends on several factors. These include Krebs cycle activity leading to NADH production and phosphate potential that depends on ATP hydrolysis (i.e. the cellular work). From these considerations it appears that a large change in flux of ATP synthesis must be accompanied by a large change in the related forces, resulting in a paradox: a high flux of ATP synthesis can be achieved only if mitochondrial ATP concentration is very low. The regulation of oxidative phosphorylation is much subtler and achieves a very large change in ATP synthesis at nearly constant forces. As an example, during myofibrillar contraction increased calcium concentration promotes energy dissipation, by simultaneously activating several dehydrogenases, particularly those involved in the Krebs cycle. Hence, the increase in calcium results in coordinated changes affecting energy metabolism via a simultaneous increase in both the NADH supply system (Krebs cycle) and the ATP consuming processes (muscle contraction). With this mechanism of a simultaneous push and pull, a large change in the oxygen consumption–ATP synthesis pathway is possible without a major change in the related forces: redox or phosphate potentials.

Yield of ATP synthesis (ATP/O ratio)

The yield of oxidative phosphorylation can be expressed as the ratio between ATP synthesis rate and the number of atoms of oxygen consumed (ATP/O). This ratio is of major importance to life and it can be modified by several parameters. Therefore, its regulation is finely tuned. Three main mechanisms modify the fluxes of oxidation and phosphorylation; although both oxidation and phosphorylation are considered as one pathway, they can be independently and differentially regulated by:

- the number of coupling sites at the level of the respiratory chain
- the stoichiometry of the coupling process at the level of the proton pumps (slipping)
- the proton permeability across the mitochondrial inner membrane (proton leak).

The number of coupling sites located on the electron pathway towards molecular oxygen depends on the nature of the redox carrier (NADH or $FADH_2$). For NADH three coupling sites are successively involved (complexes 1, 3 and 4), while there are only two coupling sites for $FADH_2$ (complexes 3 and 4). Hence, the yield of ATP synthesis is roughly 30% lower when $FADH_2$ is oxidized, compared with NADH. The glycolytic pathway results in NADH formation, while the fatty acid β-oxidation results in equimolar formation of NADH and $FADH_2$. Hence, the stoichiometry of ATP synthesis to oxygen consumption is lower when lipids are oxidized, compared with carbohydrates.[3] Since the mitochondrial inner membrane is impermeable to NADH, cytoplasmic NADH donates reducing equivalents to the mitochondrial electron transport chain through two shuttle systems, the malate/aspartate shuttle and the

glycerol-3-phosphate/dihydroxyacetone-phosphate shuttle. Although the first one gives electrons to complex I (i.e. as NADH), the second shuttle gives electrons directly to complex II. Subsequently, by tuning the respective proportion of flux through the two shuttles, the yield of oxidative phosphorylation can be regulated. This target is one of the major effects of thyroid hormones on mitochondrial energy metabolism. These hormones affect the transcription of mitochondrial glycerol-3-phosphate dehydrogenase, which regulates the flux through the glycerol-3-phosphate/dihydroxyacetone-phosphate shuttle.

The modulation of the coupling between proton transport (proton pump slipping) and redox reaction (respiratory chain) or ATP synthesis (ATP synthase) is another possibility to adjust the flux of oxidation and phosphorylation. The coupling between the two vectorial reactions (proton transport and oxidation or phosphorylation) is not fixed and several experiments have shown some variations in this coupling. For example, general anesthetics or the lipid composition of the mitochondrial membrane can alter this.

The inner mitochondrial membrane is not completely impermeable to protons, and proton leak results in uncoupling between respiratory rate and phosphorylation. This energy is dissipated as heat. This phenomenon, first described in brown adipose tissue, is probably a general feature of all kinds of mitochondria. It results in slight disconnection between the rate of oxidation and phosphorylation, and therefore alters the yield of oxidative phosphorylation. This mechanism should not be viewed as a negative event leading to less efficient ATP synthesis. It allows independent adaptation of oxygen consumption/reoxidation of reducing equivalents and ATP synthesis. Indeed, the discovery of this function in brown adipose tissue in mammals, which is related to an uncoupling protein (UCP), has opened a new era in our understanding of the regulation of oxidative phosphorylation by describing a physiological role for energy wastage. Several other UCPs have been described recently, and UCP1 mediates this effect in brown adipose tissue. Homologs including UCP2 and UCP3, are expressed in most tissues, including white adipose tissue, muscle, macrophages, spleen, thymus and Kupffer's cells. However, their role in energy metabolism is less defined than that for UCP1. The complementary DNA (cDNA) encoding brain mitochondrial carrier protein has also been cloned. This protein (BMCP1), is also homologous to the UCPs; when expressed in yeast it is a potent uncoupler, so it could be a new member of the UCP family. The physiological function of UCP1 in brown fat is well recognized as a heat-producing mechanism. The presence of homologous uncoupling proteins (UCP2 and UCP3) in white adipose tissue and skeletal muscle suggests that they may also influence whole-body energy metabolism and may play a role in the pathogenesis of obesity. However, not all studies support this hypothesis. For example, overexpression of UCP3 in skeletal muscle reduces white adipose tissue mass, but adipose tissue is not altered in UCP2 and UCP3 knockout mice. It has also been proposed that mitochondrial uncoupling regulates mitochondrial ROS production. Moreover, it is becoming clear that the mitochondrial membrane potential plays a role in the regulation of many important cellular functions, including calcium signaling, permeability of the transitional mitochondrial pore [permeability transition pore (PTP)], fatty acid oxidation and apoptosis. Therefore, it is likely that the role of mitochondrial uncoupling in cellular homeostasis is not limited to energy metabolism.

ATP distribution: cellular energy circuits

It is not yet known how ATP distribution among the different cellular sites of energy dissipation (e.g. biosynthetic pathways, muscle contraction, metabolite transport and membrane potential maintenance, gene transcription and translation, protein synthesis and degradation) is regulated. Indeed, all of these processes compete with each other, and a very precise regulation of energy distribution is mandatory. In many textbooks it is tacitly supposed that ATP and ADP simply diffuse in the cell, except for crossing intracellular membranes where specific carriers are involved. Such a simple view cannot hold when considering that a simple diffusion through the cytoplasm would not be compatible with a specific energy supply to a given step. Several experimental studies have addressed this problem, and investigated the role of the phosphocreatine/creatine shuttle in the transfer of energy in muscle and cardiac cells. It was proposed that cytosolic and mitochondrial creatine kinases act as an energy shuttle (see Figure 3.4), permitting the channeling of energy from one cellular location (a part of the mitochondrion membrane) to a precise site of energy utilization (myofibrillar ATPase, Na^+/K^+-ATPase, endoplasmic reticulum ATPase, biosynthetic pathway, etc.). In such a view the 'energy-rich bond' is

transported rather than ATP or creatine phosphate molecules per se. Hence, by playing with the location of creatine kinase (e.g. by the transcription of different isoforms), the cell can build several tracks for energy channeling that can be used according to the cellular priorities for energy.

Mitochondrial metabolism and cell signaling

Mitochondria have many specific functions related to some peculiar enzymic equipment. For instance, they play a major role in fatty acid β-oxidation, as well as in urea synthesis and gluconeogenesis. Recently, the role of mitochondria in cellular calcium homeostasis has been extended by the discovery of transitional permeability, mediated by the PTP, which mediates calcium uptake across the inner mitochondrial membrane. This phenomenon, which is blocked specifically by cyclosporin A, appears to be involved in the trigger of cellular death pathways, necrosis or apoptosis. Mitochondria regulate cell death, or apoptosis, by releasing cytochrome c into the cytosol when mitochondria swell after PTP opening. Mitochondria also play a major role in cellular calcium homeostasis, by a mechanism called calcium uptake–calcium release. Mitochondria achieve this because they are able to take up free calcium from the cytoplasm, owing to their specific channels and very high membrane potential, and to release it when the PTP opens.

The mitochondrion has other effects on cellular signaling. It is a major site for ROS formation. Indeed, two specific complexes of the respiratory chain are largely recognized as sites for ROS production: complex 1 or NADH reductase and complex 3 or bc_1-complex, with the latter being quantitatively the most important site. The production of mitochondrial ROS seems to represent not only a negative event leading to irreversible mitochondrial DNA damage and to aging, but also a main signaling pathway both in physiology (oxygen and substrate sensing) and in pathology.

Cellular anaerobic metabolism

In the absence of oxygen, there are in principle three possibilities for ATP synthesis:

- adenylate kinase
- creatine kinase
- lactate production from glucose.

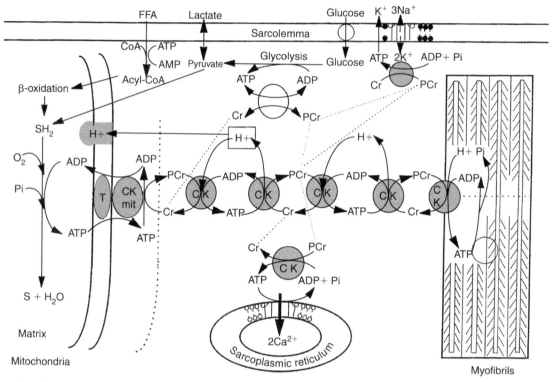

Figure 3.4 Channeling of energy in a cardiac cell. The pathway for intracellular energy transport and the corresponding feedback signal conduction in muscle, brain and many other types of cells (but excluding liver cells) is the phosphocreatine pathway (energy circuit or energy shuttle). This chaneling enables a wave of energy to be transferred from a precise location in the mitochondrial membrane to a precise site of dissipation (myofibrils, Ca^{2+} ATPase in the sarcoplasmic reticulum, sodium ATPase, etc.). Conversely, the signal given by a rise in ADP, due to mechanical work for instance, is channeled to the mitochondrial matrix without effective transportation of the ADP molecule. From this picture it is clear that the meaning of an average cellular ATP or ADP concentration becomes limited. (From Saks *et al.* (1994) with permission of Kluwer Academic Publishers.)

Although the first two possibilities are qualitatively important as ATP synthetic pathways, their significance is quantitatively very limited, and could only meet the energy needs for a few seconds or minutes. Conversely, glycolysis is a more powerful and sustained pathway for ATP synthesis in the absence of oxygen when substrate supply (glucose) and wastage disposal (reducing equivalent and proton) as lactate are sufficient. In this pathway, two ATPs are produced from one glucose molecule, whereas three ATPs are formed when glucose is provided from glycogen stores. The net result of glycolysis is the formation of pyruvate, ATP, NADH and H^+. The pool of NAD^+–NADH is very small, so the maintenance of a sustained glycolytic flux even in the presence of sufficient amounts of glucose is possible only when NAD^+ is regenerated from NADH reoxidation. Since in the absence of oxygen this cannot be achieved by mitochondrial metabolism, the

unique way to remove the excess of reducing equivalents, in lactic organisms, is to convert pyruvate into lactate (yeast can produce ethanol or glycerol for the same purpose). Lactic acid production allows the release of reducing potential, together with protons and carbons. Hence, ATP production by anaerobic glycolysis is mainly controlled by:

- the phosphate potential [ATP/(ADP · Pi)]
- the pH
- the level of cytosolic redox state (NADH/NAD ratio).

Adaptation to energy deficit

The consequences of cellular energy deficit and the mechanisms underlying adaptation to this situation can be understood from the results of numerous studies, both in hypoxia and in ischemia. Such adaptation must rely on a permanent adjustment between energy demand and

ATP synthesis. When oxygen and ATP are decreasing, energy dissipating processes must also be reduced to the same extent and according to several priorities. Therefore, energy demand has to adapt to match oxygen supply and ATP production capacity. This needs a sensitive oxygen-sensing system, associated with the possibility of a cellular metabolic conformance to oxygen disposal. Oxygen conformance means that cells can probably anticipate any possible lack or excess of oxygen by sensing the oxygen tension in the surroundings. The pathway of cellular oxygen signaling is now understood, especially the role of ROS production on gene expression. The adaptive changes related to hypoxia or energy deficit have been divided into defense and rescue phases. The defense phase occurs immediately after a decline in oxygen and consists of channel arrest, decreased Na^+/K^+-ATPase activity, urea synthesis, gluconeogenesis, protein synthesis and proteolysis (a highly ATP-consuming process), in such a way that ATP demand equals ATP production. Then, the rescue phase involves transcriptional effects [hypoxia-induced factor (HIF)], HIF-mediated activation of genes for sustained survival at low ATP turnover (increased glycolytic enzymes, decreased enzymes involved in aerobic-linked metabolism) and, finally, production of tertiary cell signaling messengers (fos and jun).

3.3 Energy metabolism in the body as a whole

General considerations

Energy in the body is mainly utilized for active transport across cellular membranes, synthesis of new molecules and contraction of contractile fibers. Whole-body energy metabolism is expressed as resting energy expenditure (REE), which is much easier to determine than the classical basal energy expenditure (BEE). In healthy adults, it is estimated as $40\,kcal\,h^{-1}\,m^{-2}$, the body surface being determined as follows:

$$S\,(m^2) = 71.84 \times H^{0.725}(cm) \times W^{0.425}(kg)$$

As shown in Table 3.1, REE is predominantly related to the metabolism of four main organs: liver, brain, heart and kidneys. Although these organs represent only 5.5% of total body mass, they account for almost 60% of total body energy expenditure. REE is influenced by many factors, such as age ($55\,kcal\,h^{-1}\,m^{-2}$ for

Table 3.1 Respective contribution of the different organs to oxygen consumption and body mass

	Oxygen consumption (%)	Mass (%)
Liver	20	2.5
Brain	20	2.0
Heart	10	0.5
Kidneys	10	0.5
Muscles	20	40.0
Others	20	54.5

the newborn versus $35\,kcal\,h^{-1}\,m^{-2}$ in the elderly), gender (10% higher in males as compared to females), food intake, pregnancy and several diseases.

Energy metabolism can be investigated by several means. The most common way to determine the energy expenditure is based on measurements by indirect calorimetry that assess energy dissipation from oxygen consumption (V_{O_2}). Moreover, by determining the respiratory quotient (RQ = V_{CO_2}/V_{O_2}, where V_{CO_2} is carbon dioxide production) and the excretion of urea, it is possible to determine the nature of the oxidized substrates (carbohydrates versus lipids).[4] As described above, energy metabolism (i.e. the transduction of energy contained in nutrients to ATP synthesis) involves many steps, and some of them can be investigated in clinical practice by measuring lactate/pyruvate or β-hydroxybutyrate/acetoacetate ratios and oxygen consumption. The other methods are limited to clinical research. Examples of these include intracellular ATP by NMR or by biopsy, infrared spectroscopy for *in situ* redox potential determination and doubly labeled water.

Interplay between aerobic and anaerobic energy metabolism

The amount of ATP produced from nutrients by mitochondrial oxidative phosphorylation is far higher than that occurring in anaerobic conditions. A healthy adult human produces, and therefore consumes, a mass of ATP approximately equivalent to his or her body mass every day. Total ATP body content is about 100–200 g. Assuming for simplification that ATP synthesis is achieved only from glucose metabolism, 650 g of glucose is required for the aerobic synthesis of 70 kg of ATP. In comparison, 13 kg of glucose would be necessary to produce the same quantity of ATP by the anaerobic pathway. But, besides the indisputable quantitative advantages of aerobic metabolism, the anaerobic pathway is qualitatively of great importance.

Tissue anaerobic metabolism

In several tissues anaerobic energy metabolism is predominant even in the presence of a sufficient oxygen concentration. This is the case in red blood cells, which completely lack mitochondria. It is interesting to consider that although these cells contain probably the highest amount of oxygen, their energy needs are completely met anaerobically. Erythrocyte anaerobic energy metabolism is not marginal, when considering that red blood cells represent a completely anaerobic organ of almost 2.5 kg ($\approx$40 g of glucose-lactate/day, i.e. 20% of total glucose turnover). Epithelial cells of the cornea are also dependent on anaerobic glycolysis as their unique energy source. The kidney medulla is another example of a physiological advantage of anaerobic energy production despite the low rate of ATP synthesis. In this tissue a very high osmotic pressure is maintained in the extracellular fluid as the result of tubular cell activity of ion transport. A rich vascularization would lead to a high energetic cost to maintain such a gradient because of efficient exchanges between cells and plasma. However, owing to the poor blood supply to these cells, the energy metabolism of these cells is achieved mainly via the anaerobic pathway occurring from the glucose present in the tubular ultrafiltrate.

Energy metabolism is compartmentalized in the cell. Glycolytic ATP resulting in lactate formation even in fully aerobic experimental conditions probably predominantly supports the plasma membrane-linked ATPase activities. Hence, in cardiac cells, which are fully aerobic in physiological conditions, lactate release is very low or absent, but a specific role of glycolytic ATP meets the energy requirements of plasma membrane active transport, while the energy required for contraction comes from mitochondrial oxidative phosphorylation. This example illustrate the complementary aspects of aerobic and anaerobic energy metabolism even in a well-oxygenated organ.

Energy metabolism in the brain: neurone astrocyte cooperation

The brain is very sensitive to hypoxia, because of its high metabolic rate. A moderate degree of hypoxia results in brain lactate accumulation. Some recent experimental data lead to a very fascinating hypothesis, known as the activity-dependent astrocyte–neurone lactate shuttle. It is proposed that the main energy substrate for neurones is not glucose but lactate, provided by astrocyte anaerobic glycolysis. In astrocytes, ATP provided by glycolysis is functionally linked to the plasma membrane Na-ATPase. After glutamate activation, the reuptake of glutamate by astrocytes is associated with sodium, and the active pumping of sodium out of the cell is then linked to glycolysis activation. The lactate produced is used as the energy substrate for activated neurones. In this view there is a functional coupling between astrocyte and neurone energy metabolism. The upper part of glucose oxidation (i.e. from glucose to lactate) occurs in astrocytes, while the lower part (i.e. pyruvate oxidation) occurs in neurones, in such a way that brain metabolism as a whole is permitted by complete glucose oxidation into water and carbon dioxide.

Aerobic–anaerobic metabolism: perspectives in whole-body integrated metabolism

Except for the initial substrates (nutrients, oxygen) and the final waste products (water, carbon dioxide, urea, etc.), every metabolite is a substrate for some cells, while it is a product for others. Hence, although anaerobic ATP production is a reality at cellular level, this is not the case when the whole-body integrated metabolism is considered at steady state. In this latter case, energy metabolism is always purely aerobic. Indeed, anaerobic metabolism implies that the end-product of glycolysis must be excreted as lactate in human cells, or as ethanol or glycerol in yeast, for instance. This can be the case for isolated cells or organs, but since lactate excretion from the body is negligible, lactate is ultimately metabolized or oxidized. Therefore, when considering the body as a whole, energy metabolism is fully aerobic and lactate is not a waste end-product, but a metabolite that is an alternative substrate and product. When lactate accumulates in the body, such as during a short-bout of high-intensity exercise, anaerobic metabolism contributes to net ATP synthesis. However, during the recovery process, lactate is metabolized and disappears from the body without significant net excretion. Accordingly, when considering both exercise and recovery periods, energy metabolism is completely aerobic. Similarly, in pathological diseases, if blood lactate concentration is stable, whatever its concentration, energy metabolism is fully aerobic.

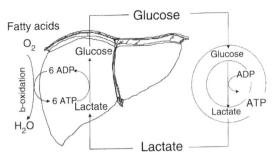

Figure 3.5 Combination of anaerobic and aerobic pathways results in a fully aerobic life. The glucose recycled via lactate creates a futile cycle between 3- and 6-carbon compounds. On the one hand this dissipates directly two-thirds of the energy as heat (since 6 ATP are needed to build 1 glucose from 2 lactate, whereas only 2 ATP are produced when splitting glucose into lactate), but on the other hand, the source of energy in liver mainly comes from fatty acid oxidation. Hence, glucose recycling provides 'glycolytic ATP' to several peripheral cells (e.g. erythrocytes) while this ATP is formed from energy coming from lipid oxidation. In other words, one can say that 'the liver respires for anaerobic tissues like erythrocytes'.

> All metabolism is ultimately aerobic, and anaerobic metabolism exists in certain tissues and in certain metabolic states for defined and logical reasons.

The glucose–lactate cycle, initially described by Cori as substrate recycling between erythrocytes and the liver, can be extended to nearly all organs and cells. This recycling has important metabolic implications for both qualitative and quantitative aspects of whole-body energy homeostasis. On the one hand, only 2 moles of ATP result from the fermentation of 1 mole of glucose, whereas 6 moles of ATP are needed to give back 1 mole of glucose (Figure 3.5). Hence, when considering the *overall yield*[5] of glucose–lactate cycling, one-third of the ATP synthesized aerobically in the liver is used anaerobically in the erythrocytes. On the other hand, glycolysis provides glycolytic ATP to cells, whereas glucose was built with an energy source provided by fatty-acid aerobic oxidation, since this source is largely predominant, if not exclusive, in the liver.

Hence, the metabolic result of glucose–lactate recycling is the transfer of aerobically synthesized ATP from lipid oxidation in the liver, to anaerobic glycolytic ATP in peripheral cells. This is achieved by a decrease in *efficiency* (but see Note 5), which is compensated by qualitative metabolic advantages. The large mass of lipid stores compared with the limited amount of carbohydrates or the metabolic cost of the use of gluconeogenic

amino acids provided from protein breakdown might represent one of these advantages. A second advantage is related to the possibility of sharing between organs or cells a part of the aerobic energy metabolism pathway. For example, erythrocyte energy metabolism is entirely anaerobic owing to the lack of mitochondria, but since lactate is further metabolized by the liver, the erythrocyte and liver work as a fully aerobic system. Hence, the liver respires for red blood cells and, except for the situation when lactate is accumulating or excreted, energy metabolism is entirely aerobic whatever the lactate concentration. Therefore, lactate plays a pivotal role not only in anaerobic metabolism but also in aerobic metabolism by providing reduced substrates from one cell to the respiratory chain of another. Lactate–pyruvate interconversion may also be viewed as a shuttle for transporting reducing equivalents from one organ to another or from one cell to another, as it has been described during prolonged submaximal exercise. Such redox shuttle is not limited to interorgan exchanges but also concerns intraorgan metabolism; that is, intercellular shuttle (Figure 3.6), and any reduced compound released by one cell and taken up by another can play the role of a redox shuttle. A large increase in the interconversion of lactate to pyruvate and pyruvate to lactate has been recently reported in type 2 diabetes. Such a phenomenon could explain a regional lactate production and utilization in critically ill patients.

Role of lactate in ischemia–reperfusion injury

The succession of aerobic–anaerobic phases that results in deleterious events is known as ischemia–reperfusion injury. This occurs in various cell types, but some, including the brain, are especially sensitive to this kind of injury. In experimental conditions, as well as in clinical practice, an increased brain lactate is always interpreted as proof of brain hypoxia. It is believed that lactate is not only a marker of hypoxia but also a causal pejorative event. Lactic acid is interpreted as a toxic metabolite for neurons. This leads to the acceptance that hyperglycemia exacerbates the brain ischemia–reperfusion injury. It was recently proposed that lactate is in fact an adequate substrate for aerobic energy production during the initial stage of recovery after transient ischemia or hypoxia: 'brain lactate production is not a suicide note, it is a survival kit!' Monocarboxylate anions (i.e. lactate or ketones) prevent cerebral dysfunction during hypoglycemia and the protective effect of lactate is also present in patients with insulin-dependent diabetes.

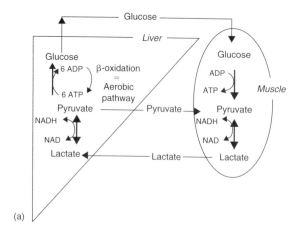

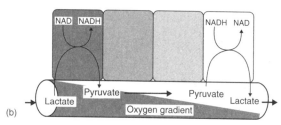

Figure 3.6 Role of lactate/pyruvate interconversion as a reducing equivalent shuttle. Lactate-to-pyruvate exchange and vice versa could be viewed as a reducing equivalent shuttle (a) from one organ to another, or (b) from one cell to another, depending on the oxygen tension in the immediate cell vicinity. This mechanism enables the oxidative energy metabolism to be shared between cells, one cells being able to respire for another.

3.4 Perspectives on the future

Several key questions regarding cellular energy metabolism are still poorly understood as yet and further investigations are mandatory for a better understanding of the pathogenesis of several diseases. So far, our view of the mechanisms and the consequences of the metabolic compartmentation is very limited. It is probable that this field of investigations will explode in the future. The relationship between cellular death and mitochondrial metabolism represents a new direction that might lead to significant therapeutic advances. Nevertheless, it is clear that the most difficult achievement is to obtain a real integrative view of the energy metabolism. How are the hierarchy and priorities of the different ATP-utilizing pathways defined? Shall we be able to manipulate this hierarchy by using new drugs in the future?

Notes

[1] The complete oxidation of one acetyl-CoA in the Krebs cycle results in three $NADH,H^+$ and one $FADH_2$, leading to the formation of $(3 \times 3$ ATP$) + 2$ ATP $= 11$ ATP; since pyruvate oxidation results in the formation of one $NADH,H^+ (=3$ ATP$)$ the net result of pyruvate oxidation is 14 ATP, while glycolysis produces 4 $NADH,H^+ (=12$ ATP$)$. Hence, the result of the complete oxidation of one glucose molecule is $(2 \times 14) + 12 + 2$ (produced at the levels of the Kreb's cycle). Hence, the ATP actually produced at the level of the Krebs cycle represents only 2/38, i.e. 5% of total ATP. It must be realized that these calculations require a fixed stoichiometry of ATP synthesis from respiration, which is not completely true (see below).

[2] Plasma lactate/pyruvate and 3-hydroxybutyrate/acetoacetate ratios reflects schematically cytoplasmic and mitochondrial redox states, respectively. They can be used to assess disorders in the redox pathway: lactate/pyruval increase may indicate a deficit in oxidation and 3-hydroxybutyrate/acetoacetate a deficit in liver mitochondrial function, since the liver plays a major role in ketone metabolism. However, it must be kept in mind that these parameters in the blood reflect an averaged value between several tissues, organs, cells and mitochondria (see *milieu intérieur*) and therefore one value may hide the opposite change in the various organs.

[3] When a fatty acid is oxidized through mitochondrial β-oxidation (1 $NADH,H^+$ and 1 $FADH_2 = 5$ ATP) and acetyl-CoA in the Krebs cycle $(11 + 1$ ATP$)$ it leads to the formation of 17 ATP per two-carbon fragment, but since fatty acids require an activation (ATP $\rightarrow$ AMP) it represents a cost equivalent to 2 ATP per chain of fatty acid. This explain why the actual yield of ATP production is dependent on the length of the chain (see Note 1).

[4] The actual metabolic reflect of the respiratory quotient is limited by the fact that the kinetics of the changes are not of the same order of magnitude between oxygen and carbon dioxide. Indeed, oxygen storage is very limited in the body and any metabolic change at the level of cellular respiration is reflected by the body respiratory exchanges. By contrast, regarding carbon dioxide, owing to extremely broad storage, mainly as bicarbonate, there is latency between the changes occurring at the cellular level and the total body respiratory exchanges. Therefore, any statement concerning non-steady state conditions must be interpreted with extreme caution. This is the reason why some authors propose calling the parameter respiratory exchange ratio (RER) rather than respiratory quotient (RQ).

[5] The notion of yield in this sense is not really proper. Indeed, *sensu stricto* yield means the proportion of energy converted from one form to another. For example, one can speak of the yield of mechanical work, which is the percentage of energy converted to work, the difference being heat loss in this example. Concerning the body as a whole in steady state, if no net mechanical or biological (pregnancy, lactation, growth, increase in body weight, etc.) work is achieved, the actual yield is always zero: the entirety of energy is dissipated as heat. In the case of glucose–lactate cycling, yield is taken is the sense of metabolic efficiency: only one-third of the energy derived from aerobic ATP synthesis is ultimately used in erythrocyte metabolism.

Further reading

Boss O, Muzzin P, Giacobino J-P. The uncoupling proteins, a review. Eur J Endocrinol 1998; 139: 1–9.

De Duwe CR. Vital Dust. Life as a Cosmic Imperative. Glasgow: Harper Collins, 1995.

Newsholme E, Leech A. Biochemistry for the Medical Sciences. Chichester: John Wiley, 1983.

Nicholls DG. Bioenergetics: An Introduction to the Chemiosmotic Theory. London: Academic Press, 1982.

Saks, VA *et al.* Metabolic compartmentation and substrate channeling. Mol Cell Biochem 1994; 133(134): 155–192.

Westerhoff HV, Groen AK, Wanders RJ. Modern theories of metabolic control and their applications (Review). Biosci Rep 1984; 4: 1–22.

4

Integration of Metabolism 2: Protein and Amino Acids

JT Brosnan and VR Young

Key messages

- Protein and amino acid metabolism are large-scale, dynamic and regulated processes that accomplish a variety of physiological functions. Their measurement, in living animals, requires the application of sophisticated methodology involving isotopic tracers. In a healthy adult human, some 300 g of protein is synthesized and degraded each day; some 100 g of amino acids are consumed, as dietary protein, on a typical Western diet.
- Protein synthesis and degradation (or turnover) play a critical role in determining the levels of the many proteins in organisms, e.g. enzymes, contractile proteins, membrane proteins, plasma proteins, peptide hormones and regulatory proteins. Protein synthesis and turnover are, therefore, of the most fundamental importance.
- The synthesis of different proteins is primarily regulated by the expression of individual genes, but there is also a variety of other regulatory processes, especially at the initiation of messenger RNA translation.
- Protein breakdown is a random process, such that newly synthesized proteins are as likely to be degraded as older proteins. Protein degradation has the additional function of promptly removing damaged or mutant proteins. The rate of protein turnover is heterogeneous; thus, different proteins are degraded at varying rates, from a half-life in minutes for ornithine decarboxylase to a half-life of years for mature collagen.

- Muscle, the largest protein mass in the body, plays an important role as a source of amino acids in a number of situations, e.g. as a source of amino acids for gluconeogenesis during starvation and for the synthesis of defense proteins (acute phase proteins, immunoglobulins) during catabolic illness.
- Amino acids are the most versatile of nutrients. In addition to their primary role as precursors for protein synthesis, they play a variety of other roles such as serving as neurotransmitters (e.g. glutamate and glycine) and precursors for neurotransmitters (e.g. serotonin and dopamine), for signaling molecules (e.g. nitric oxide and epinephrine) and for the synthesis of a variety of small molecules (e.g. creatine and glutathione). The metabolic disposal of dietary amino acids and, in particular, of the nutritionally indispensable (or essential) amino acids, is tightly regulated.
- There is a considerable flux of amino acids between tissues. This interorgan metabolism is facilitated by amino acid transporters and accomplishes a variety of physiological roles such as supplying amino acids to the liver for gluconeogenesis, to the kidney for acid–base balance, and the synthesis of dispensable amino acids. This interorgan amino acid metabolism can vary during development and between species.

4.1 Introduction

This chapter is concerned with the integration of amino acid and protein metabolism within the organism. Chapter 4 of the first volume of this series (*Introduction to Human Nutrition*) deals, in large part, with the dietary requirement for protein and amino acids, determination of their requirements, as well as the means of meeting them. The present chapter builds on these themes and examines the functions, mechanisms, and regulation of protein and amino acid metabolism that underlie their nutritional requirements. It also attempts to integrate this metabolism so as to provide an understanding of the roles played by different tissues in different circumstances.

Proteins are major functional molecules of cells and it follows that normal body function depends, in a profound way, on the expression of a myriad of specific proteins. The precise quantity of each protein in a cell depends on its rate of synthesis and degradation. Accordingly, the mechanisms and regulation of protein synthesis and turnover are major topics in this chapter. Furthermore, it is clear that although the outlines of these processes are common, from tissue to tissue, their regulation occurs in a tissue-specific and protein-specific manner. Thus, during catabolic illnesses there is a net loss of muscle protein; at the same time, there is an increased hepatic synthesis of a set of defense molecules, known as positive acute-phase proteins. Decreased availability of a specific amino acid will result in a generalized decrease in protein synthesis, although the synthesis of the specific amino acid transporter that imports this amino acid into cells may be enhanced. Indeed, an appreciation of the differences between the metabolism of amino acids and protein metabolism in different tissues is key to an understanding of the integration of this process within the body. Amino acid metabolism provides one of the best examples of an interorgan process in which events in different tissues combine and collaborate to bring about overall physiological goals. Thus, there is a maintenance of concentrations of amino acids circulating in the blood, normally within certain limits, and this ensures a supply of these key substrates for protein synthesis to all tissues and organs. The synthesis of individual amino acids is the responsibility of specific tissues. During starvation, amino acids released as a result of muscle proteolysis are converted to glucose in the liver and, thus, provide a key energy fuel to the brain. The earlier view of the role of the intestine in amino acid metabolism has been transformed from an organ that is involved only in digestion and absorption to one that obtains a substantial fraction of its metabolic energy from the catabolism of dietary amino acids and undertakes a significant metabolic processing of absorbed amino acids before their entry into the portal circulation. The liver is the major organ for the catabolism of amino acids and in the regulation of amino acid catabolism plays a major role in determining dietary amino acid requirements. The fact that the rate of amino acid catabolism is never zero is one of the principal reasons why adults require a continuous supply of dietary nitrogen and of indispensable (essential) amino acids.

This chapter provides the reader with an understanding of the nature and regulation of protein synthesis and turnover and an appreciation of how these occur in a tissue-specific manner. It will also discuss the techniques that are available to determine the rates of protein synthesis, protein turnover and amino acid oxidation, both on a whole-body basis and in some individual organs, and give an appreciation of the magnitude of these fluxes. The regulation of amino acid metabolism will be discussed, in particular, amino acid catabolism and the many metabolic roles played by amino acids. Hopefully, at the end of reading this chapter you will have an understanding of how these different processes occur in an organ-specific manner (including amino acid fluxes between organs) and appreciate the integration of amino acid and protein metabolism, both under physiological situations (e.g. fed versus fasted states) and during pathological challenges (e.g. catabolic illnesses and genetic diseases of amino acid transport).

4.2 Protein and amino acid turnover

The proteins of cells and organs and those in the circulation play various roles (Table 4.1); they are the 'workhorses' and serve in such roles as biological catalysts (enzymes), regulators of gene expression, components of molecular structures, such as the cell membrane, endoplasmic reticulum, the contractile apparatus of smooth, striated and cardiac muscle and the multifunctional proteolytic complex (proteasome) that is responsible for a major fraction of cellular protein breakdown. In most cells and tissues proteins are being continually synthesized and degraded. The overall process of

Table 4.1 Some functions of proteins

Function	Examples
Enzymic catalysis	Branched-chain ketoacid dehydrogenase
Plasma transport	B_{12} binding proteins, ceruloplasmin, apolipoproteins, albumin
Membrane transport	Na^+/K^+-ATPase, glucose transporters
Messengers/signals	Insulin, growth hormone
Movement	Kinesin, actin
Structure	Collagens, elastin
Protein folding	Chaperonins
Storage/sequestration	Ferritin (for iron), metallothionein (for zinc)
Immunity	Antibodies, tumor necrosis factor, interleukins
Growth, differentiation, gene expression	Peptide growth factors, transcription factors

synthesis and degradation, or of anabolism and catabolism, is referred to as protein turnover. Each component of turnover consists of a complex organization of proteins and other molecules that are subject to regulation. Hence, rates of synthesis and degradation of proteins may vary depending on the intracellular and extracellular environmental conditions. These include the availability and balance of nutrients to which cells are exposed, and the hormones and other peptide factors that bind to receptors in cell surfaces, or within the cell, causing turnover to change. This continuous, variable-rate, cycle of protein synthesis and breakdown permits:

- the organism to adjust to changes in the internal environment
- tissue remodeling during growth or repair
- selective removal of mutant, damaged and misfolded proteins.

About 30% or more of protein production is faulty and these defective products are removed by the mechanisms described below. Turnover serves a critical role in multiple cell functions, including cell cycle progression, oncogenesis, apoptosis (programmed cell death), regulation of gene expression, inflammation and immune surveillance, and the regulation of metabolic pathways. It is not surprising, therefore, that malfunctions in protein turnover are associated with human diseases, including neurodegenerative disorders and cancer. For example, what if apoptosis, or cell death, was prevented owing to a defect in the turnover of one or more of the many enzyme proteins involved in this process, such as the caspases (a group of cysteine proteases that are one of the main effectors of apoptosis), and where mitosis (cell division) proceeded at a normal rate? It could be estimated that an 80-year-old person would have 2 tonnes of bone marrow and lymph nodes and a gut that was about 16 km long!

The amino acids serve as the currency of protein metabolism. In addition to serving as the building blocks for proteins they meet many other functions (Table 4.2), some of which will be considered later in this chapter. However, at this stage it is important to appreciate that there is an intimate relationship between the rates of protein synthesis and breakdown and the status of cellular and organ amino acid metabolism, making it somewhat difficult to separate a discussion of each of these major components of the nitrogen economy of the organism. Nevertheless, the mechanisms of protein synthesis and degradation or breakdown will be considered

Table 4.2 Some biochemical functions of amino acids

Amino acid	Functions
Alanine	Nitrogen transport in blood
Arginine	Urea cycle intermediate
	Substrate for nitric oxide synthesis
	Substrate for creatine synthesis
Aspartate	Nitrogen donor for urea synthesis
	Substrate for purine and pyrimidine synthesis
Cysteine	Substrate for glutathione synthesis
	Substrate for taurine synthesis
Glutamate	Partner in transamination reactions
	Neurotransmitter
	Substrate for glutathione synthesis
	Precursor for GABA synthesis
	Agonist for umami taste receptor
Glutamine	Nitrogen donor for purine, pyrimidine and amino sugar synthesis
	Acid–base balance: source of urinary ammonia
	Metabolic fuel for enterocytes and cells of the immune system
	Nitrogen transport in blood
	Substrate for citrulline and arginine synthesis
Glycine	Bile salt synthesis
	Substrate for heme synthesis
	Neurotransmitter
	Source of methylene groups for one-carbon pool
	Substrate for creatine synthesis
Histidine	Precursor of histamine
Methionine	Major methyl donor via S-adenosylmethionine
	Major substrate for polyamine synthesis via decarboxylated S-adenosylmethionine
Serine	Source of hydroxymethylene groups for the one-carbon pool
	Precursor in phospholipid and sphingosine biosynthesis
Tryptophan	Precursor for serotonin synthesis
Tyrosine	Precursor for epinephrine (adrenaline), norepinephrine (noradrenaline) and dopamine synthesis

first. A examination of how these processes are regulated will follow, before turning to the metabolism of amino acids. Subsequently, those factors of nutritional importance that influence the rates of protein synthesis and breakdown, the mechanisms involved, the organs affected and the impact of these factors on and interactions with amino acid metabolism will be considered.

4.3 Protein synthesis

In a healthy adult human, about 300 g of new protein is synthesized per day and, for a maintenance condition, an equivalent amount of protein is degraded to their amino acids. The synthesis of proteins consists of many different patterns and amounts depending on the type of cell and its condition at that time. The production of proteins follows the synthesis of messenger RNA (mRNA) via the process of *transcription* of a gene's nucleotide sequence, which involves several steps. The first is transcription initiation and elongation. This is followed by RNA-processing reactions such as capping and splicing and the transcription termination. With the appearance of the mRNA in the cytosol the *translational* phase of protein synthesis takes place, although it might be noted that about 23 proteins are made within the mitochondrion. All mammalian organisms initially construct proteins from a set of 20 amino acids (the only variants being

formyl-methionine and selenocysteine) via the translation of mRNA that codes for a predetermined sequence of amino acids in the polypeptide chain. The three major stages of translation are:

1. initiation
2. elongation
3. termination.

Initiation

The *initiation* of translation occurs via a complex process in which initiator transfer RNA (tRNA), 40S and 60S ribosomal subunits are assembled, with the aid of eukaryotic initiation factors (eIFs), into an 80S ribosome at the initiation codon of the mRNA (Figure 4.1).

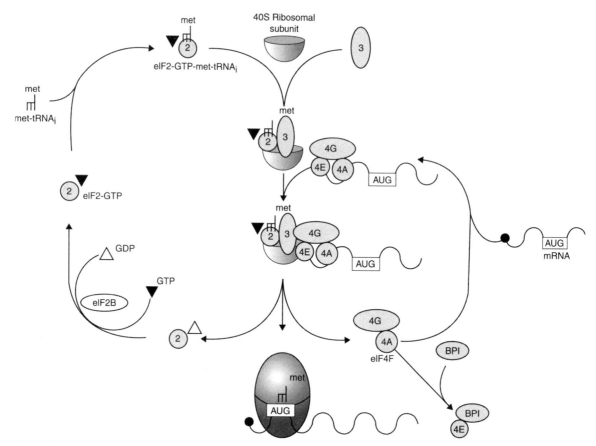

Figure 4.1 Translation initiation pathway in mammalian cells. The figure depicts the methionyl-transfer RNA (met-tRNA) binding step (left side) and the mRNA binding (right side) in translation initiation. The various eukaryotic translation initiation factors (eIF) and their roles in mRNA translation are described in greater detail by Jefferson and Kimball (2001). mRNA translation begins with the binding of met-tRNA to the 40S ribosomal subunit, a reaction mediated by eIF2. The binding of mRNA to the 40S ribosomal subunit occurs through the interaction of the eIF4E component of the eIF4F complex with the m⁷GTP cap structure at the 5′-end of the mRNA and the association of eIF4G with the eIF3 already bound to the 40S ribosomal subunit. Initiation ends when the initiation complex scans to the initiator AUG start codon and assembles with the 60S ribosomal subunit. At this point, initiation factors are thought to be released from the complex. (From Jefferson and Kimball, 2001, with permission.)

There are several linked stages involved in this process:

1. selection of initiator tRNA from the pool of tRNAs by eukaryotic initiation factor (eIF)2 and binding of an eIF2/GTF/Met-tRNA, ternary complex and other eIFs to the 40S ribosomal subunit, with the formation of a 43S preinitiation complex
2. binding of the 43S complex to mRNA, which in most instances occurs by a mechanism that involves initial recognition of the m^{7}G cap at the mRNA 5′-terminus by the eIF41 (cap-binding) subunit of eIF4F
3. movement of the mRNA-bound ribosomal complex along the 5′-non-translated region (5′NTR) from its initial binding site to the initiation codon, to form a 48S initiation complex, where the initiation codon is base-paired to the anticodon of initiator tRNA
4. displacement of factors from the 48S complex and the joining of the 60S ribosomal subunit to form an 80S ribosome, leaving Met-tRNA in the ribosomal P site.

Elongation

The *elongation* phase proceeds following the formation of the initiation complex. It involves three distinct steps that are repeated many times during the formation of a polypeptide. These include:

1. transfer of an appropriate aminoacyl-tRNA from cytoplasm to the A-site of the ribosome
2. covalent linkage of a new amino acid to the growing polypeptide chain, or peptidyl transfer
3. movement of tRNA from the A-site to P-site and with simultaneous movement of mRNA by three nucleotides, or a translocation.

The formation of the aminoacyl-tRNA involves the hydrolysis of high-energy phosphate bonds and the cycle is repeated and proceeds at a rate of about 18–20 amino acids incorporated per second. The binding of the aminoacyl-tRNA to the ribosome and the translocation of the peptidyl-tRNA require energy that is obtained via the hydrolysis of two guanosine triphosphates (GTPs) per cycle.

Termination

The final step is of *termination*. This involves the release of the polypeptide chain from the mRNA. It requires

three so-called STOP codons (UAA, UAG or UGA), a eukaryote release factor (eRF) and one GTP.

This integrated process of initiation, elongation and termination is the *translational phase* of protein synthesis. The *transcriptional phase*, as noted above, involves the earlier reading-out of the genetic blueprint of the protein in the form of the messenger molecule (mRNA). Both of these phases are regulated, where the latter involves the regulation of gene expression. This is discussed in Chapter 2 of this volume.

4.4 Regulation of the translation phase of protein synthesis

Our bodies are composed of more than 200 distinct types of differentiated cells and, with few exceptions, all cells contain identical genetic information. Thus, at the most basic level, the pattern and content of the different proteins in cells are determined by their patterns of gene expression, with regulation of transcription. However, an important site of regulation also occurs at the level of mRNA translation.

The rate-limiting step in translation is usually, but not always, located within the initiation phase, with the intrinsic activity or strength of most mRNAs determined by:

- the accessibility of the capped 5′-terminus to initiation factors,
- the ability of the 40S ribosomal subunit to bind and scan the mRNA distally,
- the frequency of recognition of the initiator codon and surrounding context.

In addition, an important regulator of the expression of specific mRNAs is the mobilization of mRNAs from repressed mRNPs into active polysomes through controls that are separate from those involving ribosome initiation on polysomes.

The dominant mechanism of control of global protein synthesis is via phosphorylation/dephosphorylation of the translation components, primarily of initiation and elongation factors. Thus, a major target of phosphorylation is eIF-4F (the mRNA cap-binding protein complex), although phosphorylation of other proteins such as eIF-3, eIF-4B and ribosomal protein S6 are also important in regulation. Phosphorylation may also cause a repression of protein synthesis, normally by modifying the α-subunit of initiation factor eIF-2 or the elongation factor eEF-2. Indeed, phosphorylation of eIF-2α appears to be a general mechanism for inhibiting initiation of translation, whereas EF-2 phosphorylation affects elongation rates and may be used less frequently. Thus, a complex set of interactions, some redundant or overlapping, serve to link the rate of translation to the overall metabolic needs and state of the cell.

4.5 Post-translational events

While the process of polypeptide synthesis, as outlined above, is limited essentially to the incorporation of the common 20 amino acids, chemical analysis of proteins for their constituent amino acids often reveals many more than just these 20 amino acids. Although it is impossible to propose a precise number of amino acids

Table 4.3 Examples of common post-translational modifications

Modifiation	Normal form		Modification form	
Additions[a] Glycosylation	NH_3, O; $^-OOC-C-CH_2CNH_2$; H	Asparagine	NH_3, O; $^-OOC-C-CH_2CN-GlcNAc-GlcNAc^b-$; H	N-linked oligosaccharide
	COO^-; H_3N^+-C-H; CH_2OH	Serine	COO^-; H_3N^+-C-H; $CH_2O-GalNAc-Gal-Nan$; Nan	O-linked oligosaccharide
Phosphorylation	COO^-; H_3N^+-C-H; CH_2OH	Serine	COO^-; H_3N^+-C-H, O; CH_2O-P-O^-; O^-	O-phosphoserine
Methylation	NH_3^+, H; $^-OOC-C-CH_2CH_2CH_2-N-C-NH_2$; H, $^+NH_2$	Arginine	NH_3^+, H CH_3; $^-OOC-C-CH_2CH_2CH_2-N-C-NH$; H, N; CH_3	Dimethylarginine
Acylation	COO^-; $H_3N-C-CH_3$; H	Alanine	O COO^-; $H_3CC-N-C-H$; CH_3	N-acetylalanine
Conversions Deamidation/ citrullination	NH_3, O; $^-OOC-C-CH_2CNH_2$; H	Asparagine	NH_3; $^-OOC-C-CH_2COO^-$; H	Aspartic acid[b]
Isoaspartyl	O; CH_2COH; $NH-CH-C-NH-CH_2C-$; O	Isoaspartic acid	O; $CH_2C-NH-CH_2-C-$; $NH-CH-C-O^-$, O; O	Aspartic acid–glycine
Deimination	H; $H_2N-C-NH-CH_2CH_2CH_2-C-COOH$; $^+NH_2$, NH_3^+	Arginine	$H_2N-C-NH-CH_2CH_2CH_2CH-COOH$; O, NH_2	Citrulline

Reproduced from Doyle and Mamula (2001) with permission of Elsevier Science. GlcNAc: N-acetyl-D-glucosamine; GalNac: N-acetyl-D-galactosamine; Gal: D-galactose; Nan: N-acetyl-neuraminic acid.

[a] The majority of these modifications are mediated by specific enzymes, which for the sake of clarity are omitted from this table.

[b] The major product (60–85%) of aparagine deamidation is isoaspartic acid, with the remainder of the product being aspartic acid (see the isoaspartyl reaction). For the sake of clarity, deamidation is classified as a separate reaction in this table.

and their derivatives actually present in proteins in the biosphere, the number may be quite high. There are about 1000 amino acids or more in nature, although not all of these are found as protein-bound amino acids. Furthermore, the final polypeptide produced may differ from that specified by the gene through modifications of the number of peptide bonds. Shortening of the polypeptide chain by proteolytic cleavage or, in other cases, lengthening of the chain by addition of amino acids to the carboxy- (C-) or amino- (N-)terminal ends may occur.

The secondary, or derived, amino acids found in proteins arise by chemical modification of the primary amino acid during, or after, its gene-specified insertion into the polypeptide. This process is termed the 'post-translational' phase and it has been estimated that 50–90% of the proteins are modified in this way. Together with the highly specific processes by which proteins are folded and delivered to their sites of action, they represent additional critical steps in the synthesis and positioning of functional proteins in all living cells.

The post-translational modifications of most proteins may be classified into one of three major categories:

- modifications that involve peptide bond cleavage and formation
- modifications that involve N- or C-terminal amino acids
- modifications that involve specific amino acid side-chain moieties.

Some of the more common post-translational modifications are listed in Table 4.3. These modifications are achieved by the involvement of specific enzyme activities, or they can occur spontaneously, as in the deamidation reaction that converts aspargine to aspartic acid or isoaspartic acid (Table 4.3).

Post-translational events can often carry the same significance for production of functional proteins as do the transcriptional and translational phases that are responsible for the formation of proteins in the first instance.

4.6 Protein degradation

As already implied, the breakdown of tissue and organ proteins is an extensive, continuous and regulated process. In association with protein synthesis, the degradation or breakdown of proteins determines the qualitative and quantitative nature of the cellular protein profile.

In mammalian cells, there are separate lysosomal and non-lysosomal mechanisms that are involved in different aspects of protein degradation (Figure 4.2); proteins that enter the cell from the extracellular milieu (such as via receptor-mediated endocytosis and pinocytosis) are degraded in lysosomes. Lysosomal degradation of intracellular protein occurs mostly under stressed conditions, such as in starvation, and this process is activated by glucocorticoids and suppressed by insulin or by a dietary protein deficiency.

Non-lysosomal mechanisms are responsible for the selective turnover of intracellular proteins that occurs under basal metabolic conditions and for many of the changes that occur in response to diet and hormones. The proteolytic system that degrades the bulk of cell proteins, including the rapid elimination of abnormal proteins and short-lived regulatory polypeptides, is non-lysosomal and ATP dependent. It occurs in a large multiple-protein complex, the 20S proteosome, consisting of at least 50 subunits, which in total might account for as much as 1% of the total cell protein. Proteins are degraded within the central core of the proteosome, the 20S particle, which contains different

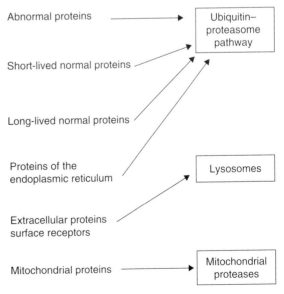

Figure 4.2 Substrates of different proteolyic pathways in mammalian cells. (Reproduced with permission from Lecker *et al*. 1999.)

proteolytic activities (two chymotrypsin-like, two trypsin-like and caspase-like active sites). Protesomes hydrolyze most peptide bonds and generate peptides that are typically 3–22 amino acids long, which results in a loss of the biological properties of the proteins, except in the case of antigen presentation.

An initial step in the hydrolysis of many such proteins is a 'marking' reaction involving their covalent conjugation by the 76-residue polypeptide ubiquitin, via a multistep process; the C-terminus of ubiquitin becomes attached by an isopeptide bond to ε-amino groups on lysine residues of the protein substrate. Much of the selectivity for proteolysis resides in this conjugation step involving several families of enzymes, which may comprise hundreds of members to achieve

high selectivity. It is thought to be rate limiting and requires adenosine triphosphate (ATP). Figure 4.3 shows a proposed sequence of events in the conjugation and degradation of protein via this system. The proteosome also recognizes and degrades some non-ubiquitinylated proteins and there seem to be multiple ubiquitin- and proteosome-dependent pathways.

4.7 Selectivity of protein turnover

The proteins of a single tissue (e.g. skeletal muscle, liver, kidney) turn over at heterologous rates. This general characteristic of protein metabolism is illustrated for the liver in Table 4.4. Not only do the cytoplasmic

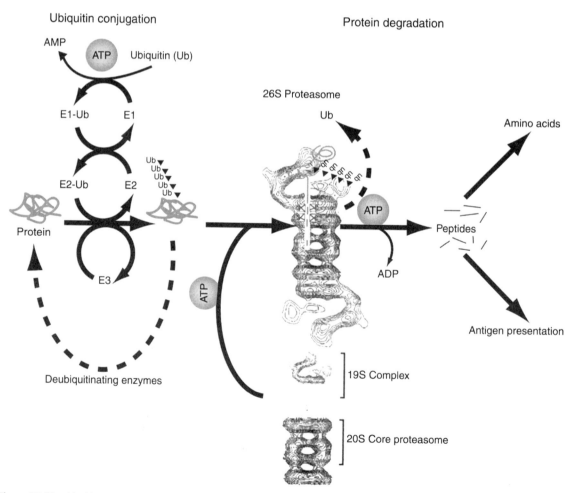

Figure 4.3 The ubiquitin–proteasome pathway of intracellular protein breakdown. Ub: ubiquitin. (Reproduced with permission from Lecker *et al.* 1999.)

proteins in a liver cell turn over at vastly different rates, by as much as 2000-fold difference, but also the proteins of the mitochondria have differential rates of turnover. Another characteristic of protein turnover is randomness of breakdown, as indicated by the first-order kinetics of degradation.

Based on their turnover, as measured most often by tracer techniques, proteins have been classified as short-lived proteins (degradation within about 1 h) and long-lived proteins (degradation takes many hours, and as long as days in some instances). Furthermore, the different subunits of a functional protein can turn over at different rates. For example, the light chain of myosin turns over about three times as rapidly as the myosin heavy chain. Finally, the mature collagen in skin does not reveal a turnover but is lost from the body by shedding of cells from the surface.

Various hypotheses have been proposed to explain the heterologous turnover of proteins and their subunits. Some of these hypotheses, usually based on physicochemical properties of the proteins, are shown in Table 4.5. In each case examples in favor of the hypothesis can be found and the reader is encouraged to consult the reading list for further details.

Table 4.4   Half-lives of some proteins

Protein type	Name	EC number	Liver half-life (h)
Cytoplasmic	1. Ornithine decarboxylase	4.1.1.17	0.2
	2. Tyrosine aminotransferase	2.6.1.5	2.0
	3. Tryptophan oxygenase	1.13.11.11	2.5
	4. HMG-CoA reductase	1.1.1.34	3.0
	5. Serine dehydratase	4.2.1.12	4.0
	6. Phosphoenolpyruvate carboxykinase	4.1.1.32	5.0
	7. Glucokinase	2.7.1.2	12
	8. Dihydroorotase	3.5.2.3	12
	9. Glucose-6-phosphate dehydrogenase	1.1.1.49	15
	10. Pyruvate kinase	2.7.1.40	30
	11. Fructose-1,6-biphosphatase	3.1.3.11	36
	12. Histidase	4.3.1.3	60
	13. Arginase	3.5.3.1	96
	14. Aldolase	4.1.2.13	118
	15. Glyceraldehyde-3-phosphate dehydrogenase	1.2.1.12	130
	16. Lactate dehydrogenase (isoenzyme 5)	1.1.1.27	144
Nuclear	17. RNA polymerase I	2.7.7.6	1.3
	18. RNA polymerase II	2.7.7.6	12
	19. Histone		432
Mitochondrial	20. δ-Aminolevulinate synthetase (matrix)	2.3.1.37	1.1
	21. Ornithine oxo-acid aminotransferase (matrix)	2.6.1.13	19
	22. Alanine transaminase (matrix)	2.6.1.2	20
	23. Glutamate dehydrogenase (matrix)	1.4.1.3	24
	24. Monoamine oxidase (outer membrane)	1.4.3.4	55
	25. Citrate synthase (matrix)	4.1.3.7	94
	26. Malate dehydrogenase (matrix)	1.1.1.40	96
	27. Glycerol-P dehydrogenase (inner membrane)	1.1.99.5	96
	28. Pyruvate carboxylase (matrix)	6.4.1.1	110
	29. Cytochrome *bc* (inner membrane)		132
	30. Cytochrome *c* oxidase (inner membrane)	1.9.3.1	134
	31. Cytochrome *c* (inner membrane)		150
	32. Carbamoyl phosphate synthetase (matrix)	6.3.4.16	185
	33. Pyruvate dehydrogenase (matrix)	1.2.4.1	194

Modified from Jennissen (1995).
HMG-CoA: 3-hydroxy-3-methylglutaryl-coenzyme A.

Table 4.5 Significant hypotheses for explaining selective degradation rates in protein turnover

---

Hypothesis

1. Coenzyme depletion (Pyridoxal-P, NAD$^+$) (apoenzyme degraded by 'group-specific proteases')
2. Molecular mass (degradation rate increases with molecular mass)
3. Isoelectric point (degradation rate increases with decrease in isoelectric point)
4. Hydrophobicity (degradation rate increases with hydrophobicity)
5. Surface polarity (charge)
6. Thermal stability (degradation rate increases with decreased thermal stability)
7. Phosphorylation (degradation rate dependent on inter-conversion state)
8. Oxidation (inactivation by oxidation marks enzyme for degradation)
9. Ubiquitylation free α-amino group N-end rule (ubiquitylation marks protein for degradation)
10. Sequence-specific degradation signals; PEST hypothesis; dipeptide hypothesis (intramolecular sequences signal rapid degradation)
11. Coproteins (specific second proteins, e.g. 'antizymes' initiate and promote degradation)

PEST: a sequence rich in proline, glutamic acid, serine and threonine. From Jennissen (1995), where original references for these hypotheses are given.

4.8 An integration of these processes of turnover with respect to amino acid metabolism

The metabolism of the amino acids that are released into the body pools during the process of protein breakdown, as described above, is determined by, and also in turn affects, the status of protein synthesis and breakdown. Also, the metabolism of amino acids differs from that of lipid and carbohydrate macromolecules in two important ways, and these determine the overall pattern of their metabolism. The first is that the body has no specific store for amino acids, in contrast to its ability, albeit limited, to store carbohydrate as glycogen and the considerable capacity to store fatty acids as triacylglycerol. It is true that, in certain circumstances, proteolysis in the liver and musculature can make amino acids available for particular purposes (e.g. acute-phase protein synthesis or gluconeogenesis), but these liver and muscle proteins, together with all other body proteins (with the exception of milk proteins), are primarily synthesized for their specific physiological function and not as a nutritional store of amino acids.

Protein synthesis requires that all amino acids must be available to tissues simultaneously; this is the basis for dietary protein complementation (see Chapter 5 in Introduction to Human Nutrition in this series). The corollary of this is that tissue amino acids in excess of the capacity and requirements for protein synthesis are very rapidly oxidized and the need for rapid metabolism of dietary protein can also be argued simply on osmotic grounds. A typical North American adult ingests about 100 g protein/day. Upon digestion and absorption, this amounts to about 1000 mmoles of amino acids (100 g of glucose is 600 mmoles). This quantity of amino acids, if distributed evenly throughout body water (about 42 liters in a 70 kg person), would increase the osmotic pressure by about 24 mOsm. Hence the need to remove these amino acids rapidly by catabolizing those that are not required for protein synthesis.

The second way in which the metabolism of amino acids differs from that of carbohydrate or of fat is in the nature of its end-products. In addition to carbon dioxide and water, amino acid catabolism produces nitrogen-containing end-products (principally urea and ammonia) and sulfur-containing end-products (principally sulfate). These, too, have important implications for shaping amino acid catabolism. Since ammonia is a potent neurotoxin, its blood concentration must be kept low (about 30 μmol in humans). Ammonia detoxification via urea synthesis is confined to the liver. Therefore, much of amino acid disposal occurs in the liver. When amino acid metabolism occurs in the periphery, mechanisms exist for transporting the nitrogen to the liver in a form that avoids elevation of the blood ammonia concentration. There are also important acid–base consequences to the catabolism of the sulfur amino acids as this involves the production of a strong metabolic acid. The elimination of this acid is also accomplished via amino acid metabolism.

4.9 Regulation of amino acid metabolism

As for the case of protein synthesis and breakdown, there is a fine regulation of amino acid metabolism, particularly in reference to the metabolism of the indispensable amino acids. Thus, a variety of mechanisms, both short and long term, come into play. These include enzyme induction and turnover, covalent modification of enzymes and control by K_m. For example, glucagon secretion is increased upon ingestion of a high-protein meal. This response plays two roles. First, a high-protein intake also stimulates insulin secretion. Insulin promotes protein synthesis from the ingested amino acids, but will also increase glucose utilization. This latter action, if unopposed, could result in hypoglycemia after the ingestion of a high-protein, low-carbohydrate meal. The increased glucagon levels prevent this by increasing hepatic glucose production. The second action of glucagon is to stimulate amino acid catabolism. That glucagon plays a major role in the catabolism of many amino acids is evident from the generalized hypoaminoacidemia in patients with a glucagonoma.

- Glucagon activates phenylalanine hydroxylase by an adenosine 3′5′-cyclic monophosphate (cAMP)-dependent mechanism.
- Glucagon activates glutaminase and the glycine cleavage enzyme, although the mechanism of this effect remains obscure.
- Glucagon and glucocorticoids can also induce the synthesis of a number of amino acid catabolizing enzymes.

In addition to hormones that stimulate the catabolism of a variety of amino acids, there must be mechanisms specific to individual amino acids that can accommodate appropriate amino acid oxidation in the face of varying amounts of different amino acids. The most obvious of these is control by K_m. Many enzymes that initiate amino acid degradation have quite high K_m values for their amino acid substrates, relative to the tissue concentrations of the amino acids. Thus, these enzymes can automatically respond to increased postprandial tissue levels of amino acids with increased catabolism. The corollary of this is that as tissue concentrations of amino acids decrease so will their catabolism. However, it is clear that control by K_m is not sufficient to protect indispensable amino acids from excessive catabolism, and a number of other mechanisms have evolved. A particularly effective mechanism is that of rapid enzyme induction and degradation. Many of the hepatic enzymes that initiate amino acid catabolism, particularly the catabolism of the indispensable amino acids, are highly inducible. Increased dietary protein brings about increased synthesis of these enzymes; these effects are often hormonally mediated. Furthermore, many of these enzymes have quite short half-lives, as already noted above. The combination of

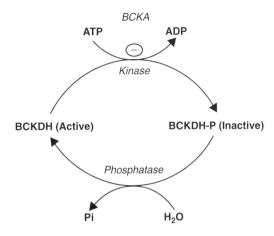

Figure 4.4 Regulation of the branched-chain α-keto acid (BCKA) dehydrogenase.

these factors means that there are quite large amplitude changes (as much as 10-fold) in the hepatic activities of enzymes such as tyrosine aminotransferase, ornithine aminotransferase, tryptophan dioxygenase, threonine dehydratase and histidase. The physiological significance of these effects is clear. The induction of the enzymes can facilitate increased catabolism when the amino acid supply is high, while the virtual disappearance of some of these enzymes when the amino acid supply is low serves to conserve these indispensable amino acids.

Finally, some of the key enzymes of amino acid catabolism are regulated by covalent modification. The branched-chain α-ketoacid dehydrogenase (BCKADH) is the controlling enzyme in the catabolism of the three branched-chain amino acids (valine, leucine and isoleucine). Existing as a multienzyme complex, similar to that of pyruvate dehydrogenase, the BCKADH complex contains a protein kinase and a protein phosphatase that can regulate its activity by reversible phosphorylation (Figure 4.4). The enzyme is inhibited by phosphorylation. The BCKADH kinase is inhibited by the branched-chain α-ketoacids (most potently by α-ketoisocaproate, the α-ketoacid derived from leucine), which results in a dephosphorylation and, hence, activation, of the BCKADH. Another striking regulatory mechanism is found in the catabolism of phenylalanine. Phenylalanine hydroxylase, the controlling enzyme in the catabolism of phenylalanine, is regulated by its amino acid substrate and by phosphorylation/dephosphorylation. Glucagon can activate the enzyme via a cAMP-dependent phosphorylation. However, the enzyme can also exist in two forms, dimeric and tetrameric, and can be converted to the more active tetrameric form in the presence of phenylalanine. These two forms of activation appear to be synergistic in that phenylalanine also increases the rate of phosphorylation by glucagon. Thus, both of these enzymes, BCKADH and phenylalanine hydroxylase, are activated by increased substrate concentrations through mechanisms that are quite different from control by K_m. However, the combination of these mechanisms and control by K_m combine to make the catabolism of these amino acids particularly sensitive to substrate concentrations and provide elegant mechanisms whereby these amino acids are readily catabolized when their supply is high and conserved when supply is low. It is conceivable that similar, but undiscovered, mechanisms may exist for some of the other indispensable amino acids.

4.10 Amino acid synthesis: the dispensable amino acids

Nutritionists pay great attention to the indispensable (essential) amino acids. It can be argued, however, that the retention, during evolution, of the synthetic pathways for the dispensable (non-essential) amino acids speaks of their importance in metabolism.

The synthesis of many of these amino acids is fairly simple; for example, alanine is synthesized in a single transamination reaction, in which glutamate provides the amino group and the carbon skeleton, pyruvate, is readily available from glycolysis. However, for other amino acids, the situation is more complex. Arginine (a conditionally indispensable amino acid) provides an excellent example of a complex synthetic pathway in which there are both developmental variations and important interspecies differences.

In many adult mammals, including humans, arginine is synthesized by a pathway that involves the small intestine and the kidney (Figure 4.5). In brief, citrulline produced in the enterocytes is added to the blood and removed by the kidneys, which convert it to arginine. This arginine is then released in the renal vein. Citrulline is produced, in the intestine, in two ways. A major portion arises from the metabolism of glutamine. A key enzyme in this pathway is pyrroline-5-carboxylate synthetase, which is found only in these cells. Proline can also be a source of citrulline (Figure 4.5). Citrulline is taken up by kidneys where it is converted to arginine, in cells of the proximal tubule, by the combined action of argininosuccinate synthetase and argininosuccinate lyase (Figure 4.5). The importance of this intestinal/renal axis for arginine synthesis is evident from the arginine deficiency that occurs when intestinal citrulline synthesis is inhibited or after massive surgical resection

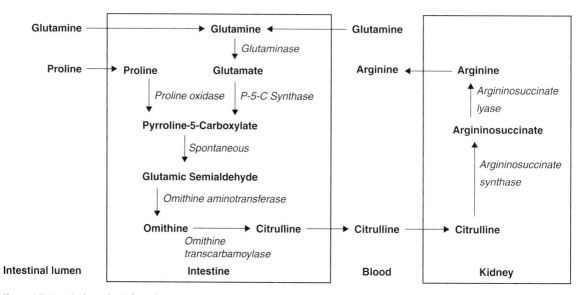

Figure 4.5 Intestinal–renal axis for endogenous arginine synthesis.

of the small intestine. A similar situation occurs in strict carnivores, such as cats and ferrets, whose intestines synthesize almost no citrulline owing to low activities of pyrroline-5-carboxylate synthetase and ornithine aminotransferase. In these animals, ingestion of a single arginine-free meal can result in hyperammonemia, convulsions and even death. Finally, it is apparent that the entire pathway for arginine synthesis is expressed in enterocytes from newborn animals and that newly synthesized arginine is released into the hepatic portal vein. However, such intestinal arginine synthesis is strictly a neonatal event, as it declines within a few days of birth (in piglets), and intestinal citrulline production is evident a few days after weaning.

The synthesis of dispensable amino acids such as arginine, as described above, glutamine, glycine and proline normally proceeds at rates commensurate with metabolic needs. However, under certain conditions, such as in prematurity or in catabolic stress, their rates may not proceed at rates sufficient to meet the metabolic requirement. In this case a dietary source of the amino acid is required and in this context these amino acids are classified as being 'conditionally indispensable' or 'conditionally essential'.

4.11 *In vivo* aspects of protein and amino acid turnover

Techniques for measurement of protein turnover

Various tracer techniques have been used to estimate amino acid fluxes and protein kinetics at the whole-body

Table 4.6 Methods of measuring protein turnover *in vivo*: whole-body, region and specific proteins

	Example of tracer
Whole body	
End-product (EP) methods	[^{15}N]glycine
Precursor methods	[^{13}C]leucine/[^{13}C] KIC
Specific proteins	
Bolus/constant infusion tracer protocols	[^{13}C]leucine, [^{2}H$_5$]phenylalanine
Region	
Constant infusion/biopsy	[^{2}H$_5$]phenylalanine
Arteriovenous difference tracer studies	[^{15}N-1-^{13}C]leucine
Multiple isotope (iv/ig-splanchnic)	[^{2}H$_3$]leucine (iv), [1-^{13}C]leucine (ig)

iv: intravenous; ig: intragastric.

level and in individual tissues and organs (Table 4.6). The different whole-body approaches may be classified into one of two major categories:

- those involving the use of ^{15}N and measurement of the label in end-products of nitrogen metabolism (end-product methods)
- those involving administration of specifically labeled amino acids and measurement of the tracer in body fluids, such as plasma or urine (plasma or precursor method).

Measurement may also be made of the appearance of the tracer in metabolic products of the amino acid metabolism, such as in expired air or in a more proximal metabolite, such as tyrosine in the case of a labeled phenylalanine tracer, or α-ketoisocaproate where labeled leucine is the tracer. This second approach may further be regarded as a substrate-specific method, especially when the major focus of interest is on the metabolism of a specific amino acid, in contrast to the case where a labeled amino acid, such as leucine, is used as an index of the overall status of amino acid and whole-body protein kinetics. The precursor method can be used to estimate rates of tissue or specific protein synthesis by determining the incorporation of the tracer into proteins isolated from suitable samples taken by biopsy. The tracer may be given as a constant infusion or as a bolus. In the latter case a modification might involve the 'flooding'-dose technique, which will be described below. Details of the various models used and of the specific analytical methodology, as well as the ways in which the data are handled, are outside the scope of this chapter, but the reader may wish to consult the further reading list for further information.

^{15}N End-product methods

The principle behind ^{15}N end-product approaches for measurement of protein (nitrogen) turnover in the whole body is depicted in Figure 4.6; it involves administration of a ^{15}N-labeled precursor (often [^{15}N] glycine) as a continuous infusion or as a single bolus and measurement of the appearance of the isotope in urinary, ammonia or total nitrogen. In its simplest form the metabolic nitrogen pool is depicted as a single homogeneous pool into which nitrogen enters from protein breakdown and from the diet. Nitrogen leaves via protein synthesis and by pathways of nitrogen excretion. This model, or modifications of it, has been used extensively by many investigators since it was first used more than 50 years ago by Schoenheimer at Columbia University in New York.

The isotopic data generated from ^{15}N-labeled tracer administration may be evaluated using a compartmental modeling approach or by applying a stochastic model in which the overall flow of nitrogen into and out of the metabolic pool is of interest, rather than the movement of nitrogen within and among the intermediate pools. The stochastic method gives less information than the compartmental modeling approach, but is obtained more easily; this might be an advantage in studies dealing with protein and amino acid turnover that are conducted under demanding experimental conditions such as in various clinical settings or even in the field. Additional details, problems and limitations of this approach are to be found by consulting the further reading list.

Precursor, plasma or substrate-specific methods

Under this general category a tracer-labeled amino acid is administered, most often by continuous intravenous infusion, often immediately preceded by a priming dose to help to achieve a rapid approach to isotopic plateau equilibrium within the sampled compartment. In human studies, the latter is most often the venous blood circulation, although urine could be sampled as a basis for the non-invasive determination of the isotopic enrichment in the free amino acid pool. Alternative procedures within this class of methods include giving the isotope tracer(s) by bolus intravenous injection or by oral administration or by both, where simultaneous doses of different specific labeled tracers of an amino acid are given via these routes.

The basic features of the precursor procedure are depicted in Figure 4.7, where enrichment of the tracer is measured in the plasma and, if appropriate, the appearance of the label in expired carbon dioxide is also monitored. Using simple dilution principles, the flux of the amino acid in the sampled compartment can be determined. Under steady-state metabolic and isotopic conditions, when a nutritionally indispensable amino acid is used as a tracer, estimates can be made of the rate of disappearance of the tracer via non-oxidative metabolism, assumed to be a measure of protein synthesis, and of the rate of appearance of the tracer into the compartment via protein breakdown. The most widely used tracer protocol in studies of human whole-body protein turnover has been L-[1-^{13}C]leucine, given as a primed continuous intravenous infusion.

Several technical and modeling issues need to be considered when using the plasma or precursor approach for measurement of amino acid fluxes and

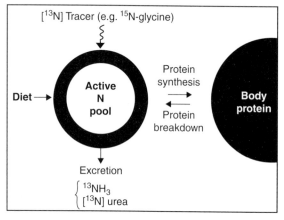

Figure 4.6 Schematic of the ^{15}N-end-product model for determination of whole-body protein turnover.

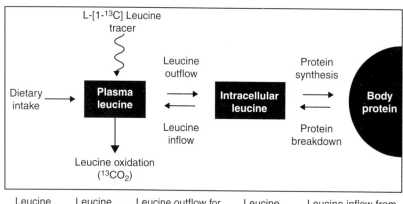

Figure 4.7 Schematic of the plasma precursor model, using ^{13}C-leucine as the example tracer, for determination of whole-body protein turnover.

for estimation of whole-body protein dynamics. For summary purposes, Table 4.7 lists some of the questions that must be answered when attempting to estimate the whole-body amino acid flux, and rate of protein synthesis in the body as a whole. A particularly important problem is that of determining isotopic enrichment of the precursor of interest in order to estimate either whole-body amino acid flux, the rate of protein synthesis or the rates of synthesis of specific proteins in its various regions. Since in most clinical investigations it would be difficult, or unethical, to sample the tissue or organ pools of interest, the problem might be overcome, at least in part, by measuring in blood the enrichment of a metabolite derived from the intracellular metabolism of the tracer and which is in rapid equilibrium with the extracellular compartment. In this context the transamination product of leucine, α-ketoisocaproate (KIC), is often used to predict intracellular leucine labeling and various studies have generally supported the validity of this approach. However, other approaches have been used for specific purposes, and that of mass isotopomer distribution analysis (MIDA) is particularly powerful; this involves quantifying precursor-product events from the distribution of mass isotopomer patterns in the labeled precursor and product.

The 'flooding'-dose technique
Finally, mention should be made of the flooding-dose method, which has been used in both experimental animals and humans to determine rates of synthesis of muscle proteins and of various blood proteins, such as albumin in humans. This approach involves giving the tracer (e.g. $[1\text{-}^{13}C]$leucine or $[^{2}H_5]$phenylalanine) together with a large amount of unlabeled amino acid to create a similar isotopic enrichment in the extracellular and intracellular compartments, including the pool supplying amino acids for tRNA charging and protein synthesis. The idea and approach is highly attractive, particularly since it involves a relatively brief study period for any one experimental subject and, therefore, is potentially applicable in complex clinical settings. Estimates of albumin synthesis obtained by this method are in general agreement with those derived from the constant tracer infusion approach, but concern has been raised about the appropriateness of the technique for estimating synthesis rates of muscle proteins. The flooding-dose approach is particularly suited to measurements made on tissues that can be taken during surgery.

4.12 *In vivo* rates of protein turnover

Whole body
The various methods summarized above have provided a picture of human protein metabolism where, for example, protein synthesis rates are high in the newborn and, per unit of body weight, these rates decline with progressive growth and development (Table 4.8). Three points emerge from the values shown in this table. Firstly, not only is the higher rate of protein synthesis in the young, compared with that for the adult, related to the net protein deposition that occurs during growth, but also there is a high rate of total protein turnover

Table 4.7 Some issues and questions related to precursor or 'plasma' approach for measurement of amino acid fluxes and whole-body and organ/tissue protein turnover

1. What model and why?
   (a) for whole-body protein turnover
   (b) for measurement of organ (regional) protein and amino acid metabolism
   (c) for study of specific amino acid metabolism; its conversions and interconversions and metabolic fate
   (d) for studying the carbon and/or nitrogen moiety and/or functional groups of the molecule
2. What is the isotopic enrichment of the 'precursor' amino acid pool(s) for accurate measurement of whole-body flux and oxidation rates?
3. What is the appropriate amount of tracer and length of infusion period, and is there a problem of recycling of label?
4. Are infusion and sampling sites important? Which are best?
5. For measurement of components of flux, what is the retention of $^{13}CO_2$?

Table 4.8 Some representative estimates of whole-body protein synthesis rates, in humans at various ages compared with dietary protein allowances

Age group	Protein synthesis (A) (g/kg per day)	Protein allowance (B) (g/kg per day)	Protein ratio A/B
Infant (premature)	11.3, 14	~3.0	4.5
Child (15 mo)	6.3	1.3	5
Child (2–8 years)	3.9	~1.1	4
Adolescent (~13 years)	~5	~1.0	5
Young adult (~20 years)	~4.6	0.75	6

From Young *et al.* (1985), where references to the original studies are given. Reproduced with permission of the *American Journal of Clinical Nutrition*. © American Society of Clinical Nutrition.

Table 4.9 Some estimates of tissue protein turnover in a 70 kg adult human

Tissue/organ	% Body weight	Total protein content (g)	Fractional synthesis rate (%/day)	Amount (g/day)	Protein synthesis (% of whole body)
Skeletal muscle	40	4200	2	84	28
Stomach	0.25	26	43	11	3.6
Small intestine	1	105	40	42	14
Colon	0.6	63	9	6	2
Liver	2.5	263	20	53	18
Heart	0.5	53	5.2	3	1
White cells			6.2		

Reproduced from Ingenbleek and Young (2002). This table was kindly constructed for the authors by Professor Peter Garlick, SUNY, Stonybrook, New York, USA.

(synthesis and breakdown), related, in part, to tissue remodeling. Hence, protein synthesis in the premature infant is about twice as high as in the preschool child and approximately three or four times as high as in the adult. Secondly, at all ages, the rates of whole-body protein synthesis and breakdown are considerably greater than intakes of dietary protein apparently necessary to meet the needs for maintenance or for the support of growth. It follows, therefore, that there is an extensive reutilization within the body of the amino acids entering tissue pools during the course of protein breakdown. Thirdly, there is a general relationship between the age- and developmental-associated changes in protein turnover and the dietary protein needs for each specific age group. This implies that when rates of synthesis and breakdown of body proteins change in response to various stimuli, such as infection and trauma, the dietary requirement for nitrogen and specific amino acids intakes will change. This prediction is consistent with the increased total protein (nitrogen) needs of patients following severe trauma.

Organs and tissues

Although whole-body rates of protein turnover change with different physiological and pathological states, these measurements do not provide information on the status of protein turnover in different tissues and organs. Hence, estimates of protein turnover by individual organs and tissues have also been made and a summary of some of these is presented in Table 4.9. The fractional rates of synthesis differ among the organs, with those for liver being about 10 times the value for skeletal muscle. However, because of the size

Table 4.10 Effects of various nutritional and pathological states on muscle and liver protein synthesis in young rats or mice

Treatment	Protein synthesis (% of control)	
	Liver	Muscle
Starvation (2 days)	71	47
Protein-free diet (9 days)	70	27
Diabetes	51	41
Malaria infection	66	49
Turpentine injection	116	66
Interleukin-1β	145	68
Cancer	126	56

Reproduced from Garlick and McNurlan (1994), where references to original sources of the data are given.

of the musculature it accounts for about 20% of whole-body protein synthesis or about the same as that for the liver.

It should now be clear that there are major differences among the various tissues and organs in their rates of protein turnover. As might be expected, therefore, the responses of different organs to nutritional and pathological stimuli also differ, and this can be with respect to the direction of change and the extent of change. To illustrate this point, Table 4.10 summarizes the responses of the liver and muscle of young rats to a variety of nutritional and pathological treatments. As shown here, the rates of protein synthesis in these rat tissues change in same direction during nutrient deprivation, but they respond differently to various disease states. Although the available data are more limited in humans the same different pattern of response appears to apply. Thus, the higher rate of whole-body protein

Table 4.11 Calculated amounts of acute phase protein synthesized in response to infection

Protein	Normal concentration (g/l)	Maximum increase in 48 h	New synthesis (g/kg per.24 h)
C-reactive protein	0.01	×1000	0.25
Serum amyloid A	0.01	×1000	0.25
α_1-Acid glycoprotein	1	×4	0.1
α_1-Antitrypsin	2	×4	0.2
Fibrinogen	2	×4	0.2
Heptoglobin	2	×4	0.2
Total			1.2

Reproduced from Waterlow (1992), where references to original observations are given.

turnover in severely traumatized patients is associated with higher rates of muscle protein breakdown and also higher rates of liver protein and immune cell protein synthesis. For example, in severely burned adult patients, rates of whole-body protein synthesis might be double those for healthy subjects. It has been estimated that in response to infection acute-phase protein synthesis might account for an additional 1 g protein synthesis/kg body weight per day (Table 4.11), which is six times the normal rate of albumin synthesis in adult humans.

4.13 Mechanisms and factors responsible for alterations in protein turnover

Protein synthesis

As is already evident, rates of protein synthesis and breakdown are not constant but change in response to different pathophysiological conditions. Among the important factors responsible for alterations in protein synthesis rates is the availability of amino acids. They regulate the expression of genes involved in growth, cellular function or amino acid metabolism. The finer details of the mechanisms involved are only now being worked out, but one mechanism appears to involve the increased expression of the genes encoding for an insulin-like growth factor binding protein, CHOP [a CCAAT/enhancer-binding protein (C/EBP)-related gene] and asparagine synthetase. This is regulation at the transcriptional level.

Changes in amino acid availability also can either up-regulate or down-regulate the translational phase of

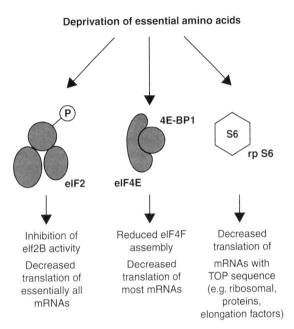

Deprivation of essential amino acids

Inhibition of elf2B activity

Decreased translation of essentially all mRNAs

Reduced eIF4F assembly

Decreased translation of most mRNAs

Decreased translation of mRNAs with TOP sequence (e.g. ribosomal, proteins, elongation factors)

Figure 4.8 Effect of deprivation of essential amino acids on translation initiation. Deprivation of essential amino acids inhibits the initiation phase of mRNA translation at one or more steps, including those involving eIF2, eIF4E and S6 (rp S6). (Reproduced with permission from Kimball, 2002.)

protein synthesis via an effect on translation initiation at various steps in the process described earlier. The response may be general, that is by affecting the translation of most mRNAs, or it may be specific, by affecting the translation of a single class or subset of mRNAs (Figure 4.8). The general response is mediated via regulation at both the initiator methionyl-RNA and mRNA binding steps, via alterations in the phosphorylation status of specific initiation factors. With respect to the more specific responses, these involve the mRNA binding step and the phosphorylation of one of the proteins (S6) of the 40S ribosomal subunit. The mode by which the cell recognizes a change in amino acid availability and sufficiency is not known precisely, but it seems that multiple recognition sites and multiple signaling pathways are involved. Figure 4.9 indicates the potential signaling pathways, with one including a protein kinase referred to as the mammalian target of rapamycin (mTOR). This appears to be a point of convergence of signals generated by the action of hormones, such as insulin, and those elicited by changes in the availability of amino acids. This mTOR-dependent pathway is specifically responsible for the responses to changes in leucine availability, whereas

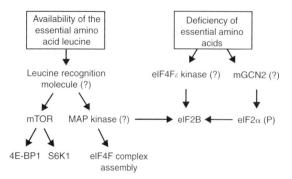

Figure 4.9 Potential signaling pathways involved in the response of translation initiation to amino acid sufficiency. At least two mechanisms exist that detect the sufficiency of essential amino acids. A recognition molecule that preferentially, but not exclusively, senses leucine sufficiency signals to S6K1 and eukaryotic initiation factor (eIF)4F complex assembly, the latter through both direct and indirect (i.e. through phosphorylation of 4E-BP1) mechanisms. The leucine recognition molecule may also signal to eIF2B. A second mechanism for detecting amino acid sufficiency involves regulation of eIF2B through changes in eIF2α phosphorylation and possibly through changes in eIF2Bε phosphorylation. (Reproduced with permission from Jefferson and Kimball, 2001.)

Table 4.12 Experimental observations in models of muscle wasting, indicating increased rates of ubiquitin-dependent proteolysis

↑ ATP-dependent proteolysis in isolated muscles
↑ Susceptibility of proteolysis to proteasome inhibitors
↑ Ubiquitin content of muscles
↑ Content of ubiquitin–protein conjugates
↑ Ubiquitin mRNA (total mRNA falls)
↑ mRNA for ubiquitin-carrier proteins (E2s)
↑ mRNA of proteasome subunits
↑ Ubiquitin conjugation to muscle proteins

Reproduced with permission from Lecker et al. (1999).

another pathway that involves an activation of the eIF2 kinase is responsive to the changes in the sufficiency of any indispensable amino acid. There is a great deal more to be learned about how the cell senses changes in amino acid availability, the basis for the specificity of the response to particular amino acids, and the nature and extent of the cooperativity between amino acids and growth-promoting hormones in the regulation, translation and initiation of protein synthesis.

Protein breakdown

A profound loss of muscle mass may occur under various experimental conditions, such as following glucocorticoid treatment, denervation and fasting. This also occurs in patients suffering from major trauma, including burn injury, sepsis and cancer. This erosion of muscle protein is due, in part, to enhanced rates of protein breakdown or proteolysis, and especially the contractile or myofibrillar proteins may be affected. In models of muscle wasting there are various changes that indicate an activation of the proteasome–ubiquitin-dependent pathway (Table 4.12). The increases in mRNA levels for polyubiquitin, of certain proteasome subunits and of specific ubiquitination enzymes suggest a coordinated series of biochemical adaptations in the atrophying muscle that enhance the activity and capacity of this pathway, leading to muscle wasting.

In contrast to the stimulation of muscle breakdown, under some conditions there are other conditions that favor conservation of muscle cell protein. Thus, if energy intake is adequate but protein or amino acid intake inadequate protein turnover muscle is reduced. In this case there is a reduced capacity to degrade proteins. This is associated with a suppression of the ubiquitin-dependent proteasome pathway as well as reduction in the activity of the lysosomal pathway.

Such adaptations to protein inadequacy are seen in humans in prolonged starvation or malnutrition, where physiological mechanisms have evolved that permit survival to continue with little or no energy and protein intake for relatively prolonged periods. However, a continued and sustained loss of cell proteins is lethal and so the capacity to mobilize protein from cells as a source of energy is limited. In the initial days of a fast or catabolic illness, muscle and skin proteins are mobilized and amino acids are metabolized for energy and/or used to meet the amino acid needs for protein synthesis in the splanchnic region and by the immune system. After several days of food deprivation, that catabolic response ceases and other mechanisms are activated to suppress muscle protein breakdown and amino acid oxidation. The conservation of muscle protein occurs concomitantly with a reduction in oxygen consumption and metabolic rate, and the overall rates of protein breakdown vary with changes in nutrient supply and endocrine factors. Thus, muscle proteolysis is controlled by several hormones, especially insulin and glucocorticoids.

The turnover of proteins and their response to changes in the internal and external environments, possibly brought about by altered substrate availability, including amino acids and energy sources, and by hormones and peptide mediators, including cytokines, occur in the context of the movement of amino acids among organs and within tissues. This aspect of the integration of protein and amino acid metabolism will be discussed in the following section.

4.14 Interorgan amino acid metabolism

Fed and fasted states

There is a considerable amino acid traffic between the various organs of the body. The principal vehicles for this transport are the free amino acids themselves. However, distribution via proteins and peptides should also be considered. The liver is the site of synthesis of a number of plasma proteins, of which albumin is quantitatively the most important. In a well-nourished healthy adult, approximately 20 g of albumin per day is synthesized by the liver and catabolized in the periphery. Albumin synthesis is sensitive to nutritional and pathological conditions, increasing with the feeding of protein-rich meals and decreasing in kwashiorkor, for example. Albumin degradation occurs in many tissues of the body, including skin, muscle, kidneys and even in the liver itself; it seems that fibroblasts in these tissues are particularly active. In terms of amino acid traffic, it can be estimated that some 20 g of amino acids per day are normally made available to peripheral tissues as a result of albumin catabolism.

Peptides have also been suggested as a vehicle for interorgan amino acid traffic. Certainly, some peptides that arise physiologically, such as the C-peptide of proinsulin or peptide products of angiotensinogen proteolysis, are very rapidly catabolized. The kidney has a high capacity for such peptide catabolism. It has also been suggested that peptides can play a major role in interorgan amino acid metabolism. However, the situation is far from clear as the existence of a significant circulating peptide pool is controversial.

The principal technique for the study of interorgan amino acid metabolism is that of arteriovenous (or A-V) difference. When combined with simultaneously measured rates of blood flow, such A-V differences provide quantitative data on the net uptake or output of amino acids across different organs. There are two important points to appreciate about this technique. First, it measures *net* metabolic exchanges. It is entirely possible that there may be simultaneous utilization and production of an amino acid across an organ (e.g. glutamine utilization in periportal hepatocytes and glutamine synthesis in perivenous hepatocytes). Delineation

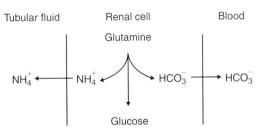

Figure 4.10 Renal glutamine uptake, ammonium excretion and bicarbonate regeneration.

of these individual processes requires the application of isotopic techniques, in addition to that of the A-V difference approach. Secondly, A-V differences are, almost always, small differences between two large numbers. As such, they require great analytical precision and it can be assumed that many small, though physiologically important, differences escape detection.

Major A-V differences for amino acids have been found across many tissues. Across the fed intestine, there is a net outflow of amino acids into the hepatic portal vein as proteins are digested and amino acids are absorbed but, in addition there is an uptake of glutamine and an output of alanine and citrulline. The carbon skeleton of alanine arises from glycolytically derived pyruvate, while the nitrogen arises from glutamine metabolism. Kidneys remove citrulline and convert it to arginine, which is released (Figure 4.5). They also remove glycine and produce serine. Kidneys also take up glutamine, for acid–base homeostasis (Figure 4.10), and this uptake increases dramatically in metabolic acidosis (e.g. diabetic ketoacidosis) or during ingestion of a high-protein diet when increased quantities of sulfuric acid are produced from methionine and cysteine oxidation. Skeletal muscle oxidizes an important proportion of dietary branched-chain amino acids. It also releases substantial quantities of alanine and glutamine. Alanine is synthesized via alanine aminotransferase; its nitrogen comes from the branched-chain amino acids and its carbon from glucose. This alanine is taken up by the liver and converted to glucose (the glucose–alanine cycle). Thus, alanine serves as an innocuous means of transferring nitrogen to the liver without increasing blood ammonia concentrations. In the fed state, more glutamine than alanine is released by muscle. The nitrogens for glutamine synthesis are derived from all three of the branched chain amino acids, but the carbon skeleton can only be provided from isoleucine and valine.

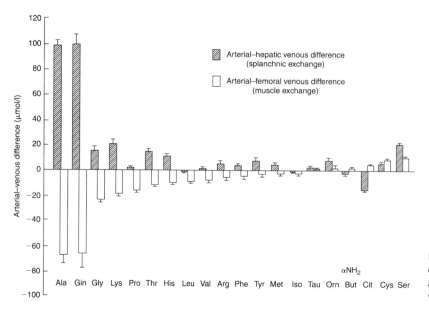

Figure 4.11 Splanchnic and leg exchange of amino acids in humans after an overnight fast. (Reproduced with permission from Felig, 1975.)

During starvation there is marked muscle proteolysis to provide amino acids to the liver for gluconeogenesis. However, the pattern of amino acids released by the liver does not correspond to the amino acid composition of muscle protein, in that alanine and glutamine comprise at least 50% of the amino acids released. Much of the alanine arises via the glucose– alanine cycle. In this case, carbon skeletons for glutamine synthesis are derived from the intramuscular metabolism of glutamate, aspartate, asparagine, valine and isoleucine. There is a remarkable concordance between the pattern of amino acids released from skeletal muscle and taken up by splanchnic tissues after an overnight fast (Figure 4.11).

4.15 Amino acid and peptide transport

Amino acid pools

Free amino acids comprise a very small portion of total body amino acids, where about 99% are found in proteins. However, the free amino acid pools are, metabolically, very dynamic. The principal extracelullar pool, that of blood plasma, is the major vehicle for interorgan amino acid exchange. Cellular amino acid pools are hetereogeneous, both between cell types and within intracellular compartments. Thus, brain contains particularly high concentrations of glutamate, an important neurotransmitter, while muscle contains the great bulk of the body's free glutamine. Cellular amino acid pools are crucial for the specific metabolic functions of individual cell types (e.g. the role of arginine, ornithine and citrulline in the liver's urea cycle) as well as, more generally, being the immediate pool of amino acids from which proteins are synthesized and to which amino acids are returned by intracellular proteolysis. Table 4.13 gives the concentrations of free amino acids in human plasma and within human muscle cells. It is apparent that there is considerable variability in the intracellular/extracellular gradients for different amino acids. These gradients are largely determined by amino acid transport mechanisms.

Amino acid transporters

Since the early 1990s enormous progress has been made in this field as many amino acid transporters have been identified, cloned and studied in detail. This new knowledge has complemented and expanded our earlier understanding, which was almost entirely derived from kinetic studies and genetic defects. Most cells contain systems A, ASC, L, y^+ and X_{AG}^- (Table 4.14), as well as tissue-specific transport systems. From the new molecular studies it is now appreciated that there are many individual transporters within these different systems. A common feature of these transporters is that, generally, they transport a number of amino acids that share common structural features.

Amino acid transporters differ in their preferred substrates and in the thermodynamic driving forces

Table 4.13 Concentrations of free amino acids in human muscle and plasma

Amino acid	Plasma (mM)	Intracellular muscle (mM)
Aspartate	0.02	
Phenylalanine	0.05	0.07
Tyrosine	0.05	0.10
Methionine	0.02	0.11
Isoleucine	0.06	0.11
Leucine	0.12	0.15
Cysteine	0.11	0.18
Valine	0.22	0.26
Ornithine	0.06	0.30
Histidine	0.08	0.37
Asparagine	0.05	0.47
Arginine	0.08	0.51
Proline	0.17	0.83
Serine	0.12	0.98
Threonine	0.15	1.03
Lysine	0.18	1.15
Glycine	0.21	1.33
Alanine	0.33	2.34
Glutamate	0.06	4.38
Glutamine	0.57	19.45
Taurine	0.07	15.44

Data from Bergstrom *et al.* (1974).

Table 4.14 Some major amino acid transport systems in mammalian cells

System	Specificity	Distribution
Na^+-*dependent systems*		
A	Small aliphatic amino acids	Widespread
ASC	Small aliphatic amino acids	Widespread
N	Glutamine, histidine, asparagine	Liver
N^m	Glutamine, histidine, asparagine	Skeletal muscle
B^o	Most neutral amino acids	Brush-border membranes of renal and intestinal epithelia
X_{AG}^-	Glutamate, aspartate	Widespread
Na^+-*independent systems*		
L	Mainly branched-chain and aromatic amino acids	Widespread
y^+	Lysine, histidine, arginine	Widespread

they use. Systems A, ASC and L transport neutral amino acids; systems A and ASC mediate transport of amino acids with small side-chains, whereas system L prefers amino acids with bulky side-chains (i.e. branched and aromatic groups). Alanine, serine and glutamine are preferred substrates for system A, and alanine, serine and cysteine for system ASC. Transport via systems A and ASC is in symport with sodium ions and uses sodium entry down its electrochemical gradient as a driving force. System L is not sodium linked and may, in many circumstances, mediate amino acid efflux from cells. System y^+ mediates high-affinity sodium-independent transport of cationic amino acids as well as sodium-dependent transport of neutral amino acids. System X_{AG}^- transports glutamate or aspartate together with sodium, when transporting into the cell, and together with potassium, when transporting out of the cell.

In addition to these fairly ubiquitous transporters, mention should be made of system B^o (and related systems), which are found on the apical poles of epithelial cells, such as in the intestine and kidney. These effect the sodium-dependent accumulation of a broad range of neutral amino acids, including those transported, in other cells, by system L. Transport of glutamine, asparagine and histidine occurs via a sodium-dependent system N in hepatocytes and system N^m in skeletal muscle. It is thought that the massive loss of glutamine from skeletal muscle during catabolic illness occurs via system N^m. It should be emphasized that the amino acid transporters described above constitute only a fraction of those that have been identified. In addition, with the application of molecular techniques it is certain that many more of these transporters will shortly be discovered. Chapter 8 of this volume deals in greater detail with amino acid transporters of importance to brain function.

Peptide transporters

Peptide transporters have been identified that transport dipeptides and tripeptides in intestinal and renal epithelia. PEPT1 is expressed in the intestine and, to a lesser degree, in the kidney. PEPT2 is found only in the kidney. These transporters have quite broad specificity with respect to the amino acid composition of the dipeptides and tripeptides transported, but they will not transport amino acids or tetrapeptides. The peptide transport occurs together with a hydrogen ion; the driving force for peptide accumulation is the transmembrane electrochemical H^+ gradient (Figure 4.12). These peptides are hydrolyzed to amino acids within renal and intestinal cells. The peptide transporters are also of considerable pharmacological importance as they transport a number of drugs, including cephalosporins and penicillins, that contain peptide-like structures.

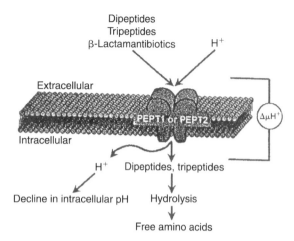

Figure 4.12 Peptide transporter function in the apical membranes of intestinal and renal cells. (Reproduced with permission from Daniel, 2000.)

Physiological function and regulation of amino acid and peptide transport

The most obvious function of the amino acid and peptide transporters is in the absorption of amino acids from the intestine, the reabsorption of filtered amino acids in the kidney, and the cellular uptake and interorgan metabolism of amino acids. Amino acid transporters also play important roles in the maintenance of cell volume. Transepithelial amino acid transport (e.g. in the intestine and kidney) requires two amino acid transporters, one on the apical (brush-border) membrane and the other on the basolateral membrane. These two transporters are, invariably, distinct. In the intestine, the combination of amino acid and peptide transporters is responsible for the absorption of about 160 g of amino acids per day, comprising about 100 g of dietary protein and about 60 g from intestinal secretions and sloughed cells. In the intestine, the peptide transporters are quantitatively more important than the amino acid transporters.

The total plasma amino acid concentration is about 2.5 mmol/l, and the glomerular filtration rate, in humans, is about 180 l/day. Therefore, it can be calculated that the renal amino acid transporters reabsorb about 450 mmoles of amino acids per day (equivalent to the amino acids in about 45 g of protein). In the absence of reliable data on the plasma concentrations of dipeptides and tripeptides a similar calculation cannot be made for the amount of peptide transport in the kidney, but it is believed to be much less than

amino acid transport. It should be noted that the brush-border membranes of the cells of the proximal tubule contain highly active peptidases that can attack larger peptides and small filtered proteins, and that these processes will make additional dipeptides and tripeptides available to the peptide transporters, but it is difficult to quantify this activity. However, it is clear that the renal peptide transport systems will play a major role in the hydrolysis of peptides provided in parenteral nutrition.

In addition to facilitating amino acid uptake and output by cells, amino acid transporters may exercise control on such amino acid traffic. It has already been indicated that the loss of glutamine from skeletal muscle during catabolic illness is attributable to the system N^m transporter. The hepatic uptake of alanine may be limited by its transport. Competition between large neutral amino acids limits their uptake into the brain (Chapter 8). The capacity of many of these transport systems is also controlled. Perhaps the best examples come from system A, whose activity, in a variety of tissues, can be made to vary markedly. For example, hepatic system A activity is up-regulated in diabetes and during starvation as well as by the administration of glucocorticoids and interleukin-6, (IL-6) and by both glucagon and insulin. Its expression is decreased by growth hormone.

There are three well-described situations where system A is markedly up-regulated in almost all cells: adaptive regulation, hypertonicity and cell proliferation. In each of these situations the up-regulation requires protein synthesis. Adaptive regulation refers to the increase in system A activity that becomes apparent when cells are placed in a medium lacking system A substrates. (Conversely, system A activity is down-regulated when cells are transferred to an amino acid-rich medium.) This mechanism relates to the fundamental nutritional needs of cells as the up-regulation helps cells to cope with a limited extracellular availability of amino acids. System A also shows remarkable sensitivity to osmotic pressure. Cells shrink when placed in a hypertonic medium but, after some time, exhibit a regulatory volume increase in which up-regulation of system A and the expansion of the amino acid pool play a key role in the restoration of cell volume. System A can also regulate cell volume during isotonic conditions. In particular, increased system A activity has been implicated in the increased cell volume associated with cell proliferation. System A is up-regulated as cells leave the G_0 phase and enter the cell cycle, while the marked increase in cell volume in the G_1 and S phases is attributable to increased accumulation of potassium and amino acids. These effects expand the role of amino acid transporters, from the simplest one of supplying cells with amino acid substrates for metabolism and protein synthesis, to a more complex and fundamental role in osmoregulation. The signaling pathway whereby system A is enhanced in these conditions is, currently, a highly active research field.

Genetic diseases of plasma amino acid transport

Various amino acid transport disorders are known. These have provided valuable knowledge about the transport process as well as providing nutritional challenges for patient care. Cystinuria is an autosomal recessive disease, often associated with increased urinary loss of cationic amino acids that share a transporter with cystine. Owing to its low solubility, cystine often precipitates to form urinary calculi. Indeed, the name 'cystine' derives from such a calculus, or cyst, studied by Wollaston in 1810. The intestinal transport mechanisms for the absorption of cystine and the cationic amino acids are, also, often defective in cystinuria; however, this appears to have no nutritional consequences owing to alternative uptake mechanisms. Hartnup disorder is an autosomal recessive impairment of neutral amino acid reabsorption in the kidney. Defective transport is also evident in the intestine. Lysinuric protein intolerance is an autosomal recessive disease associated with greatly increased urinary excretion of lysine, arginine and ornithine. These amino acids are also poorly absorbed in the intestine. The transport defect is localized in the basolateral membrane of these epithelia. The condition is associated with intolerance and rejection of high-protein food as well as hyperammonia, which has been attributed to impaired urea synthesis. Other amino acid transporter defects include iminoaciduria, characterized by increased urinary excretion of glycine, proline and hydroxyproline, and dicarboxylate aminoaciduria, characterized by massive urinary excretion of glutamate and aspartate. It is obvious that most of these genetic transporter diseases have been discovered as a result of increased urinary amino acid excretion. It may be assumed that comparable defects occur in which the lesion is exclusively expressed in internal organs but which have not yet been discovered because of the lack of so convenient a means for their identification.

4.16 Disposal of dietary amino acids and roles of specific organs

With the continuous turnover of proteins and movement of amino acids between and in and out of organs and the tissues of the body there is an inevitable and irreversible loss of indispensable amino acids and of end-products of nitrogen metabolism. Hence, a dietary supply of indispensable amino acids in adequate amounts and proportions, together with suitable carbon and nitrogen sources that can be used to synthesize dispensable and conditionally indispensable amino acids, is needed to maintain this dynamic state of protein turnover and cell and organ function. It is necessary, therefore, to consider here the metabolism of amino acids entering from the diet.

Events in the intestine

The digestion and absorption of dietary protein is dealt with in detail in Chapter 10. In terms of quantitation, it is important to appreciate that, although an adult may ingest some 100 g of protein per day, the quantity digested and absorbed is much greater than this. It is estimated that approximately another 70 g arises in the intestine as a result of the sloughing of mucosal cells and the protein content of secreted juices. Since fecal nitrogen is equivalent to some 10 g protein daily, it follows that about 160 g of protein will be digested and absorbed per day.

It is now apparent that the small intestine is a major site of amino acid catabolism and, in the fed state, can obtain a significant amount of its energy requirements from this process. As much as 90% of dietary glutamate and aspartate and much glutamine are catabolized within the small intestinal mucosa in the first pass. In addition, appreciable quantities of indispensable amino acids (isoleucine, leucine, valine, lysine, methionine and phenylalanine) are catabolized. There is also substantial metabolism of threonine, but this may be due largely to mucin synthesis rather than catabolism. In the case of many of these amino acids, as much as 30–50% does not enter the hepatic portal circulation, so that intestinal metabolism is a major determinant of whole-body amino acid requirements. In addition, this phenomenon has important implications for amino acid nutrition during parenteral feeding, as the elimination of first pass intestinal metabolism means that indispensable amino acid requirements will be decreased.

Finally, it should be noted that intestinal amino acid catabolism is often not complete, and products released into the hepatic portal vein include other amino acids such as alanine, citrulline and proline. It is clear that first pass intestinal metabolism substantially modifies the pattern of amino acids that are available to the rest of the body. Much of the recent work on intestinal amino acid metabolism has been carried out using the piglet model. It will be important to determine whether this tissue is as quantitatively important in adult animals.

Role of the liver

The liver has long been recognized as the principal organ that metabolizes dietary amino acids. It is the only organ that contains the enzymic capacity to catabolize all of the amino acids, though its ability to metabolize branched-chain amino acids is limited. It also contains the urea cycle, so that ammonia arising from amino acid catabolism can be readily detoxified. Indeed, the ammonia concentration in the hepatic venous blood that exits the liver is much lower than in the blood that enters via the hepatic portal vein, which is enriched in ammonia partly as a result of bacterial activity in the intestine. However, ammonia detoxification cannot be entirely attributed to urea synthesis. It is now apparent that there are two hepatic processes that remove ammonia: urea synthesis and glutamine synthesis. Furthermore, these two processes do not occur in the same liver cells. The enzymes of the urea cycle are found in the periportal and central hepatocytes, whereas glutamine synthetase is restricted to the perivenous hepatocytes, where it can serve as a fail-safe mechanism to scavenge ammonia that escapes

detoxification in the earlier part of the hepatic acinus (Figure 4.13). As the K_m of glutamine synthetase for ammonia is much lower than that for carbamylphosphate synthetase 1, the hepatic ammonia detoxification system can be thought of as a low-affinity, high-capacity system (urea synthesis) in series with a high-affinity, low-capacity system (glutamine synthesis). These two systems, together, are responsible for the very low levels of ammonia that are normally found in the systemic circulation.

The capacity of the liver for urea synthesis is very high, so that it can readily respond to increased substrate supply. In addition, there are important acute and long-term controls that act on this process (see also Chapter 4, Introduction to Human Nutrition in this series). The principal acute regulation occurs via changes in the concentration of N-acetylglutamate, an obligatory activator of carbamylphosphate synthetase-1, the first enzyme of urea synthesis. Levels of N-acetylglutamate can change very rapidly and are very responsive to protein intake. The mechanism by which N-acetylglutamate increases rapidly in response to a high-protein meal is not clear, but it is known that glucagon can rapidly increase the hepatic concentration of this regulator. Long-term regulation of the urea cycle occurs via alterations in the activities of its enzymes in response to changes in habitual protein intake or to endogenous protein catabolism. These enzymes are not known to be regulated by covalent modification and changes in their activities are due to corresponding changes in the amounts of the enzyme proteins. A variety of mechanisms underlies these alterations in enzyme activity. Certainly, altered rates of

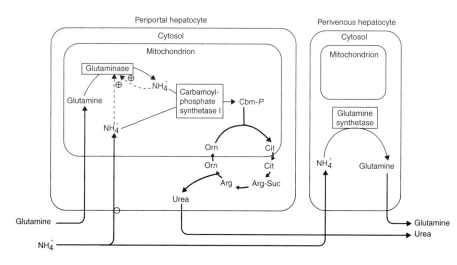

Figure 4.13 Hepatic zonation of urea and glutamine synthesis. (Reproduced from Haussinger, 1988.)

gene transcription (mediated by glucagon and gluco-corticoids) play a major role, but other mechanisms, such as alterations in mRNA translation and protein stability, may also be important.

Traditionally, urea was thought of as a classical end-product. It is now apparent, however, that there is appreciable recycling of urea nitrogen. Urea diffuses into the intestinal lumen and is also a constituent of pancreatic and biliary secretions. This urea is hydrolyzed by urease-containing gut bacteria and much of the ammonia is returned to the body in the hepatic portal vein. It is estimated that approximately 25% of total hepatic urea production is recycled in this way. As discussed in Chapter 4 of *Introduction to Human Nutrition*, the extent to which this recycled nitrogen contributes to nitrogen retention is still unclear.

Amino acid oxidation provides a substantial fraction of the body's energy. The oxidation of the amino acids in 100 g of protein requires the consumption of about 5 moles of oxygen. This compares with a consumption of approximately 3 moles of oxygen per day by the typical adult liver. Clearly, the traditional textbook description of amino acid oxidation, that dietary amino acids are almost completely oxidized in the liver, cannot be true. Even if the dietary amino acids were the liver's only fuel, their oxidation would require more oxygen than the liver actually consumes and would produce more ATP than the liver could use. The solution to this conundrum is two-fold. First, there is substantial extrahepatic amino acid oxidation and, secondly, many of the amino acids metabolized by the liver are only partially oxidized there; their carbon chains are converted to glucose or to the ketone bodies that are released and may be oxidized by other tissues. The principal extrahepatic tissues for amino acid catabolism are the small intestine (see above), skeletal muscle and kidney.

The liver removes about two-thirds of the absorbed amino acids. Of these, perhaps as much as two-thirds are metabolized and one-third is used for protein synthesis, of both plasma proteins and hepatic protein, which undergoes a temporary increase. About one-third of the absorbed amino acids, enriched in the branched-chain amino acids, reaches the peripheral tissues.

Skeletal muscle and kidney

Skeletal muscle plays a crucial role in branched-chain amino acid catabolism. The first two enzymes in their catabolism (the branched-chain aminotransferase and the branched-chain keto acid dehydrogenase) are common to the catabolism of all the branched-chain amino acids. The liver has very low activities of the aminotransferase, so that almost all dietary branched-chain amino acids are delivered to the systemic circulation. Skeletal muscle, which has substantial activities of both enzymes, is the major catabolic organ for these amino acids. The nitrogenous end-products are glutamine and alanine, which are released from muscle. In some animals (e.g. the rat) many of the branched-chain keto acids produced by transamination are released from the muscle and metabolized in the liver. However, it is evident that in humans the bulk of these ketoacids is metabolized within the muscle.

The kidney uses amino acid metabolism to maintain acid–base status. The two sulfur-containing amino acids, methionine and cysteine, generate sulfuric acid on oxidation (Equations 4.1 and 4.2).

$$2\ C_5O_2NH_{11}S\ (\text{Methionine}) + 15\ O_2 \rightarrow$$
$$(NH_2)_2CO\ (\text{Urea}) + 9\ CO_2 + 7\ H_2O$$
$$+ 4\ H^+ + 2\ SO_4^{2-} \quad\quad (4.1)$$

$$2\ C_3O_2NH_7S\ (\text{Cysteine}) + 9\ O_2 \rightarrow$$
$$(NH_2)_2CO\ (\text{Urea}) + 5\ CO_2 + 3\ H_2O$$
$$+ 4\ H^+ + 2\ SO_4^{2-} \quad\quad (4.2)$$

In an individual ingesting 100 g of protein a day this can amount to some 60–70 mmoles of hydrogen ions per day. This production of acid cannot be considered in isolation, as it will be offset by any base produced from other dietary constituents, such as from the oxidation of alkali salts of carboxylic acids, which are abundant in fruits. Most individuals on a typical Western diet will have a net daily generation of about 30 mmoles of hydrogen ions. Significant concentrations of hydrogen ions are not allowed to accumulate; they are promptly neutralized by the blood bicarbonate buffer system (Equation 4.3).

$$H^+ + HCO_3^- \leftrightarrow H_2CO_3 \leftrightarrow H_2O + CO_2 \quad (4.3)$$

However, the buffering of 30 mmoles of hydrogen ions amounts to a daily bicarbonate loss of similar magnitude. A process that can regenerate bicarbonate is necessary. Such a process, involving amino acid metabolism, is found in the kidney (Figure 4.10). The principle behind the process is simple. The kidney does not contain a urea cycle, so amino acid nitrogen gives rise to ammonium. Metabolism of a neutral amino acid to a neutral end-product (e.g. carbon dioxide or glucose) will produce, as end-products, NH_4^+ and

HCO_3^-. Transport processes within the renal tubules effect the separation of NH_4^+ from HCO_3^- such that NH_4^+ is excreted in the urine while HCO_3^- is returned to the body via the renal vein (Figure 4.10). This regenerates the bicarbonate that was lost when hydrogen ions were buffered. In addition to glutamine, glycine is used as a source of NH_4^+ and HCO_3^-. However, glutamine is the predominant substrate in situations where there is massive acid production, such as diabetic ketoacidosis. In human kidneys, the carbon skeleton of glutamine is converted to glucose via renal gluconeogenesis.

4.17 Catabolic illnesses

As mentioned above, patients suffering from burn injuries, cancer, trauma or sepsis, or who have undergone major surgery frequently have greatly increased rates of protein turnover and catabolism. The origins of these catabolic states are complex and anorexia may play a role. However, if so, anorexia only plays a minor role since the provision of nutrients by way of intravenous nutrition does not arrest the catabolism. These pathological catabolic conditions are clearly different from the physiological response to starvation, where lipid oxidation provides the bulk of the energy and protein catabolism is somewhat restrained. The pathological catabolic states are characterized by massive loss of lean body mass (muscle protein catabolism) as well as high rates of lipolysis and fat oxidation. They are also often accompanied by hypermetabolism (increased resting energy expenditure). Circulating levels of cortisol, glucagon, epinephrine and tumor necrosis factor (TNF) are invariably elevated and many of the features of the muscle protein catabolism can be reproduced by infusions of these hormones. Of these hormones, cortisol appears to be an important contributor to the catabolic state, with the protein imbalance being further increased by a decreased concentration or responsiveness to various anabolic hormones, such as growth hormone or insulin-like growth factor-1.

Thus, a high rate of protein and amino acid turnover in catabolic illness inevitably means a relatively high requirement for nitrogen and for specific amino acids. Indeed, rates of turnover (or flux) of nitrogen and indispensable amino acids as well as their oxidation rates in patients suffering from burn injury, for example, are generally much higher than in healthy adults.

For example, the turnover of protein amounts to about 7.3 g protein/kg per day in severely burned patients, in comparison with the healthy adult where turnover approximates 4 g protein/kg per day.

Another relationship of both metabolic and nutritional interest is that between energy metabolism and the rate of whole-body protein turnover. As mentioned earlier, protein synthesis, amino acid transport and protein breakdown are all energy-dependent processes. While their energy requirements differ, it can be estimated that in normal adults amino acid transport and protein synthesis alone appear to account for at least 20% of basal energy metabolism. It follows, once again, that major changes in body protein turnover due, for example, to severe infection or major trauma affect not only the protein and amino acid utilization and requirements but also the status of body energy expenditure and requirements. In adult burn patients, the increased rate of protein turnover has also been estimated to account for about 20% of the increased metabolic rate characteristic of this stressful condition.

One of the most remarkable features of muscle metabolism in these conditions is the massive loss of free glutamine. Glutamine is the most abundant free amino acid in human skeletal muscle, being present at concentrations of about 20–25 mmol. During these catabolic illnesses it can decrease to as little as 8–10 mmol. This is quite specific for glutamine; the other free amino acid pools of muscle are not comparably decreased. The importance of glutamine depletion relates to evidence, from *in vitro* studies with rat muscle, that intracellular glutamine may exert some control of protein synthesis and degradation. High glutamine concentrations favor net protein accretion and lower concentrations favor net proteolysis. The mechanism whereby glutamine may bring this about is uncertain, but it may be related to osmotically induced changes in cell volume.

The increased muscle protein catabolism and glutamine efflux seen in these catabolic conditions serve functions that are designed to improve the organism's survival. Glutamine is directed to the liver where, with other amino acids, it serves as a gluconeogenic precursor, and to rapidly dividing cells, cells of the immune system and wounded tissue, where it is used as a metabolic fuel and a precursor for nucleotide synthesis. The increased gluconeogenesis seen in these situations often leads to hyperglycemia, which may serve the physiological role of increasing the delivery of glucose to poorly perfused wounded tissue, since glucose is the preferred fuel of tissues with limiting oxygen delivery. The hyperglycemia may also maintain glucose delivery to the brain in situations where its perfusion is decreased due to shock. Arginine delivery to macrophages will be used for the synthesis of nitric oxide, which is used by these cells as a bacteriocidal agent. In addition, these amino acids will be used for repair of damaged tissue and by the liver for increased synthesis of acute-phase proteins. Despite these beneficial functions of muscle protein catabolism, it is apparent that when the catabolism is excessive it can contribute to increased mortality and morbidity. For this reason, many studies have provided substantial amounts of glutamine (either as free glutamine or in peptide form) to such patients in attempts to replace muscle glutamine and to arrest or reverse the loss of lean body mass. Beneficial results, such as improved nitrogen balance and gut integrity and reduced rates of infection while in hospital, have been reported.

Another point to note, of particular interest in surgical metabolism and nutrition, relates to the post-translational modifications of protein mentioned earlier. Thus, there is a methylation of histidine residues within actin and myosin, the major fibrillar proteins in skeletal muscle. Since the 3-methylhistidine released during the degradation of myosin and actin is not further metabolized to any extent, it is largely excreted via the urine unchanged. Hence, its rate of output via the kidney serves as an index of the approximate rate of muscle myofibrillar protein degradation. This technique offers a relatively simple *in vivo* and non-invasive index of protein breakdown, and this should aid in an understanding of the *in vivo* regulation of muscle protein degradation and its response to nutritional and pharmacological treatment. In addition, methylated derivatives of arginine occur in muscle proteins and they are also excreted in urine. It has been shown that $N^G N^G$-dimethyl-L-arginine, the dominant form of methylarginine synthesized by human endothelial cells, can be produced in quantities that may affect nitric oxide production via inhibiting nitric oxide synthase. Nitric oxide, a free radical, is a ubiquitous intracellular and intercellular messenger with multiple physiological and pharmacological functions, and it will be important to characterize more fully the mechanisms determining the intracellular and extracellular levels of these methylated arginines under various pathophysiological conditions. However, this offers another example of the intimate relationship between protein turnover, amino acid metabolism and function.

4.18 Non-proteinogenic metabolic functions of amino acids

In addition to their roles as substrates for protein synthesis and as regulators of protein turnover, amino acids display more functional diversity than any other of the major nutrients. They are extraordinarily important in the brain as neurotransmitters (glutamate, glycine) and as neurotransmitter precursors (tyrosine, tryptophan, histidine, glutamate, cysteine). These issues are discussed in Chapter 18 of this volume. In the other tissues of the body amino acids also play crucial roles in metabolism and biosynthesis (Table 4.3).

Many of the dispensable amino acids are involved in high-capacity metabolic fluxes. For example, the malate–aspartate shuttle is the principal means of oxidizing NADH generated in the cytoplasm during glycolysis and, therefore, is involved in the oxidation of some 200–400 g carbohydrate per day, in most adults. Glutamate is involved in the transamination of almost all of the amino acids and, thus, in the metabolic disposal of about 100 g protein per day (on a typical Western diet). Alanine is the major vehicle for shuttling nitrogen to the liver after amino acid catabolism in muscle or intestine. There is a very high rate of glutamine synthesis and degradation (40–80 g/day in adults), which is only partly explained by the fact that glutamine is a major fuel for intestinal cells and for cells of the immune system. Arginine is involved in the synthesis of some 30 g urea per day (on a typical Western diet). Aspartate is the immediate source of half of the nitrogen in urea. It could be argued that the magnitude of the fluxes involved in these processes obliged the retention of pathways for the synthesis of these amino acids. However, both dispensable and indispensable amino acids play key roles in many lower flux pathways. These are given in Table 4.2. Three aspects of amino acids that are of particular interest are selected here. These are the role of methionine as a methyl donor, the biosynthesis of creatine, and the synthesis and function of glutathione.

Methionine metabolism

The metabolism of methionine provides an excellent example of:

- a key amino acid function (methylation)
- the crucial involvement of vitamin-derived cofactors
- the adaptation of metabolic fluxes to nutritional conditions

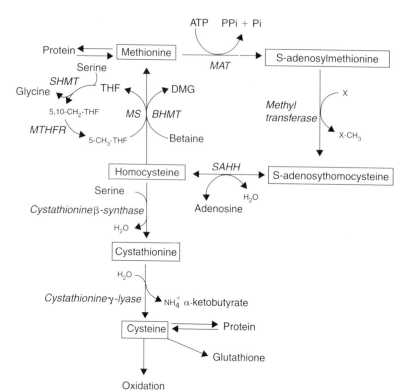

Figure 4.14 Outline of methionine metabolism. MAT: methionine adenosyltransferase; SHMT: serine hydroxymethyltransferase; MTHFR: 5,10-methylenetetrahydrofolate reductase; MS: methionine synthase; BHMT: betaine:homocysteine, methyltransferase; SAHH: S-adenosylhomocysteine hydrolase; THF: tetrahydrofolate reductase; DMG: dimethylglycine.

- the influence of a common genetic polymorphism on metabolism.

It also provides insight into factors that affect the production of homocysteine, which has been identified as an important risk factor for cardiovascular disease. Figure 4.14 shows an outline of the major pathways of methionine metabolism. In fact, Figure 4.14 depicts two separate pathways: the catabolism of methionine via the transsulfuration pathway and the methionine cycle. Probably all cells have the methionine cycle, while the transsulfuration pathway, which converts homocysteine to cysteine, is most active in the liver but is also found in the kidney, intestine and pancreas.

The methionine cycle describes the reactions whereby the methyl group of methionine is used in methylation reactions and then regenerated, while preserving the carbon skeleton of this indispensable amino acid. The reactions involve the conversion of methionine to S-adenosylmethionine, which serves as a universal methylating agent in more than 30 different methyltransferases. Examples of such methyltransferases are found in the synthesis of epinephrine, creatine and phosphatidylcholine, and in the methylation of DNA. S-adenosylhomocysteine, produced in these methylation reactions, is hydrolyzed to adenosine and homocysteine. To complete the cycle, homocysteine is remethylated to methionine by one of two enzymes: either by the ubiquitously distributed methionine synthase, which uses 5-methyltetrahydrofolate (5-methyl THF) as the methyl donor, or by betaine methyltransferase, which is restricted to the liver and the kidney. Betaine arises from the catabolism of choline. The transsulfuration pathway effects the catabolism of methionine. Homocysteine is removed from the cycle and converted to cysteine by the successive actions of cystathionine β-synthase and cystathionine γ-lyase. An important feature of these pathways is the role of vitamin-derived cofactors. Methionine synthase has methylcobalamin as its cofactor; both cystathionine β-synthase and cystathionine γ-lyase contain pyridoxal phosphate. In addition, methionine synthase utilizes a methyl group from the folic acid–one-carbon pool.

Figure 4.14 shows that homocysteine sits at a metabolic crossroads as it may be reconverted to methionine or catabolized to cysteine. Careful balance data and isotopic measurements of methionine's fate in both humans and rats show that the partitioning of homocysteine between remethylation and transsulfuration depends on the dietary supply of methyl groups. When methionine and choline intake is low, homocysteine is predominantly remethylated. However, when dietary methyl groups, in the form of methionine and choline, are abundant, remethylation is decreased and flux through the transsulfuration pathway is increased.

Since the early 1990s, convincing epidemiological evidence has accumulated to support the proposition that elevated plasma homocysteine is an important risk factor for cardiovascular disease. This has stimulated a great deal of interest in factors that affect the plasma level of homocysteine. Deficiencies in the B vitamins important in methionine metabolism (folic acid, vitamin B_{12} and pyridoxal) are all associated with elevated plasma homocysteine. Of these, it is apparent that folic acid deficiency is the most important contributor to hyperhomocystinemia. Indeed, the US 'national' plasma homocysteine level has decreased by some 5–10% since the advent of folic acid fortification. Whether or not this will result in a decreased incidence of cardiovascular disease is of great interest.

Finally, metabolism of methionine and homocysteine provides a remarkable example of the influence of common genetic polymorphisms. Methylenetetrahydrofolate reductase (MTHFR) reduces 5,10-methylene THF to 5-methyl THF, which is used by methionine synthase to remethylate homocysteine to methionine (Figure 4.14). An MTHFR polymorphism (C677T), in which alanine-222 is replaced by valine, is remarkably common. Indeed, in most populations that have been examined, homozygosity for this polymorphism varies from 4 to 24%. Individuals with this variant tend to have an increased folate requirement, as well as increased plasma homocysteine because of impaired provision of 5-methyl THF for methionine synthase. Whether or not this genetic polymorphism is a risk factor for cardiovascular disease is controversial, but there is no question that the C677T polymorphism predisposes to neural tube defects.

Creatine synthesis

Creatine synthesis provides an excellent example of amino acids as biosynthetic precursors. It is also a pathway that consumes substantial amounts of arginine and of methyl groups. An adult human loses some 1–2 g of creatinine per day in the urine. This creatinine

arises from the spontaneous breakdown of both creatine and phosphocreatine. Creatine synthesis (which replaces the loss) involves three different amino acids. It involves only two enzymes. The first step (Equation 4.4) is catalyzed by arginine:glycine transamidinase:

$$\text{Glycine} + \text{Arginine} \rightarrow \text{Guanidinoacetate} + \text{Ornithine} \tag{4.4}$$

The second reaction is catalyzed by guanidinoacetate methyltransferase (Equation 4.5):

$$\begin{aligned} \text{Guanidinoacetate} &+ S\text{-Adenosylmethionine} \\ &\rightarrow \text{Creatine} + S\text{-Adenosylhomocysteine} \end{aligned} \tag{4.5}$$

These two enzymes occur in different tissues: the transamidinase is most abundant in the kidney and absent from the liver, while the methyltransferase is restricted to the liver. Thus, creatine synthesis is an interorgan process in which guanidinoacetate is released by the kidney and taken up by the liver. Creatine synthesis makes major demands on arginine and on methyl groups. It can be calculated that an 18–29-year-old male requires about 2.5 g arginine per day for creatine synthesis. This is about 50% of dietary arginine if he ingests 100 g protein/day. Creatine synthesis is also the major consumer of methyl groups. Indeed, the methylation of guanidinoacetate uses approximately 70% of physiologically labile methyl groups.

Glutathione

Glutathione provides an excellent example of a key amino acid-derived molecule whose synthesis may be restricted, in certain nutritional and pathological conditions, by the availability of its amino acid constituents and whose function is determined by an inorganic micronutrient, selenium. Glutathione is a tripeptide (L-γ-glutamyl-L-cysteinylglycine) composed of three amino acids in which the glutamate is joined to cysteine by an unusual γ-peptide linkage. It plays a number of roles within cells in such diverse areas as:

• conjugation and elimination of xenobiotics
• covalent modification of protein via glutathionylation
• transfer of nitric oxide as S-nitrosoglutathione.

Glutathione is also the major low molecular weight thiol in animal cells and, as such, serves both as a redox buffer and as an agent for the detoxification of reactive oxygen species (ROS). The key to glutathione's function in these processes lies in its ability to undergo oxidation. Glutathione with a free thiol (GSH) can be oxidized to glutathione disulfide (GSSG). In cells almost all of the glutathione exists as GSH owing to the action of glutathione reductase (Equation 4.6):

$$NADPH + H^+ + GSSG \rightarrow NADP^+ + 2\,GSH$$
$$(4.6)$$

The NADPH is provided by the pentose phosphate pathway. Glutathione plays a major role in the destruction of hydrogen peroxide (Equation 4.7) and a variety of organic hydroperoxides (Equation 4.8) via the action of glutathione peroxidase:

$$2\,GSH + H_2O_2 \rightarrow GSSG + 2\,H_2O \qquad (4.7)$$

$$2\,GSH + ROOH \rightarrow GSSG + H_2O + ROH$$
$$(4.8)$$

Hydrogen peroxide arises from a variety of reactions, including the scavenging of superoxide radicals by superoxide dismutase. The hydroperoxides arise from lipid peroxidation of polyunsaturated fatty acids. Thus, glutathione can deal with a variety of ROS. It can also prevent lipid peroxidation because of its ability to scavenge free radicals, such as those that propagate lipid peroxidation. Glutathione, therefore, is part of the cell's defense against oxidative stress. Depletion of glutathione or excessive production of ROS is associated with peroxidative cell damage in a variety of pathological conditions.

Glutathione peroxidase contains selenium in the form of an unusual amino acid, selenocysteine. The selenium replaces the sulfur atom of cysteine. The activity of this enzyme is, therefore, greatly reduced in selenium deficiency, with a consequent increased susceptibility to an oxidative challenge. Recent work has examined red blood cell glutathione synthesis in humans. This is quite sensitive to sulfur amino acid availability. Patients infected with human immunodeficiency virus (HIV) have quite low erythrocyte GSH levels owing to decreased erythrocyte cysteine concentrations: cysteine supplementation leads to an increased rate of GSH synthesis and an increase in the erythrocyte GSH concentration. Thus, precursor amino acid availability can determine the concentration of this key molecule.

4.19 Perspectives on the future

Protein synthesis, protein turnover and amino acid metabolism play major roles in the bodily economy. Isotopic and other techniques have revealed the magnitude of these fluxes. In a healthy adult human, some 300 g of new protein is synthesized each day and a comparable quantity of protein is catabolized. This compares with approximately 100 g of protein consumed, per day, on a typical Western diet. Protein synthesis and turnover are major components of resting energy expenditure. Such a high metabolic price underlies important functions, including adjusting to changes in the internal environment, tissue remodeling and the removal of mutant or damaged proteins. A crucial feature of these processes is their physiological selectivity, with regard to both individual proteins (rates of turnover of individual proteins vary by factors of over 1000) and individual tissues (e.g. catabolic illnesses are associated with a marked loss of muscle protein but with net increases in the rates of protein synthesis in cells of the immune system). Both protein synthesis and degradation are regulated, in complex ways, by amino acid availability and by hormones.

Amino acids serve as the building blocks of proteins and they also serve other functions. Thus, amino acid metabolism is an intimate component of the protein and nitrogen economy of the body. The catabolism of dietary amino acids is finely regulated by a variety of mechanisms. This is critical as the rate of amino acid catabolism is an important determinant of amino acid requirements. Gluconeogenesis, from muscle-derived amino acids, is a major component of the physiological response to starvation. Certain tissues have a specific requirement for certain amino acids. For example, intestinal cells and cells of the immune system require glutamine, as does the kidney for acid–base homeostasis; cells that produce nitric oxide, such as endothelial cells and macrophages, require arginine; the brain requires amino acids as neurotransmitter precursors; the kidney and liver combine to produce creatine from glycine, arginine and methionine; glutathione serves as a defense against ROS. Interorgan amino acid metabolism integrates these different tissue amino acid requirements. These interorgan amino acid fluxes are facilitated by, and in some cases regulated by, specific amino acid transporters.

The study of proteins and amino acids continues to provide novel insights and stimulation for the nutritionist. Scarcely a year goes by without some major discovery that forces us to look at things in a new light. One of the most extraordinary of discoveries has been that of the production of nitric oxide from arginine and of its many biological functions. It is now also understood that a retrovirus (the murine leukemia virus) uses the y^+ amino acid transport system as its cell-surface receptor. Recently, it has been discovered that the brain contains a serine racemase that converts L-serine to D-serine, which may be used as a coagonist of the N-methyl-D-aspartate receptor. Clearly, it is a certainty that there will be more surprises. The completion of the sequencing of the human genome and that of other organisms will accelerate the pace of discovery and there can be no doubt that we will uncover spectacular new vistas in the field of amino acid and protein nutrition. There is also the possibility of genetic engineering. Will mammals or species of agricultural importance always require the same spectrum of indispensable amino acids? Genes that encode for threonine synthesis in bacteria have already been introduced into mouse cells such that these cells, in culture, no longer require exogenous threonine. Could a similar approach be taken with intact animals, say with poultry, so that they could be fed a lower quality protein ration? Such approaches may be limited more by ethical and regulatory constraints than by technical ones.

Further reading

Bergstrom *et al.* J Appl Physiol 1974; 36: 693–697.

Daniel, H. Nutrient transporter function studied in heterologous expression systems. Ann NY Acad Sci 2000; 915: 184–192.

Davis TA, Reeds PJ. Of flux and flooding: the advantages and problems of different isotopic methods for quantifying protein turnover in vivo: II. Methods based on the incorporation of a tracer. Curr Opin Clin Nutr Metab Care 2001; 4: 51–56.

Doyle HA, Mamula MJ. Post-translational protein modifications in antigen recognition and autoimmunity. Trends Immunol 2001; 22: 443–448.

Fafournoux P, Bruhat A, Jousse C. Amino acid regulation of gene expression. Biochem J 2000; 351: 1–12.

Garlick PJ, McNurlan MA. Isotopic methods for studying protein turnover. In: Protein Metabolism During Infancy (NCR Railia, ed.). Nestlé Nutrition Workshop Series Vol. 33, pp. 29–42. New York: Raven Press, 1994.

Hellerstein MK, Neese RA. Mass isotopomer distribution analysis: A technique for measuring biosynthesis and turnover of polymers. Am J Physiol 1992; 263: E998–E1001.

Ingenbleek, Y. and Young, V.R. Significance of transthyretin in protein metabolism. Clin Chem Lab Med 2002; 40(12): 1281–1291.

Jefferson LS, Kimball SR. Amino acid regulation of gene expression. J Nutr Soc 2001; 1: 246OS–2466S.

Jennissen HP. Ubiquitin and the enigma of intracellular protein degradation. Eur J Biochem 1995; 231: 1–30.

Jogoe RT, Goldberg AL. What do we really know about the ubiquitin-proteasome pathway in muscle atrophy? Curr Opin Clin Nutr Metab Care 2001; 4: 183–190.

Kimball SR. Regulation of global and specific mRNA translation by amino acids. J Nutr 2002; 132: 883–886.

Krebs HA. Some aspects of the regulation of fuel supply in omnivorous animals. Adv Enz Regul 1972; 10: 397–420.

Lecker SH, Solomon V, Mitch WE, Goldberg AL. Muscle breakdown and the critical role of the ubiquitin-proteasome pathway in normal and disease states. J Nutr 1999; 129: 227S–237S.

Millward DJ. Methodological considerations. Proc Nutr Soc 2001; 60: 3–5.

Reeds PJ, Davis TA. Of flux and flooding: the advantages and problems of different isotopic methods for quantifying protein turnover in vivo: 1. Methods based on the dilution of a tracer. Curr Opin Clin Nutr Metab Care 1999; 2: 23–28.

Rucker RB, McGee C. Chemical modifications of proteins in vivo: Selected examples important to cellular regulation. J Nutr 1993; 123: 977–990.

Waterlow JC. Metabolic adaptation to low intakes of energy and protein. Annu Rev Nutr 1986; 6: 495–526.

Waterlow JC. Protein energy malnutrition. London: Edward Arnold, 1992.

Waterlow JC. Whole-body protein turnover in humans – past, present and future. Annu Rev Nutr 1995; 15: 57–92.

Waterlow JC, Garlick PJ, Millward DJ. Protein turnover in mammalian tissues and in the whole body. Amsterdam: North Holland, 1978.

Young VR, Meredith C, Hoerr R, Bier DM, Matthews DE. Amino acid kinetics in relation to protein and amino acid requirements: the primary importance of amino acid oxidation. In: Substrate and Energy Metabolism in Man (JS Garrow, D Halliday eds), pp. 119–133. London: John Libbey, 1985.

5
Integration of Metabolism 3: Macronutrients

KN Frayn and AO Akanji

Key messages

- We take in carbohydrate, fat and protein; ultimately (if we are not growing) we oxidize them, liberating energy, but they may be directed to storage pools before this happens.
- The metabolism of each of these macronutrients is highly regulated, partly by direct metabolic interactions between them, but largely through the secretion of hormones.

- In particular, the metabolic fates of fat and carbohydrate are intimately related: when one is predominant, the other tends to be minimized. This is achieved both by hormonal effects (e.g. insulin suppresses fat mobilization) and by metabolic interaction (e.g. fatty acids tend to inhibit glucose oxidation in muscle).
- Interplay of these various regulatory systems in different tissues enables humans, as intact organisms, to adapt to a wide variety of metabolic demands: starvation, overfeeding or a sudden increase in energy expenditure during exercise.

5.1 Introduction: fuel intake and fuel utilization

The human body as a machine

The human body is a type of machine. It takes in fuel (chemical energy in food) and converts this to useful forms of energy: heat, physical work, and other forms of chemical energy including biosynthesis and pumping of substances across membranes. The chemical energy is liberated from the fuels by oxidation.

The fuels that we take in are the macronutrients: carbohydrate, fat and protein. Each of these may be burned in a bomb calorimeter. The products are carbon dioxide, water and oxides of nitrogen from the nitrogen content of the protein. Their combustion also liberates heat. Similarly, after their oxidation in the body, waste products are excreted. These are essentially carbon dioxide, water and urea (which contains the nitrogen from the protein). Within the body these macronutrients may be partially oxidized (e.g. glucose to pyruvic acid) or converted to other substances, but essentially in the end they are either oxidized completely

in the body or stored: humans do not excrete significant amounts of lactate, ketone bodies, amino acids or other products of their metabolism. It is often useful to maintain this 'global' view of the body's metabolic activities (Figure 5.1).

The pattern of energy intake is sporadic: people usually take in regular, discrete meals, which are digested and absorbed into the circulation over discrete periods. Even though the pattern of food consumption in developed countries may be approaching one of continuous 'grazing', the pattern of energy intake is not geared in general to the pattern of energy expenditure. Therefore, the body must be able to take in fuels (macronutrients), store them as necessary and oxidize them when required. This clearly requires control mechanisms that are similar to the throttle that determines when gasoline (petrol) is used from the storage tank in a car. The situation is more complex than the flow of gasoline, however. In the car there is just one engine demanding fuel. In the human body there are multiple organs, each with its own requirements that vary with time on an individual basis. Furthermore, whereas we fill up

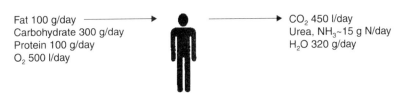

Figure 5.1 Global view of the body's macronutrient utilization. Figures are very approximate and refer to a 70 kg person. Note that, ultimately, combustion of the dietary macronutrients is complete except for the conversion of protein-nitrogen to urea and ammonia.

Table 5.1 The body's macronutrient stores in relation to daily intake

Macronutrient	Total amount in body (kg)	Energy equivalent (MJ)	Days' supply if the only energy source	Daily intake (g)	Daily intake as % of store
Carbohydrate	0.5	8.5	<1	300	60
Fat	12–18	550	56	100	0.7
Protein	12	200	(20)	100	0.8

These are very much typical, round figures. Days' supply is the length of time this store would last if it were the only fuel for oxidation at an energy expenditure of 10 MJ/day: the figure for protein is given in parentheses since protein does not fulfill the role of energy store in this way.

our car tank with just one fuel, as humans we take in the three macronutrients. Each of the body's organs has its own particular requirements for these macronutrients, and so the flow of individual substrates into and out of storage pools must be regulated in a complex, highly coordinated way. This regulated flow of 'energy substrates', and the way in which it is achieved, is the theme of this chapter.

Macronutrient stores and the daily flow of fuel

The body's macronutrient stores are summarized in Table 5.1. Also summarized are the daily intakes (in very round figures) of the macronutrients, for comparison. It will immediately be obvious that the store of carbohydrate, glycogen, is very limited in relation to the daily turnover. In comparison, most people have vast stores of fat and protein.

The concept of energy balance was introduced in Chapter 3. Here, the concept of substrate balance is introduced (Figure 5.2). It is less clear-cut than that of energy balance, because of potential interconversion of substrates. However, if someone is in a steady state of body weight, then the amount of each macronutrient completely oxidized each day must equal that ingested (on average: there will be fluctuations from day to day).

It is useful here to think of the body's 'strategy' in using its fuel stores. The term 'strategy' has to be interpreted

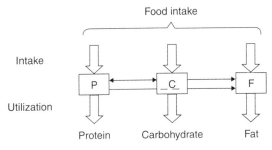

Figure 5.2 Concept of macronutrient balance. As with energy balance, what goes in must come out, with the exception of what is stored. In the case of macronutrients, however, some interconversions are possible. (Based on Frayn 1995.)

carefully. It does not imply that someone is directing substrate flows: rather, that these are the patterns that have evolved because they have survival benefits. Some important organs can, under normal circumstances, only use carbohydrate as a fuel source. The brain is the best example. The adult brain requires about 100 g glucose per day, close to the amount of glycogen stored in the liver. (As we will see, glycogen stored in skeletal muscles has a local role as a fuel source for the muscles themselves.) Therefore, the glycogen store may be regarded more as a daily buffer than as a long-term fuel reserve. Although there appears to be plenty of protein, there is no specific storage form of protein. All

Table 5.2 Fat and carbohydrate as fuel stores

	Energy liberated on oxidation (kJ/g)	Water associated (g/g of fuel)	Energy stored (MJ)/kg carried
Carbohydrate	17	3	4.3
Fat	37	0.2	31

Carbohydrate (glycogen) is stored with about three times its own weight of water; fat with only a small amount of adipocyte cytoplasm.

proteins in the body have a defined role: structural, enzymic, and so on. Therefore, to use protein as a fuel involves some loss of bodily function. Hence, it is not surprising that protein is relatively well protected and the body's protein is not, in general, used as a fuel for energy beyond an amount equivalent to the daily intake. In contrast, the body's fat stores are there primarily as a source of energy. There is a very clear reason why fat (triacylglycerol) is the major energy store in mammals. Because triacylglycerol molecules are hydrophobic, they coalesce into lipid droplets that are stored, in adipocytes, with only a small amount of cytoplasm. The efficiency of energy storage in terms of kilojoules stored per gram is around eight times that for carbohydrate (Table 5.2). Protein is similar to carbohydrate, although some proteins may be less heavily hydrated. During starvation, the body's strategy is to minimize the use of carbohydrate and protein, and to obtain as much energy as possible from fat stores.

5.2 Regulatory mechanisms

The body needs mechanisms for regulating the flow of individual macronutrients in and out of storage pools. There are various ways in which this regulation is achieved.

It is useful to think of short-term and longer term mechanisms. Short-term means minutes or hours and covers what might pass in between meals or during a bout of exercise. Longer term is taken to mean a period of several hours or days.

Short-term regulation of macronutrient flux

In the short term, some regulation is achieved simply by substrate availability affecting rates of reaction by 'mass action' effects. There is an old observation that if an unusual excess of protein is ingested, it will be oxidized over the next 24 h or so. Krebs investigated the means by which this is achieved, and concluded that it reflects the kinetic properties of the initial enzymes of amino acid degradation, including the aminotransferases (transaminases), which have a high K_m (typically several mmol/l, but for alanine aminotransferase 34 mmol/l). A high K_m means that the higher the concentration of substrate, the faster will be the reaction. Similarly, the first steps in glucose uptake and metabolism in the liver, transport across the cell membrane by the facilitated transporter GLUT2, and phosphorylation by hexokinase IV (glucokinase), are both characterized by a high K_m and high capacity. Therefore, glucose will be taken up and enter metabolic pathways in the liver according to its extracellular concentration. As glucose is absorbed from the small intestine and reaches the liver via the hepatic vein, so it will be taken out of the bloodstream (thus helping to minimize fluctuations in blood glucose concentration). Another example is that of ethanol: the first enzyme in the metabolism of ethanol has a low K_m but high capacity, and ethanol will be oxidized at a constant rate when it is available from the diet.

Beyond that, many pathways are regulated by the effects of pathway products or intermediates on the enzymes of that pathway. Often this is achieved by binding of substrates to enzymes, causing allosteric effects that regulate enzyme activity. One example is that of phosphofructokinase in the pathway of glycolysis. The activity of this enzyme is regulated by a number of compounds related to the pathway, including activation by adenosine monophosphate (AMP) and inhibition by adenosine triphosphate (ATP) and citrate. It is also activated by the compound fructose-2,6-bisphosphate, a by-product of the pathway of glycolysis (note that fructose-1,6-bisphosphate is the product of phosphofructokinase), generated by a separate enzyme apparently purely for regulatory purposes.

These examples help to explain the regulation of pathways within cells. When considering the regulation of macronutrient-derived substrates in the body, one often has to think of effects that involve more than one tissue. For instance, the use of fatty acids as a fuel by skeletal muscle during exercise requires that adipocytes increase the release of fatty acids as muscle uses them. Such intertissue coordination is brought about largely through the nervous and hormonal systems. Hormones are released from the endocrine glands in response to some signal, transmitted either through the blood

Table 5.3 Some response elements in genes regulating macronutrient metabolism that are affected by dietary nutrients

Response element	Examples of genes with this element	Notes
Carbohydrate response element	Pyruvate kinase (glycolysis) Pyruvate dehydrogenase E1 subunit Fatty acid synthase	Glucose-6-phosphate may be the signaling molecule; nature of the transcription factor is not yet clear
Insulin response element	Hexokinase II ($+$ve) Acetyl-CoA carboxylase ($+$ve) Glucose-6-phosphatase ($-$ve) Carnitine palmitoyltransferase ($-$ve)	May be positive (stimulates transcription) or negative (suppresses transcription)
PPAR-response element (α and γ isoforms)	α: Enzymes of peroxisomal fatty acid oxidation in liver γ: Factors leading to adipocyte proliferation	Ligand for PPAR is probably a fatty acid derivative, perhaps an eicosanoid
Sterol regulatory element	LDL receptor HMG-CoA reductase (cholesterol synthesis)	The transcription factor is SREBP; it is activated by a low cellular cholesterol concentration

PPAR: peroxisome proliferator-activated receptor; acetyl-CoA: acetyl-coenzyme A; LDL: low-density lipoprotein; HMG-CoA: 3-hydroxy-3-methylglutaryl-coenzyme A; SREBP: sterol regulatory element binding protein.

(e.g. an increase in the blood glucose concentration stimulates insulin secretion from the pancreas) or through the nervous system [e.g. release of epinephrine (adrenaline) from the adrenal medulla is brought about by nerve stimulation]. The hormone travels through the circulation to transmit a signal to another tissue, by binding to a specific receptor (a protein), which may be on the cell surface (this is the case for epinephrine, and for peptide hormones such as insulin and glucagon) or within the cell (steroid hormones, thyroid hormones). Binding of hormone to receptor brings about changes in signal transduction pathways, often involving reversible phosphorylation of proteins, and ultimately changes in enzyme activity. Short-term changes in enzyme activity are themselves often the result of reversible phosphorylation or dephosphorylation (e.g. epinephrine stimulates fatty acid release from adipocytes by phosphorylation of the enzyme hormone-sensitive lipase, causing its activity to increase many-fold).

Longer term regulation of macronutrient flux

In the longer term, regulation is achieved in many cases by alteration of gene expression, usually increased or decreased transcription, but sometimes via alterations in the stability of messenger RNA (mRNA). This would

be the case, for instance, if someone switches from a high-fat to a high-carbohydrate diet. Adaptation, through alterations of gene expression, will occur over a period of days. This form of regulation will also operate during a normal day – for instance, the expression of the lipoprotein lipase gene alters during the day in response to fasting overnight and feeding during the day – but usually the acute effects of hormones are more dominant over this period.

Alterations in gene expression can be brought about by both substrates and hormones. This a field where knowledge has expanded rapidly in recent years. It is now recognized that the genes for many enzymes concerned with energy metabolism have specific promoter sequences that recognize the availability of carbohydrate, fatty acids and related hormones (e.g. insulin-response elements). Some of these response elements are listed in Table 5.3.

5.3 Hormones that regulate macronutrient metabolism

Pancreatic hormones

The pancreas is mainly an exocrine organ, producing digestive juices that are discharged into the small intestine. Only 1–2% of the volume of the pancreas is occupied by endocrine (hormone-producing) cells,

Table 5.4 Macronutrients in the circulation and their effects on insulin and glucagon secretion

	Insulin	Glucagon	Comments
Glucose	Stimulates	Inhibits	
Amino acids	Stimulates	Stimulates	Some amino acids are more potent than others
Non-esterified fatty acids	Short-term: potentiates glucose stimulation Long-term: inhibits glucose stimulation	No effect	

arranged in groups (the islets of Langerhans) surrounded by exocrine tissue. Nevertheless, the products of these endocrine cells are of enormous importance for the regulation of macronutrient metabolism according to nutritional state. Each islet is supplied with blood through a small arterial vessel, and drained by veins that lead to the hepatic portal vein. Therefore, the islet cells can respond to changing concentrations of substrates in the blood (e.g. blood glucose), and the hormones they release act first upon the liver. The liver extracts a large proportion (40–50%) of insulin and glucagon, so other tissues are exposed to lower concentrations.

Insulin

Insulin is produced by the β-cells of the pancreatic islets. The insulin molecule is synthesized as one polypeptide chain, but during processing in the β-cell it is cleaved to produce two peptide chains linked by disulfide bonds. Although the β-cell responds to concentrations of various macronutrients in the blood (Table 5.4), the major factor regulating insulin secretion under most circumstances is the blood glucose concentration. Thus, insulin responds to nutritional state: in the fed state, since most meals contain carbohydrate, insulin secretion is stimulated, and during fasting, when glucose concentrations fall, insulin secretion is low.

Insulin exerts its effects on other tissues by binding to specific receptors in the plasma membrane. These receptors are composed of four protein subunits, two α- and two β-subunits. (The α- and β-subunits are synthesized initially as one polypeptide chain.) When insulin binds to the cytoplasmic face of the insulin receptor, the intracellular domains become activated and initiate phosphorylation of tyrosine residues, both in themselves and in other proteins. Among these other proteins are a family known as insulin receptor substrate (IRS) proteins, particularly IRS-1 and IRS-2. This initiates a chain of events, which for metabolic signals includes activation of the enzyme phosphatidylinositide-3-kinase. The signal passes via other steps to the enzyme to be regulated. Enzymes are regulated in the short term by insulin, usually by dephosphorylation. Insulin also brings about longer term regulation by alteration of gene transcription. Some of the important effects of insulin on macronutrient metabolism are summarized in Table 5.5.

Overall, the metabolic effects of insulin may be summarized as anabolic. It brings about a net deposition of glycogen in liver and muscle, a net storage of fat in adipose tissue, and a net synthesis of protein, especially in skeletal muscle. Note that these effects are brought about at least as much by inhibition of breakdown as by stimulation of synthesis: in the case of muscle protein, this is probably the major mechanism for the anabolic effect of insulin. Patients with untreated type I diabetes mellitus, who lack insulin, display marked wasting, which is reversed when insulin is given.

Glucagon

Glucagon is a single polypeptide chain of 29 amino acids, secreted from the α-cells of the islets. Its main metabolic effects are on the liver: in fact, it is debatable whether glucagon has metabolic effects outside the liver. Its major role is to maintain glucose output during fasting, and its secretion is stimulated when the plasma glucose concentration falls. In many respects hepatic glucose output is regulated by the ratio of insulin to glucagon (insulin/glucagon high, glucose output suppressed; insulin/glucagon low, glucose output increased). Glucagon secretion is also stimulated by amino acids (Table 5.4). It has been suggested that this is important if a meal of pure protein is eaten (as might have been the case after a hunt, for our hunter–gatherer

Table 5.5 Major metabolic effects of insulin

Tissue	Pathway/enzyme	Short or long term?	Key enzyme	Comments
Liver	Stimulation of glycogen synthesis/suppression of glycogen breakdown	Short	Glycogen synthase/ glycogen phosphorylase	Regulates glucose storage in liver
	Stimulation of glycolysis/ suppression of gluconeogenesis	Short and long	Short term mainly via fructose 2,6-bisphosphate Long term via altered expression of a number of enymes	Regulates hepatic glucose output
	Stimulation of *de novo* lipogenesis	Short and long	Acetyl-CoA carboxylase	*De novo* lipogenesis does not (under most circumstances tested) make a major contribution to triacylglycerol synthesis in liver, but this pathway is important for regulation of fatty acid oxidation
	Stimulation of triacylglycerol synthesis	Short and long	Phosphatidic acid phosphohydrolase, diacylglycerol acyltransferase (and others)	
	Stimulation of cholesterol synthesis	Short and long	3-Hydroxy-3-methyl-glutaryl-CoA reductase	
	Suppression of fatty acid oxidation/ketogenesis	Short	Carnitine palmitoyl transferase-1	Via malonyl-CoA (product of acetyl-CoA carboxylase)
Skeletal muscle	Stimulation of glucose uptake	Short	Glucose transporter GLUT4	Regulates glucose uptake by muscle
	Stimulation of glycogen synthesis	Short	Glycogen synthase	
	Net protein anabolic effect	Short	Not clear	Insulin may suppress protein breakdown more than stimulation of protein synthesis
Adipose tissue	Activation of triacylglycerol removal from plasma	Short and medium	Lipoprotein lipase	'Medium term' is during periods between meals, by increased transcription + altered intracellular processing
	Stimulation of triacylglycerol synthesis	Short and long	Phosphatidic acid phosphohydrolase, diacylglycerol acyltransferase (and others)	
	Suppression of fat mobilization	Short	Hormone-sensitive lipase	Suppresses release of non-esterified fatty acids

ancestors), as glucagon would then prevent hypoglycemia caused by amino acids stimulating insulin secretion.

Catecholamines

The catecholamines that are relevant to macronutrient metabolism are epinephrine (adrenaline) and norepinephrine (noradrenaline). Epinephrine is a hormone released from the central part (medulla) of the adrenal glands, which sit over the kidneys. Its release is initiated by nervous signals that come from the hypothalamus, the integrating center of the brain. Stimuli for epinephrine release include stress and anxiety, exercise, a fall in the blood glucose concentration and a loss of blood. Epinephrine acts on tissues through adrenergic receptors (sometimes called adrenoceptors) in cell mem-

Table 5.6 Adrenergic receptors

	Receptor subtype		
	β	α₁	α₂
Second messenger system	Adenylate cyclase/cAMP	Phospholipase C/intracellular [Ca²⁺]	Inhibition of adenylate cyclase
Metabolic effects	Glycogen breakdown	Glycogen breakdown	Inhibition of lipolysis
	Fat mobilization		

There are at least three subtypes of β-adrenergic receptor, not distinguished here.
Based on Frayn (2003).

branes. These receptors are again proteins. The family of adrenergic receptors is summarized in Table 5.6. They are linked with metabolic processes through a signal chain. For certain types of adrenergic receptor, the first step is the interaction of the receptor with a trimeric protein that can bind guanosine triphosphate, called a G-protein. There are inhibitory and stimulatory G-proteins, named for their effects on the next step in the sequence, the enzyme adenylate cyclase. Adenylate cyclase produces cyclic 3′,5′-adenosine monophosphate (cAMP), which then acts on the cAMP-dependent protein kinase (protein kinase A) to bring about phosphorylation of key proteins, including glycogen phosphorylase and hormone-sensitive lipase. (In the case of glycogen phosphorylase, there is another step: protein kinase A phosphorylates phosphorylase kinase, which then acts on glycogen phosphorylase.) Therefore, epinephrine acting on β-receptors will cause mobilization of stored fuels, glycogen and triacylglycerol, raising plasma concentrations of glucose and non-esterified fatty acids. This was termed by the American phys-iologist Walter Cannon in 1915 the 'fight or flight' response, implying that epinephrine, released in response to stress or anxiety, produces fuels that may be used to run away or stand up to an aggressor.

The inhibitory effects of epinephrine, mediated by α₂-adrenergic receptors, may be seen as moderating the effects of overstimulation via β-receptors. For instance, adipocytes have both β- and α₂-adrenergic receptors, the latter presumably opposing excessive lipolysis that might be brought about by high concentrations of (nor)epinephrine.

Norepinephrine is not strictly a hormone, at least under normal circumstances. It is a neurotransmitter. It is released at the ends of sympathetic nerves (nerve terminals) in tissues. It acts on adrenergic receptors, which are identical to those acted upon by epinephrine, and listed in Table 5.6. The stimuli for norepinephrine release are similar to those for epinephrine, and in many cases it is not clear which exerts the more important effect. Most of the norepinephrine released from sympathetic nerve terminals is taken up again by the nerve ending for degradation or resecretion, but some always escapes or spills over, and may reach the plasma. Plasma concentrations of norepinephrine are usually higher than those of epinephrine, and when norepinephrine is present at elevated concentrations (e.g. during strenuous exercise) it is believed to act as a hormone as well.

Cortisol

Cortisol is a steroid hormone, released from the outer layer (cortex) of the adrenal glands. It responds to stress in a similar way to epinephrine. Its secretion is stimulated by another hormone, adrenocorticotrophic hormone (ACTH), which in turn is released from the pituitary gland at the base of the brain. About 95% of circulating cortisol is bound to plasma proteins, especially cortisol binding globulin (CBG or transcortin). Thus, only a relatively small fraction (~5%) circulates free; however, it is this free fraction that is the physiologically active form. As will be discussed in further detail later, in relation to thyroid hormones, the highly significant protein binding of cortisol has important implications.

Cortisol acts on receptors, but these are not in the cell membrane: they are within the cell, and once cortisol is bound, they migrate and bind to the chromosomes where they regulate gene transcription. Therefore, the metabolic effects of cortisol are all long term, mediated by increased gene expression. Its metabolic effects are generally catabolic, including increased fat mobilization, stimulation of gluconeogenesis and increased breakdown of muscle protein.

Growth hormone and insulin-like growth factors

Growth hormone is a peptide hormone released from the pituitary gland, and has some direct metabolic effects on tissues. These include increased fat mobilization and stimulation of hepatic glucose output. Its secretion is stimulated by stress, including a fall in the plasma glucose concentration. However, the main effect of growth hormone, as its name suggests, is an anabolic one, promoting growth, especially through increased cartilage synthesis, an important aspect of longitudinal growth (lengthening of bones). It was shown in the 1960s that this is not a direct effect; rather, growth hormone acts on the liver to stimulate production of further peptide hormones, the insulin-like growth factors (IGF-1 and IGF-2) that directly mediate these effects. IGF-1 and -2 have structural similarities to insulin, as their name suggests, and they act via similar (but specific) receptors. However, it has been proposed that when insulin is present at abnormally high concentrations, it can bind to and activate IGF receptors, and vice versa.

Thyroid hormones

The thyroid hormones, thyroxine (also known as T_4 since it contains four atoms of iodine per molecule) and triiodothyronine (T_3), are produced by the thyroid gland in the neck, responding in turn to the peptide hormone thyroid-stimulating hormone (TSH) released from the pituitary. Most (about 80%) of the circulating T_3 concentration is derived from deiodination of T_4 in peripheral tissues, especially the liver and the kidney. T_3 is a significantly more potent thyroid hormone than T_4; many would indeed consider T_4 as only a prohormone for T_3. Deiodination may also produce another thyroid hormone, called reverse tri-iodothyronine (rT_3); this hormone is essentially metabolically inactive. Its levels increase particularly during stressful situations as with major surgery, starvation and severe sepsis. Increased production of rT_3 in these situations may be considered part of the adaptive energy-conserving response to stress.

More than 99% of the circulating thyroid hormones, T_3 and T_4, is bound to plasma proteins, especially thyroxine binding globulin (TBG), thyroxine binding prealbumin (TBPA) and albumin. Only a tiny fraction (<1%) circulates free; however, it is this free fraction, designated as free T_4 or free T_3, that is the physiologically active form that promotes thyroid hormone activity at the peripheral tissues. The highly significant protein binding of the thyroid hormones (as with cortisol) has two important implications: (1) variations in plasma protein concentrations will affect the plasma levels of these hormones; for example, the hypoproteinaemia of severe protein malnutrition is associated with low total thyroid hormone levels; free hormones are, however, retained at normal levels by the action of pituitary TSH; and (2) certain important drugs such as salicylates and phenytoin can displace thyroid hormones from binding sites on plasma proteins; this may also reduce the total but not free hormone levels.

The action of free thyroid hormones on other tissues is mediated via nuclear receptors, as described for cortisol, and therefore again thyroid hormones have long-term rather than short-term effects. Their effects are again mainly catabolic, and include net breakdown of muscle protein. However, their most important metabolic effect is a stimulation of energy expenditure. People with elevated thyroid hormone concentrations have elevated metabolic rate and may become thin, whereas people deficient in thyroid hormone concentrations have a low metabolic rate and easily gain weight. It should be added here that alterations in thyroid function are not considered to be responsible for the vast majority of cases of human obesity, and treatment with thyroid hormones is not useful in weight reduction (unless there is a deficiency) as the system is highly regulated, and administration of thyroid hormones simply leads the thyroid gland to produce less.

The metabolic explanation for the increased energy expenditure brought about by thyroid hormones is not entirely clear, but is usually considered to represent some effect on the efficiency of coupling respiration with ATP synthesis in mitochondria.

Leptin

The peptide hormone leptin was only discovered at the end of 1994, although its existence had been postulated much earlier. It is produced almost exclusively by adipocytes in white adipose tissue. Traces are produced in other tissues, including placenta and stomach, but their function is not clear and they do not appear to contribute significantly to plasma concentrations. It is secreted in amounts that correspond to the degree of fat storage in the adipocyte: bigger fat cells secrete more leptin. It acts on receptors that are present in a number of tissues, although probably the most important are in the brain, particularly the hypothalamus. A short isoform of the leptin receptor is expressed in the choroid

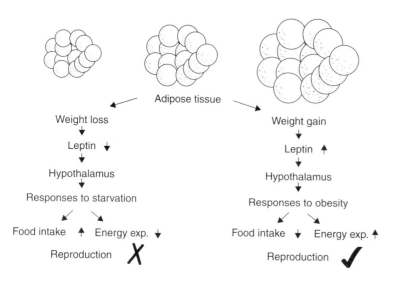

Figure 5.3 Leptin system and energy balance. Well-filled adipocytes secrete leptin, which signals to the hypothalamus to decrease food intake and increase energy expenditure (the latter only in rodents, not humans). They also signal to the reproductive system that energy reserves are sufficient. (Reproduced with permission from Friedman 1997.)

plexus, the region that governs the blood–brain barrier, and is believed to transport leptin into the brain.

In the brain, leptin signals a decrease in appetite and, in small animals, an increase in energy expenditure. The latter does not seem to be true in humans. This constitutes an important system for regulation of energy stores. When fat stores are low, leptin levels are low, and this alters signals in the hypothalamus with the net result of an increase in appetite. When fat stores are high, leptin levels are increased and the hypothalamic signals tend to lead to a net reduction in food intake. The system is summarized in Figure 5.3.

The power of this system is seen when it is disturbed. It was discovered through genetic work on the *ob/ob* mouse, a mutant mouse with spontaneous high food intake, low energy expenditure and massive obesity that leads to diabetes. This mouse is homozygous for a mutation in the *ob* gene, now known to code for the protein leptin. Treatment of *ob/ob* mice with synthetic leptin leads to a reduction in body weight through decreased food intake and increased energy expenditure. The *db/db* (diabetic) mouse is another mutant with identical phenotype: it has a mutation in the leptin receptor and cannot be treated with synthetic leptin. A few people have been found with mutations in either the leptin gene or the leptin receptor. They all display massive obesity, associated with an intense drive to eat. Two children with mutations in the leptin gene have now been treated with synthetic leptin and are showing reductions in weight for the first time in their lives. However, the vast majority of obese humans have a normal leptin gene, and leptin secretion that appears to be operating normally, in that they have high levels of leptin in the blood. It has been postulated that these people suffer from 'leptin resistance', implying that there is some problem with access of leptin to the brain, or with its function within the brain. In one sense this must be true, but a precise molecular explanation has not yet been found.

The leptin system also appears to have an important role in reproduction. The *ob/ob* mouse is sterile, and people with mutations in leptin or its receptor have delayed sexual maturity. Leptin seems to be a signal from adipose tissue to the reproductive organs, relaying that there are sufficient energy reserves to begin the energy-demanding processes of reproduction and nurturing children (Figure 5.3).

5.4 Macronutrient metabolism in the major organs and tissues

As mentioned in the Introduction, different tissues have their own characteristic requirements, or preferences, for metabolic fuels, and their demand for fuel may vary from time to time. Some of the major consumers of metabolic energy will be discussed in this section. Many of these tissues or organs also play roles in energy metabolism other than simply consuming fuel. Often they need energy derived from oxidative metabolism to support these activities.

Brain

The brain is a large organ (1.5 kg in an adult) and has a high requirement for oxidative metabolism to support its continuous electrical activity. This is usually met almost entirely by glucose. Fatty acids cannot cross the blood–brain barrier in significant amounts for use as an energy substrate, although the brain also has a large need for fatty acids for structural purposes, especially during development. Brain glucose consumption has been estimated by drawing blood from the carotid artery (supplying the brain) and the jugular vein (draining the brain). It is around 100–120 g/day. In the overnight fasted state the liver produces about 2 mg glucose/kg body weight per minute which, for a 70 kg person, is equivalent to about 200 g/24 h. Thus, the brain would consume about half of the liver's glucose output after an overnight fast.

The brain can use other water-soluble fuels, notably the ketone bodies, 3-hydroxybutyrate and acetoacetate. When their concentration rises during starvation, they displace glucose as a fuel, and can sustain about two-thirds of the brain's oxidative fuel requirement during prolonged starvation.

Liver

The adult human liver weighs about 1.5 kg and is a highly active organ in the regulation of carbohydrate, fat and amino acid metabolism. To support its metabolic activities, it has a large requirement for oxidative fuel metabolism (its oxygen consumption is about 20% of the whole body's at rest, the largest of any single organ or tissue, excluding skeletal muscle during exercise). The fuels used by the liver are amino acids, fatty acids and glucose, usually in that order of importance.

However, the liver's importance in energy metabolism is more as a regulatory organ, controlling the uptake and release of compounds to maintain homeostasis. The best example is that of blood glucose. When the glucose concentration in the blood is high, the liver takes up glucose and phosphorylates it to glucose-6-phosphate. The fate of that glucose-6-phosphate is determined by hormones, particularly the balance of insulin and glucagon, which stimulate glycogen synthesis and degradation, respectively. When the glucose concentration is low, the liver will release glucose, formed from glycogen breakdown and from gluconeogenesis. The liver is the major organ releasing glucose into the blood, although the kidney plays an increasing role during starvation. Thus, the liver plays a major role in keeping blood glucose concentrations relatively constant throughout the day. Major control points for glucose metabolism in the liver are illustrated in Figure 5.4.

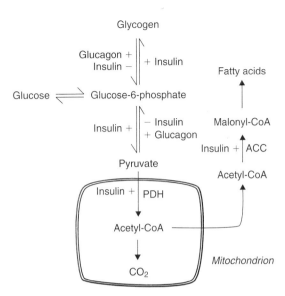

Figure 5.4 Regulation of glucose metabolism by the liver. When blood glucose concentrations are elevated, the liver extracts glucose from the circulation and phosphorylates it to glucose-6-phosphate. The metabolic fate of glucose-6-phosphate is determined by the balance of insulin and glucagon. Conversely, when blood glucose levels fall, the liver releases glucose from stored glycogen or from gluconeogenesis. PDH: Pyruvate dehydrogenase; ACC: acetyl-coenzyme A carboxylase.

The liver is a major site for fatty acid oxidation. It derives fatty acids from plasma non-esterified fatty acids (released from adipose tissue) and from the uptake of lipoprotein particles that carry triacylglycerol and cholesteryl esters. Fatty acid oxidation leads directly to production of acetyl-coenzyme A (acetyl-CoA), but in the liver this may be converted to ketone bodies, 3-hydroxybutyrate and acetoacetate. The liver is the only organ producing ketone bodies which, as mentioned above, are an important fuel for the brain during starvation. The alternative fate for fatty acids in the liver is esterification, especially to form triacylglycerols. The balance between fatty acid oxidation and esterification is regulated by the mechanism shown in Figure 5.5. This mechanism, involving malonyl-CoA, is central to the integration of carbohydrate and fat metabolism in liver and skeletal muscle.

The liver is the only site of urea production. Amino acids derived from dietary protein, and from protein breakdown in peripheral tissues, are oxidized and their nitrogen is transferred to the urea cycle. As well as providing a route for disposal of excess amino acids and their nitrogen content, this provides the major source of oxidative fuel for the liver under most circumstances. The rate

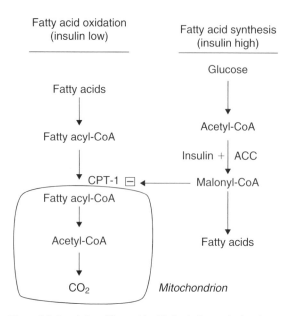

Figure 5.5 Regulation of fatty acid oxidation in liver and other tissues by malonyl-Coenzyme A (CoA). Insulin stimulates synthesis of malonyl-CoA (see Figure 5.4) and this inhibits fatty acid entry into the mitochondrion for oxidation. In tissues other than liver (e.g. skeletal muscle) this system operates to regulate fatty acid oxidation, although the later part of the pathway of fatty acid synthesis (beyond malonyl-CoA) is absent. ACC: acetyl-CoA carboxylase; CPT-1: carnitine-palmitoyl transferase-1 (sometimes called carnitine-acyl transferase-1).

of amino acid oxidation is largely determined by amino acid availability, as mentioned earlier.

Kidneys

Each kidney, weighing about 150 g in an adult, is composed of many cell types. However, a broad distinction can be made between the outer layer, or cortex, and the inner part or medulla. Most of the metabolic activity involved in pumping substances back from the tubules after filtration goes on in the cortex. The cortex, therefore, has a larger requirement for oxidative fuel, and appears able to oxidize most fuels (fatty acids, ketone bodies, glucose). It has a correspondingly high blood flow and oxygen consumption; the oxygen consumption of the two kidneys is about 10% of the whole body's at rest. The major role of the renal cortex in energy metabolism in the body is as a relatively large consumer. The medulla, in contrast, has a rather poor blood supply and an anaerobic pattern of metabolism.

The kidneys also play a specific role in amino acid metabolism. Glutamine is used by the kidney, especially during starvation, and ammonia is liberated during its metabolism and excreted into the renal tubules. Ammonia will sequester hydrogen ions (to form NH_4^+ ions), so achieving a loss of hydrogen ions from the body into the urine. This can be an important means of reducing an acid load in the circulation which, as shown later, is a potential problem during starvation.

Adipose tissue

There are two types of adipose tissue, white and brown. The metabolic function of brown adipose tissue is to generate heat, largely by oxidation of fatty acids. It is important in small animals, especially the newborn, and in animals that hibernate, but it does not play a significant role in adult humans. This section will therefore concentrate on white adipose tissue, the major site for storage of excess dietary energy in the form of triacylglycerol. The amount of triacylglycerol stored within each adipocyte is large in comparison to daily turnover, so the half-life for turning over adipocyte triacylglycerol stores is around 1 year. This, coupled with the fact that the requirement of white adipose tissue for oxidative fuel consumption is very low, led to the view that white adipose tissue is rather inert metabolically. It has been recognized in recent years, however, that white adipose tissue has a highly active pattern of metabolism. It is the only site of release of non-esterified fatty acids, a major metabolic fuel for many tissues, into the circulation, and it controls the flow of non-esterified fatty acids on a minute-by-minute basis. To match this, it is also responsible for a large proportion of the uptake of dietary fatty acids via the enzyme lipoprotein lipase (LPL), situated in adipose tissue capillaries, and the pathway of triacylglycerol synthesis within adipocytes. All this is achieved with a very small consumption of fuel, which in white adipose tissue appears to be mainly glucose. Regulation of the major pathways of fat mobilization and storage is shown in Figure 5.6.

Skeletal muscle

Skeletal muscle constitutes typically 40% of body weight. Resting muscle has a rather low blood flow and metabolic activity, but because of its bulk, it makes a significant contribution to whole-body fluxes of the macronutrients. During exercise, however, the metabolic activity of skeletal muscle can increase 1000-fold, and it may dominate the body's metabolic activities.

Skeletal muscle is composed of fibers, or multinucleate cells. There are different types of fiber, adapted for either short-duration, rapid contractions, using

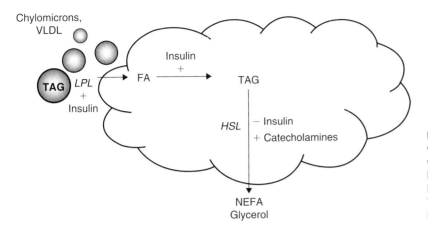

Figure 5.6 Regulation of the major pathways of fat mobilization and storage in white adipose tissue. FA: fatty acids; HSL: hormone-sensitive lipase; LPL: lipoprotein lipase; NEFA: non-esterified fatty acids; TAG: triacylglycerol; VLDL: very low-density lipoprotein particles.

Table 5.7 Metabolic characteristics of different muscle fiber types

	Type I Red	Type IIa White	Type IIb White
Other names	Slow-twitch oxidative (SO)	Fast-twitch oxidative/glycolytic (FOG)	Fast-twitch glycolytic (FG)
Speed of contraction	Slow	Fast	Fast
Myoglobin content	High	Low	Low
Capillary density	High	Low	Low
Mitochondrial (oxidative) enzyme activity	High	Low	Low
Triacylglycerol content	High	Low	Low
Myofibrillar ATPase activity	Low	High	High
Glycogenolytic enzyme activity	Low	High	High

fuels present within the fiber, or slower, rhythmic contractions that can be continued for long periods, largely using fuels and oxygen supplied from the blood. The differences between these fiber types are summarized in Table 5.7.

The oxidative fuels used by skeletal muscle are mainly fatty acids and glucose. Amino acid oxidation typically accounts for around 15% of muscle fuel oxidation, similar to the whole body, and this figure does not increase appreciably with exercise. Skeletal muscle plays important roles in whole-body macronutrient metabolism, both as a consumer (glucose, fatty acids, amino acids) and as a supplier (lactate, particular amino acids, especially glutamine and alanine).

The main factors regulating muscle fuel utilization are nutritional state (feeding and fasting) and exercise. In the fed state, insulin stimulates glucose uptake and utilization, by recruitment of the insulin-regulated glucose transporter GLUT4 to the cell membrane and by activation of glycolysis and glycogen synthesis. When fatty acids are available at high concentrations (e.g. during fasting, when insulin concentrations will also be low), they will be used as the preferred fuel. The reciprocal utilization of glucose and fatty acids by muscle is therefore determined partly be extracellular factors (substrate availability, insulin), but also by mechanisms within the cell. Oxidation of fatty acids, when available, will suppress glucose oxidation, but a high rate of glucose utilization (and high insulin) will suppress fatty acid oxidation via the malonyl-CoA/CPT-1 system, which also operates in muscle (see Liver, above).

The store of glycogen in muscle is large, typically 300–500 g in the whole body, compared with 100 g or so in the liver. However, because muscle lacks the enzyme glucose-6-phosphatase, this cannot be delivered as glucose into the blood. It cannot therefore be used as a fuel by the brain, for instance, except by conversion to lactate and export to the liver where lactate can be converted to glucose. It seems to be present primarily as a fuel for local utilization, especially in the fast-twitch (type II) fibers.

There are different patterns of macronutrient utilization in skeletal muscle during brief, intense exercise (anaerobic exercise, involving mainly the type II fibers) and during sustained exercise (aerobic exercise, involving mainly the type I fibers). In either case the primary requirement of metabolism is to generate ATP, which fuels the sliding of myosin along actin filaments, which underlies muscle contraction.

Aerobic metabolism (e.g. oxidation of glucose or fatty acids) is efficient: about 30 ATP molecules are produced per molecule of glucose completely oxidized. In contrast, anaerobic metabolism is inefficient (3 molecules of ATP per molecule of glucose from glycogen). One might imagine that skeletal muscle would only use the former, but aerobic metabolism requires the diffusion of substrates and oxygen from the blood into the muscle fibers, and the diffusion of carbon dioxide back to the blood. The rates of these diffusion processes are low in comparison with the need to generate ATP during intense exercise. Therefore, during brief, intense (anaerobic) exercise (e.g. weight-lifting, high-jumping, sprinting 100 m), ATP is generated by anaerobic metabolism of glucose-6-phosphate derived from intracellular glycogen. The stimulus for glycogen breakdown is not initially hormonal (that would also require time for movement through the blood): instead, the processes of muscle contraction and glycogen breakdown are coordinated. The mechanism is release of Ca^{2+} from the sarcoplasmic reticulum, which initiates muscle contraction and also activates glycogen breakdown. At the same time, allosteric mechanisms activate glycolysis, and the net flux through this pathway may increase 1000-fold within a few seconds.

Despite the rapid utilization of ATP during intense exercise, the concentration of ATP in muscle only falls slightly. This is because of the existence of a reservoir of energy in the form of creatine phosphate (also called phosphocreatine). There is about four times as much creatine phosphate as ATP in skeletal muscle. As ATP is hydrolyzed, so it is re-formed from creatine phosphate (with the formation of creatine). The activity of the enzyme concerned, creatine kinase, is high and it operates close to equilibrium. At rest, creatine phosphate is re-formed from creatine and ATP. Gradual non-enzymic breakdown of creatine forms creatinine, which is excreted in the urine at a remarkably constant rate, proportional to muscle mass.

During sustained exercise, blood-borne fuels and oxygen are used to regenerate ATP through aerobic metabolism. This requires coordinated adjustments in other tissues (e.g. adipose tissue must increase fatty acid release; the heart must deliver more blood) and this is brought about by the hormonal and nervous systems. Fatty acids predominate as the oxidative fuel in low- or moderate-intensity sustained exercise, but carbohydrate is the predominant fuel for high-intensity exercise (e.g. elite long-distance running). Although most of the fuel is blood-borne, still the intramuscular glycogen store seems essential for maximal energy output, and when this is depleted, the athlete feels a sensation of sudden intense fatigue or 'hitting the wall'. Dietary preparation to maximize muscle glycogen stores before an event is now common practice.

Gut

The primary role of the intestinal tract in macronutrient metabolism is to ensure the uptake of dietary nutrients into the body. However, the intestinal tract has its own requirements for energy. There is a high rate of cell turnover, especially in the small intestine, and this requires a supply of amino acids to act as substrates for protein synthesis and for purine and pyrimidine synthesis (to make DNA and RNA). In addition, there are active transport mechanisms (e.g. for glucose absorption) that require energy. A major metabolic fuel for the small intestine appears to be the amino acid glutamine. This can be partially oxidized to produce ATP, and at the same time acts as a precursor for purine and pyrimidine synthesis. In fact, glutamine appears to be a major fuel for most tissues that have the capacity for rapid rates of cell division (e.g. lymphocytes and other cells of the immune system).

In the colon the situation is somewhat different. Bacterial fermentation of non-starch polysaccharides and resistant starch in the colon produces the short-chain fatty acids, acetic, propionic and butyric acids. Acetic and propionic acids are absorbed and used by tissues in the body (propionic mainly in the liver), but a large proportion of the butyric acid is used as an oxidative fuel by the colonocytes. The supply of butyric acid to the colonocytes appears to protect them against neoplastic change.

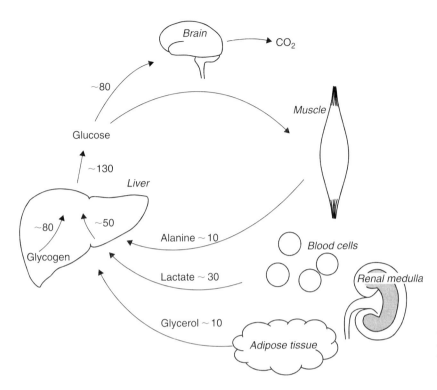

Figure 5.7 Carbohydrate metabolism after an overnight fast. Numbers are approximate values in mg/min for a typical person. (Redrawn from Frayn 2003.)

5.5 Substrate fluxes in the overnight fasting state

The nutritional state of the human body typically cycles through feeding and fasting over each 24 h period. The macronutrients of the three or more meals eaten during the day enter the system over a period of several hours, and are either oxidized or sent into stores. By about 8 h after a meal (variable, depending on the size and the nature of the meal) the macronutrients have been fully absorbed from the gastrointestinal tract and the body enters the postabsorptive state. This lasts until a further meal is eaten; or, if no further food is forthcoming, the body gradually enters a state of early starvation. Many studies of nutritional physiology are conducted after an overnight fast (typically around 10 h after last eating), when there is a relatively steady metabolic state.

The regulation of macronutrient flux through the circulation during these different periods of the 24 h cycle is brought about by a number of mechanisms, as outlined in Section 5.2. After an overnight fast, the concentration of insulin will be relatively low, and the glucagon/insulin ratio reaching the liver will be high.

Carbohydrate metabolism after an overnight fast

After an overnight fast, no new dietary glucose is entering the circulation, and yet the glucose in the blood is turning over, at a rate of about 2 mg/min per kg body weight (equivalent to around 200 g/24 h, see Section 5.4). The concentration will be steady at about 5 mmol/l. New glucose is coming almost entirely from the liver, partly from glycogen breakdown (stimulated by the high glucagon/insulin ratio reaching the liver) and partly from gluconeogenesis. Substrates for the latter will include lactate and pyruvate coming from blood cells and from peripheral tissues (muscle, adipose tissue), the amino acid alanine released from muscle and adipose tissue, and glycerol, released from adipose tissue as a product of lipolysis. A major consumer of glucose at this time will be the brain, with skeletal muscle, renal medulla and blood cells also using significant amounts. (Skeletal muscle glucose utilization after an overnight fast, at rest, is low per gram of muscle, but because of its large mass this becomes significant.) The pattern of glucose metabolism is illustrated in Figure 5.7.

Note that, of the tissues using glucose, only those carrying out complete oxidation lead to irreversible loss

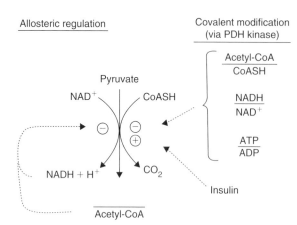

Figure 5.8 Summary of regulation of pyruvate dehydrogenase (PDH). PDH is a multienzyme complex associated with the inner mitochondrial membrane. The dehydrogenase subunit is subject to both allosteric and covalent regulation in accordance with nutritional state. Covalent modification is brought about by reversible phosphorylation, catalyzed by the enzyme PDH kinase. PDH is inactivated by phosphorylation by PDH kinase, which occurs when cellular energy status is high (e.g. during rapid oxidation of fatty acids). PDH is activated by dephosphorylation, brought about by a specific PDH phosphatase, stimulated by insulin.

of glucose from the body. In other tissues a proportion (muscle, kidney) or all (red blood cells) of the glucose is released again as three-carbon compounds (mainly lactate) and can be taken up by the liver for gluconeogenesis. This gives the enzyme pyruvate dehydrogenase (PDH) a key role in regulating loss of glucose from the body. Not surprisingly, perhaps, PDH is controlled by many factors reflecting the nutritional state of the body, including insulin, which activates it (Figure 5.8).

There is a potential metabolic cycle between peripheral tissues and the liver: muscle, for instance, releases lactate, the liver converts it to glucose, muscle can take this up and produce lactate. This is known as the Cori cycle, after its discoverer. It will be discussed again and illustrated below.

Fat metabolism after an overnight fast

Fatty acids in the circulation are present in a number of forms: non-esterified fatty acids (NEFA), triacylglycerols (TG), phospholipids and cholesteryl esters. In all cases these molecules are hydrophobic or at most somewhat amphipathic (having both hydrophobic and hydrophilic qualities). Therefore, they cannot circulate in solution in the blood plasma.

NEFAs are carried bound to albumin. Each molecule of albumin has around three high-affinity binding sites

for fatty acids. It may be imagined that albumin, in a partially delipidated state, arrives in the capillaries of adipose tissue, and picks up NEFA released from adipocytes. It arrives in the capillaries of another tissue (e.g. skeletal muscle or liver) and, because of a concentration gradient between plasma and tissue, fatty acids tend to leave it and diffuse into the tissue. A typical plasma albumin concentration is 40 g/l; with a relative molecular mass of 66 kDa, that is about 0.6 mmol/l. Therefore, there is an upper limit under many physiological conditions of about 2 mmol/l for NEFA. After an overnight fast their concentration is typically 0.5–1.0 mmol/l. They enter the circulation only from adipose tissue, where fat mobilization is stimulated after overnight fast mainly, it seems, by the fall in insulin concentration compared with the fed state. Catecholamines and other hormones, such as growth hormone and cortisol, may exert short- or longer term stimulatory effects.

NEFA are removed from the circulation by tissues that can use them as an energy source, such as liver and skeletal muscle. Fatty acid utilization in these tissues is stimulated after an overnight fast (compared with the fed state) by the increased NEFA concentration in plasma. Within the tissues, fatty acid oxidation is stimulated by the low insulin concentration and low glucose utilization, leading to a low intracellular malonyl-CoA concentration, so that fatty acids enter mitochondria for oxidation (see Figure 5.5).

The other forms of fatty acids in the circulation, TG, phospholipids and cholesteryl esters, are transported in specialized particles, the lipoproteins. Phospholipids are also carried as components of blood cell membranes. The lipoprotein particles are like droplets in an emulsion. They consist of a core of hydrophobic lipid (TG and cholesteryl esters) stabilized by an outer shell, which is a monolayer of phospholipid molecules with their polar head groups facing outwards into the aqueous plasma and their tails pointing into the hydrophobic core. There are various classes of lipoprotein particle. A detailed description is outside the scope of this chapter but important characteristics are given in Table 5.8. Phospholipids and cholesteryl esters will not be discussed further because they are not directly relevant to macronutrient metabolism, although cholesteryl esters are highly relevant to cardiovascular disease.

In the overnight fasted state most TG are carried in the very low-density lipoprotein (VLDL) particles secreted from the liver. A typical concentration would

Table 5.8 Major lipoprotein fractions in plasma

	Density range (g/ml)	Major lipids	Function, comments
Chylomicrons	<0.950	Dietary TAG	Transport dietary TAG from small intestine to peripheral tissues
Very low-density lipoproteins (VLDL)	0.950–1.006	Endogenous TAG	Transport hepatic TAG to peripheral tissues
Low-density lipoproteins (LDL)	1.019–1.063	Cholesterol/cholesteryl esters	Remnants remaining after removal of TAG from VLDL: main carriers of cholesterol in the circulation; elevated levels are a risk factor for atherosclerosis
High-density lipoproteins (HDL)	1.063–1.210	Cholesteryl esters/ phospholipids	Transport of excess cholesterol from peripheral tissues back to liver for excretion (protective against atherosclerosis)

TAG: triacylglycerol.

be 0.5–1.5 mmol/l in plasma, but this is very variable from person to person. Since each TG molecule contains three fatty acids, this is potentially a much greater source of energy than the plasma NEFA pool (TG-fatty acid concentration 1.5–4.5 mmol/l). However, the turnover is slower, and in practice plasma NEFA are the predominant substrate for fatty acid oxidation in tissues.

VLDL-TG derives within the liver from a number of sources: plasma NEFA taken up by the hepatocytes, plasma cholesteryl esters and TG taken up by the hepatocytes, and TG stored within the cells. Under many circumstances plasma NEFA are a major source, and the rate of VLDL-TG secretion is closely related to the concentration of plasma NEFA.

VLDL particles give up their TG-fatty acids to tissues through the action of the enzyme LPL. LPL is expressed in many extrahepatic tissues, especially muscle, adipose tissue and mammary gland, where it is increased enormously during lactation. Within these tissues it is bound to the luminal aspect of the capillary endothelium. Here it can interact with the VLDL particles as they pass through the capillaries, hydrolyzing their TG and releasing fatty acids that diffuse into the tissues, down a concentration gradient. There is no evidence for active transport of fatty acids into cells; instead, a powerful concentration gradient is generated by the binding of fatty acids to intracellular fatty acid binding proteins, and then their subsequent metabolism. After hydrolysis of some of its core TG, the VLDL particle may recirculate a number of times through capillary beds, losing TG until it has a core composed almost entirely of cholesteryl esters. Then it is called a low-density lipoprotein (LDL) particle.

The distribution of TG-fatty acids to tissues is regulated by the tissue-specific regulation of LPL expression in the capillaries. In turn, this is achieved through effects on gene transcription (mRNA abundance) and on intracellular, post-translational processing of the immature enzyme. In adipocytes in particular, a significant proportion of LPL molecules is degraded without reaching the capillary endothelium, and nutritional regulation of adipose tissue LPL expression largely involves switching between these pathways. A summary of tissue-specific regulation of LPL is given in Figure 5.9. It is relatively inactive in adipose tissue after an overnight fast, which makes good sense because in that state adipose tissue is a net exporter of NEFA and has no need to take up additional fatty acids.

Amino acid metabolism after an overnight fast

There is a complex pattern of flow of amino acids into and out of the circulation, but some general points can be made. In classic experiments in the early 1970s, Felig and colleagues at Yale University found that the release of amino acids from skeletal muscle after an overnight fast demonstrated a characteristic pattern (Figure 5.10). Glutamine and alanine predominated, much more than would have been predicted from the abundance in muscle protein. This implies that other amino acids are 'donating' their amino groups to form glutamine and alanine, which are exported from the muscle. Similarly, the uptake of amino acids across the abdominal tissues (liver and gut) showed almost the exact counterpart: the greatest removal was of glutamine and alanine. Hence, muscles and probably other tissue including adipose tissue, are using glutamine and alanine as 'export vehicles' for their amino acid nitrogen, sending it to the liver, where urea can be formed.

The pathway whereby alanine comes to play such a prominent role will be outlined here, since it is relatively well understood. Alanine is formed by transamination of pyruvate (Figure 5.11). Hence, other amino acids can donate their amino group to pyruvate, a substantial proportion of which is formed from the pathway of glycolysis. The remaining carbon skeleton can be

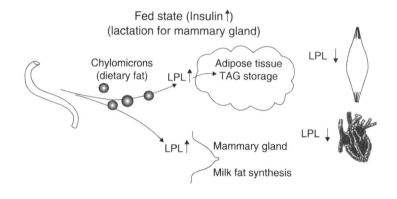

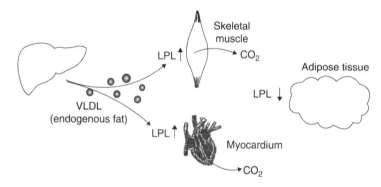

Figure 5.9 Tissue-specific regulation of lipoprotein lipase (LPL) according to the needs of the tissue for fatty acids. LPL: lipoprotein lipase; TAG: triacyl glycerol; VLDL: very low-density lipoprotein. (Reproduced from Gurr *et al.* 2002.)

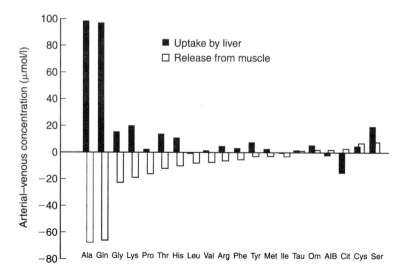

Figure 5.10 Pattern of amino acid metabolism in different tissues. The data are differences in concentration between arterial and venous blood, in normal human subjects after an overnight fast. Open bars represent arteriovenous differences across skeletal muscle; negative values imply venous concentrations greater than arterial, i.e. net release from muscle. Solid bars represent arteriovenous differences across the splanchnic bed (intestine and liver), and show net uptake of most amino acids, in amounts that correspond closely to their release from muscle. Note the predominance of alanine (Ala) and glutamine (Gln). (Redrawn from Felig 1975.)

oxidized in the muscle. The branched-chain amino acids (leucine, isoleucine, valine) play a predominant role in skeletal muscle amino acid metabolism. Their corresponding carbon skeletons, the branched-chain 2-oxo acids, are oxidized by an enzyme, the branched-chain 2-oxo acid dehydrogenase, that is similar in many ways to PDH (which is also a 2-oxo acid dehydrogenase). Thus, they contribute to oxidative fuel metabolism in muscle.

The production of alanine by transamination of pyruvate gives rise to a metabolic cycle that has been termed the glucose–alanine cycle. It operates in parallel with the Cori cycle, as illustrated in Figure 5.12.

5.6 Postprandial substrate disposal

This section examines how the relatively steady metabolic state after an overnight fast is disturbed when macronutrients are ingested and enter the circulation.

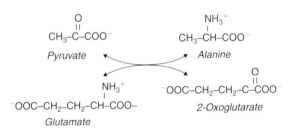

Figure 5.11 Transamination (aminotransferase) reaction involving pyruvate/alanine and 2-oxoglutarate/glutamate. All amino acids can participate in transamination reactions, which are usually the first step in their degradation.

This will demonstrate clearly some of the ways in which the metabolism of the different macronutrients is coordinated. It is unusual to eat a meal that contains only fat, and since both glucose and amino acids will stimulate the secretion of insulin, this is an important signal of the transition from postabsorptive to fed, or postprandial, state.

Impact on endogenous metabolism

Among the most rapid changes detectable in macronutrient metabolism following ingestion of a meal is the suppression of mobilization of endogenous fuels. The production of glucose by the liver is switched off, as is the release of NEFA from adipose tissue. Therefore, the body preserves its endogenous macronutrient stores, and switches to using incoming macronutrients and storing any excess.

Glucose

Glucose enters the circulation through the hepatic portal vein. Hence, it reaches the liver in high concentrations: concentrations of almost 10 mmol/l have been measured in the portal vein when the systemic concentration is still only 4–5 mmol/l. Glucose will enter hepatocytes and be phosphorylated, as described in Section 5.4. Nevertheless, despite a high capacity of the liver for soaking up glucose, some will still pass through into the systemic circulation, otherwise there would be no rise in glucose concentration and no stimulation of insulin secretion. Within the liver, the rise in insulin/glucagon ratio switches off gluconeogenesis and glycogenolysis, and stimulates glycogen synthesis.

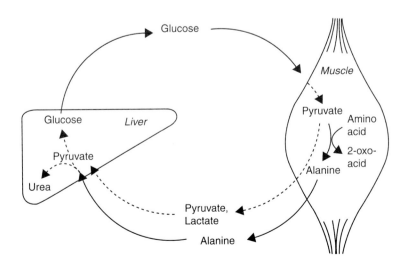

Figure 5.12 The glucose–alanine and Cori cycles operate in parallel. Note that peripheral tissues other than muscle may be involved (e.g. adipose tissue). (Reproduced from Frayn 2003.)

Until recently these were considered as 'on–off' switches: either gluconeogenesis or glycolysis operated; glycogen synthesis and glycogen breakdown operated at different times. Now it is recognized that the system is more fluid; there appears always to be some glycogen synthesis and breakdown, so there is cycling between glycogen and glucose-6-phosphate. The nutritional state determines which pathway predominates. Similarly, it is now recognized that gluconeogenesis must continue in the postprandial period. Studies with isotopic tracers show that a significant proportion of liver glycogen laid down in the period following a meal is not synthesized directly from blood glucose. Instead, the glucose is first converted to three-carbon compounds (lactate, pyruvate, alanine) and then, via pyruvate, converted by the gluconeogenic pathway to glycogen. The latter is known as the indirect pathway for glycogen synthesis and, depending on the experimental design, accounts for around 25–40% of liver glycogen synthesis.

Skeletal muscle will also take up glucose, insulin activating the glucose transporter GLUT4 (recruiting it to the plasma membrane) and, within the cell, insulin stimulating both glycogen synthesis and glucose oxidation. This is aided by the fall in plasma NEFA concentration (see below), so removing competition for oxidative disposal. There is no indirect glycogen synthesis in muscle since the gluconeogenic pathway does not operate. Other insulin-responsive tissues such as adipose tissue also increase their glucose uptake: although this does not make a major contribution to glucose disposal from the plasma, it has important effects within the adipocytes (Section 5.3). The brain, and the red blood cells, continue to use glucose at the same rate as before, since their glucose uptake is not regulated by insulin.

Lipids

NEFA release from adipose tissue is suppressed very effectively by insulin. Thus, the body's fat stores are 'spared' at a time when there are plenty of dietary nutrients available. This suppression is brought about by dephosphorylation of the enzyme hormone-sensitive lipase in adipocytes, which catalyzes the hydrolysis of stored TG. Because the flux of NEFA to muscle is reduced, competition for glucose uptake is removed. The reduced delivery of NEFA to the liver will tend to suppress the secretion of VLDL-TG. In addition, insulin seems to suppress this directly. However, the short-term regulation of VLDL-TG secretion is not clearly understood *in vivo*; it has been studied mainly in isolated hepatocytes.

Dietary TG is absorbed into the enterocytes, and packaged into large, TG-rich lipoprotein particles, the chylomicrons. These enter the circulation relatively slowly (peak concentrations after a meal are typically reached at 3–4 h) and give the plasma a turbid appearance (postprandial lipemia). It seems beneficial for the body to be able to remove chylomicron-TG from the circulation quickly; there is considerable evidence that delayed removal of chylomicrons is associated with an increased risk of developing coronary heart disease. Rapid removal is achieved by insulin activation of adipose tissue LPL. Chylomicrons and VLDL compete for clearance by LPL, but chylomicrons are the preferred substrate, perhaps because their larger size enables them to interact with a larger number of LPL molecules at once. Nevertheless, it would make good physiological sense if VLDL-TG secretion were suppressed after a meal, as discussed above, to minimize competition and allow rapid clearance of chylomicron-TG. Because of the tissue-specific activation of LPL by insulin (Figure 5.9), adipose tissue plays an important role in clearance of chylomicron-TG, although muscle, because of its sheer mass, is also important; and in a physically trained person, muscle LPL will itself be up-regulated (compared with a sedentary person), so making a greater contribution to minimizing postprandial lipemia.

Within adipose tissue, the fatty acids released from chylomicron-TG by LPL in the capillaries diffuse into the adipocytes: this is aided by the suppression of hormone-sensitive lipase, reducing intracellular NEFA concentrations. Insulin also acts to stimulate the pathway of TG synthesis from fatty acids and glycerol phosphate. The precise steps at which insulin acts are not entirely clear, but it may be that a number of enzymes of fatty acid esterification are activated. In addition, increased glucose uptake will produce more glycerol-3-phosphate (from dihydroxyacetone phosphate, an intermediate in glycolysis), and this itself will stimulate TG synthesis. Thus, dietary fatty acids can be stored as adipose tissue TG by a short and energy-efficient pathway (Figure 5.13).

Amino acids

Again, the pattern of amino acid metabolism is complex (with 20 different amino acids, each having its own pathways), but some generalizations can be drawn. The small intestine itself may remove some amino acids

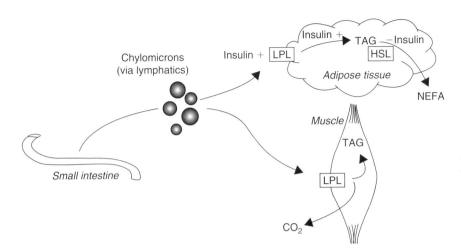

Figure 5.13 Most direct pathway for storage of dietary fat as adipose tissue triacylglycerol (TAG). Skeletal muscle is also shown as this will be the destination of some of the dietary fat. HSL: hormone-sensitive lipase; LPL: lipoprotein lipase; NEFA: non-esterified fatty acids.

such as glutamine for use as a metabolic fuel. A further selection of amino acids is removed by the liver, and the mixture of amino acids entering the systemic circulation is depleted of glutamine and enriched in the branched-chain amino acids. These will be taken up largely by muscle, where they play a special role in oxidative metabolism. Amino acids are secretagogues for (i.e. they stimulate secretion of) both insulin and glucagon (Table 5.4).

The rate of protein synthesis in muscle, the largest single reservoir of protein in the body, is regulated by many factors, including anabolic hormones (androgens, growth hormone), physical activity of the muscle and catabolic hormones (e.g. thyroid hormones, cortisol). In the short term, insulin also has a net anabolic effect. Measurements made using isotopic tracers suggest that this reflects not so much a stimulation of muscle protein synthesis as an inhibition of muscle protein breakdown. Nevertheless, the net effect is an increased sequestration of amino acids in muscle in the fed state.

Cardiovascular changes

The regulation of the metabolic disposal of the macronutrients in the period following a meal was discussed above. It is important to realize that eating a meal leads to a series of coordinated changes. As well as the purely metabolic responses, there are changes in the cardiovascular system. Cardiac output will rise (slightly, this a relatively small effect compared with physical exercise) and the distribution of blood flow to different tissues will change. There is an increase in blood flow to the abdominal viscera, to help in the process of absorption and transport of nutrients into the circulation. The blood flow through certain tissues also increases: skeletal muscle blood flow is stimulated by insulin (there is some debate about the physiological relevance of this, although it is certainly seen when insulin is infused at high concentrations) and adipose tissue blood flow rises after a meal. These changes may help to deliver substrates to the tissues where they will be used.

5.7 Short-term and longer term starvation

Starvation: general aspects

Earlier, the postabsorptive state was defined as that in which the absorption of nutrients from the gastrointestinal tract is essentially complete, and the body is in a relatively stable metabolic state (typically, after an overnight fast in humans). In addition, the events were described that occur when this state is interrupted, as it usually is, by ingestion of a meal. Another possible outcome is that no meal is forthcoming, perhaps because of food shortage, or for therapeutic reasons (to achieve rapid weight loss, or in preparation for surgery), or perhaps because the individual chooses not to eat, for instance for religious reasons. In that case the body gradually enters a state of early starvation, progressing eventually to a relatively steady metabolic state of complete starvation, which can last for a matter of several weeks. Some initially obese people, starved under close medical supervision and with supplementation with vitamins and minerals, have survived several months of starvation. The ability of the human body to cope with long periods of starvation illustrates perfectly the interaction and coordination of metabolism in different organs and tissues.

Starvation may be total or partial (when energy intake is not sufficient to maintain a steady body mass). Our understanding of complete starvation largely comes from detailed studies carried out in the 1960s on obese women fasting under medical supervision to lose weight. There is a worry that the responses observed may not be typical, because the excess initial fat stores of the subjects may have produced a different set of responses from those of initially slimmer people. There are some observations of normal-weight people starved for various reasons: during periods of famine in Europe in World War II, during periods of famine elsewhere in the world today, and people who have chosen to starve themselves, for instance, for political reasons. Tragic though these cases are, the observations that have been made help us to understand the adaptations of the body to deprivation and may in the future help those whose access to food, or ability to consume it, is limited. Our understanding of partial starvation was increased enormously by studies carried out in Minnesota, USA, during World War II, by the celebrated nutritionist Ancel Keys. The volunteers were conscientious objectors. They were fed for a period of 24 weeks on about 40% of their estimated energy requirements and they were carefully monitored during this time. Noticeable features of starvation were lethargy and depression. These were rapidly reversed when full feeding was resumed. The data from these studies were published in full, and papers are still being written on them today. The responses to partial starvation seem essentially to be similar to those to total starvation, albeit somewhat less marked.

If no carbohydrate is entering the body from the gut, then the body's limited carbohydrate reserves (Table 5.1) become very precious, and much of the metabolic pattern in starvation can be understood in terms of preservation of carbohydrate. Some tissues have a continual need for glucose. If the glucose is oxidized, specifically if its carbon atoms in the form of pyruvic acid go through the PDH reaction, then it is irreversibly lost to the body. Glucose can then be generated *de novo* only from non-carbohydrate precursors: glycerol from lipolysis, and the carbon skeletons of some amino acids. While triacylglycerol stores may be used without detriment to the organism, all the body's protein, as discussed earlier, has some specific function other than as a fuel for oxidation. As discussed later, the pattern

of metabolism adapts to starvation in such a way that protein oxidation is minimized, so far as possible, and as much energy as possible derived from fat.

Short-term starvation

A rapid response to starvation is loss of the liver glycogen store: this is virtually completely depleted within 24 h. At this stage there is still a need for generation of glucose at a high rate for oxidation in the brain. Net protein breakdown may be relatively rapid. This is sometimes called the gluconeogenic phase (e.g. until 2–3 days of complete starvation). Because of the lack of incoming glucose, plasma glucose concentrations will fall slightly, insulin concentrations will fall and glucagon secretion will increase. These changes reduce glucose utilization by tissues such as skeletal muscle, which can use fatty acids instead, and in particular suppression of PDH activity in tissues that are responsive to insulin will reduce irreversible disposal of glucose. There will be stimulation of lipolysis in adipose tissue, and of hepatic glucose production through gluconeogenesis. At this stage gluconeogenesis is largely proceeding at the expense of muscle protein. This phase may last for 3–4 days.

Longer term starvation

At around 1 week, short-term starvation merges into a period when glucose and insulin concentrations fall further, lipolysis increases still further and a sparing of protein breakdown is observed. This sparing of protein oxidation is reflected in a gradual decrease in the excretion of nitrogen in the urine. It is understandable in terms of the body's need to protect its protein, but the mechanism is not fully clear. Some features of this phase are clear. Increased lipolysis leads to increased delivery of non-esterified fatty acids and glycerol from adipose tissue. Since glycerol is a gluconeogenic precursor, the need for amino acids is reduced. Further, the oxidation of fatty acids within the liver is increased by the high glucagon/insulin ratio, and ketone bodies are produced in high concentrations in the circulation. Although the brain cannot use non-esterified fatty acids, it can use the water-soluble ketone bodies that are derived from them. In the phase of adapted starvation, say from 2–3 weeks of starvation onwards, ketone bodies reach a relatively steady concentration around 7–9 mmol/l (compared with less than 0.2 mmol/l typically after an overnight fast) and largely replace glucose as the oxidative fuel for the brain: they have been shown to meet about two-thirds of brain oxidative fuel requirements. Therefore, the need for protein breakdown to feed gluconeogenesis is again reduced. Because of the inactivation of pyruvate dehydrogenase (by the low insulin concentration), the glucose that is used by tissues outside the brain is largely only partially broken down, to pyruvate and lactate, which can then be recycled in the liver through gluconeogenesis. Thus, red blood cells, for instance, which have an obligatory requirement for glucose, are not depleting the body of glucose.

Although this shows how the need for protein oxidation is reduced, the cellular mechanism by which this is achieved also needs to be understood. There are several suggestions. Energy expenditure (metabolic rate) falls during starvation, sparing the body's fuel stores for as long as possible. The main mechanism is a fall in concentration of the active thyroid hormone, T_3 (with increased production of the inactive form, rT_3; see Section 5.3). The reduction in protein breakdown has been suggested simply to reflect this overall slowing of metabolism. Since thyroid hormones have a catabolic effect on muscle protein, the fall in their concentration may in itself spare muscle protein. In addition, it has been suggested that the high concentrations of ketone bodies exert a protein-sparing effect, possibly through suppression of the activity of the branched-chain 2-oxo acid dehydrogenase in skeletal muscle that is responsible for irreversible breakdown of the branched-chain amino acids.

The high concentrations of non-esterified fatty acids and ketone bodies (note that both 3-hydroxybutyric acid and acetoacetic acid are acids) might cause a metabolic acidosis (low blood pH), but this is corrected in part by the mechanism described earlier, whereby glutamine is metabolized in the kidney, releasing ammonia that is excreted along with H^+ ions. Urinary nitrogen excretion is normally largely in the form of urea, but during starvation the relative amount of ammonia increases, as does the contribution of the kidney to gluconeogenesis (the carbon skeleton of glutamine will contribute to this).

Ultimately, the body's fat store limits the length of survival. It appears that once the fat store is essentially depleted, then there is a phase of rapid protein breakdown that leads quickly to death. Thus, fatness is a useful adaptation when food is plentiful, if there are likely to be long periods of famine. In present-day industrialized societies, the latter is not a feature of life, but it may explain why there is such a strong tendency for people to become obese.

5.8 Perspectives on the future

The Human Genome Project has now produced the first draft of the DNA sequence making up the entire human genome. It encodes about 30 000–40 000 genes, each of which may lead to several different protein products by differential splicing and post-translational modifications. The function of most of these proteins is unknown. A major challenge for the next few decades will be to bridge the gap between molecular biology and whole-body function. Many new techniques will be required. For instance, proteomics is the determination of the proteins expressed in any one cell or tissue: the proteome is the protein equivalent of the genome. No-one has yet deciphered the proteome of any human cell. Once this has been done, it will be an enormous task to determine how all these proteins interact within one cell, and then to determine how cells interact within tissues and how tissues and organs interact in the whole body. The science of integrative physiology, well known in the early to middle part of the twentieth century, will have to be resurrected to make this possible.

Nutrition is a prime example of a science in which an integrated approach is necessary. We can study the nutritional needs of a single cell, although not in any real sense of a molecule, but most cells require a constant supply of nutrients to keep them alive in cell-culture systems. They will die within a day or two if nutrients are not provided. A human being, in contrast can survive for perhaps 2 months without food, because of the coordination that occurs between different cells. This chapter has described metabolism at the level of the cell, the tissues and organs, and the whole body. It is hoped that this approach will help the reader to see the grander picture of life: there is more to it than molecules!

Further reading

Felig P. Amino acid metabolism in man. Annu Rev Biochem 1975; 44: 933–955.

Frayn KN. Physiological regulation of macronutrient balance. Int J Obes 1995; 19 (Suppl 5): S4–S10.

Frayn KN. Metabolic Regulation: A Human Perspective, 2nd edn. Oxford: Blackwell Publishing, 2003.

Friedman JM. The alphabet of weight control. Nature 1997; 385: 119–120.

Friedman JM, Halaas JL. Leptin and the regulation of body weight in mammals. Nature 1998; 395: 763–770.

Gurr MI, Harwood JL, Frayn KN. Lipid Biochemistry: An Introduction, 5th edn. Oxford: Blackwell Science, 2002.

Murray RK, Granner DK, Mayes PA, Rodwell VW. Harper's Biochemistry, 25th edn. Stamford: Appleton and Lange, 2000.

Salway JG. Metabolism at a Glance, 2nd edn. Oxford: Blackwell Science, 1999.

6
Pregnancy and Lactation

JMA van Raaij and CPGM de Groot

Key messages

Pregnancy

- The crucial role of nutrients at various stages of pregnancy is evident, but still little is known about the quantitative needs of the individual nutrients. Even nutritional interventions in later pregnancy may have beneficial effects on the growth performance of the fetus.
- The approach to nutritional needs in pregnancy is mainly focussed on the amount and composition of the pregnancy weight gain and on the increased metabolism. A desirable weight gain over pregnancy is a weight gain that results in a desirable pregnancy outcome (in general, birth weight between 3 and 4 kg).
- The value for a desirable weight gain depends on the woman's pre-pregnancy weight and height. For well-nourished women of 60–65 kg and a body mass index (BMI) within the normal range, a reference pregnancy can be projected with a weight gain over pregnancy of 12.5 kg, an infant birth weight of 3.4 kg and an increased maternal fat stores of 2.0–2.5 kg.
- For such a reference pregnancy a total energy cost has been projected of 300 MJ or 1.1 MJ/day, which is only 10–15% above pre-pregnancy energy intake. To learn more about the nutritional needs of pregnancy, longitudinal studies are needed which include baseline measurements before or in early pregnancy.
- Methods of measuring body composition which rely on assumptions that might not be valid in pregnancy, should be modified for application in pregnancy. Physiological and metabolic adaptations in pregnancy have no or small effects on needs for energy and macronutrients, but for several micronutrients increased absorption rates have been found in pregnancy. Whether this depends on the level of maternal nutritional status remains to be clarified.
- Food consumption data indicate that in most studies the cumulative increase in food intake over pregnancy shows enormous variation between individuals, but on average it was not more than 25% of the estimated energy needs. Since mothers have several options to meet the energy and nutrient needs of pregnancy; by increasing intakes, by decreasing physical activity or by limiting storage, there are good arguments against setting one specific recommendation for increased intake for all pregnant women.

Lactation

- Estrogens and progesterone in the circulation during pregnancy inhibit prolactin from being effective. Following delivery of the infant and placenta, a sharp fall in maternal estrogen and progesterone levels occurs, prolactin is released and breast milk flow begins.
- Maintenance of milk production appears to be under feedback control, presumably by an inhibitor of milk secretion which enables women to adjust milk synthesis to the amount withdrawn by their infants.
- Breast milk changes in consistency during time. Initially, colostrum is produced, low in macronutrients but high in immunoglobulins. The concentrations of fat and lactose increase over time with transitional milk and mature breast milk.
- Breast-feeding confers several benefits on the infants and is considered the perfect food for the normal infant as long as the maternal system can sustain lactation and as long as there are no contraindications, such as the use of certain drugs by the mother.
- In well-nourished women, little relationship exists between maternal diet and milk production: mothers appear to protect breast-feeding through the depletion of their own body stores.

Section I: Pregnancy

6.1 Introduction

Nutrition before and during pregnancy and during lactation can have a significant effect on the long-term health of infants and their mothers. The potential impact of nutrition is greater at this time than during any other stage of life. A woman who enters pregnancy in an inadequate nutritional status has a risk of having inadequate pregnancy performance, of depleting her own body stores of nutrients, and of entering lactation in a state of suboptimal nutrition status that could deteriorate further as lactation progresses. Infants who are undernourished in the womb are at risk of a variety of adverse outcomes, ranging from low birth weight to severe mental and physical retardation and even death.

The effect of undernutrition before pregnancy and during pregnancy and lactation depends on the nutrient or nutrients involved and the stage at which undernutrition occurs. Each stage of this part of the life cycle has specific tissue needs for nutrients and shortcomings in tissue supply of these nutrients may have undesirable consequences. The success of pregnancy and lactation involves other factors such as the mother's age, the intake of substances such as alcohol, nicotine and drugs, the physical and emotional stresses to which she is subjected, and the presence of any infections or other diseases. This chapter, however, will mainly concentrate on the nutritional aspects.

6.2 Physiological stages of pregnancy and their nutritional demands

Pregnancy can be divided into three main physiological stages: implantation, organogenesis and growth.

Implantation

The implantation stage includes the first 2 weeks of gestation, when the fertilized ovum becomes embedded in the wall of the uterus. The nutrients provided by the secretions of the uterine gland pass directly into the fertilized ovum and developing embryo.

Organogenesis

The next 6 weeks of pregnancy are known as the period of organogenesis or embryogenesis. During this stage the cells of the embryo begin to differentiate into distinct tissues and functional units that later become organs, such as heart, lungs and liver. The development of the skeleton also begins at this time. During organogenesis the fetus obtains nourishment mainly from the mother's blood. When organogenesis is complete, the fetus weighs about 6 g and is less than 3 cm long.

Evidence from animal studies indicates that the presence of particular nutrients at specific times is crucial for the normal development of various tissues. There are critical periods of organogenesis during which the absence of certain nutrients can cause specific congenital abnormalities. For example, riboflavin deficiency during a critical period has been associated with poor skeletal formation, pyridoxine and manganese deficiencies with neuromotor problems, and vitamin B_{12}, vitamin A, niacin and folate deficiencies with defects in the central nervous system. Not surprisingly, little information is known on nutrient deficiencies and critical periods of organogenesis in humans. There is some information with respect to folate. Recently, it has become clear that folate is important for the prevention of neural tube defects (NTD). The critical period for the formation of the neural tube is from day 17 to day 30 of pregnancy. It has been shown that ample folate intake before and in early pregnancy may significantly reduce the risk of this form of fetal abnormality, and so nowadays an extra folate intake of 400 µg/day is recommended from before conception and for the first 3 months of pregnancy.

Growth

The remaining 7 months of pregnancy are known as the growth period. Most of the nutrients for growth are delivered through the placenta. Blood does not flow directly from the mother's circulation to the fetal circulation. Altogether about 10–11 m^2 of surface area are available for the transfer of materials between the placental circulation and the fetal circulation. Free fatty acids and cholesterol can be transferred across the placenta by simple diffusion, carbohydrates (mainly glucose) cross by facilitated diffusion (diffusion assisted by the presence of a protein embedded in the membrane) and amino acids by active transport (transport against a concentration gradient powered by the release of cellular energy). Most water-soluble vitamins are present in the fetal circulation at higher concentrations than in the maternal circulation and so presumably enter the fetus by active transport. Fat-soluble vitamins are present at lower concentrations in the fetus than in the mother and probably enter the fetus by passive diffusion. Both calcium and iron cross the placenta by active transport via mechanisms that are not well understood.

During the period of growth the tissues and organs formed during organogenesis continue to grow and mature. Growth of the fetus occurs in three phases. During the first phase, known as hyperplasia, there is a rapid increase in the number of cells. The large numbers of cell divisions involved require sufficient supplies of folate and vitamin B_{12}. In the next phase, cellular replication continues with hypertrophy, when cells are growing in size. This requires sufficient supplies of amino acids and vitamin B_6. In the final phase of growth, hypertrophy or cellular growth predominates, whereas cellular division ceases. Just as with the phase of organogenesis, also with respect to the growth phase little is known of the consequences of specific nutritional deficiencies in humans. What we do know is that inadequate nutrition during the growth phase may cause intrauterine growth retardation (IuGR) and a low birth weight, but at this stage it will not cause the more serious abnormalities associated with deficiencies at earlier times. This is certainly not to say that IuGR can be considered as a problem of minor importance. On the contrary, it should be clearly recognized that infants with low birth weights show higher rates of morbidity and mortality, probably because of infectious diseases and impaired immunity, and they are at increased risk of growth failure and abnormal cognitive development as infants. It should, however, be noted that a depression of growth during a temporary period of undernutrition is often compensated by an increased growth when nutrition becomes adequate again. This means that nutritional interventions in pregnancy during the growth phase of the fetus may still have beneficial effects on the growth performance of the fetus.

In summary, variation in the nutritional demands throughout pregnancy are evident. Inadequate food intakes in pregnancy, quantitatively and/or qualitatively, have obvious effects on pregnancy performance in terms of pregnancy weight gain and pregnancy outcome, but little is known of the consequences of deficiencies of individual nutrients. Therefore, it is not surprising that in the approach of the nutritional needs in pregnancy much attention is focussed on the amount and composition of the pregnancy weight gain and on the increased metabolism.

6.3 Principles for estimating nutritional needs in pregnancy

The commonly used approach to estimate energy and nutrient needs during pregnancy is the factorial approach. This implies consideration of the extra energy and nutrient needs imposed by pregnancy above the baseline needs for non-pregnant, non-lactating women. Thus, the extra needs related to deposition of new tissues and to maintaining of these new tissues should be taken into account. These needs will depend on the amount and composition of the weight gain over pregnancy.

If recommendations have to be set up then a decision has to be made on what should be considered, as this implies some concept of an appropriate or desirable pregnancy weight gain. A desirable weight gain should result in a desirable pregnancy outcome, for example a term infant weighing between 3 and 4 kg. But the size of the desirable weight gain will also depend on the woman's pre-pregnant weight. For a woman who is clearly underweight a higher desirable weight gain should be projected than for an overweight woman of the same height.

Reference weight gain over pregnancy

In well-nourished women from affluent countries with a pre-pregnant body weight between 60 and 65 kg, an average weight gain over pregnancy of 12.5 kg is observed and an average infant birth weight of 3.4 kg. The components of weight gain can be divided into three categories: the products of conception (the fetus, the amniotic fluid and the placenta), the increased amounts of maternal tissues other than fat (extracellular fluid, uterus, breasts, blood) and the increased amount of fat stores. A representative proportion of the total weight gain over pregnancy that can be attributed to each of the components is shown in Table 6.1. The distribution of the total weight gain of 12 500 g over the four quarters of pregnancy is calculated on 650, 3350, 4500 and 4000 g, respectively.

This typical pregnancy weight gain and composition of weight gain was first described in the 1960s by Hytten and Leitch, who derived theoretical estimates of the extra nutritional needs from this outline. Since

Table 6.1 Components of weight gain over pregnancy

Products of conception	4850 g
Fetus	3400 g
Amniotic fluid	800 g
Placenta	650 g
Maternal tissues (excluding fat stores)	4305 g
Extracellular fluid	1680 g
Uterus and breasts	1375 g
Blood	1250 g
Maternal fat stores	3345 g
Fat stores	3345 g
Total weight gain	12 500 g

then, many national and international bodies have adopted this as a reference pregnancy for developing recommended intakes in pregnancy.

Although specific nutrient deficiencies may restrict gestational weight gain, energy is the main determinant of this weight gain. For that reason, the principles of approaching nutritional needs during pregnancy will be worked out in more detail using energy as example.

Energy cost of pregnancy

The average extra energy costs of the reference pregnancy as given in Table 6.1 were estimated to be about 350 MJ over the 9 month period. These costs can be divided into three main components:

- the energy deposited in fat stores: about 150 MJ (154 MJ based on 3345 g fat; at an energy cost of 46 kJ/g fat)
- the energy deposited in other tissues such as fetus, placenta, uterus, breasts, amniotic fluid and blood: about 50 MJ (47 MJ based on 440 g fat and 925 g protein; at an energy cost of 46 kJ/g and 29 kJ/g)
- the energy required to maintain the new tissues at about 150 MJ. The gain in fat stores and the increased metabolism are by far the largest components of the energy costs of pregnancy.

It is important to verify the theoretical estimates of Hytten and Leitch against what is really happening in various populations and under various conditions. Therefore, since the 1980s several appropriate longitudinal studies on pregnancy have been performed in a broad range of settings and in both developing and developed communities. These studies included measurements in the second and third trimesters of pregnancy as well as baseline measurements performed

before pregnancy or in the first trimester of pregnancy. Sometimes these studies were also complemented with measurements throughout the first 1 or 2 months postpartum, which may also help to derive quantitative estimates of increments throughout pregnancy. In the following paragraphs the main findings with respect to the increase in maternal fat stores and in maintenance metabolism will be presented.

Increase in maternal fat stores

The change in maternal fat stores can be obtained by taking the difference between late pregnancy fat mass and pre-pregnancy (or early pregnancy) fat mass, and by subtracting about 0.4 or 0.5 kg for assumed fat deposition in the fetus. The observed variation in changes in maternal fat stores is large and ranges from no increase at all in some developing countries to more than 5 kg in more affluent countries. For women with a pregnancy weight gain of 12.5 kg an increase in maternal fat stores of about 2.0 kg (equivalent to 92 MJ: 2000 g × 46 kJ/g) to 2.5 kg (115 MJ) was found, which is about 1 kg less than the previous theoretical derived estimate (see Table 6.1). The actual energy costs for the deposition of the maternal fat stores will therefore be closer to 100 MJ than to 150 MJ.

To obtain valid estimates of gain in maternal fat mass, it is not enough to use an appropriate longitudinal study design, it is also important to be aware of the strengths and weaknesses of the various methods to estimate fat mass in pregnancy. The most commonly used methods to estimate fat mass are based on measuring skinfold thicknesses, total body water (TBW), body density (D_{body}) or bioimpedance. Sometimes combinations of these measurements are used. It should be noted that all these methods are based on assumptions that may not be valid in pregnancy. For example, the method to derive fat-free mass (FFM) from TBW is based on an assumed water content for FFM of 73%. However, in late pregnancy, the water content of maternal FFM is higher than 73% because of the higher water content of the fat-free part of maternal weight gain over pregnancy. Equally, the method used to derive fat mass from D_{body} is based on the assumption that the density of maternal FFM is 1.1 kg/dm^3. However, again in late pregnancy, the density of maternal FFM will be lower, because of the higher water content of the fat-free part of pregnancy weight gain. Applying the usual assumption in the TBW method will result in an overestimation of the mother's actual fat mass in late pregnancy, whereas application of the usual assumption in the D_{body} method will result in an underestimation of the mother's actual fat mass.

Increase in maintenance metabolism

The increase in maintenance metabolism over pregnancy is approached by studying basal metabolic rate (BMR) throughout pregnancy. Measurements are made under standardized conditions (rest, postabsorption and thermoneutrality) and gaseous exchange is measured using a Douglas bag, ventilated hood or respiration chamber. The increase in maintenance metabolism is calculated as the cumulative area under the curve represented by the rise in a mother's BMR above the pre-pregnancy baseline metabolic rate. Examples of the cumulative changes in basal metabolism are given in Figure 6.1.

There is a wide variability in cumulative increases in maintenance metabolism over pregnancy between populations. These costs may range from +210 MJ in Swedish women to −45 MJ in unsupplemented Gambian women. The Swedish mothers also show a much larger weight gain over pregnancy than the Gambian mothers. When results from all available studies are combined, a good correlation appears between pregnancy weight gain and cumulative increase in maintenance metabolism over pregnancy. For the

reference weight gain of 12.5 kg the increase in BMR is estimated to be about 160 MJ, which is very close to the estimate based on theoretical calculations (150 MJ).

In summary, for a reference pregnancy a total energy cost has been estimated to be about 300 MJ or 1.1 MJ/day. If this has to be completely covered by food intake, then the additional energy intake would be only 10–15% more than the pre-pregnant energy intake, which can be estimated for these women to be between 8.4 and 9.0 MJ/day. In other words, to meet to extra energy needs of pregnancy, there is no need for large increases in food intake.

6.4 Physiological adjustments that may effect energy and nutrient needs of pregnancy

Section 6.3 sets out how estimates of the extra energy costs of pregnancy can be calculated. Whether these needs should be fully covered by increased foods intakes depend on whether certain physiological or metabolic adjustments occur.

Basal metabolism

As previously discussed, one of the main components of the energy cost of pregnancy is the increase in maintenance metabolism. This can be estimated from the cumulative area under the curve represented by the rise in a mother's BMR above the pre-pregnancy rate. As shown in Figure 6.1 however, such curves might be very different. In well-nourished women BMR usually begins to rise soon after conception and it increases continuously until delivery. In women from developing countries with weight gains over pregnancy of about 8 kg and infant birth weights around 3 kg, the BMR does not begin to rise before the second half of pregnancy. In contrast, in undernourished Gambian women a pronounced suppression of metabolism has been demonstrated that persisted well into the third trimester of pregnancy. As a result, the cumulative area under the curve might become negative, indicating that the average maintenance metabolism in pregnancy is even lower than before pregnancy. This is remarkable since there has been a gain in weight and thus a larger body to maintain. This finding suggests an increase in efficiency of basal metabolism, but more studies in very undernourished women should be performed to confirm the finding in other populations.

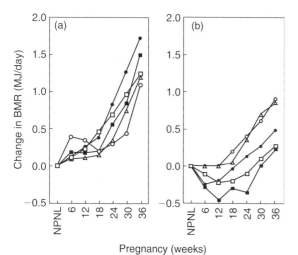

Figure 6.1 Mean changes in basal metabolic rate (BMR) measured longitudinally throughout pregnancy. (a) Developed countries: △: Scotland; ○: The Netherlands; ●: Sweden; ■: England; □: The Netherlands; (b) developing countries: □: The Gambia–supplemented; ■: The Gambia–unsupplemented; △: Thailand; ○: The Philippines; ●: The Gambia. (Reproduced with permission from Prentice et al., 1996.)

Diet-induced thermogenesis

Diet-induced thermogenesis (DIT) refers to the increase in energy expenditure above basal metabolism following the ingestion of food. It is due mainly to the energy costs of digestion, absorption, transport and storage, and averages approximately 10% of the daily energy intake. It has been hypothesized that energy expenditure in pregnancy might be lowered through a reduction in DIT, for example due to another metabolic substrate routing. However, well-controlled human trials revealed only small or no changes in DIT in pregnancy.

Metabolic efficiency of performing physical activities

It has been hypothesized that the metabolic efficiency of performing physical activities might be increased in pregnancy. However, studies in pregnancy on weight-bearing activities such as treadmill walking or non-weight-bearing activities as cyclometer activities, failed to demonstrate relevant improvements in metabolic efficiency.

Protein metabolism

Shifts in protein metabolism are complex and change gradually throughout gestation, so that nitrogen conservation for fetal growth achieves full potential during the last quarter of pregnancy. Nitrogen balance studies in pregnant and non-pregnant women revealed that there is no evidence that women deposit nitrogen in early pregnancy to be mobilized later. However, nitrogen retention is increased in late pregnancy and is due to a reduction in urinary nitrogen excretion. A decrease in urea synthesis seems to account for this reduction in urinary urea nitrogen and suggests that amino acids are conserved for tissue synthesis. Because there is no evidence that pregnant women store protein in early pregnancy for later fetal demands, the increased requirements of late pregnancy might, at least in part, be met by these physiological adjustments that enhance dietary protein utilization. If the dietary supply is low, a greater change in the physiological adjustments is needed to meet fetal needs than if dietary intake is liberal. However, the extent to which low intakes of dietary protein may affect urea synthesis or circulating concentrations of amino acids is yet to be established in pregnant women. Presumably, maternal protein status at conception also influences the physiological adjustments made in nitrogen metabolism. Future studies of nutrient metabolic adjustments in women consuming marginal to adequate diets are needed to understand fully the interactions among the physiology of pregnancy, nutrient metabolism and maternal nutritional status.

Micronutrient metabolism

Although fetal demand for nutrients occurs primarily during the latter half of gestation, when >90% of the fetal growth occurs, adjustments in nutrient metabolism are apparent within the first weeks of pregnancy. The concentration of serum lipids increases during pregnancy while circulating concentrations of most other nutrients decrease by the end of the first 10 weeks of gestation and remain lower than non-pregnant values until term. The decrease starts before there is an increase in plasma volume and the reduction in later stages is less than the change in plasma volume. Thus, the total amount of vitamins and minerals in circulation increases during pregnancy.

For many nutrients an increased absorption rate in pregnancy has been found. The mechanisms underlying this increased absorption are still to be clarified.

Total plasma calcium levels fall very early in pregnancy, mediated by a fall in plasma albumin as part of the process of hemodilution. However, ionized calcium levels and phosphate levels remain normal throughout pregnancy. Plasma levels of 1,25-dihydroxy-D are elevated early in pregnancy and remain elevated throughout pregnancy. Intestinal calcium absorption doubles in pregnancy, probably owing to the changes in vitamin D status. The earliest study of calcium absorption was at 12 weeks and, as early as then, this very dramatic rise in calcium absorption was noted. The observed elevation in 1,25-dihydroxy-D_3 is associated with an observed rise in calcium binding protein $_{9K}$-D. Given that the fetal need for calcium does not arrive until later in pregnancy, it is possible that the increased calcium flow from the gut leads to storage in the skeletal pool. Indeed, increased bone density has been observed in animal models.

In contrast, there are conflicting schools of thought on the possible adaptive response in iron absorption in pregnancy. However, since the cessation of menstrual losses saves some 0.5–1.0 g of the body iron pool, that represents a very significant part of the increased requirements of pregnancy, accounting for as much as one-third of needs.

Folate and neural tube defects

Neural tube defects (NTDs) are severe congenital malformations of the central nervous system that occur as a result of the failure of the embryonic neural tube to close normally within the first 4 weeks postconception. Folate has been implicated in the formation of NTDs from an early stage, because of its critical role in cell division coupled with the historical observations of increased incidence of NTDs during times of decreased nutritional status. Furthermore, NTDs have also been demonstrated to have strong genetic factors, with differences in the prevalence of NTDs across different ethnic groups and also the increased risk of a mother having recurring NTD births.

The main metabolic function of folate is its coenzyme role, which carries one-carbon units and thereby acts as a cofactor to specific enzymes, allowing them to carry out their specific functions. One-carbon reactions include those involved in purine and pyrimidine synthesis, amino acid metabolism and the formation of the primary methylating agent S-adenosyl methionine (SAM). A defective folate metabolism or folate shortage in the mother may also lead to a shortage of folate in the developing embryo, which could result in a defective DNA synthesis or an impaired transcription of genes involved in the neurulation process. Additional folate intake may overcome impaired DNA synthesis or DNA methylation.

Initially, several studies examined the effect of folic acid supplementation on the ability to prevent recurrence of NTDs in women who already had a previously affected pregnancy. The results of these studies demonstrated impressive reductions in the recurrence rates, but the study design came under scrutiny and it became apparent that a randomized trial was needed. In 1983 the British Medical Council undertook the first randomized double-blind study examining the supplementation of folic acid and other vitamins on recurrence of NTD. The results showed conclusively that 72% of recurring NTD could be prevented by periconceptual ingestion of 4 mg of folic acid in a supplement form. It also showed the 'other' vitamins did not reduce the incidence of recurrence, thus underlying the importance of folate status in NTDs. Further studies such as the Budapest Trial then examined the effects of folic acid supplementation on the occurrence of NTDs and reached similar conclusions. However, the amount of folic acid taken in these trials varied considerably, from 360 µg to 4 mg. Examination of the results of these studies led to the consensus that supplementation of 400 µg periconceptually could afford optimum protection from the occurrence of an NTD.

Such studies have now led to the recommendation that women of childbearing age should consume a 400 µg folic acid supplement daily periconceptually for at least 1 month and then 12 weeks postconception to prevent an NTD. Furthermore, it is recommended that 4 mg should be taken to prevent a recurrence of an NTD pregnancy.

Serum micronutrient levels may decrease gradually throughout pregnancy, the absolute amounts in serum will not change. This is explained by the fact that the extracellular fluid volume expands in pregnancy, causing hemodilution and the dilution of the components in blood. When adjustments are made for the expansion of blood plasma, the absolute amounts of micronutrients in circulation are often increased in pregnancy. It is important that the fall in serum nutrient concentration caused by hemodilution should not be interpreted as a sign of nutritional deficiency. Assessment of the micronutrient status of the pregnant woman can thus only be done validly if appropriate pregnancy standards are being used.

In summary, there are several physiological adjustments in pregnancy, which may have beneficial effects on energy or nutrient utilization, but they do not have substantial effects on the extents of the projected energy and nutrient needs. It is conceivable that in undernourished mothers some more profound energy and nutrient-saving mechanisms exist, but so far this has not really been supported by experimental evidence.

6.5 Ways in which mothers may deal with the energy and nutrient needs of pregnancy

Mothers have two behavioral options to deal with the energy and nutrient needs in pregnancy. They may (1) eat more and/or eat other types of food products; or (2) change their level of physical activity.

Amount of food consumed and food choice

The energy needs over pregnancy have been estimated to be in the region of 300 MJ over the 9 month period, or 1.1 MJ per day. This is about 10–15 % of the dietary reference value for energy for non-pregnant, non-lactating women (for Europe 8.4–9.0 MJ/day). Most studies in well-nourished women revealed either no change, or only minor increases in the amount of energy and nutrients consumed in pregnancy, and if an increased intake was found, then the observed level of increment would only partly cover the energy cost of pregnancy. An analysis of available data from longitudinal studies in populations with average birth weights >3 kg revealed a cumulative intake of only 85 MJ over the whole of pregnancy or only 0.3 MJ/day, which is only 25% of the estimated needs. The possibility of underestimation with longitudinal comparisons should be considered. However, most studies provide little support for the contention that the low intakes observed during pregnancy might be due to measurement fatigue, that is, continued measurement of food intake over a pregnancy. It is also possible that the expected increment in energy intake (15% above pre-pregnant level) would be too small to be detected by the commonly used food consumption methods. Well-designed studies using appropriate methodologies and including appropriate numbers of subjects can detect increments in energy intake of 5–10%.

Beliefs about prenatal diets and food cravings or food aversions may influence food choices in pregnant women. Knowledge of the individual's total dietary intake is necessary before the nutritional effect of food cravings or aversions can be assessed. Food cravings and aversions do not necessarily have a deleterious effect on the quality of the diet.

Level of physical activity

The energy costs for a person's daily physical activity depend on:

- the time–activity pattern (amount of time spent on various activities)
- the pace or intensity of performing the various activities
- body weight.

Since body weight increases over pregnancy, an increase in energy costs might be expected, at least for weight-bearing activities. However, a mother may compensate for this by reducing the pace or intensity with which the activity is performed. A pregnant woman may also choose to change her activity pattern and, for example, reduce the amount of time spent on weight-bearing activities. However, this assumes that mothers will be more or less free to change their daily activities or to change the pace or intensity of the work performed. This

might be the case for many women from affluent societies, but it certainly does not hold for all societies. For example, low-income women from developing countries often have to continue their strenuous activity pattern until delivery, and so for them the option to save energy by reducing physical activity is not available. Also, for mothers who enter pregnancy with an existing light daily activity pattern (not uncommon in affluent societies), the possibilities to save energy by reducing physical activity are limited. It should also be realized that even if women voluntarily decrease their pace and consequently the energy expenditure per minute, the energy cost to complete a task may be unchanged or even increased. Longitudinal time–motion studies provide valuable information, but since the type and intensity of activities within an activity category may change, such studies cannot give conclusive data on how much energy is saved by changing activity patterns throughout pregnancy. The answer might come from measurements of total daily energy expenditure using the doubly labeled water method. However, at present, only a few longitudinal studies, including pre-pregnancy measurements, have been performed, but these studies showed an increase in energy cost for physical activity in the second half of pregnancy and not a lowering.

6.6 Dietary recommendations for pregnancy

The increased demands of pregnancy may be met in a variety of ways. Some mothers will meet the demands by increasing intake, others by decreasing level of physical activity or by limiting storage (e.g. fat storage), and still others by a combination of these options. It is not possible to advise women before pregnancy about the most appropriate strategies to balance intake and expenditure. With respect to the option of increasing food intake, it is clear that adequate and appropriate foods must be available to and accessible by the women. With respect to the option of changing level of physical activity, it should be recognized that sometimes the activity levels are already very low and that in situations where the levels might be high, the women do not have always the social or economic freedom to reduce that level. Finally, the option of limiting storage clearly depends on the pre-pregnant nutritional status of the mother. Mothers with no or low reserves should be able to build up an appropriate reserve to enter lactation in an appropriate nutritional status, and mothers who already have ample reserves before pregnancy probably do not need to create an additional reserve.

Thus, there are good arguments against setting a specific recommendation for increased intake for all pregnant women. A policy might be to permit considerable freedom in food intake recommendations on the basis of individual preferences and to monitor weight gain carefully and make adjustments in food intake only in response to deviations from the normal pattern of gain.

To estimate energy and nutrient needs during pregnancy the factorial approach is commonly used. This means that the extra energy and nutrient needs imposed by pregnancy are added to the baseline estimates for non-pregnant, non-lactating women.

Energy

The reference pregnancy, assuming an increase in maternal fat stores of 2.0–2.5 kg, takes about 290–310 MJ extra over the whole of pregnancy or about 1.1 MJ/day. The dietary reference value (DRV) value of the World Health Organization (WHO) of 0.8 MJ/day (Table 6.2) is based on an assumed reduction in physical activity in pregnancy.

Protein

Recommendations for protein intake during pregnancy are based on the estimated 925 g of protein deposited during pregnancy in the fetal, placental and maternal tissue. About half of the protein gained is in the fetal tissues. Most of the additional protein in maternal tissues is accumulated in early pregnancy, during the growth of the uterus, placenta and mammary glands. If protein intake is restricted during pregnancy the amount stored in the mother's body, rather than the amount transferred to the fetus, is reduced. The reference additional protein intake in pregnancy (mean protein requirement +2 SD) is established by WHO as 6 g/day.

Fat-soluble vitamins

Although it is well established that adaptive mechanisms improve the body's use of minerals during pregnancy, there is no evidence of similar mechanisms for adapting to vitamin needs. Dietary reference values for pregnancy include substantial increases for vitamins D, a small increase for vitamin A, and no increments for vitamin E and K.

Little is known about the need for vitamin A during human pregnancy. However, if the mother is adequately nourished, her infant will be born with a reserve of

vitamin A in the liver, even if the mother did not increase her vitamin A intake during pregnancy. It is important to note that high intakes of vitamin A can be damaging for the developing fetus and should be avoided.

Both active forms of vitamin D readily cross the placenta to play an active role in the metabolism of calcium in the fetus. The need for vitamin D during pregnancy is estimated to be 10 μg/day, which is substantially more than the DRV for the non-pregnant adult female (2.5 μg/day). Mothers who consume enough milk to meet the calcium needs do not need an additional source of vitamin D.

Water-soluble vitamins

DRVs in pregnancy for water-soluble vitamins are increased by 10–100% or more above those for non-pregnant women.

Minerals

Mineral needs in pregnancy are estimated from the amounts transferred to the fetus. These amounts might come from the mother's stores, from an increased consumption or from an increased absorption rate. The extent to which these various options may contribute probably depends on maternal pre-pregnancy nutritional status and the mother's access to food. Calcium, iron and zinc are the main minerals of interest during pregnancy. DRVs for these minerals during pregnancy are given in Table 6.2.

The mother transfers about 30 g of calcium to her infant before birth, most of it in the last trimester of gestation. A well-nourished woman has more than

Table 6.2 Some dietary reference values for pregnant women

Energy	+0.8 MJ/day (last trimester)	EAR
Protein intake	+6 g/day[a]	RNI
Vitamin A (retinol equivalent)	600 μg/day	Safe level
Vitamin D	10 μg/day	RNI
Thiamin	+0.1 mg/day	RNI
Riboflavin	+0.2 mg/day	RNI
Folate	370–470 μg/day	Safe level*
Calcium	1000–1200 mg/day	RNI
Iron	No increment	
Zinc	7.3–13.3 mg/day	Normative
Iodine	200 μg/day	Normative

[a] Based on egg and milk protein; assuming complete digestibility.
EAR: estimated average requirement; RNI: reference nutrient intake, 2 SD above EAR; Safe level: upper end of normative storage requirement; Safe level*: normative storage requirement plus 2 SD; Normative: population mean intake sufficient to meet normative requirements.

1000 g of stored calcium from which she can draw. Part of the 30 g of calcium provided to the fetus comes from the stores in the mother's bones; the rest comes from mother's diet and the increased efficiency with which she absorbs calcium in pregnancy. It is assumed that the enhanced calcium absorption in early pregnancy provides part of the calcium that is transferred to the fetus in the latter half of gestation. The current DRV for pregnant women is 1000–1200 mg/day, which is substantially more than the value for non-pregnant, non-lactating women (400–500 mg/day).

Infants are born with a supply of iron stored in the liver sufficient to last for 3–6 months. To achieve this storage, the mother must transfer about 200–400 mg of iron to the fetus during gestation. In addition, the pregnant woman requires additional iron for the formation of the placenta, for the hemoglobin required by the expansion of blood volume, and to compensate for the loss of blood during delivery. Once this is taken into account, the total requirement for iron over the course of pregnancy amounts to 800–900 mg. Therefore, each day, the diet or maternal iron stores must supply approximately 3 mg of iron. However, many young women enter pregnancy with practically no reserves of iron. Fortunately, the efficiency of iron absorption may increase from 10% to 30% in the second half of pregnancy.

The amount of iron that must be absorbed by the pregnant woman amounts to 3 mg/day. This figure is substantially more than the amount of iron that must be absorbed by menstruating women. Menstrual iron losses vary greatly among women, but they usually amount to about 0.5–1 mg/day when averaged over the whole menstrual cycle. Thus, the cessation of menstrual iron losses can contribute between one-sixth and one-third of the iron requirements in pregnancy.

A total of 100 mg of zinc is estimated to accumulate within fetal and maternal tissues during pregnancy. Assuming 25% absorption, approximately 3 mg of additional dietary zinc per day is required during the last trimester, in addition to the 6.5 mg DRV for non-pregnant, non-lactating women. It is unknown whether the efficiency of zinc absorption increases in human pregnancy.

6.7 Perspectives on the future

It is well established that adequate nutrient provision before and during pregnancy and during lactation can have a significant effect on the long-term health of both infant and mother. Experimental studies designed to examine intervention strategies to improve maternal weight gain with the objective of optimizing health outcomes for mother and baby would be invaluable in this regard.

Different ethnic groups have been shown to have widely variable energy requirements during pregnancy. Observational studies in a variety of ecological and ethnic settings on the relationship between pregnancy, body mass index (BMI) and maternal energy needs are necessary to explain this variability. In addition, further work would be valuable in assessing the causes and consequences of extremes of weight gain in pregnancy. Dietary studies would be useful in looking at the influences of diet on the prevalence of low birth weight. It is clear that many women gain excessive weight during pregnancy and yet low birth weight of infants still occurs in this group.

Many physiological adaptations occur during pregnancy to supply the growing fetus with its increasing requirements for macronutrients and micronutrients. This increase in nutrient bioavailability manifested by an increase in gastrointestinal absorption has not been fully elucidated and work in this area is required.

As shown in the next section, breast-feeding instills many benefits to the infant and mother, but insufficient information is available regarding the consequence of inadequate gestational nutrition on lactation.

Section II: Lactation

6.8 Regulation of milk production

Lactation is an integral part of the reproductive cycle. During pregnancy the alveolar system of the mammary gland develops (mammogenesis) under the combined action of estrogen and progesterone, supplemented by greatly increased amounts of prolactin from the mother's anterior pituitary gland. Estrogens and progesterone in the circulation during pregnancy inhibit prolactin from being effective. Following delivery of the infant and placenta, a sharp fall in maternal estrogen and progesterone levels occurs, prolactin is released and breast milk flow begins. Suckling from the infant induces a variety of hormonal responses. In the mother it stimulates the continued production of prolactin and induces the release of oxytocin from the hypothalamus. Oxytocin is essential for the milk letdown reflex. This reflex initiates the release of milk from the alveoli into the ducts and to the nipple. Milk is then withdrawn by the infant's suckling.

Following the birth of the infant, the prolactin level starts to return to the non-pregnant level. Hereby it remains one of the two major hormones involved in initiating and sustaining milk secretion. Each time the mother nurses the infant, nerve impulses from the nipples to the hypothalamus increase the release of prolactin-releasing hormone, resulting in a 10-fold increase in prolactin secretion by the anterior pituitary that lasts for about 1 h. Concurrently, the oxytocin response is transient and intermittent rather than sustained. Plasma levels often return to basal between milk ejections even though suckling continues.

Maintenance of milk production appears to be under feedback control, presumably by an inhibitor of milk secretion, which enables women to adjust milk synthesis to the amount withdrawn by their infants. Key factors in the regulation of milk synthesis are the frequency and completeness of milk removal. Thus, for mothers it is essential to be adequately instructed on the art of breast-feeding. Most commonly, the cause of poor lactational performance is either the infant's lack of access to the breast or inappropriate suckling behavior.

6.9 Colostrum, transitional and mature milk

During late pregnancy and the first 2 days after birth, the mammary glands secrete around 30 ml/day of fluid called colostrum. This volume increases following suckling-induced milk production, which also stimulates the synthesis of lactose and attracts water osmotically. Though colostrum contains relatively little water, lactose and fat, it is rich in constituents that enhance the neonate's immune system and protect the infant during the first few months of life (Table 6.3). During the colostral period, concentrations of fat and lactose increase, while those of protein and minerals decrease. Thus, colostrum serves adequately until the appearance of transitional milk (days 7–21 postpartum), which gradually changes to become mature over the first 2 weeks of breastfeeding.

6.10 Protective aspects of human milk

There is a complex system of antimicrobial factors in human milk. These include:

- carbohydrates that inhibit binding of certain bacterial pathogens to epithelial cells
- nitrogen-containing sugars that promote growth of beneficial lactobacilli and bifidobacteria in the lower intestinal tract
- antibodies such as secretory immunoglobulin A (IgA, and to some extent serum IgG), which prevent binding and proliferation of pathogens and may actively prime the newborn's immune system
- anti-inflammatory agents
- antioxidants
- white blood cells
- lactoferrin, an iron binding protein that inhibits proliferation of iron-requiring bacteria
- lysosyme, an enzyme that attacks microbial pathogens
- antiviral lipids
- antiprotozoan factors.

These interacting factors can be characterized as:

- biochemically heterogeneous
- produced throughout lactation

Table 6.3 Concentrations of selected immunological factors in human several phases of lactation

	2–3 days	1 month	6 months	1 year
Lactoferrin (ng/ml)	5.3 ± 12.9	1.9 ± 0.3	1.4 ± 0.4	1.0 ± 0.2
Serum immunoglobulin A (ng/ml)	2 ± 2.5	1 ± 0.3	0.5 ± 0.1	1.0 ± 0.3
Lysosyme (ng/ml)	0.09 ± 0.03	0.02 ± 0.03	0.25 ± 0.12	0.2 ± 0.1

Data are shown as mean $\pm$ SD
Source: Goldman and Goldblum (1989).

- relative resistant to digestive processes
- protective, by non-inflammatory mechanisms, principally in the digestive tract and the respiratory system of the infant.

Breast-feeding confers several benefits to the infant and is considered the perfect food for the normal infant as long as the maternal system can sustain lactation and as long as there are no contraindications, such as the use of certain drugs by the mother. Thus, for normal full-term infants breast-feeding is generally considered the preferred method of feeding for the first 4–6 months of life, not only because human breast milk provides all of the nutrients needed by the infant. In March 2001 a WHO expert consultation on the optimal duration of exclusive breast-feeding recommended exclusive breast-feeding for 6 months, applying this to populations, recognizing that some mothers are unable to, or choose not to follow this recommendation. These mothers should also be supported to optimize their infants' nutrition. Despite the numerous recognized advantages of breast-feeding, no more than an estimated 35% of the world's infant population are exclusively breast-fed between 0 and 4 months of age (WHO Global Data Bank on Breastfeeding, 2001). As a substitute for breast milk, cow's milk is considered inadequate owing to its high contents of protein, sodium, calcium, phosphate and chloride, whereas concentrations of iron and copper are too low. Based on the current knowledge of infant requirements and the composition of breast milk, industries nowadays modify the composition of cow's milk and put a variety of formula milks on the market.

6.11 Maternal nutrition and lactational performance

Milk volume

In well-nourished women, little relationship exists between maternal diet and milk production: mothers appear to protect breast-feeding through the depletion of their own body stores. Actual measurements of milk yield from groups of women from a wide range of nutritional and cultural conditions revealed that breast-milk output was similar in early lactation (Figure 6.2).

Thus, even small, undernourished women are able to produce about 700 ml of breast milk/day early in lactation as long as they are not actually starving. Following the introduction of formula feeding and of solid foods, milk production tends to fall to approximately 600 ml/day in full breast-feeders and to 50% of this amount in partial breast-feeders. Although the mother's level of food intake does not seem to affect milk yield, the quality of the mother's diet can influence the secretion of specific components of breast milk.

Energy and macronutrient content of breast milk

As in the case of milk volume, the macronutrient content of human breast milk (Table 6.4) appears rather insensitive to differences in maternal nutrition. Estimates of the gross energy content of milk vary from 2.55 to 3.00 kJ/g, with 2.80 kJ/g as a compromise.

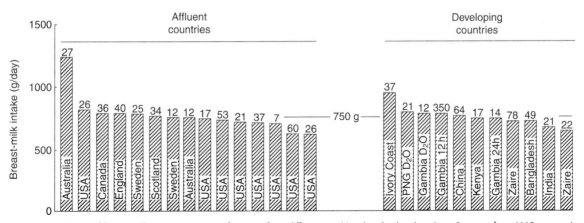

Figure 6.2 Similarity of breast-milk output in groups of women from different nutritional and cultural settings. Data are from 1118 women in 26 studies. (Reproduced with permission from Prentice *et al.*, 1996.)

Table 6.4 Estimates of the mean concentration of nutrients per liter of mature human milk

Nutrient	Amount	Unit
Lactose	72.0 ± 2.5	g
Protein	10.5 ± 2.0	g
Fat	39.0 ± 4.0	g
Minerals		
Calcium	280 ± 26	mg
Phosphorus	140 ± 22	mg
Magnesium	35 ± 2	mg
Iron	0.3 ± 0.1	mg
Zinc	1.2 ± 0.2	mg
Copper	0.25 ± 0.03	mg
Iodine	110 ± 40	μg
Selenium	20 ± 5	μg
Manganese	6 ± 2	μg
Fluoride	16 ± 5	μg
Chromium	50 ± 5	μg
Vitamins		
A^-	670 ± 200	RE
E	2.3 ± 1.0	mg
D	0.55 ± 0.10	μg
K	2.1 ± 0.1	μg
C	40 ± 10	mg
Thiamin	0.21 ± 0.03	mg
Riboflavin	0.35 ± 0.025	mg
Niacin	1.5 ± 0.2	mg
B_6	93 ± 8	mg
Folate	85 ± 37	μg
B_{12}	0.97	μg

Adapted from Institute of Medicine (1991).

Protein

Compared with the milk of other mammals, human milk contains a very low concentration of protein. It declines from 20–30 g/l at 1–5 days of lactation to 8–9 g/l at 1 month and to about 7 g/l at 3.5–6.5 months of lactation. Human milk proteins consist mainly of caseins (60%) and whey proteins (40%, mostly α-lactalbumin). Proteins in human milk have multiple functions:

- they supply the essential amino acids
- they protect against infection (sIgA, lactoferrin and lysosyme)
- they are components of lactose synthesis within the mammary gland
- they carry metals (calcium, zinc and magnesium).

The exact functions of non-protein nitrogen in human milk are mostly unknown. These compounds contribute about 25% to total nitrogen and include nitrogen-containing oligosaccharides ('bifidus factor'). Together with lactose, the principal carbohydrate (80%) in human milk, they enhance colonization of the intestine with *Lactobacillus bifidus*. In established lactation, the concentrations of lactose (70–74 g/l) and oligosaccharides (about 12 g/l) are high.

Fat

Fat is the most variable milk component. The lipid fraction not only contributes to the energy content of human milk, but also serves as a carrier of fat-soluble vitamins and certain fat-soluble hormones. In well-nourished women, milk fat averages about 37–40 g/l. A positive correlation exists between the milk fat concentration and measures of the mother's body fatness. More importantly, the nature of the fat consumed by the mother influences the fatty acid composition of milk, which provides the essential fatty acids linoleic acid (C18:2n-6) and linolenic acid (C18:3n-3), from which long-chain (20- and 22-carbon) polyunsaturated metabolites (LCPUFAs, e.g. docosahexaenoic acid, C22:6n-3) can be derived. These LCPUFAs have profound biological activity and, as structural component of membranes, they may affect cognitive development and visual acuity. Though human milk contains small amounts of LCPUFAs, these may benefit the psychomotor and visual development of the infant (see Chapter 9).

Vitamins and minerals

The water-soluble vitamins in milk are all linked to the current dietary intake of the mother. Thus, they respond quickly to supplementation of the mother's diet. Fat-soluble vitamins are less responsive, since maternal stores and carrier proteins are able to buffer the effects of inadequate postpartum intakes. Also, breast-milk concentrations of iron, zinc, chromium, copper, sodium, calcium and magnesium do not appear to be related to dietary intake. In general, it seems that milk nutrient levels are well protected, if necessary, through depletion of the mother's own body stores.

6.12 Recommended intakes during lactation

The total amount of nutrients secreted in milk is directly related to the extent and duration of lactation. Thus, nutrient needs during lactation depend primarily on the volume and composition of milk produced, and on the mother's initial nutrient needs and nutritional status. Severe effects on milk production occur when poor intakes in pregnancy are followed by poor intakes in lactation.

Table 6.5 Suggested figures for energy requirements during lactation

Period (month)	Milk volume (g/day)	Energy requirement (kJ/day)	
		Full costs	Allowing for fat loss
All women			
0–1	680	2380	1730
1–2	780	2730	2080
2–3	820	2870	2220
Full breast-feeders			
3–6	820	2870	2220
6–12	650	2275	2275
12–24	600	2100	2100
Partial breast-feeders			
3–6	410	1430	780
6–12	325	1140	1140
12–24	300	1050	1050

Reproduced with permission from Prentice *et al.* (1996).

Micronutrient intakes that often are of concern to lactating women include vitamin A (in developing countries), calcium, zinc, folate, and vitamins E, D and B_6.

Energy

There is a wide range of variability in breast-milk volume among women. This may vary from about 550 g to over 1000 g/day. Accordingly, energy needs can vary considerably between women. Average energy costs of lactation can be calculated as the sum of:

- maternal requirements, including non-pregnant, non-lactating requirements ± changes in activity; any effects of possible changes in physical activity are thus included in the maternal requirements
- breast milk volume × energy density × conversion efficiency
- ±changes in body fat.

Table 6.5 summarizes supplemental requirements, assuming

- energy density of milk to be 2.80 kJ/g
- a dietary milk energy conversion efficiency of 80%
- an allowance for fat loss of 500 g/month up to 6 months postpartum and nothing thereafter.

Amounts to be added to maternal requirements range from 1050 to 2870 kJ/day as full costs or from 1050 to 2275 kJ/day allowing for fat loss. There is little evidence of energy-sparing adaptations in BMR or dietary-induced thermogenesis, which have been suggested to compensate for part of the energy demand of lactation.

Lactating women predominantly meet the energy costs of lactation by increasing their energy intake. Some studies show that next to mobilization of body fat they tend to decrease their physical activity. The fat loss allowance is not considered obligatory, depending on the initial stores of the mother. In overweight women weight losses of approximately 2 kg/month do not seem to affect milk production or infant growth adversely. For undernourished, stressed women the fat loss allowance should probably not be assumed, particularly when pregnancy fat gain has been minimal.

Protein

Additional recommended protein intakes (FAO/WHO/UNU, 1985) during lactation amount to:

- 16–17 g/day for 0–6 months of lactation
- 12.3 g/day for 6–12 months of lactation
- 11.3 g/day for 12–24 months of lactation.

As yet, there is no clear evidence that low maternal protein intake compromises milk volume, although some short-term studies suggest an impact on the milk nitrogen fraction.

Vitamin A

Estimates of vitamin A requirements during lactation have been based on calculations of how much would be needed to replace that excreted daily in breast milk (Table 6.6). There is a relatively wide range of recommended daily allowances, from 850 IU/day (WHO/FAO) to 1300 IU/day (US), related to the extent of inadequate vitamin A status, vitamin A availability and the socioeconomic constraints of the community. Useful specific guidelines for supplementation have been published by WHO. In industrialized countries there is no need for vitamin A supplementation. In areas of endemic vitamin A deficiency caution should be applied regarding vitamin A supplementation, given the potential risk of teratogenesis.

Folate

The folate concentration of human milk remains relatively constant. The average daily amount secreted in human milk is estimated to be 85 μg/l. The additional dietary intake needed to provide this amount is 133 μg/day. Women who are only partially breast-feeding would need less.

Table 6.6 Recommended levels for micronutrient intake during lactation

Micronutrient	Food and Nutrition Board, National Academy of Sciences–Institute of Medicine (1998–2001)			WHO
	EAR	RDA		
Thiamin (mg/day)	1.2	1.5	+0.2	1970, RNI
Riboflavin (mg/day)	1.3	1.6	+0.4	1965, RNI
Niacin (mg/day)	13	17	+3.7	1970, RNI
Vitamin B_6 (mg/day)	1.7	2.0		
Folate (μg/day)	450	500	270	1988, safe level
Vitamin B_{12} (μg/day)	2.4	2.8	1.3	1988, safe level
Pantothenic acid (mg/day)[a]	7			
Biotin (μg/day)[a]	35			
Choline (mg/day)[a]	550			
Iron (mg/day)	7/6.5 (14–18/19–50 years)	10/9 (14–18/19–50 years)	10.5	Median basal requirement
Calcium (mg/day)[a]	1000		1000–1200	1961, RNI
Phosphorus (mg/day)	580/1055 (19–50/14–18 years)	700/1250		
Magnesium (mg/day)	265/255/300 (31–50/19–30/14–18 years)	320/310/360		
Vitamin D (μg/day)[a]	5.0		10	1970, RNI
Fluoride (mg/day)	2.9/3.1 (14–18/19–50 years)			
Vitamin A (μg/day)	880/900 (14–18/19–50 years)	1200/1300 (14–18/19–50 years)	850	1988, safe level
Vitamin C (mg/day)	96/100 (up to 18/19–50 years)	115/120	50	1970, RNI
Vitamin E (α-tocopherol) (mg/day)	16	19	0.15–2 mg/kg	1987, ADI
Selenium (μg/day)	59	70		40, normative requirement

[a] AI: adequate intake; instead of RDA if sufficient scientific evidence is not available.
EAR: estimated average requirement; RNI: reference nutrient intake, 2 SD above EAR; RDA: recommended dietary allowance, 2 SD above EAR; Safe level is the upper end of normative storage requirement.

Vitamin D and calcium

Available data indicate that vitamin D requirements are not increased during lactation. Concentrations of vitamin D in breast milk are low, between 12 and 60 IU/l. Although the milk 25-hydroxy-vitamin D [25(OH)D] concentration correlates with maternal 25(OH)D concentration and maternal vitamin D intake, infant 25(OH)D concentrations do no not correlate with milk 25(OH)D, unless the mother receives high doses of supplemental vitamin D (e.g. 2000 IU/day). Within 8 weeks of delivery, vitamin D stores are depleted in vitamin D-replete mothers. Therefore, just after birth vitamin D should be administered to newborns when maternal vitamin D status is poor, and dietary guidance for lactation women should include recommendations for good sources of calcium. Daily supplementation with 10 μg/day should be considered for mothers who avoid

milk, eggs and fish, as well as for populations with limited sunshine exposure.

As is the case in pregnancy, lactation is a period of high calcium requirement. If milk products are not a major part of the diet it is difficult for many lactating women to consume the recommended amount. During lactation physiological adaptive processes ensure that calcium is provided for milk production. Thus, although there are wide differences among women, the concentration of calcium in breast milk is not influenced by the calcium intake of the mother during the breast-feeding period. Furthermore, calcium nutrition does not influence the changes in bone mineral status and calcium and bone metabolism, and these changes are not responsive to an increase in calcium intake by breast-feeding women. This recent scientific evidence supports the view that calcium increments are no longer necessary in lactation, despite the current poor understanding of mechanisms involved in calcium regulation in lactation.

6.13 Energy and nutrient inadequacies

In general, lactating women are considered at high risk of energy and nutrient inadequacies. Selected groups of lactating women may need special nutritional attention, including:

- groups with restricted eating patterns
- complete vegetarians
- women who diet to lose weight
- women who avoid dairy products
- women on a low income.

Vegetarian mothers

In vegetarian women, vitamin D and calcium status may be low and vitamin B_{12} deficiency has been reported in their offspring. Given sufficient sunlight exposure, supplemental vitamin D does not appear to be necessary and the low calcium intake in vegetarian women does not result in a lower milk calcium content. One of the major nutritional concerns for vegetarian women is vitamin B_{12}, a lack of which leads to elevated methyl malonic acid levels in both mothers and infants.

Mothers with insulin-dependent diabetes mellitus

The goal of treatment of insulin-dependent diabetes mellitus (IDDM) during lactation is to decrease infant mortality and morbidity as well as the sequelae of the disease in the mother. Extra needs of lactation must be recognized, and both energy and insulin dose adjusted to meet those needs. To ensure adequate infant nutrition, mothers with IDDM should receive lactation counseling, addressing all factors that may influence the success of lactation: hyperglycemia, hypoglycemia, method of delivery, feeding frequency, fetal condition, gestational age, incidence of mastitis, metabolic control and maternal dietary intake.

Maternal caloric restriction and exercise during lactation

Following lactation many women in affluent populations are eager to return to their pre-pregnancy weight. To achieve this goal they may restrict energy intake or increase exercise. For women with adequate reserves milk energy output is maintained even if they are losing weight up to 0.5 kg/week. Only when women with low energy reserves are in negative energy balance does milk energy output decrease. The threshold at which low energy reserves and negative energy balance affect milk energy output is, however, yet to be identified.

6.14 Perspectives on the future

Research is needed to identify the threshold of nutritional status at which mothers can no longer sustain lactation. Cross-cultural comparisons that suggest that lactational performance is remarkably unaffected by environmental factors need further confirmation since many possible confounding differences may exist between cultures.

More research is required to define whether low nutrient intakes before or during pregnancy can have deleterious effects on lactational performance.

Supplementation studies in undernourished mothers are needed to confirm the ecological studies and to explore the impact of supplementation practices on lactational performance. So far there have been few studies to show that improving maternal dietary intake increases infant milk intake. Such studies might also add to the little information available on the relationship between maternal nutrition and the well-being of lactating women.

Further reading

Pregnancy

Abrams B, Altman SL, Pickett KE. Pregnancy weight gain: still controversial. Am J Clin Nutr 2000; 71 (Suppl): 1233S–1241S.
Dewey KG. Energy and protein requirements during lactation. Annu Rev Nutr 1997; 17: 19–36.
FAO/WHO/UNU. Energy and Protein Requirements. Geneva: World Health Organization, 1995.
King JC. Physiology of pregnancy and nutrient metabolism. Am J Clin Nutr 2000; 71 (Suppl): 1218S–1225S.
National Academy of Sciences. Dietary Reference Intakes for Thiamin, Riboflavin, Niacin, Vitamin B_6, Folate, Vitamin B_{12}, Pantothenic Acid, Biotin and Choline. www.nap.edu 2000

Lactation

Bates CJ, Prentice A. Breast milk as a source of vitamins, essential minerals and trace elements. Pharmacol Ther 1994; 62: 193–220.
Dewey KG. Energy and protein requirements during lactation. Annu Rev Nutr 1997; 17: 19–36.
Institute of Medicine. Nutrition During Lactation. Washington, DC: National Academy Press, 1991.
Prentice AM, Spaaij CJK, Goldberg GR et al. Energy requirements of pregnant and lactating women. Eur J Clin Nutr 1996; 50 (Suppl 1): S82–S111.
Wilde CJ, Prentice A, Peaker M. Breast-feeding: matching supply with demand in human lactation. Proc Nutr Soc 1995; 54: 401–406.

7
Growth and Aging

ML Wahlqvist, A Kouris-Blazos, KA Ross, TL Setter and P Tienboon

Key messages

- Growth provides an indication of nutritional status in preadult years.
- Changes in body composition and anthropometry reflect changes in growth and thus nutritional status.
- Nutritional needs change in accordance with the demands of growth throughout the different stages of life.
- The interplay of genetic and environmental factors determines growth outcomes and disease risk.
- Undernutrition during the early years of life can drastically impair growth, and can affect stature and health outcomes in later life.
- Catch-up growth is a phenomenon that compensates for deviations in growth from the genetic trajectory.
- Maximal height may not be equivalent to 'optimal' height with respect to positive health outcomes.

- Obesity and overweight in early life, and especially during adolescence, increase the likelihood of obesity and associated risk factors in adult life.
- Chronological and biological age do not necessarily correlate.
- Energy requirements generally decrease with age; however, nutrient needs remain relatively high; animal studies suggest that energy restriction promotes longevity, but human studies suggest that 'eating better not less' is desirable.
- Physical activity can improve health and well-being, and reduce morbidity risk at any stage of the lifespan.
- Many health problems commonly associated with older age are not necessarily products of 'aging'; instead they can be prevented or delayed by consuming a nutritionally adequate diet and engaging in regular physical activity.

7.1 Introduction

Nutrition plays an important role in human growth and development throughout life. Infancy and childhood are important times for nutrition and growth as they strongly predict health outcomes later in life. Nutrition once again plays an important role in later life, when prevention of chronic disease and system degeneration becomes a major priority. All people require the same nutrients to maintain health and well-being, but these are required in differing amounts according to their stage of life. Optimal growth and healthy aging will occur if nutritional requirements are met and environmental influences are conducive to health throughout life.

7.2 Growth and development

'Growth' may be defined as the acquisition of tissue with a concomitant increase in body size. 'Development' refers to changes in the body's capacity to function both physically and intellectually through increased tissue and organ complexity. Different individuals experience these processes at different rates.

There are five stages under which major growth and developmental changes occur in humans:

- infancy
- childhood
- adolescence
- adulthood
- late adulthood.

These stages can be distinguished by changes in growth velocity and distinct biological and behavioral characteristics. Nutritional needs change in response to the demands that these stages of growth place on the body. If nutritional needs are met and adverse social circumstances or disease are not encountered, optimal growth will occur.

Cellular aspects of growth and death

Cell division

Cells are subject to wear and tear as well as to accidents and death. Therefore, we must create new cells at a rate as fast as that at which our cells die. As a result, cell division is central to the life of all organisms. Cell division or the M phase (M = mitotic) consists of two sequential processes: nuclear division called mitosis and cytoplasmic division called cytokinesis. Before a cell can divide it must double its mass and duplicate all of its contents to ensure that the new cell contains all the components required to begin its own cycle of cell growth followed by division. Preparation for division goes on invisibly during the growth phase of the cell cycle, denoted as interphase. Cells spend 90% of their lifetime in interphase, during which cell components are continuously being made. Interphase can last for up to 16–24 h, whereas the M phase lasts for only 1–2 h. Interphase starts with the G_1 phase (G = gap) in which the cells, whose biosynthetic activities have been slowed during the M phase, resume a high rate of biosynthesis. The S phase begins when DNA synthesis starts, and ends when the DNA content of the nucleus has doubled and the chromosomes have replicated. When DNA synthesis is complete the cell enters the G_2 phase, which ends when mitosis starts. Terminally differentiated and other non-replicating cells represent a quiescent stage, often referred to as G_0 phase (Figure 7.1).

In multicellular animals, like humans, the survival of the organism is paramount, not the survival of any of its individual cells. As a result, the 10^{13} cells of the human body divide at very different rates depending on their location and are programmed and coordinated with their neighbors. Something in the order of 10^{16} cell divisions take place in a human body in the course of a lifetime. Different cell types have given up their potential for rapid division so that their numbers can be kept at a level that is optimal for the organism as whole. Some cells, such as red blood cells, do not divide again once they are mature. Other cells, such as epithelial cells, divide continuously. The observed cell-cycle

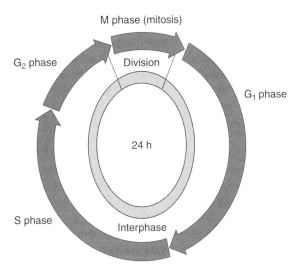

Figure 7.1 Cell growth and division: the four successive phases of a typical cell cycle.

times, also called generation times, range from 8 h to 100 days or more. Cells that are not actively proliferating have a reduced rate of protein synthesis and are arrested in G_1 phase. Once a cell has become committed to divide by passing a special restriction point (R) in its cycle in G_1, it will make DNA in the S phase and proceed through to the next stages. Cells arrested at R stop growing but do not stop biosynthesis. This growth-control mechanism involving a specific restriction point may have evolved partly because of the need for a safe resting state (at R) for cells whose growth conditions or interactions with other cells demand that they stop dividing. Cells that have been arrested at this stable resting state are said to have entered a G_0 phase of the cell cycle. Whether or not a cell will grow and divide is determined by a variety of feedback control mechanisms. These include the availability of space in which a cell can flatten (contact inhibition of cell division) and the secretion of specific stimulatory and inhibitory factors (peptides, steroids, hormones, short-range local chemical mediators and others still to be identified) by cells in the immediate environment.

Cancer cells have escaped from or respond abnormally to many of these control mechanisms that regulate cell division. Cancer cells require fewer protein growth factors than do normal cells in order to survive and divide in culture; in some cases this may be because they produce their own growth factors. A second fundamental difference between normal and cancer cells is that the latter can go on dividing indefinitely. For example, cells taken from older animals will divide fewer times in culture than the same cells taken from young animals, suggesting that older cells have used up many of their alloted divisions while in the animal. As cells differentiate they become programmed to die after a certain number of divisions. This programmed cell death is an additional safeguard against the unbridled growth of one particular cell. However, cancer involves something more than just abnormalities of proliferation and programmed senescence; it requires the coincidental occurrence of several specific mutations in a single cell, enabling it to proliferate in disregard of the usual constraints and to invade regions of the body from which it would normally be excluded.

Cell death

Apoptosis is an active process in which cells undergo genetically programmed death. Apoptosis occurs when a calcium-dependent enzyme (endonuclease) fragments the genome of the cell into approximately 180 base pairs. The dead cells are then removed by phagocytosis. It is still unclear how many mechanisms are involved in causing cell death, but it is known that alterations in intracellular calcium levels can trigger apoptosis. Cell death appears to be activated by special genes in dying cells. For cell death to occur, genes identified as *ced-3* and *ced-4* must be expressed in a dying cell. A third gene, *ced-9*, is a major control factor, which negatively regulates the *ced-3* and *ced-4* genes. Animal studies have shown that mutations to *ced-9* inactivate the gene, causing the death of cells that were otherwise intended to survive, and thereby killing the animal under study. Cell senescence occurs when the cell does not divide or proliferate and DNA synthesis is blocked. Cells are programmed to carry out a finite number of divisions, which is called the Hayflick limit. If cells do not reach senescence they continue to divide, in effect becoming immortal. Immortal cells eventually form tumors, so this is an area where aging research and cancer research intersect. It is thought that senescence may have evolved because it protected against cancer. Cells exhibiting evidence of DNA damage and oxidative stress may recover from those stresses, provided they are equipped with an adequate DNA repair system and an adequate level of stress-response proteins, and/or antioxidant defenses. Most theories that aim to explain the aging process suggest that senescence results from the accumulation of unrepaired

damage. Telomeres (the sections of DNA at the end of chromosomes) shorten with each division of the cell, resulting in a set lifetime for each normal cell. Inhibition of telomerase is thought to reduce cellular aging. Although genes play an important role and can be an indicator of disease risk in later life, environmental factors also strongly influence the development of disease. The general degenerative properties of aging are also a factor in disease development. Greater understanding of the molecular events regulating cell progression and apoptosis is rapidly emerging. The non-nutritional and nutritional factors affecting cell division and growth are outlined below.

Non-nutritional factors affecting growth

Growth is influenced by a number of important factors including genetics and endocrine control, and also by the surrounding environment, such as nutritional factors, social factors (socioeconomic status and cultural practice) and psychological factors. For example, physical growth of school children aged 6–9 years is the result of both environmental and genetic factors and the interaction between these two factors. It is too simplistic to think that these factors affect growth in isolation, as ultimately, it is the interaction of all of these factors that will affect growth. It is often difficult to isolate the effects on growth of these individual factors as they are often closely linked.

Genetic factors

Genetic factors play arguably the most important role in determining growth and development outcomes. It is clear that the genetic make-up of the individual and what is inherited from previous generations greatly influence how they advance through life. Studies of twins have shown that patterns of growth, age of menarche, body shape, composition and size, and deposition of fat are all closely linked to genetic factors. Many studies support a genetic component in obesity-related traits. Height is influenced strongly by genetic predisposition, whereas weight appears to be mostly influenced by environment. The effects of genetic control are often quite explicit and limited in terms of their action. Dental maturation, for example, appears to be independent of skeletal maturation, and some evidence suggests that genes regulating the growth of different sections of limbs are also independent. Evolution and genetic factors largely explain racial differences, although the role of socioeconomic and educational advantage and disadvantage, and of living conditions, including food, is likely to be underestimated. For example, skeletal maturation and growth rates differ between white American children and black African–Americans in the first few years of life. While this is largely attributed to genetic factors, increasing evidence for intragenerational and intergenerational effects of intrauterine nutrition and early childhood rearing are important qualifiers.

Gender differences are predominantly explained by genetic factors, such as differences in both the timing of the adolescent growth spurt and the sex-specific changes that occur during puberty. At the age of 10 years, males and females are of a similar height, weight and body fatness. However, after puberty major differences are evident. Although the timing of the growth spurt is largely genetically controlled, hormonal factors are thought to control its intensity and duration, while environmental factors also play an important role. Females typically achieve skeletal maturation at an earlier age than males. Genes on the Y chromosome, which are found only in males, are thought to retard skeletal maturation relative to females. A disturbance in the expression of a single gene or group of genes can have widespread and drastic effects leading to compromised growth and development. Insults to gene expression during intrauterine life, in particular, can have important consequences in later life in terms of growth and development, and even in the formation of degenerative diseases. Inborn errors of metabolism such as phenylketonuria, galactosemia and hereditary fructose intolerance are all genetic conditions that require vigilant dietary management to avoid deficiencies of essential nutrients.

Hormones and growth factors

Hormones are responsible for coordinating much of the appropriate timing and rates of growth. There are many hormones that have recognized effects on growth. There are generally three distinct endocrine phases of linear growth: infancy (including fetal growth), childhood and puberty. Each of these phases is regulated by different endocrine growth-promoting systems. Thyroid and parathyroid hormones, through thyroxine and triiodothyronine, stimulate general metabolism. Other hormones and growth factors include epidermal growth factor (important in actions in the epidermis), platelet-derived growth factor (involved in blood clots and possibly cell division) and melatonin (has a role in regulating puberty and possibly growth

velocity). Hormones are largely responsible for many of the changes in body composition and the development of secondary sexual characteristics that occur as individuals age. The effects of hormones are often influenced and regulated by other hormones and growth factors.

One of the most important hormones that regulates growth is human growth hormone (GH). GH exerts a powerful effect on growth, at least in part, through somatomedins or insulin-like growth factors (IGF-I, IGF-2). IGF acts by stimulating muscle cell differentiation and is therefore important in fetal and postnatal growth and development. GH is important in regulating protein synthesis and cellular division, and is thus thought to be the major regulator of the rate of human growth and development from the latter few months of the first year of life. Synthetic forms of GH are regularly used in a clinical setting to encourage growth in children of a small stature. It is thought that sex steroids, which are active around puberty, may trigger significant secretions of GH, and thus IGF. Hormones such as thyroxine and cortisol may also influence IGF plasma levels. Disturbances to genetic programming *in utero* during critical phases of fetal development may result in impairment of the endocrine factors responsible for growth in later life. Studies have reported associations between growth retardation and abnormalities in levels of hormones such as GH and hormone-mediated factors such as IGF.

Neural control

It has been proposed that within the brain there is a central 'growth centre' that is responsible for regulating growth. The hypothalamus has been implicated as a possible growth centre owing to its close association with the anterior pituitary, a hormonal gland closely involved in growth. By this action, any deviation of growth from its predetermined genetic pathway will be identified by the hypothalamus, and compensated for the subsequent release of growth specific hormones from the anterior pituitary gland to compensate for any growth or developmental impairment. The peripheral nervous system may also play an important role in growth. This effect is thought to be through the secretion of neural chemicals that can then influence growth.

Local biochemical control

Areas of localized growth rely on complex regional influences, whether they are mechanical or chemical stimuli, for optimal growth. These can be paracrine factors, such as neighboring proteins acting as local signaling and growth factors, or autocrine factors, such as hormones or growth factors, that influence the growth of quite localized areas despite being secreted from a more distant position. These mechanisms appear to be responsible for the growth of specific tissue. Furthermore, the age of groups of cells or a specific tissue can determine the amount of cell replication and division that is possible. This is the case where cells undergo a finite number of mitotic divisions.

Social and cultural factors

The major social factors affecting growth are culture, age, family, gender and socioeconomic status. Emotional disorders have also been related to growth abnormalities. Different countries or regions may exhibit their own cultures and cuisines, which reflect a mixture of geographical, agricultural, historical, religious and economic factors, among others. These factors may either directly or indirectly affect growth through their influence on a number of factors such as health, nutrition, food selection and cooking methods. Infants and children who emigrate to other areas may often experience changes to growth patterns. Generational differences in stature, for example, often reflect changing environments. Many adolescents eagerly seek independence, and factors associated with this have an effect on nutritional status. Physical activity levels, peer pressure, self-esteem and distorted body image, chronic dieting and disordered eating, and substance abuse are all factors that can affect nutritional status and thus growth. Chronic dieting, in particular, can also place an individual at risk of many micronutrient deficiencies, compromised immune function, infertility, long-term degenerative diseases such as osteoporosis and a compromised immune system, which can negatively affect growth and health outcomes.

Family factors that have been associated with compromised growth and development include single-parent families, family conflict, and disturbance to the family unit such as divorce and separation. Growth retardation in conflict situations may partly be a result of stress, which is thought to affect GH levels. The amount of care and attention that an infant receives will also have an important impact on growth. This can be related to the number children and birth position in the family. Various cultures may practice a gender bias, and favor one gender over the other. This can be

seen to a larger degree in developing countries where boys may be more favored and thus receive more care and nourishment. In both developing and industrialized countries, socioeconomic status is associated with many behavioral, nutritional and health outcomes which can influence growth. Usually children of a higher socioeconomic class are taller, display faster growth rates and become taller adults. Children of lower classes are typically smaller at birth, shorter and, particularly in industrialized countries, have higher levels of body fat. Socioeconomic status is also a strong predictor of certain micronutrient deficiencies, such as vitamin A and iron deficiencies.

Independently, educational attainment and income have been positively associated with growth and development, mainly through the alleviation of poverty. Females, in particular, benefit from schooling, as they are able to exert greater control over their environment and show improved growth and pregnancy outcomes. Typically, as income increases a larger amount of money will be spent on animal products such as meat owing to the prestige factor associated with such foods. The inclusion of greater amounts of animal protein in the diet can influence growth and development. Infant feeding practices, such as breast-feeding and weaning, may also follow culturally or socially acceptable patterns of a region. Women of higher socioeconomic status are known to breast-feed for longer periods than women of lower classes. This can have important growth and development outcomes on the infant. Dental caries are common in both developing and industrialized countries where dental hygiene is inadequate and in areas where water fluoridation is absent. Dietary factors associated with increased dental caries under such conditions include the regular consumption of foods high in sucrose, particularly sticky sweet forms.

7.3 Nutritional factors affecting growth

In order for growth to proceed at its predetermined genetic rate, adequate nutrition is essential. Food supplies the individual with the required energy, nutrients and food components to influence growth. The strong link between food intake and growth was supported from studies of food intake patterns during famines encountered at the time of the two world wars. Children of Dutch and German families living in these areas exhibited impaired growth, while in Japan, a reduction in the mean height of adults was observed between 1945 and 1949. Nutrition affects all body systems and factors influencing growth. For example, a compromised nutrient intake can influence gene replication and expression, hormonal control, neural control and other environmental factors that are important for growth.

Inadequate nutrition is the predominant factor leading to malnutrition, which can be expressed as either undernutrition or overnutrition. Undernutrition occurs when there is not only inadequate energy but also a lack or imbalance of specific food components and nutrients. Chronic energy deficiency, commonly referred to as protein–energy malnutrition (PEM), occurs in both developing and industrialized countries; however, it is more prevalent in the former. Characteristic features of PEM include stunted growth, delayed maturation, reduced muscle mass and decreased physical working capacity.

In addition to sufficient energy, adequate supplies of macronutrients and micronutrients are required to promote optimum growth. The proportions and amounts of these nutrients may change according to the various stages of growth. For example, protein is a prerequisite for optimal growth at all life stages, while fat may arguably have its most important role during infancy and childhood as a major supplier of energy and long-chain polyunsaturated (n-3) fatty acids, which are important in neural development. Components of certain foods, called growth factors, may have powerful effects on growth. For example, some of the proteins present in milk are thought to promote growth. Population groups that consume large amounts of milk also typically exhibit taller statures.

Nutritional status is found to affect greatly hormonal status. GH, for example, will not stimulate linear growth unless there is adequate nutrition. IGF plasma levels appear to respond closely to acute directional changes in the body's nitrogen balance. This suggests that the ingestion of several dietary components, such as essential amino acids, adequate energy and optimal nitrogen balance, may be critical for optimal hormonal control. When this is not the case, it may have negative effects on growth and development. Food and its components, such as metabolites of vitamins A and D, fatty acids, some sterols and zinc, can directly influence gene expression and thus growth. Components of dietary fiber are thought to influence gene expression indirectly by a number of pathways,

Table 7.1 Micronutrients affecting growth

Children	Adolescents
Iodide	Calcium
Zinc	Folate
Iron	
Vitamin A	
Riboflavin	
Vitamin C	
Vitamin D	

including altering hormonal signaling, mechanical stimulation and through metabolites produced by flora of the intestine. The micronutrients that are frequently held responsible for much of the functional impairment and growth retardation experienced globally are shown in Table 7.1.

Iodide

Iodide deficiency at different life stages produces differing health outcomes. Its intake is of most critical importance *in utero* and during the first 2 years of life, when neural cells in the brain undergo major cellular division. Adequate iodide intakes during these times are therefore essential for mental and cognitive growth and development. The extent of mental dysfunction may be lessened if sufficient dietary iodide levels are administered in the early years of life. Complications associated with iodide deficiency in childhood and adolescence may appear as goiter, hypothyroidism, mental dysfunction, retarded mental and physical growth and reduced school performance.

Vitamin A

Severe deficiency in vitamin A is commonly associated with impaired vision, retarded growth and development, poor bone health, compromised immune functioning, and complications with reproductive health and outcomes. In industrialized countries, vitamin A deficiency is rare. Too much vitamin A in the diet can also slow growth. Subclinical vitamin A deficiency greatly increases the risk of morbidity and mortality in vulnerable population groups. Reductions in mortality rates of around 20–25% can be achieved by improving the vitamin A status in young children in populations where deficiency has been identified.

Zinc

Zinc is of crucial importance in over 200 enzyme reactions. It is of structural and functional importance in biomembranes, DNA, RNA and ribosomal structures. Zinc deficiency has been linked with disturbed gene expression, protein synthesis, immunity, skeletal growth and maturation, gonad development, pregnancy outcomes, behavior, skin integrity, eyesight, appetite and taste perception. Zinc deficiency can cause major intrauterine growth retardation (IUGR) if the maternal diet provides inadequate sources of zinc. It is therefore of great importance for linear growth as well as the development of lean body mass.

Iron

In industrialized countries, iron represents the major micronutrient deficiency; however, in developing countries iron deficiency occurs on a much larger scale. Although iron is important at all life stages, iron deficiency commonly affects preschool and school-aged children who as a consequence face compromised growth if dietary intake is inadequate. Iron is very important in pregnant women, as low intakes can have wide implications for the newborn infant born with limited iron stores. The effects of iron deficiency are varied; however, a major effect is its impairment of cognitive development in children. Other consequences of iron deficiency include a reduced work capacity and a decreased resistance to fatigue.

Other nutrients

Other nutrients of importance to growth include vitamin B_2, which affects general growth, vitamin C, which is important in bone structure, and vitamin D, which is involved in calcium absorption from the intestines. Chronically low dietary intakes of these vitamins can greatly impair growth and bone health. Calcium and folate appear to be micronutrients of importance for growth during adolescence.

Phytochemicals

There is emerging evidence that certain phytochemicals, such as the isoflavones genistein and daidzein (found in legumes, especially soy), may help to inhibit tumor formation by regulating cell-cycle progression, by promoting cell differentiation and apoptosis (cell death). Formation of new vasculature is required for a cancer to grow and metastasize; isoflavones have also been identified as antiangiogenic agents that inhibit the formation of new vasculature and thus the development and dissemination of tumors.

7.4 Nutrition and the life cycle

Energy and nutrient needs differ according to the different life stages and it is important for food intake to reflect these changing demands. Inadequate nutrition exerts its most detrimental impact on prepubertal growth. Supplementation programs and interventions that are provided before this time will have the most beneficial growth and development outcomes. Nutrient needs during infancy are influenced by length of gestation, the newborn's nutrient reserves, body composition, growth rate, activity levels, and the length and duration of breast-feeding. An infant is wholly dependent on a carer for some or all nourishment, ideally via breast milk.

The essential long-chain fatty acids (LCPUFA), such as the n-3 fatty acids docosahexaenoic acid (DHA) and arachidonic acid (AA), are important structurally in cell membranes, particularly in the central nervous system. Most infant formulae contain only the precursor essential fatty acids, α-linolenic acid (ALA, the n-3 precursor) and linoleic acid (LA, the n-6 precursor), from which infants must assemble their own DHA and AA, respectively. Studies have suggested that such formulae may not be effective in meeting the full essential fatty acid requirements that are needed by most infants. Reduced cognitive, motor and visual acuity outcomes have been reported in formula-fed infants compared with their breast-fed counterparts; however, not all studies have reported such findings. From 6 to 24 months of infant life, breast-feeding alone cannot provide all of the nutrients and energy needed to promote and sustain adequate growth. Therefore, complementary feeding is necessary. If complementary feeding is introduced too late there is a risk of impaired growth, macronutrient deficiency, impaired cognitive and physical development, and stunting as a result of PEM.

Early weaning (4 months or earlier) has been associated with negative health outcomes, such as the formation of allergies, diarrhea and even death. Chronic or episodic diarrhea may affect the absorption of nutrients which, if not addressed, may lead to growth impairment. Common reasons for introducing complementary feeding with formula milk or solids include a perceived inferior quality of milk, poor weight gain, difficulties or pain with feeding, mother's employment, refusal by the infant to feed and lack of mother's confidence. Many people perceive formula to be of higher quality than breast milk, particularly as a result of aggressive marketing strategies from infant formula manufacturers. This may cause the mother to abandon exclusive breast-feeding from an early age. In 2001 the World Health Organization (WHO) released a systematic review on the optimal duration of exclusive breast-feeding. These results indicate that breast-feeding should be exclusive for the first 6 months of life (http://www.who.int/inf-pr-2001/en/note2001-07.html).

Some individuals experience erratic growth during childhood, largely reflecting changes in appetite and food intake, or even an underlying illness. Nutrient needs increase throughout childhood, reflecting the continuing growth of all body systems. Children can exhibit good growth and thrive on most lacto-ovo vegetarian and vegan diets provided they are well planned and supplemented. Growth delays have occasionally been reported in children fed severely restricted diets (primarily macrobiotic, Rastafarian and fruitarian forms). However, by school age, the growth of vegetarians and non-vegetarians becomes more alike. Few differences have been found in the timing of puberty or completed adult growth. Little effect is evident on intelligence quotient (IQ), assuming a reasonably adequate vegetarian diet. Typically, girls tend to consume less than boys at all ages. However, it is during adolescence that males begin to increase their intake to levels well above that of most females. Adolescence is a time that requires the greatest total energy intake of all of the life stages, as a result of the body being in a highly metabolically active state. Inadequate intakes of nutrients and energy during this time can potentially impede growth and delay sexual maturation. Pregnancy during adolescence has many increased risks for both the mother and the child, as the fetus and the mother must compete for nutrients to maintain and promote their respective growth. This is of even greater concern if the adolescent is malnourished. Calcium is of particular concern, as it is needed for continuing bone development in the mother while also being required in large quantities by the developing fetus. Birth and maternal complications during adolescent pregnancy are greater than those for older women of similar nutritional status. For example, adolescent mothers face increased risks of infant and maternal mortality, preterm delivery and giving birth to babies prematurely and of a low birth weight. The Australian dietary guidelines for children and adolescents and the American dietary guidelines for healthy people over 2 years old are shown in Tables 7.2 and 7.3.

Table 7.2 Australian dietary guidelines for children and adolescents, 1995

1. Encourage and support breastfeeding
2. Children need appropriate food and physical activity to grow and develop normally. Growth should be checked regularly
3. Enjoy a wide variety of nutritious foods
4. Eat plenty of breads, cereals, vegetables (including legumes) and fruits
5. Low-fat diets are not suitable for young children. For older children, a diet low in fat and in particular, low in saturated fat, is appropriate
6. Encourage water as a drink. Alcohol is not recommended for children
7. Eat only a moderate amount of sugars and foods containing added sugars
8. Choose low-salt foods

Guidelines on specific nutrients
1. Eat foods containing calcium
2. Eat foods containing iron

Source: National Health and Medical Research Council (1995). © Commonwealth of Australia. Reproduced with permission.

Table 7.3 American dietary guidelines for healthy people over 2 years old, 2000

Aim for fitness
Aim for a healthy weight
Be physically active each day

Build a healthy base
Let the pyramid guide your food choices
Choose a variety of grains daily, especially whole grains
Choose a variety of fruits and vegetables daily
Keep food safe to eat

Choose sensibly
Choose a diet that is low in saturated fat and cholesterol and moderate in total fat
Choose beverages and foods to moderate your intake of sugars
Choose and prepare foods with less salt
If you drink alcoholic beverages, do so in moderation

Source: USDA (2000).

The guidelines are listed in descending order of priority.

7.5 Effects of undernutrition

Identifying the cause of undernourishment is not always an easy task. Inadequate dietary intake may not be the sole cause. Social, cultural, genetic, hormonal, economic and political factors may also be important. Underlying health problems and inadequate care and hygiene may also be contributing factors to undernourishment.

The outcomes of undernutrition are largely determined by its severity and duration. Consequences of undernutrition include death, disability, and stunted mental and physical growth. Poor nutrition often commences *in utero* and in many cases extends into adolescence and adult life. Females in particular are affected by lifelong poor nutrition. Evidence from epidemiological studies from both developing and industrialized countries now suggests a causal relationship between fetal undernutrition and increased risks of impaired growth and various adult chronic diseases. This is the basis of the fetal origins of disease hypothesis. Wasting is often one of the earliest signs of acute undernutrition. Wasting can be detected by reduced measures of weight-for-age and skinfold thickness, reflecting a loss of weight or a failure to gain weight. In severe cases of undernourishment, individuals may exhibit other clinical symptoms such as hair loss, skin discoloration or pigmentation (in marasmus) and edema (in kwashiorkor), and evidence of deficiencies that are characteristic of specific nutrients. Stunting reflects chronic undernutrition and is detected as impaired linear growth. However, where stunting and wasting are both present, as in chronic cases of undernourishment, growth charts may not detect abnormal weights (or heights)-for-length owing to proportional growth retardation of both weight and height (or length). A stunted infant is likely to remain stunted throughout childhood and adolescence and is likely to become a stunted adult, particularly if the individual continues to live in the same environment that instigated the stunting. Adult stunting and underweight have direct effects not only on a woman's health and productivity, but also by increasing the risks of pregnancy complications such as gestational diabetes and the likelihood that her offspring will be born of a low birth weight (LBW); thus, stunting commonly spans generations.

Most growth impairment, of which underweight and stunting are outcomes, occurs within a relatively short period, from before birth until about 2 years of age. Severe undernutrition during infancy can be particularly damaging to the growth of the brain. This can result in major retardation of cognitive growth and functioning. Delayed intellectual development is a risk factor for absenteeism from school and poor school performance. Infants born of LBW who have suffered IUGR are born undernourished and face a greatly increased risk of mortality in the neonatal period or later infancy. Suboptimal intakes of energy, protein, vitamin A, zinc and iron during the early years of life may exacerbate the effects of fetal growth retardation. There is a cumulative negative impact on the growth and development of an LBW infant if undernutrition continues during childhood, adolescence and pregnancy. The LBW infant is thus more likely to be underweight or stunted in early life. Undernourished girls tend to have a delayed menarche and grow at lower velocities but for longer periods compared with their better nourished counterparts. This means that they may attain similar heights to better nourished girls, if undernutrition is limited to adolescence. However, if childhood stunting was also experienced, undernourished adolescent females are unlikely to reach similar heights to well-nourished girls. Optimal development during adolescence is reliant on both the present and past nutritional intake. Malnourishment and impaired growth during infancy and early childhood can greatly affect an individual's attainment of height.

Catch-up growth

Catch-up or catch-down growth is a phenomenon that appears to compensate for retarded or accelerated intrauterine growth, whereby children return to their genetic trajectory. Many studies have suggested that the potential for catch-up growth and reversal of cognitive impairment among children who have suffered growth retardation during infancy and/or early childhood is thought to be limited after the age of 2 years, particularly when children remain in poor environments. However, other studies have shown that undernourished children in poor environments can display spontaneous catch-up even without environmental change. As adolescence is a time of rapid growth, this provides an opportunity for further catch-up growth. It is thought, however, that the potential for significant catch-up during this time is limited. Reversed stunting in women may reduce the risk of pregnancy outcomes that are commonly associated with women of small stature. However, in most cases, regardless of whether growth catch-up has occurred, problems associated with reduced cognitive function remain. Females appear to display greater catch-up than males. Zinc deficiency, of which growth retardation is an outcome, is a commonly reported reason why males may be less able to catch up. At all ages, zinc requirements are very much higher for males than females and therefore a zinc limitation may explain restricted growth in males to a much greater extent than females, and explain why males are unable to catch up to the same extent as females. Catch-up growth has been associated with a number of adverse outcomes in later life. It is not known why catch-up growth is detrimental; however, one theory involves IUGR restricting cell numbers; therefore, ensuing catch-up growth is achieved by the overgrowth of a restricted cell mass.

Short stature and plant food environments

Many populations in developing countries exist on diets that are predominantly plant based. Such diets are commonly associated with micronutrient deficiencies, chronic energy deficiency and poor growth outcomes. Thus, populations who consume a predominantly plant-based diet are often seen to exhibit short stature. In addition to containing fewer kilojoules, plant-based diets are thought to contain large amounts of protective phytochemicals that may act to limit the amount of 'metabolic dysregulation' that can lead to the development of degenerative diseases, and the antinutrients may also act to limit growth. It has been suggested that short stature and micronutrient deficiencies may represent adaptations for group survival in adverse environmental conditions. For example, slow growth rates associated with zinc deficiency may represent an adaptation to situations where this is a survival advantage.

Maximal versus optimal height

As undernutrition and stunting during infancy and early childhood have been consistently found to affect detrimentally both the short- and long-term health of an individual, much of the public health focus has been on encouraging secular growth or the trend towards more rapid growth and larger attained size. Secular growth is apparent in many cultures. There is evidence, however, that secular growth in many developed countries, such as North America, Western Europe and Australia, is slowing and reaching a plateau. Current nutrition theory holds that an individual should achieve their maximal height potential in order to achieve the best health outcomes. Recent studies, however, have questioned this theory and have introduced the concept of 'optimal' rather than 'maximal' stature. It has been suggested that smaller stature confers many health benefits and represents an adaptive response to an individual's environment. Although small stature carries with it an increased risk of abdominal obesity and heart disease, tall stature increases the risk of developing cancer and degenerative diseases.

7.6 Effects of overnutrition

Obesity is of global epidemic proportions, affecting children, adolescents and adults in growing numbers. In some countries over half of the adult population is affected, thus leading to increasing death rates from heart disease, hypertension, stroke and diabetes. It is the growing prevalence of obesity in younger age groups that has raised alarm. Obesity is multifactorial and is a problem of both nutrient imbalance and insufficient physical activity levels. Declining physical activity levels have been associated with television viewing and other modern technological advances. Children who watch large amounts of television are particularly at risk of becoming overweight or obese.

Effects of overweight and obesity

Being overweight or obese as a child and adolescent has many associated health, social and psychological implications. Overweight and obese children may suffer from impaired social interaction and self-esteem. They are often taller than their non-overweight peers and are often viewed as more mature. This is an inappropriate expectation that may result in adverse effects on their socialization. Obese individuals at all ages often do less well academically, leading to higher rates of poverty, and have poorer job prospects in later life. Being overweight or obese can negatively affect mobility and physical fitness. Serious physical complications associated with high weights in children are rare, but include cardiomyopathy, pancreatitis, orthopedic disorders, and respiratory disorders such as upper airway obstruction and chest wall restriction. These are largely restricted to the severely obese and are of low prevalence. In adolescents, obesity confers significant cardiovascular risks, abnormal glucose tolerance, hypertension and lipid profile abnormalities. Furthermore, a greater percentage of abdominal fat in children of both genders is associated with early maturity. Few studies have investigated the long-term effects of childhood obesity on adult health outcomes, but obesity experienced during childhood or adolescence seems to increase the risk of adult morbidity and mortality.

Age of onset and obesity in later life

Differences exist in the prevalence of obesity between boys and girls, between men and women, and between social classes. Social factors were a predominant determinant of body fatness and thus obesity. Obesity is, however, also a familial condition. It has been reported that less than 10% of obese children have both parents of a normal weight, with 50 and 80% of obese children having one and two obese parents, respectively. Obese children are more likely to remain obese as adolescents and as adults. The age of the onset of obesity strongly influences this risk. The older the obese child, the more probable it is that he or she will be become an obese adult. The correlation between adult and childhood obesity rises with age and with the severity of childhood obesity, while the rate of spontaneous weight reduction decreases with age. The proportion of overweight or obese in adults who had been overweight or obese in adolescence ranges from 20 to 45%, while from 25 to 50% of overweight or obese adolescents had been overweight or obese in early childhood. Obese adolescents have significantly more abdominal fat than the non-obese. Obesity that begins during or close to adolescence is often characterized by the abdominal type of fat distribution. In the 1960s it was reported that both hypermasculine and hyperfeminine types of body fat distribution in women often began prior to adulthood, with the hyperfeminine variety tending to originate prepubertally and the hypermasculine tending to originate during adolescence. Adolescence may thus be a sensitive period for the development of android or abdominal obesity in both males and females.

Predictors of body size and fatness in adolescence

The interaction of both genetic and environmental factors appears to determine human body fatness. Measures that predict body size and fatness in adolescence have been identified. Predictors in early life of body size and fatness in adolescence include birth weight, anthropometric measures at 12, 50 and 80 months, weight and height velocities during the first year, the presence of a major illness, and parental socioeconomic status in early life. Tienboon *et al.* (1992) found that the consumption of fish oil [high in eicosapentaenoic acid (EPA) and DHA] in early life lowered the risk of developing obesity, particularly abdominal obesity. Self-reported measures of exercise, appetite and consumption of some specific food items correlated more closely with contemporary predictors of adolescent body size and fatness when measured at adolescence.

Factors affecting weight status in children and adolescence

Many factors, including season, geographical region, population density, ethnicity, socioeconomic status, family size, gender, parental education, physical activity levels, maternal age and maternal preference for a chubby baby, have been reported to affect the development of obesity in children and adolescents. Weight status may differ between children and adolescents living in rural and urban areas. Adolescents from urban areas may be significantly taller and heavier, and have more superficial fat and longer legs than adolescents from rural areas.

Rate of weight gain and mode of feeding in early life

Early feeding experience is related to development of excess weight in infancy. Both breast-feeding and the delayed introduction of solid foods appear to exert a protective effect against adiposity up to 2 years of age and probably in later life. However, not all studies have shown this effect. The ages where most obesity arises before adulthood are between 0 and 4 years, 7 and 11 years and during adolescence. During infancy, rapid increases in weight have been associated with obesity at adolescence in boys. Early catch-up growth, between the ages of 0 and 2 years, has been frequently reported as a predictor of childhood obesity, particularly for central or abdominal obesity.

Familial aggregation of weight status

In the 1920s one the first and more detailed of the early genetic studies was conducted and it was found that alleles for obesity tended to be dominant, and thus more likely to be expressed compared with non-obese alleles. Slender individuals tended to be homozygous, whereas obese persons were often heterozygous for these alleles. Overweight or obese individuals generally have at least one overweight or obese parent. Between 49 and 69% of overweight or obese children have at least one obese parent, with a fat mother (26–43%) being more common than a fat father (12–16%). When all other family members are obese, the likelihood of children being obese is very high (24–28%).

Many studies have investigated the relationship between body fatness and fat distribution among families. The effects of environmental factors with respect to weight status have been demonstrated in studies of twins and siblings. Both genetic and environmental factors appear to play a role in total body fat levels and distribution patterns. Measures of body mass index (BMI) for immediate family members are often highly correlated. In addition, it appears that people living together can have similar degrees of fatness. Under shared environmental conditions, both genetically related and unrelated household members show similar amounts of total body fatness. In this sense genetically unrelated subjects are about as similar, fat-wise, as genetically related individuals. However, studies have found that genetic rather than environmental factors may be more influential in determining the fat distribution pattern. Spouses who do not share genetic make-up often show little relationship in fat distribution, even after 20 years of cohabitation. However, family members of shared genetic origin show similarities in fat distribution patterns, and the degree of correlation is gender specific.

7.7 Growth during childhood and adolescence

The most rapid periods of growth take place during the first few months of life and during adolescence. Growth velocity slows significantly after the first year of life. The growth rate accelerates again as an individual enters puberty in adolescence over a period of 1–3 years. After the peak growth velocity of puberty has been attained, the growth rate slows considerably

until growth in height ceases at around 16 years of age in girls and 18 years in boys (Figure 7.2).

During the first year of life, a well-nourished infant will ideally increase in length by 50% and in weight by 300%. Rapid and essentially linear growth occurs in well-nourished infants, with rates of weight and height keeping pace with each other. Infants have a high surface area to body weight, which means that their energy and nutritional needs are much higher than adults on a per kilogram of body weight basis. Infants are prone to heat stress and dehydration because of this; however, the ratio of surface area to body weight decreases with age. The period of infancy ends when the child is weaned from the breast (or bottle), which in pre-industrialized societies occurs at a median age of 36 months, and less in more developed countries. During early childhood, height and weight increase in an essentially linear fashion. Steady growth necessitates a gradual increase in the intakes of most nutrients to support growth and development. It is thought that the age of 6–7 years is a critical period for determining future weight and height status. During childhood, an individual is still largely dependent on the caregiver for providing nourishment, but this begins to change during late childhood when a child begins to develop increased control over his or her food intake and relies less on caregivers.

During adolescence the body undergoes a large number of changes as a result of puberty. Once puberty is reached, an individual is capable of sexual reproduction.

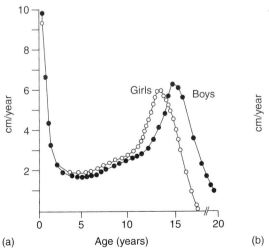 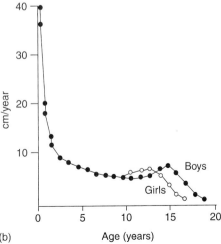

(a)   Age (years)

(b)   Age (years)

Figure 7.2   Growth velocities through childhood and adolescence: (a) 50th centile weight velocities; (b) 50th centile height velocities. (Reproduced with permission from Gracey *et al.*, 1989.)

The onset of puberty is characteristically earlier in females than in males (10.5–11 years and 12.5–13 years, respectively). As males reach puberty later than females, they experience on average 2 more years of prepubertal growth than females, resulting in typically higher statures going into puberty than females.

Before puberty, there are no significant height differences between girls and boys. It is during the adolescent growth spurt that major skeletal differences between males and females become apparent. In males, there is a widening of the shoulders with respect to the pelvis, while the opposite is seen in females. Typically, height gains of approximately 20 and 15 cm are realized in males and females, respectively.

In both genders, a sequential pattern of growth is observed: the feet and hands, the calves and forearms, the hips and chest, and the shoulders, followed by the trunk. Skeletal growth ceases once the epiphyses, the active area of bone at the end of long bones, have closed. Once this occurs bones are unable to achieve further length and are largely unresponsive to exogenous GH administration. In males, puberty is marked by growth of the sexual organs, followed by changes in the larynx, skin and hair distribution. The growth of the ovaries signifies the beginning of puberty in females. Fat is deposited in the breasts and around the hips, dramatically changing the female body shape. Menarche coincides with the peak adolescent growth spurt, after which growth decelerates.

Body composition changes during childhood and adolescence

Growth and development in children and adolescents are associated with changes in body composition that affect body fatness and leanness. Body composition is used as one of the measures of growth. It also provides an indication of both nutritional status and physical fitness.

Changes in fat-free mass and body water content

Lean body mass (LBM) includes all non-lipid body constituents as well as essential fats and phospholipids. In adolescence, LBM increases to a much greater extent in males than in females, with muscle and bone representing the largest gains in growth. Fat-free mass (FFM) is similar to LBM, but it excludes all essential fats and phospholipids. FFM density (effectively lean mass) increases from the first year of life through to 10 years of age, and then again dramatically during

puberty. Both males and females show a linear increase in FFM mineral content from the age of 8–15 years. The body's water content, measured as FFM–water content, decreases from birth to adulthood, from 81 to 72%. This drop in water content coincides with the abrupt rise in the mean FFM density seen between these ages.

Changes in body fat

Full-term infants have 10–15% body fat. In infancy, the amount of fat is correlated with body weight. Body fat shows a remarkable increase during the first year of life. By the end of this year it is estimated that body fat represents 20–25% of total body weight. Thereafter, there is a decline in the percentage of body fat, to its lowest level in the mid-childhood years, and then an increase in adolescence. Girls experience a much larger increase in body fat than boys during adolescence. Adolescent boys typically have significantly less superficial fat, less total body fat and less percentage body fat than adolescent girls. Further, adolescent boys have a significantly higher abdominal or central fat distribution than girls, as shown by waist–hip ratio and subscapular–triceps skinfold thicknesses ratio.

Fat patterning in children and adolescents

The waist-to-hip circumference ratio (WHR) measures the predominance of fat storage in the abdominal region relative to the gluteal region. A high WHR is indicative of excess abdominal fat, that is, a central fat distribution. In adults, the WHR has been related to a number of metabolic diseases and is a strong predictor of mortality; however, the implications of a high WHR in children are not clear. WHR is significantly influenced by age and gender. Boys generally have higher measures of WHR than girls. The WHR decreases with age from about 1.1 in the youngest children to about 0.8 in pubertal children. From puberty onwards, the WHR approaches the values reported for adults. In children, WHR is more or less independent of the total body fatness, whereas in adults the WHR is positively correlated with body fatness, as measured by BMI. In general, subcutaneous adipose tissue is distributed peripherally for most children up until puberty. For most boys but only a few girls, fat begins to be stored more centrally. The rate of change towards a more central fat distribution decreases in girls after about 13–14 years of age, but continues in boys. In adults, a central fat pattern is common in men, but not in women.

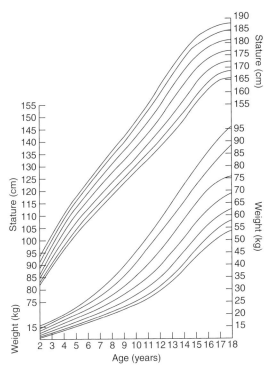

Figure 7.3 Growth chart (attained): boys 2–18 years. (Source: Lee and Nieman, 1996.)

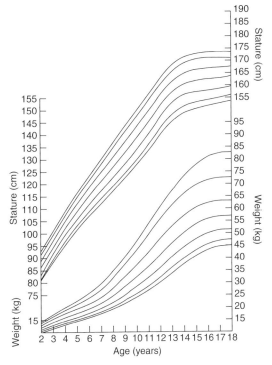

Figure 7.4 Growth chart (attained): girls 2–18 years. (Source: Lee and Nieman, 1996.)

However, a central fat pattern is more prevalent in elderly women than in younger adult women.

Assessment of growth

Growth charts are routinely used to assess growth and are used in diagnosis and management of diseases and in monitoring the efficacy of therapy. Chronic undernutrition or overnutrition is typically reflected in growth rates and therefore the monitoring of growth is used as an integral part of nutritional assessment. Common growth charts include weight-for-age, length-for-age (for children below 2 years of age) and height-for-age (for children 2 years and over) (Figures 7.3 and 7.4).

Although growth charts that show attained growth may show a steady progressive increase in anthropometric body measures with age, growth velocity charts reveal the changing rates of growth more visibly (see Figure 7.2). The growth charts may suggest that an infant or child who is above the 97th centile or below the third centile is unusually large or small; however, such a conclusion is not always appropriate. The growth of a well-nourished individual will typically follow a

growth curve and therefore an individual who is considered small or large from a growth chart may simply reflect that the infant or child's growth is a result of individual variation. A greater cause for alarm is when an individual crosses centiles, particularly if this happens over a short period. This may indicate inappropriate weight gain or acute growth failure or retardation, such as wasting or stunting, as a result of chronic undernutrition due to either chronic malnourishment or an underlying disease condition. Wasting is detectable on weight-for-age growth charts and by reduced skinfold measures, while stunting is seen as impairment of linear growth as detected by length- or height-for-age growth charts. It should be noted, however, that there are large variations between individuals in rates and patterns of growth, and these variations must be taken into consideration when determining whether a child's growth is abnormal.

Appropriate measures must be used for specific population groups. Growth charts based on Caucasian bottle-fed babies are unlikely to be appropriate for use in certain developing countries, as using such charts may misclassify an individual or population group as

Table 7.4 International cut-off points for body mass index (BMI) for overweight and obesity by gender between the ages of 2 and 18 years

Age (years)	Overweight		Obese	
	Males	Females	Males	Females
2	18.41	18.02	20.09	19.81
2.5	18.13	17.76	19.80	19.55
3	17.89	17.56	19.57	19.36
3.5	17.69	17.40	19.39	19.23
4	17.55	17.28	19.29	19.15
4.5	17.47	17.19	19.26	19.12
5	17.42	17.15	19.30	19.17
5.5	17.45	17.20	19.47	19.34
6	17.55	17.34	19.78	19.65
6.5	17.71	17.53	20.23	20.08
7	17.92	17.75	20.63	20.51
7.5	18.16	18.03	21.09	21.01
8	18.44	18.35	21.60	21.57
8.5	18.76	18.69	22.17	22.18
9	19.10	19.07	22.77	22.81
9.5	19.46	19.45	23.39	23.46
10	19.84	19.86	24.00	24.11
10.5	20.20	20.29	24.57	24.77
11	20.55	20.74	25.10	25.42
11.5	20.89	21.20	25.58	26.05
12	21.22	21.68	26.02	26.67
12.5	21.56	22.14	26.43	27.24
13	21.91	22.58	26.84	27.76
13.5	22.27	22.98	27.25	28.20
14	22.62	23.34	27.63	28.57
14.5	22.96	23.66	27.98	28.87
15	23.29	23.94	28.30	29.11
15.5	23.60	24.17	28.60	29.29
16	23.90	24.37	28.88	29.43
16.5	24.19	24.54	29.14	29.56
17	24.46	24.70	29.41	29.69
17.5	24.73	24.85	29.70	29.84
18	25	25	30	30

Reproduced with permission of BMJ Publishing Group from Cole *et al.* (2000) British Medical Journal; 330: 1240.

underweight. New international growth references are being developed based on pooled data from seven countries, combining measurements from over 13 000 breast-fed healthy infants and children. This will provide a more scientifically reliable tool for use in all countries to monitor growth and nutritional status. Other anthropometric measures that are routinely used to monitor growth and nutritional status include head circumference, which is used in young infants, mid upper arm circumference, which is widely used in developing countries as a measure of muscle and fat in both children and adults, and skinfold thicknesses, which measure subcutaneous fat. BMI centiles (Table 7.4),

using Quetelet's ratio (weight in kilograms divided by the square of height in meters) have recently been developed to detect overweight and obesity in children.

Both GH and IGFs can be measured in the plasma and their levels are thought to reflect changes in growth and cellular activity. IGF plasma levels are considerably more stable and do not display as large fluctuations as GH exhibits. Because of this greater stability, plasma levels of IGF can provide a sensitive measure of growth. Growth is a process that is multifactorial. The relative contributions of genetic and environmental factors to growth and development outcomes of an individual are still under investigation. Both overnutrition and undernutrition exert negative and often irreversible impacts on growth at all life stages, and unless addressed in the early years life, long deficits may result.

7.8 Aging

Aging is not a disease. Nor are the so-called diseases of aging – cancer, heart disease, arthritis and senility – the inevitable consequences of advancing years. If we live long enough, changes in body composition, physical function and performance will occur in all of us. Many of these changes, as well as health problems which become more common in old age, have long been attributed to the 'normal aging process'. This section will highlight that these health problems can be delayed to the last few years of life (i.e. compression of morbidity).

Sociodemography

Humans are living longer than ever before with several population life expectancies at birth now exceeding 80 years. Since the early 1970s, life expectancies have increased globally by about 1 year every 3 years. The elderly today are living almost 20 years longer than their ancestors at the beginning of the twentieth century. At present, the proportion of centenarians is also increasing (upwards of 1 in 1000 of the population in economically advantaged countries); however, individuals do not appear to exceed a maximal lifespan of about 120 years. Maximal lifespan may yet increase as biotechnology, lifestyle and health care develop in favor of greater longevity.

Adults are reaching older age in better health and the majority will live independently. Life expectancy is increasing for men and women alike. Between 1981 and 2001 the number of older people in the population increased by 50%, with an even greater increase in those aged over 70. Although maximum life expectancy has not increased over the past century, average life expectancy has changed substantially. Men born in 2020 can expect to live to 79, and women to 87. Our ability to live longer is, in part, attributable to better nutrition and to other lifestyle changes (e.g. reduced substance abuse, greater recreational opportunities), to improved health care (e.g. reduced infant and maternal mortality, earlier diagnosis and management of cancers and heart disease), to educational and economic improvements, and to better housing (especially less crowding) and social support systems. But as we live longer, our nutritional needs may change, either with 'healthy' aging or because of the advent of disease. Keeping an elderly population well is of great importance for the individuals themselves, for the well-being of society in general (the transfer of knowledge and skills to younger people, especially descendants and a reduced burden on others), and for reasons of available resources to care for the aged. Remarkably, the numbers of elderly people in developing countries now approach and will exceed those in developed countries (Table 7.5), so that the problem is global.

Biological and chronological age and compression of morbidity

Biological and chronological age

Aging may be defined as chronological age (a person's age in years since birth) or biological age (the decline in function that occurs in every human being with time). Some elderly people look and function as though they were older and others as though they were younger at the same 'chronological age'. Prospective studies, where some assessment of biological age has been made during the twentieth century in Sweden, indicate that people are less biologically old at the same chronological age than they used to be, and that this difference may be as much as 10 years of biological age. This is a rather remarkable change and some of it is likely to be attributable to improved lifelong nutrition. It may well be that much of what we currently regard as aging is preventable by nutritional means. In other words, even though genes have a strong influence on biological age, it is now believed that lifestyle factors also have a strong influence. You may be able to remain biologically younger if you look after yourself in your younger adult years. The question is, what aspects of aging are biologically inevitable, having to do, for example, with the programmed death of cells (apopotosis), and how

Table 7.5 Proportion of the population aged 65 years and over, selected countries 1985 and 2005

	% of population aged 65+	
	1985	2005
Europe		
France	12.4	14.8
Germany (FRG)	14.5	18.9
Greece	13.1	16.9
Hungary	12.5	15.0
Italy	13.0	16.9
Poland	9.4	12.3
Sweden	16.9	17.2
UK	15.1	15.3
North America		
Canada	10.4	12.5
USA	12.0	13.1
Other developed countries		
Australia	10.1	11.4
Japan	10.0	16.5
Less developed countries		
Brazil	4.3	5.8
China	5.1	7.4
India	4.3	6.1
Kenya	2.1[a]	2.1
Mexico	3.5	4.6

Reprinted from Grundy (1992) with permission from Elsevier Science.
[a]1988.

much is it age related? While the clock cannot be turned back in terms of chronological age, the search for prolonging youth continues to invoke much interest and research. The older people are, the more dissimilar they become from others of the same chronological age. Some of this variability may reflect heterogeneity in true rates of aging, but other factors that accompany aging also seem to be of major importance. These include lifestyle factors such as poor eating habits, a sedentary lifestyle and smoking, and the development of disease. Each of these factors can contribute to deterioration in cardiovascular, lung or endocrine functions, thereby accelerating one's apparent rate of aging. For example, declining cardiovascular function was observed in the Baltimore Longitudinal Study of Aging. However, after careful exclusion of those with heart disease, no consistent declines in function with age remained. Thus, the apparent declines in the study group members as they aged were due to inclusion of people with defined disease rather than to the aging process per se. As discussed later in this chapter, the

and physiological reserves to prevent major health problems
- engaging in social activity
- avoiding substance abuse (including alcohol, tobacco, excessive caffeine intake and unnecessary intake of medications).

By focussing on the complete lifestyle rather than on just one component such as nutrition, elderly people can enjoy life without experiencing major consequences of nutritional error.

Food variety

Research has shown that food variety has an important role to play in the prevention of onset of diseases such as diabetes, cancer and cardiovascular disease. A varied diet, ideally containing 20–30 biologically distinct foods a week, is seen to be beneficial in the prevention of certain disease states. Specifically, an association between increased food variety and lower glycemic response in both insulin-dependent and non-insulin-dependent diabetes mellitus (IDDM and NIDDM) has been found. Greater dietary diversity has also been found to be predictive of less morbidity and greater longevity in people aged over 70 years. Mortality follow-up studies of elderly people aged 70 and over in Australia, Greece, Spain and Denmark have found that more varied food patterns, even as late as 70 years and onwards, could reduce the risk of death by more than 50%. To obtain this mortality advantage, the elderly in these studies had to have food patterns consistent with the following food groups, giving a score ranging from 0 to 8: (1) high in vegetables (>300 g/day); (2) high in legumes (>50 g/day); (3) high in fruits (>200 g/day); (4) high in cereals (>250 g/day); (5) moderate in dairy products (<300 g of milk/day or equivalent in cheese/yogurt); (6) moderate in meat and meat products (<100 g/day); (7) moderate in alcohol (<10 g/day); (8) high in monounsaturated fat (mainly from olive oil) and low in saturated fat (i.e. high monounsaturated:saturated fat ratio). This food pattern is consistent with food patterns prevalent in Greece in the 1960s, when Greeks enjoyed the longest life expectancy in the world. The subjects achieved greater mortality advantage if they followed the entire food pattern (i.e. had high dietary variety scores ≥4) as opposed to just achieving the required amount for one or two of the food groups (Figure 7.5).

This suggests that there may be synergy between the food groups and that we need to follow dietary

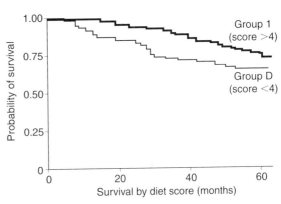

Figure 7.5 Kaplan–Meier survival curves for individual subjects with diet score up to 3 and 4 or more. (Source: Trichopoulou *et al.*, 1995.)

recommendations as a whole rather than focussing on just one food group or nutrient.

Physical activity

Ageing as we know it in modern society is, in many ways, an exercise deficiency syndrome, implying that we may have far more control over the rate and extent of the ageing process than we previously thought (Fiatarone, 1996).

Some of the most dramatic changes that we see with age are changes in body composition. A decline in muscle mass and increases in body fat tend to occur as people grow older. What is often not appreciated, however, is that these too cannot be blamed on the aging process per se. A major contributor to these changes is the increasingly sedentary nature of people's lifestyles as they grow older. Reduced physical activity leads to loss of muscle, and as a direct consequence basal metabolic rate (BMR) falls. A lower metabolic rate means that we need to eat less in order to maintain the same body weight. If one does indeed eat less to avoid weight gain, rather than remaining (or becoming) active, it becomes increasingly difficult to meet the needs for essential nutrients. Without doubt, it is preferable to keep physically active, maintain muscle mass and continue to enjoy eating.

Physical activity has been associated with greater energy intakes and subsequently nutrient intakes and quality of life in the aged. This results in a higher plane of energy nutrition. This runs counter to the disturbing advocacy that energy restriction prolongs life. These studies were conducted on rats and have no direct application to humans. To suggest that elderly people restrict their food intake to prolong life is absurd when this may contribute to frailty and loss of lean mass. The evidence is, however, that any extra energy intake must be from nutrient (and phytochemical)-dense foods, without excessive abdominal fatness. Many studies have shown energy intake declines with age, making a nutritionally adequate diet more difficult to achieve. Older men consume about 800 kcal less than younger men, and older women consume about 400 kcal less than younger women. A reduction in BMR is partly responsible for this decline in energy intake, but physical inactivity appears to be the major cause. Prospective studies show that increased energy intakes in the order of 300–500 kcal/day, which is balanced with increased physical activity to avoid fat gain, confer either decreased cardiovascular or total mortality and improve life expectancy. Physical activity also seems to protect against osteoporosis and fractures, diabetes, and breast and colon cancers, to improve mental health and cognitive function, reduce symptoms of anxiety and depression and enhance feelings of well-being in older people. An exercise intervention study in mid-life has been shown to compress morbidity (measured with disability score) towards the end of life. The subjects who belonged to a 'runner's club' in mid-life had significantly less disability in their eighties compared with control subjects. While the evidence points to the value of early and lifelong regular physical activity, recent evidence underlines just how much survivors can gain from the combination of endurance and strength training well into later life, with studies available on people well into their eighties. In other words, physical activity in old age can defer morbidity and mortality, and compress the morbidity period before death.

Social activity

Social activity is now thought to be one of the most important determinants of longevity. Participation in fewer social activities outside the home and limited social networks have been linked with higher mortality in old age. The impact of social activity on longevity could be through its impact on psychological well-being and nutrition. For example, elderly people who are socially isolated, lonely, institutionalized, recently bereaved and socially inactive have been found to have inadequate food intakes. Glass *et al.* (1999) examined associations between social (e.g. church), productive (e.g. shopping) and physical/fitness activities (e.g. walking)

at baseline and 13 year survival in 3000 older people. Social and productive activities were found to be as effective as fitness activities in lowering the risk of death. Further studies of this kind indicate the importance of social activity to the health and mortality of older people and perhaps younger people as well.

Effects of aging on physiological function

Physiological changes that occur with aging contribute to the body's declining function which, in turn, influences nutritional status just as growth and development do in the earlier stages of the life cycle. Among physiological changes, hormone activity alters body composition, immune system changes raise the risk of infections and some chronic diseases, atrophic gastritis interferes with nutrient digestion and absorption, and tooth loss and depression can adversely influence food choice. Animal studies suggest that energy restriction promotes longevity, but human studies suggest that 'eating better, not less' is desirable.

Theories of aging and energy restriction

There are three main theories of aging which predict the role that genes play in the aging process:

- programmed aging
- error theory
- free radical theory.

The theory of programmed aging suggests that the body has a built-in clock that begins ticking at birth. This theory is supported by the discovery that normal cells have a limited capacity to divide, because telomeres (the sections of DNA at the end of chromosomes) shorten at each division, resulting in a fixed lifespan for each normal cell. Furthermore, the aging process accelerates so rapidly in some individuals that they become biologically 'old' in their teens. The error theory attributes aging to increasing damage of DNA, and the progressive decline in the function of specialized enzymes that repair DNA. It is thought that diseases such as cancer, heart disease, osteoporosis and diabetes may be the result of accumulation of errors. The free radical theory proposes that free radicals (highly reactive oxygen molecules) are produced by oxygen-consuming biological reactions in the body. Free radicals damage cells and have been implicated in the development of cancer and heart disease. There is no evidence that taking antioxidants will improve longevity, but antioxidants consumed from food may have an indirect effect by reducing the damage produced by free radicals. A free radical is a molecule with an unpaired, highly reactive electron which is often associated with the development of cancer, arteriosclerosis, autoimmune diseases and aging. Antioxidants include phytochemicals (flavonoids) and nutrients (vitamins C and E and β-carotene), as well as enzymes such as superoxide dismutase (SOD), catalase and glutathione peroxidase. These prevent most, but not all, oxidative damage. Bit by bit, the damage mounts and contributes, so the theory goes, to deteriorating tissues and organs. Antioxidants may reduce the risk of cancer by protecting cellular DNA from free radical damage.

There has been a popularized view, derived mainly from rodent experiments, which has argued that energy restriction may decrease the cancer risk and increase longevity. Most of these studies are flawed insofar as extrapolation to humans is concerned because either they are conducted from early life with excessive early mortality, or they do not account for energy expenditure, and therefore energy balance, reflected in body fatness and/or its distribution. Where the full energy equation is available, increased energy throughput (e.g. higher energy intakes with no increase in body fatness) has been associated with decreased cancer risk and/or increased life expectancy. Increased energy intake (and possibly its frequency) has in its own right been associated with increased cancer risk at several sites. Again, the quality of extra food intake seems important. The Zutphen prospective study in the Netherlands showed that increased energy intake, which included relatively more plant-derived food and fish, was associated with lower cancer and total mortality over 10 years.

Body composition

Some of the most dramatic changes seen with age are changes in body composition. A decline in muscle and bone mass and increases in body fat tend to occur as people grow older, and subcutaneous fat is redistributed from limbs to the trunk. Some of these changes occur because of the activity of some hormones that regulate metabolism decreases with age (e.g. insulin, GH, androgens), while the activity of others increases (e.g. prolactin): the former contribute to a decrease in lean mass and the latter to an increase in fat mass. However, what is often not appreciated is that these cannot be blamed entirely on the aging process per se. A major contributor to these changes is the increasingly sedentary nature of people's lives as they grow older. Reduced physical activity leads to loss of muscle, and as a direct consequence BMR falls. A lower metabolic rate means that older people need to eat less energy in order to maintain the same body weight, but should ensure that this does not lead to a decrease in micronutrient intake. The incidence of people becoming underweight has been shown to increase with age. A lower body weight has been more strongly linked with morbidity in the elderly than mild to moderate excess weight, and the problem is often insidious. Survival rates in Finnish elderly (85 years and over) over a 5 year period showed the highest mortality to be in those with a BMI less than $20\,kg/m^2$ and the lowest mortality to be in the group with a BMI of 30 or more. Other studies have shown that elderly with BMIs below $27\,kg/m^2$ lived shorter lives than those with higher BMIs. Weight change and especially weight loss are of greater concern in the elderly than over-fatness. In developed countries 30–50% of older adults have been reported to be at high risk of developing health problems as a result of an inadequate food and nutrient intake.

Immune system

Both physical stressors (e.g. alcohol abuse, other drug abuse, smoking, pain, heat, illness) and psychological stressors (e.g. divorces, exams, migration, loss of a loved one) elicit the body's stress response: the classic fight-or-flight response. Stress that is prolonged or severe can drain the body of its reserves and leave it weakened, aged and vulnerable to illness. As people age, their ability to adapt to both external and internal stressors, especially via the immune system, is diminished owing to physiological changes that occur with aging. The immune system can also be compromised by nutrient deficiencies (see below), and so a combination of age and subclinical nutrient deficiencies makes older adults vulnerable to infectious diseases, including chronic diseases where the immune system is involved, such as arthritis and cancer.

Gastrointestinal tract

The intestine loses strength and elasticity with age; this slows motility and increases the risk of developing constipation (which is four to eight times more common in the elderly than in younger adults). Atrophic gastritis is also more common among older adults; about 30% of adults aged over 60 have this condition. It is a condition characterized by chronic inflammation of the stomach, accompanied by a diminished size and functioning of the mucosa and glands, resulting in less hydrochloric acid being secreted and increased levels of bacteria. These changes in the stomach can impair digestion and absorption of nutrients, especially vitamin B_{12}, biotin, calcium and iron.

Tooth loss

Chewing can be painful or difficult in old age as a result of tooth loss, gum disease and ill-fitting dentures. This can result in a reduced variety of foods consumed and an increased risk of developing nutrient deficiencies.

Sensory loss

Changes in taste and smell are variable and are often associated with lifelong cigarette smoking, poor dental hygiene and disease. Nevertheless, this phenomenon may make eating less enjoyable and may partly explain why older people tend to increase salt intake and use caffeinated beverages (caffeine also increases their appetite). Aging is associated with a decrease in the opioid (dynorphin) feeding drive and an increase in the satiety effect of cholecystokinin. Recent studies suggest that the early satiety in older persons may be caused by a nitric oxide deficiency, which decreases the adaptive relaxation of the fundus of the stomach in response to food.

Psychological changes

Depression is common among older adults, but is not an inevitable component of aging. It is frequently accompanied by loss of appetite and of motivation to cook.

Nutritionally vulnerable older adults

Contrary to the popular 'tea 'n' toast' myth, it appears that many older adults outside institutions eat reasonably well. The dietary patterns of older adults have generally been found to be similar to or healthier than those of their younger counterparts. Nevertheless, their intakes of cereals, fruit, vegetables and milk products are still below the recommended amounts. Some older people may consume a higher calorie diet without adverse health effects, which may be attributed to higher physical activity levels or intake of protective nutrients such as phytochemicals. Aging is often associated with less efficient processing of some essential nutrients, so older people may require higher intakes of particular nutrients, while requiring lower intakes of others.

As a general guide, adult energy requirements decline by an estimated 5% per decade. In developed countries energy intakes fall with advancing age (from 2800 to 2000 kcal for men and from 1900 to 1500 kcal for women), but average intakes of protein, total fat, polyunsaturated n-6 linoleic acid, vitamin A, thiamin, riboflavin, niacin, vitamin C, iron and phosphorus remain adequate in the 65-plus age group. Saturated fat and refined carbohydrates (high sugar content) continue to be consumed in excess of the recommended levels, and monounsaturated fats, n-3 fatty acids (from plants and fish), unrefined carbohydrates, fiber, folate, vitamin B_6, calcium, magnesium and zinc tend to be below the recommended intakes. These intakes may not result in the appearance of any diagnostic features or symptoms of true deficiency, but may result in subtle or subclinical nutrient deficiencies. In developed countries mild vitamin and mineral deficiencies are very common in older people, particularly those in institutions; 30–50% of older adults have been reported to be at high risk of developing health problems as a result of an inadequate food and nutrient intake, including cognitive impairment, poor wound healing, anemia, bruising, and an increased propensity for developing infections, neurological disorders, stroke and some cancers (e.g. vitamin A deficiency is associated with lung cancer).

Nutritionally vulnerable 'at-risk' groups

Some subgroups within older populations appear more likely to be consuming inadequate diets (e.g. less regular consumption of cooked meals). In Australia in 1998, 50% of older people lived with their partner and 63% lived with at least one relative; 28% lived alone and 6% in cared-for accommodation. Providing nutritious food via a Meals-on-Wheels program may not overcome the associated problem of social isolation, a risk factor for poor nutrition. This may be overcome by encouraging the individual to eat with family or friends, as this has been shown to increase food intake. An elderly person may eat less food for several reasons.

Nutritionally vulnerable 'at-risk' groups within older populations who are more likely to be consuming inadequate diets (e.g. less regular consumption of cooked meals) and to be at risk of protein–energy malnutrition include those who are:

- institutionalized
- older men living alone
- from low socioeconomic status groups

- socially isolated and lonely
- recently bereaved
- depressed or cognitively impaired
- physically and socially inactive

and those with:

- physical handicaps, impaired motor performance and mobility
- presence of chronic diseases (e.g. arthritis, diabetes, hypertension, heart disease, cancer)
- polypharmacy (unnecessary intake of medications, drug–nutrient interactions; some drugs affect appetite/mood and cause nausea)
- sensory impairment: taste/smell (reduction in taste), eyesight (cataracts)
- reduced sense of thirst (hypodypsia)
- problems with chewing (loss of teeth and poorly fitting dentures)
- limited food storage, shopping difficulties, inadequate cooking skills
- erroneous beliefs and food fadism, food preferences.

Medications, depression, dementia, chronic illness, disability, loneliness and diminished senses of smell and taste may decrease the pleasure of eating. Food beliefs in relation to health can be strongly held among elderly people and lead to both food faddism and undesirable food avoidance. There may be a significant association between food beliefs and food habits, as evidenced in studies of various elderly communities around the world. Nutrients at greatest risk of inadequate intake in 'at-risk' elderly groups are:

- energy
- protein
- folate
- vitamin B_6
- vitamin B_{12}
- vitamin D
- zinc
- calcium
- magnesium
- phytonutrients
- water.

Low intakes of these nutrients have important implications for bone health (calcium), wound healing (zinc, protein, energy), impaired immune response (zinc, vitamin B_6, protein, energy) and vascular disease via elevated homocysteine levels (folate, vitamin B_6).

Risky food patterns

When older people are physically active, marginal food patterns are less likely to lead to problems of the aged such as:

- frailty
- protein energy dysnutrition
- micronutrient and phytochemical deficiency, because greater amounts of nutritious food can be eaten without positive energy balance
- chronic metabolic disease (NIDDM, cardiovascular disease, osteoporosis) and certain cancers (breast, colonic, prostate)
- depression (there is growing evidence that n-3 fatty acid deficiency can contribute to depression in some individuals, and that exercise can alleviate it)
- cognitive impairment with the apoE4 genotype; excess dietary saturated fat is likely to increase the risk of Alzheimer's disease; and some antioxidants such as vitamin E and glutathione may reduce the risk.

Specific risky food patterns in later life include:

- large rather than smaller frequent meals or snacks, because of the inability of insulin reserve to match the carbohydrate load in those proven to have impaired glucose tolerance (IGT) or in those with NIDDM; or because, where appetite is impaired, nutritious snacks can help to avoid chronic energy undernutrition
- alcohol excess, no alcohol-free days and/or alcohol without food (since food reduces the impact of alcohol ingestion on blood alcohol concentration and its consequences)
- eating alone most of the time (since social activity encourages interest in food and, usually, healthy food preferences)
- use of salt or salty food rather than intrinsic food flavour (especially as taste and smell tend to decline with age), as excess sodium contributes to hypertension through an increased Na/K molar ratio, and to salt and water retention in cardiac decompensation, and promotes urinary calcium loss.

Nutrients at risk of inadequate intake

Protein–energy dysnutrition

It is usual to speak about protein–energy malnutrition (PEM), otherwise known as protein–calorie malnutrition (PCM), but in the aged, the body compositional disorder may be rather more complex. The most common nutritional scenario in the aged is for there to be a decrease in lean mass (comprising water and protein-dominant tissues such as muscle, organs such as liver, and also bone) and an increase in abdominal fat. This disorder could not be described as PEM, but can be described as protein–energy dysnutrition (PED). Illness or inadequate food intake may result in PED, a condition more common among elderly adults, especially in institutionalized care. It is associated with impaired immune responses, infections, poor wound healing, osteoporosis/hip fracture and decreased muscle strength (frailty), and is a risk factor for falls in the elderly. About 16% of elderly people living in the community consume <1000 kcal/day, an amount that cannot maintain adequate nutrition. Undernutrition also occurs in 3–12% of older outpatients, 17–65% of older people in acute-care hospitals and 26–59% of older people living in long-term care institutions. Studies show that being underweight in middle age and later places a person at greater risk of death than being overweight. Marasmus is a condition of borderline nutritional compensation in which there is marked depletion of muscle mass and fat stores but normal visceral protein and organ function. Because there is a depletion of nutritional reserves, any additional metabolic stress (e.g. surgery, infection, burns) may rapidly lead to kwashiorkor (hypoalbuminemic PEM). Characteristically, elderly people deteriorate to this state more rapidly than younger people, and even relatively minor stress may be the cause. Usually, susceptible elderly people are underweight, but even those who appear to have ample fat and muscle mass are susceptible if they have a recent history of rapid weight loss. The protein requirements of older people seem to be similar to or higher than those of younger people. The current dietary recommendation of protein for adults is 0.75–0.8 g/kg, whereas the recommendation for the elderly is slightly higher at 0.91 g/kg. In elderly people with PEM, edema is usually absent, and serum albumin and hemoglobin levels, total iron-binding capacity and tests of cell-mediated immune function are usually normal. When hypoalbuminemic PEM occurs, the serum albumin level is <3.5 g/dl, and anemia, lymphocytopenia and hypotransferrinemia (evidenced by a total iron-binding capacity <250 µg/dl) are likely. Often, anergy and edema are present. Albumin has a 21 day half-life, and is an excellent measure of protein status, except in people suffering from illness or trauma and after surgery. Normal, able-bodied elderly people

should have serum albumin levels >4 g/dl; only when a person is recumbent do fluid shifts result in a normal albumin level of 3.5 g/dl. Albumin levels <3.2 g/dl in hospitalized older people are highly predictive of subsequent mortality. Cholesterol levels <160 mg/dl in nursing-home residents predict mortality, presumably because such levels reflect malnutrition. Acute illness associated with cytokine release can also lower cholesterol levels. Anergy (failure to respond to common antigens, such as mumps, injected into the skin) can occur in healthy as well as malnourished older people. The combination of anergy and signs of malnutrition correlates more strongly with a poor outcome than either one alone.

Folate

Before mandatory folate fortification of cereals in several developed countries such as America and Australia, many older adults did not consume enough folate. This was compounded by the fact that folate absorption appears to be affected by atrophic gastritis, which is common in older adults. Elevated homocysteine levels have recently been defined as a marker of poor folate status in older people, and elevated levels of the former have been linked with an increased risk of heart disease and strokes. Folate metabolism may also be altered by the ingestion of antacids, anti-inflammatory drugs and diuretics commonly used by older adults. Several governments have legislated for the fortification of grain products with artificial folate since about 1998. The aim of this fortification exercise was to reduce birth defects of the spine, called spina bifida. Pregnant women need enough folate early in pregnancy to prevent most cases of spina bifida. A study in Framingham, Massachusetts, USA, studied folate levels in over 1100 people, before and after fortification was mandated. The folate levels in blood more than doubled, and the percentage of people, including older adults, with low folate levels dropped by more than 90%. This is partly explained by the greater bioavailability of artificial folate in fortified foods. For example, only about half of the folate found naturally in food is available for use in the body; in contrast, the folate found in fortified foods is nearly all absorbed.

Can folate fortification have any adverse effects on elderly people? Vitamin B_{12} deficiency is quite common in older adults owing to inadequate absorption (see below). Vitamin B_{12} is needed to convert folate to its active form. Therefore, one of the most obvious vitamin B_{12} deficiency symptoms is the anemia of folate deficiency (megaloblastic anemia). Vitamin B_{12}, but not folate, is also needed to maintain the sheath that surrounds and protects nerve fibers. Either B_{12} or folate will clear up the anemia, but if folate is consumed via fortified foods when a B_{12} supplement is needed instead, the result is devastating owing to permanent nerve damage and paralysis. In other words, folate 'cures' the blood symptoms of a vitamin B_{12} deficiency, but allows the nerve symptoms to progress, so that folate can mask a vitamin B_{12} deficiency. With sufficient folate in the diet, the neurological symptoms of vitamin B_{12} deficiency can develop in older adults without evidence of anemia. This highlights some of the safety issues surrounding the fortification of the food supply.

Vitamin B_6

During the course of life, plasma vitamin B_6 falls by approximately $3.6 \, \mu mol/l$ per decade. A number of studies suggest that age-related changes occur in both the absorption and metabolism of this vitamin, and as a consequence aged adults may have a higher requirement. Studies also show that vitamin B_6 deficiency results in decreased immune response. Vitamin B_6 deficiencies (as well as vitamin B_{12} and folate) also result in higher concentrations of homocysteine. Supplementation of vitamin B_6 in healthy elderly has been found to improve immune function and long-term memory.

Vitamin B_{12}

The prevalence of pernicious anemia increases with age, as does atrophic gastritis, and the absorption of vitamin B_{12} is reduced in individuals with either condition. The prevalence of *Helicobacter pylori* also increases with age and has been shown to be associated with vitamin B_{12} malabsorption, possibly because it contributes to gastric atrophy. As the likelihood of vitamin B_{12} deficiency is more common among older adults this not only increases the risk of irreversible neurological damage but is likely also to contribute to megaloblastic anemia and homocysteine concentrations associated with vascular disease (see Folate).

Vitamin D

Older adults are at greater risk of vitamin D deficiency than are younger people, and therefore at greater risk of exacerbated bone health decline (and resulting osteopenia and osteoporosis).

Risk factors for vitamin D deficiency include:

- lack of exposure to sunlight (may be due to less physical activity or sunscreen use)
- decline in renal function
- impaired skin synthesis (may be due to aging skin)
- low fish intake (especially fatty fish)
- low intake of egg yolks, butter, vitamin D-fortified margarine and cheese.

The diet becomes an important source of vitamin D in people who do not receive enough sunlight. Diets of elderly people are often deficient in vitamin D-rich foods such as oily fish, and fat-soluble vitamin absorption may be impaired. This is thought to contribute to the high incidence of vitamin D deficiency in older people. It appears that in the USA and Great Britain, some 30–40% of older patients with hip fractures are vitamin D deficient. However, even during old age, improving vitamin D status can provide profound benefits for bone health. In a Finnish study of outpatients over the age of 85 years and municipal home residents aged 75–84 years, those randomly assigned to receiving an annual vitamin D injection had significantly fewer fractures over a 5 year follow-up period. Probably the most striking and impressive study is one by Chapuy *et al.* (1992) of a nursing-home population of 3270 women, with an average age of 84 years. In a randomized, controlled trial of vitamin D ($20 \, \mu g/day$) and calcium ($1200 \, mg/day$), those receiving the supplement experienced 43% fewer hip fractures and 32% fewer non-vertebral fractures over an 18 month period. If blood levels of vitamin D are not reduced, vitamin D resistance may occur. Vitamin D resistance is relatively common because of impaired renal function in later life and the best indicator of this is an elevated parathyroid hormone (PTH) concentration in blood, a phenomenon referred to as secondary hyperparathyroidism. Vitamin D is important not only for bone, but also for immune function and muscle strength, and as a cell differentiator to reduce the risk of neoplastic disease.

Zinc

Plays an important role in wound healing, taste acuity and normal immune function, and may affect albumin status in older adults. It is a crucial element in numerous metalloenzymes, and its intake is dependent on foods such as meat, and limited from plant foods, in which it is bound to phytic acid, oxalate and dietary fiber. It is more bioavailable in cereals that are leavened because of the presence of phytase in yeast, which breaks down phytic acid. Low zinc intakes are associated with low energy and meat intakes. Older adults may absorb zinc less effectively than younger people, and so a diet including zinc-rich foods is important in later life. Zinc deficiency in older people is likely to be an important contributor to proneness to infection, in particular respiratory infection, such as pneumonia. Some of the symptoms of zinc deficiency are similar to symptoms associated with normal aging such as diminished taste and dermatitis, so it is difficult to determine whether to attribute these symptoms to zinc deficiency or simply to the aging process.

Calcium

Aging is associated with a decrease in calcium absorption, which is probably due to alterations in metabolism of vitamin D. However, calcium is a very important nutrient in older age, as osteoporosis becomes a problem. Postmenopausal women not on hormone replacement therapy (HRT) have higher calcium needs. Many women do not meet the current Australian recommended calcium intake for postmenopausal women (1000 mg/day). Recent studies suggest that postmenopausal women need 1500 mg calcium/day. It is recommended that elderly people who suffer from a milk allergy or are lactose intolerant seek calcium from non-milk sources or supplements to help them to meet their daily requirements.

Phytonutrients

Phytochemicals (from the Greek *phyto*, meaning plant) are unlike vitamins and minerals in that they have no known nutritional value. Phytochemicals are naturally occurring plant secondary metabolites that plants produce to protect themselves against bacteria, viruses and fungi. Many phytochemicals function as antioxidants, which protect cells from the effects of oxidation and free radicals within the body. They have been recognized only recently as potentially powerful agents that may offer protection from diseases and conditions such as heart disease, diabetes, some cancers, arthritis, osteoporosis and aging. They are present in a number of frequently consumed foods, especially fruits, vegetables, grains, legumes and seeds, and in a number of less frequently consumed foods such as licorice, soy and green tea. Phytonutrients may play a protective role in cardiovascular

disease, certain cancers and menopausal symptoms. Phytonutrients are likely to contribute to protection against many of the diseases associated with aging. A diet rich in phytoestrogens (isoflavones, lignans) may lessen the symptoms and impact of the menopause by improving vaginal health, reducing the incidence of hot flushes and improving bone mineral content (BMC). Food sources of phytoestrogens include soy, chickpeas, sesame seeds, flax seed (linseed) and olives.

One study in particular has shown that ingestion of soy may be more effective than HRT in improving BMC and therefore reducing the risks of osteopenia and osteoporosis.

In studies looking at the effect of HRT on BMC, it took 36 months to achieve an increase of just under 4%. In another study, however, an increase of 5.2% in BMC was detected after just 12 weeks of soy consumption.

Water

Total body water declines with age. As a result, an adequate intake of fluids, especially water, becomes increasingly important in later life, as thirst regulation is impaired and renal function declines. Dehydration is a particular risk for those who may not notice or pay attention to thirst, or who may find it hard to get up to make a drink or reach the bathroom. Older people who have decreased bladder control may also be at risk because they may be afraid to drink too much water.

Dehydrated elderly people appear to be more susceptible to urinary tract infections, pressure ulcers, pneumonia and confusion. Recommended intakes for the elderly are approximately 6–8 glasses of fluid a day, preferably water.

Nutrition-related health problems in the aged

There is growing awareness that the major health problems, and even mortality, in the aged have nutritional contributors and can be (in part) prevented by food intake. These health problems do not necessarily need to occur with aging, and death can be delayed. As the number of chronic conditions increases with age they contribute to disability and frailty, which in turn reduces a person's level of independence, sometimes resulting in institutionalization. The primary nutritional problems affecting the elderly are:

- protein–energy dysnutrition
- subclinical/mild vitamin deficiencies and trace mineral deficiencies
- obesity

all of which can contribute to the development of chronic conditions seen with aging. Some common nutrition-related problems in the aged are outlined below.

Sarcopenia

The condition or state of sarcopenia is specifically involuntary loss of flesh or muscle that occurs with age, and is more marked in women. It has been demonstrated that reduced muscle mass and body cell mass is associated with a loss of muscle strength, and impaired immune and pulmonary function. Furthermore, this decline in muscle strength is responsible for much of the disability observed in older adults, and in the old elderly, as muscle strength is a crucial component of walking ability. It is thought that human life cannot be sustained if levels of body cell mass fall below 60% of the normal levels of young adults. The prevalence, incidence and etiology of sarcopenia are currently unknown, and therefore require further study. Decreasing physical activity and GH levels are two likely contributing factors to the advancement of sarcopenia, along with poor nutrition (especially inadequate energy and protein intakes, which may be due to poor food intake or disease), disease and the aging process.

Obesity

Overweight and obesity are common problems in the aged, not because they are an inevitable part of growing older, but because of the associated sedentary lifestyle. Though a less serious problem in older persons than PEM, obesity can impair functional status, increase the risk of pulmonary embolus and pressure sores, and aggravate chronic diseases such as diabetes mellitus and hypertension. Greater body fatness, especially if centrally distributed, increases the risk of insulin resistance, hypertension and hypercholesterolemia in the aged. In contrast, heavier women have a lower risk of hip fracture. This is partly due to 'padding' and better muscle development, but may also be due to maintenance of higher estrogen levels from the conversion of precursor steroids to estrogen in adipose tissue. Abdominal obesity is defined as an abdominal circumference of greater than 102 cm and 88 cm for men

and women, respectively. However, abdominal obesity can be reduced in old age by engaging in some form of daily physical activity. An appropriate body weight is a protective factor in older people with advancing age. Body weight maintenance at a suitable level is desirable to maintain physical strength and activity, resistance to infection and skin breakdown, and quality of life.

Immune function

Infections are a common cause of illness and death among the aged. Aging adults are more susceptible to infection and this is probably due, in part, to the age-associated decline in immune function, but this decline may be preventable with good nutrition and physical activity. A decline in immunity may also increase the risk of cancer and arthritis. The observed decline in immune function with aging may be prevented with nutrient intakes greater than those currently recommended for 'normal' health. Nutrients important in immune function include protein, zinc, vitamin A, vitamin C, pyridoxine, riboflavin and tocopherols. Other food components not considered to be essential for health in earlier life may become more important with age.

The non-essential amino acid glutamine has an important role in DNA and RNA synthesis. It is stored primarily in skeletal muscle, and is utilized by intestinal cells, lymphocytes and macrophages. Because the contribution of skeletal muscle to whole-body protein metabolism declines with age, the rate of glutamine formation and availability may be impaired. As such, it may compromise immune function, resulting in a suboptimal response to infection or trauma. Glutamine can be synthesized from glutamic acid, which is found in wheat, soybeans, lean meat and eggs. Glutathione (a tripeptide) and phytochemicals such as flavonoids and carotenoids also appear to play a role in immune function. Meat is a good source of glutathione, with moderate amounts being found in fruits and vegetables. Whey proteins, although low in glutathione, are capable of stimulating endogenous glutathione production.

Osteoporosis and fractures

Old age is associated with decreased bone mass, and osteoporosis is one of the most prevalent diseases of aging. The incidence of osteoporosis is increasing with the aging population, with females most affected. It has been estimated that about 25% of the female population over 60 years is affected by osteoporosis, and 70% of the fractures that occur annually in Australia can be attributed to osteoporosis. In 1986, 10 000 hip fractures were recorded in Australia, and this rate is expected to rise to 18 000 per year by 2011. Hip fractures result in both mortality and morbidity. Two types of osteoporosis have been identified. Type I involves the loss of trabecular bone (calcium containing crystals that fill the interior of the bone). Women are more affected by this type of osteoporosis, with the most effective preventive measure being the administration of estrogen for at least 7 years after menopause. Type II osteoporosis progresses more slowly than type I, and involves the loss of both cortical (the exterior shell of the bone) and trabecular bone. As the person ages, the disease becomes evident with compressed vertebrae forming wedge shapes, into what is commonly referred to as 'dowager's hump'. Once again, women are more affected by this disease than men. Women are more prone to osteoporosis than men for two reasons: bone loss is accelerated after menopause, and women have a lower bone mineral density than men. A large study of elderly men and women conducted in Australia found that after the age of 60 years about 60% of women and 30% of men would sustain an osteoporotic fracture. A high intake of calcium appears to prevent or reduce bone loss in postmenopausal women. While adequate intakes of calcium appear to be protective against osteoporosis, other potentially protective factors include vitamins C, D and K, protein, boron, copper and possibly phytoestrogens. Recent evidence indicates that soy consumption may also provide benefits to bone health. A vitamin D supplement from fish liver oil has also been shown to reduce fracture rates in later life. While nutrition and physical activity can maximize peak bone mass during growth, other factors such as excess sodium, caffeine, smoking and alcohol can accelerate bone loss in later life.

Cardiovascular disease

Cardiovascular disease is the most common cause of death and disability in the developed world. Dietary habits may contribute to or provide protection against risk factors associated with cardiovascular disease. In a longitudinal health survey of elderly people living in the Netherlands, an inverse relationship was found between fish consumption and coronary heart disease mortality. Elevated serum homocystine concentrations have been identified as an independent risk factor for cardiovascular disease. In the Framingham study, elderly adults with better folate status had lower homocystine concentrations. Inadequate intake of folate and vitamins B_6 and B_{12} can lead to homocystinemia, and then to vascular damage and proneness to thrombosis.

Cancer

Specific dietary patterns that protect against cancer remain unclear. However, certain food groups are associated with a reduced risk of cancer; for instance, a high intake of fruit and vegetables appears to be associated with a reduced risk of cancer at many sites. Fruit and vegetables are excellent sources of antioxidants, phytochemicals and dietary fiber. Particular foods that may protect against prostate cancer include soy products, tomatoes and pumpkin seeds. Foods high in resistant starch, dietary fiber and salicylates may protect against colorectal cancer. Foods that appear to increase risk of cancer at specific sites include salt and smoked/cured foods (stomach cancer) and alcohol (esophageal cancer). Factors that occur early in life may affect the risk of breast cancer in later life. For instance, rapid early growth, greater adult height and starting menstruation at a younger age are associated with an increased risk of breast cancer. Although it is unlikely that appropriate interventions could be undertaken to avoid these, other nutritional and lifestyle factors are amenable to change and may reduce the risk of breast cancer. These include consuming diets high in vegetables and fruits, avoiding alcohol, maintaining a healthy body weight and remaining physically active throughout life. There is some evidence that phytoestrogens (compounds found in plants that possess mild estrogenic properties) may reduce the risk of breast cancer. Soy and linseed are two excellent sources of phytoestrogens and recently Australian food manufacturers have been adding soy and linseed to a variety of breads and cereals. The increase in prevalence of nutritionally related immunodeficiency with aging is likely to contribute to the development of neoplastic disease.

Diabetes

Aging is associated with an increased prevalence of NIDDM and glucose intolerance. Two risk factors associated with the development of both these conditions include obesity and physical inactivity. In older adults, modest weight reductions can contribute to improvements in diabetic control. This is important as retrospective studies indicate that good blood glucose control reduces the likelihood and severity of stroke, cardiovascular disease, visual impairment, nephropathy, infections and cognitive dysfunction. Dietary modification can reduce cardiovascular disease risk; even a relatively small reduction in salt and saturated fat intake can have a substantial effect on cardiovascular disease.

Endocrine function

Aging sees a decline in hormone secretion throughout the body. The decline in the level of human GH seems to play a role in the aging process in at least some individuals. GH also plays a role in body composition and bone strength. Estrogen levels also drop with age. Low levels of estrogen are associated with bone thinning, frailty and disability. Low testosterone levels in the body may weaken muscles and promote frailty and disability. Melatonin responds to light and seems to regulate seasonal changes in the body. As melatonin levels decline with age other changes in the endocrine system may be triggered. Dehydroepiandrosterone (DHEA) is being studied for its effects on immune system decline and its potential to prevent certain chronic diseases such as cancer and multiple sclerosis.

Cognitive function

Prevention of cognitive loss or dementia poses a particular challenge in older people. Some deterioration can be attributed to atherosclerotic disease and thus interventions such as aspirin or particular dietary patterns that reduce cardiovascular risk may also prevent dementia. High educational status early in life and continued mental stimulation may also be protective. Living alone has recently been reported to increase the risk of dementia. It is generally accepted that dementing illnesses and depression have a strong genetic background. However, the genetic susceptibility to a certain disease is strongly influenced by environmental factors. Thus, it may be possible to delay the onset of poor cognitive function in old age if food intake is adequate. For example, cognitive status assessed in a group of older adults from Madrid using Folstein's Mini-Mental State Examination and Pfeiffer's Mental Status Questionnaire was found to be better in those who consumed a more satisfactory global diet. This diet was characterized by a greater intake of total food, fruit and vegetables. Dementia can result in forgetting to eat, indifference to food, failure to see the need to eat, and behavioral

abnormalities such as holding food in the mouth. Changes in smell and taste may also lead to weight loss, which is common in older adults with dementia, or even anorexia in older adults. Long-term moderate (subclinical) nutrient deficiencies are now believed to produce memory impairments and declining immunity in older adults. Certain nutrients or toxic substances may directly affect brain development (e.g. alcohol, folic acid deficiency) or brain function (e.g. alcohol, vitamins B_1, B_2, B_6, B_{12}, C and E, and zinc deficiencies). Brain aging is associated with oxidative stress; thus, antioxidants and pro-oxidants (such as iron) are of particular interest. There is some epidemiological evidence that the antioxidants carotene and carotenoids, ascorbic acid and α-tocopherol may delay brain aging and iron may accelerate it. Vitamin K may also be protective against cognitive decline and Alzheimer's dementia. Depression in the elderly is a very common symptom. There is a growing body of evidence to suggest that n-3 polyunsaturated fatty acids may play an important role in the etiology of depression. Caffeine ingested as either tea or coffee has also been shown to improve mood and reduce anxiety.

Nutritional assessment of the aged

One of the greatest difficulties in making any assessment of the aged is the biological heterogeneity ('biological age'). There are clearly many health problems seen in the aged in some communities that are not seen in others, making them more age related than aging. Nutritional assessment of the aged needs to pay attention to a number of sociodemographic variables and the food culture in which the elderly person has lived. Another challenge for nutritional assessment in the aged is the question as to when nutritional factors will have operated during the lifespan to have had consequences on health in later life. With these considerations taken into account, the areas of nutritional assessment to consider are:

- food and nutrient intake
- anthropometry and body composition
- laboratory investigations by way of biochemistry, hematology and immunology
- nutritionally related risk factors for various health problems in the aged.

In Australia a tool has been developed which identifies older adults at risk of poor nutritional health by giving warning signs (Figure 7.6).

DETERMINE YOUR NUTRITIONAL HEALTH

The Warning Signs of poor nutritional health in the older person are often overlooked. Use this checklist to find out if you or someone you know is at nutritional risk.

Read the statements below. Circle the number in the column that applies to you or the person you know. For each answer, score the number in the box. Total your nutritional score.

	YES	NO
I have an illness or condition that made me change the kind and/or amount of food I eat	2	0
I eat at least 3 meals per day	0	3
I eat fruit or vegetables most days	0	2
I eat dairy products most days	0	2
I have 3 or more glasses of beer, wine or spirits almost every day	3	0
I have 6 to 8 cups of fluids (e.g. water, juice, tea or coffee) most days	0	1
I have teeth, mouth or swallowing problems that make it hard for me to eat	4	0
I always have enough money to buy food	0	3
I eat alone most of the time	2	0
I take 3 or more different prescribed or over-the-counter medicines every day	3	0
Without wanting to, I have lost or gained 5 kg in the last 6 months	2	0
I am always able to shop, cook and/or feed myself	0	2
TOTAL		

Add up all the numbers you have circled. If your nutritional score is ...

0–3	**Good!** Recheck your nutritional score in 6 months
4–5	**You are at moderate nutritional risk.** See what can be done to improve your eating habits and lifestyle. Your Council on Ageing or health care professional can help. Recheck your nutritional score in 3 months.
6 or more	**You are at high nutritional risk.** Bring this checklist the next time you see your doctor, dietitian or other qualified health or social service professional. Talk with them about any problems you may have. Ask for help to improve your nutritional health.

Source: These materials were developed and distributed by the Australian Nutrition Screening Initiative, a project of RACGP, Council on the Ageing, Dietitians Association of Australia, and Self Care Pharmacy, a joint program of the Pharmaceutical Society of Pharmacy Guild of Australia.

Figure 7.6 Example of a checklist to identify older persons at risk of poor nutritional health.

Food and nutrient intake

Assessment of food and nutrient intake is an important tool in health assessment in the aged. Because of a positive decline in memory, instruments used for food intake assessment should be as simple and practical as possible and should involve corroboration from other observers, such as family or friends. Knowing about appetite, the special senses for smell and taste, and the overall food patterns, facilitates an understanding of the various factors that may affect food intake. Food and nutrient intake can alert the healthcare worker to possible nutritionally related disease, for example, osteoporosis, by asking 'What do you have in the way of dairy products, fish, sesame based foods?' as sources of calcium. A systematic inquiry about food intake usually requires asking about each episode of eating during the day, the main meals and the snacks.

Anthropometry and body composition

Anthropometry is a simple, non-invasive, quick and reliable form of obtaining objective information about a person's nutritional status.

- **Weight**: Ambulatory elderly persons are weighed on an upright balance beam scale or microprocessor-controlled digital scale. A movable wheelchair balance beam scale can also be used for those elderly who can only sit. A bed scale should be available in geriatric hospitals for measuring the weight of bed-ridden elderly patients. Weights less than 20% of the ideal body weight indicate a significant loss of total body protein requiring immediate investigation and action. They are associated with reduced tolerance to trauma and an increased risk of morbidity, infection and mortality. Low body weight and/or unintended weight loss are significant risk factors as the aging process progresses and require careful intervention and monitoring. General guidelines requiring action would be:

  - a 2% decrease in body weight in 1 week
  - a 5% decrease in body weight in 1 month (3.5 kg in a 70 kg man)
  - a 7% decrease in body weight in 3 months
  - a 10% decrease in body weight in 6 months.

Interpretation of the weight of elderly people should be done with circumspection. Increases in body weight may indicate overweight/obesity or edema. Decreases in body weight can signify the correction of edema, development of dehydration or emergence of a nutritional disorder.

- **Height:** For the elderly who are agile and without stooped posture, height should be measured in an upright position. When this cannot be measured, *knee height* (using a knee height calliper) in a recumbent position can be used to estimate stature. The following formulae are used to compute stature from knee height:

$$\text{Stature for men} = (2.02 \times \text{knee height}) - (0.04 \times \text{age}) + 64.19$$

$$\text{Stature for women} = (1.83 \times \text{knee height}) - (0.24 \times \text{age}) + 84.88$$

The knee height measurement in these equations is in centimeters, and the age is rounded to the nearest whole year. The estimated stature derived from the equation is in centimeters. These equations are derived from observations which presume that elderly people will have lost some height, an inevitability that may not always continue as healthcare improves.

- **Arm span** is another substitute for height and happens to be the same as maximal height achieved. It is sometimes necessary to ask for maximum adult height to be recalled by the subject or by a carer. Gradual reduction in height may be an indicator of vertebral crush fractures due to osteoporosis, or it may be due to loss of vertebral disk space.

- **Mid-arm circumference (MAC):** Combined with triceps skinfold (TSF), MAC (taken at the mid-point between the acromion and olecranon) can be used to calculate mid-arm muscle area (MAMA), which is an index of total body protein mass. The equation to estimate MAMA is:

$$\text{MAMA} = [\text{MAC} - (3.14 \times \text{TSF/10})]^2/12.56$$

The MAC measurement in this equation is in centimeters and the TSF is in millimeters. The calculated MAMA derived from the equation is in centimeters squared. MAMA of less than 44 cm^2 for men and less than 30 cm^2 for women may indicate protein malnutrition.

- **Calf circumference:** Calf circumference (taken at the largest circumference using inelastic flexible measuring tape) in the absence of lower limb edema can be used to calculate weight in a bed-ridden patient.

Several anthropometric measurements, apart from calf circumference itself (Calf C), are required to compute weight. They are knee height (Knee H), MAC and subscapular skinfold thickness (Subsc SF) (taken at posterior, in a line from the inferior angle of the left scapula to the left elbow). There are separate equations for men and women:

Body weight for men
$$= (0.98 \times \text{Calf C}) + (1.16 \times \text{Knee H})$$
$$+ (1.73 \times \text{MAC}) + (0.36 \times \text{Subsc SF})$$
$$- 81.69$$

Body weight for women
$$= (1.27 \times \text{Calf C}) + (0.87 \times \text{Knee H})$$
$$+ (0.98 \times \text{MAC}) + (0.4 \times \text{Subsc SF})$$
$$- 62.35.$$

All measurements should be in centimeters and the resulting computed weight is in kilograms. Calf circumference is expected to have increasing application for assessment of lean mass. It can also be used as a measure of physical activity in the aged.

- **Anthropometric indices:** BMI has been used widely to estimate total body fatness. BMI can be obtained by using the formula: BMI = Weight (kg)/Height (m^2). BMI can be calculated to help classify whether the subject is in the reference range. Interobserver errors are possible. Height and weight have coefficient of variations in the order of less than 1%, may be altered by kyphosis in the aged and make interpretation of BMI invalid. The *abdominal* (taken at the midpoint between lower ribcage and iliac crest) and *hip* (taken at the maximal gluteal protrusion) *circumferences ratio (AHR)* is another anthropometric index to estimate fat distribution and the one now recommended by the WHO. It is fat distribution reflected in abdominal fatness, which may account for a number of chronic non-communicable diseases in the elderly if the ratio is above 0.9 for men and 0.8 for women. Several studies are now showing that umbilical measurements alone can be used to safely decide whether weight loss is necessary to reduce the risk from diseases such as heart disease and diabetes. Statistical analyses of umbilical circumferences of Caucasian men and women aged 25–74 years indicated that the ideal circumference for men is less than 102 cm and for women less than 88 cm. These conclusions are drawn from Caucasian subjects and thus may not apply in ethnic groups where the build is slight, such as in many Asian countries, and where a lesser degree of abdominal fatness may still put the person at risk of developing chronic diseases.

Laboratory investigations by way of biochemistry, hematology and immunology

Biochemical, hematological and immunological assessments are useful to confirm nutritional disorders and to identify specific complications that accompany them in the elderly (see also the chapter on metabolic and nutritional assessment in *Clinical Nutrition* in this series).

Various nutritionally related risk factors for health problems in the aged

Elderly people tend to have different degrees of risk factors (see section on Nutritionally vulnerable 'at-risk' groups).

7.9 Guidelines for healthy aging

Sometimes the assumption is made that, after we turn 65 or 70 years, perhaps lifestyle changes will no longer confer significant benefits. Are the remaining years sufficient to reap the benefits of modifications to food choice or exercise patterns? Several recent intervention and survival studies reveal that improvements in nutrition and regular exercise can benefit health even in advanced old age. For example, older muscles are just as responsive to strength-training exercises as are young muscles. Nonagenarians have shown impressive increases in muscle mass, muscle strength and walking speed with weight-training programs. Chronological age is, in itself, clearly no justification for deciding whether it is worthwhile to pursue lifestyle change. Behavioral risk factors (e.g. regularly not eating breakfast, lack of regular physical activity, overweight, smoking) have been shown to remain predictors of 17 year mortality even in people aged over 70. If elderly people pay attention to aspects of their lifestyle (physical and social activity) other than eating, they may be able to make nutritional errors with less consequence.

Physical activity

The type of physical activity can play an important role in the health of older people. The two principal forms of physical activity or exercise important in promoting health and well-being are endurance/aerobic exercise and strength training. Endurance activities improve heart and lung fitness and psychological functioning, while strength training enhances muscle size and strength, thus preventing muscle atrophy. The level of physical activity required for older adults to achieve optimal health benefits has not yet been established. Resistance (or strength) training prevents lean muscle atrophy more effectively than aerobic activity, especially during weight loss, whereas aerobic exercise may be more involved in improving psychological functioning in older people (although group membership may also be a factor). Strength training in older adults seems particularly promising in reducing or preventing the decline in muscle mass observed with aging. It can improve walking ability and balance and its associated risk for falls. Strength training also contributes to improved tendon and ligament strength, bone health and improvements in blood sugar levels. The benefits of physical activity such as strength training should make activities of daily living easier for older people. Such activities might include climbing stairs, getting out of a chair, pushing a vacuum cleaner, carrying groceries and crossing a road with sufficient speed. Research suggests that endurance activities should be performed daily (e.g. a walk of 30 min duration or three bouts of 8–10 min), along with some strength training. Endurance activities do not have to be continuous but can be accrued throughout the day through short bursts of activity.

Protective foods and food variety

The first consideration when it comes to nutritional matters is that enough food is available for basic energy and nutritional needs. Food variety is another important consideration in terms of nutritional adequacy and health outcomes. Food variety has been demonstrated to be an accurate predictor of the nutritional adequacy of the diet, and is invariably linked to food availability. Consuming a wide variety of foods (especially plant foods) has been associated with longevity. It is suggested that an ideal way to increase variety in the diet is to choose foods from across all five food groups, and a wide selection within each of these groups. Several studies have shown that energy and total food intakes decline with age, making a nutritionally adequate diet more difficult to achieve. Older men consume about 800 kcal less than younger men and older women about 400 kcal less than younger women. A reduction in BMR is partly responsible for this decline, but physical inactivity appears to be the major cause for reduced food intake. Compared with younger adults, older adults need to reach at least the same levels of intake (and in some cases, higher levels) of most vitamins, minerals and protein. Since this usually needs to be obtained from substantially lower overall food intakes, however, a nutrient and phytochemically dense diet becomes a high priority in later life. In other words, given the tendency for activity levels to decline and total food intakes to fall with advancing years, there is less room for energy-dense foods (e.g. indulgences, treats) which supply few of the essential nutrients that our bodies continue to need. Therefore, older adults need be selective about what they eat to avoid excessive fat gain and to prefer foods that are nutrient dense and high in protein (e.g. nuts, lean red meat, low-fat dairy products, legumes, seeds). This principle also applies to younger adults who are sedentary. Eating in a traditional food culture context can provide a measure of food security for the aged. This is one of the arguments for Food-based Dietary Guidelines (FBDGs) for the aged. The consumption of nutrient-dense foods reduces the risk of essential nutrient deficiencies. These foods include:

- eggs (little if any effect on serum cholesterol if not eaten with saturated fat)
- liver
- lean meat
- meat alternatives such as legumes (especially traditional soy products, e.g. tofu and tempeh) and nuts
- fish
- low-fat milk and dairy products
- fruits, vegetables, plant shoots
- wholegrain cereals
- wheat germ
- yeast
- unrefined fat from whole foods (nuts, seeds, beans, olives, avocado, fish)
- refined fat from liquid oils (cold pressed, from a variety of sources, predominant in n-3 and/or n-9 fatty acids).

The protective nutritional value of fruits and vegetables is derived particularly from their content of phytochemicals, which are multifunctional compounds, usually of health benefit (antioxidant, antimutagenic, antiangiogenic, immunomodulatory, phytoestrogens). In late 1999, the Australian government, based on the National Health and Medical Research Council report, released a set of dietary guidelines for older Australians (Table 7.6).

Table 7.6 Dietary guidelines for older Australians, 1999

1. Enjoy a wide variety of nutritious foods
2. Keep active to maintain muscle strength and a healthy body weight
3. Eat at least three meals every day
4. Care for your food: prepare and store it correctly
5. Eat plenty of vegetables (including legumes) and fruit
6. Eat plenty of cereals, breads and pastas
7. Eat a diet low in saturated fat
8. Drink adequate amounts of water and/or other fluids
9. If you drink alcohol, limit your intake
10. Choose foods low in salt and use salt sparingly
11. Include foods high in calcium
12. Use added sugars in moderation

Source: National Health and Medical Research Council (1999). © Commonwealth of Australia. Reproduced with permission.

The FBDGs were also recently published in conjunction with the WHO. They address traditional foods and dishes and most importantly cuisine, making such guidelines more practical and user-friendly at the individual level. These principles will need to be addressed by the various countries around the world when developing their own country/culture-specific FBDGs.

To summarize, the nutritional factors involved in healthy aging include food variety, nutrient and phytochemical density. A 'Mediterranean' food pattern may also reduce the risk of death in older adults. In the frail elderly there should be more emphasis on the need for support and increased nourishment and the prevention of malnutrition. The best and main message for an older person at home is to be well nourished, to be as active as possible without overdoing it, to eat better, not less, to keep their weight up and to drink plenty of fluids every day.

7.10 Perspectives on the future

While maximal lifespan is probably genetically determined, the probability of reaching that lifespan in good health seems largely determined by environmental and lifestyle factors. Thus, if humans are to continue to increase their lifespan and associated quality of life, they will most likely have to make alterations, even if very small, in the way they live their day-to-day life. This may take the form of consuming more fruit and vegetables, reading or taking a daily walk. Owing to decreased energy requirements in old age, diet plays an integral part in maintaining health and vitality. The quality of the diet is critical in ensuring that nutritional needs are met. The diet should consist of nutrient rich, low energy dense foods, which are generally low in fat.

There is not much room for indulgences in an elderly person's diet, especially if they are sedentary. Even though energy requirements are lower, nutrient needs are the same as or higher than those in younger adults. To reduce abdominal obesity and the development of subclinical deficiencies, older adults must choose foods wisely and maintain appropriate physical activity levels.

Further reading

Growth

Cole TJ, Bellizzi MC, Flegal KM, Dietz WH. Establishing a standard definition for child overweight and obesity worldwide: international survey. BMJ 2000; 320: 1240. http://www.bmj.com/cgi/content/full/320/7244/1240

Gracey M, Hetzel B, Smallwood R *et al.* Responsibility for Nutritional Diagnosis: A Report by the Nutrition Working Party of the Social Issues Committee of the Royal Australasian College of Physicians. London: Smith-Gordon, 1989.

Lee RD, Nieman DC. Nutritional Assessment, 2nd edn. Sydney: McGraw-Hill, 1996.

National Health and Medical Research Council. The Australian Dietary Guidelines for Children and Adolescents. Canberra: Australian Government Publishing Service, 1995. On-line scientific background papers for each guideline. Http://www.health.gov.au:80/nhmrc/publications/synopses/n1syn.htm

Tienboon P, Rutishauser IHE, Wahlqvist ML. Early life factors affecting body mass index and waist-hip ratio in adolescence. Asia Pacific J Clin Nutr 1992; 1: 21–6.

USDA, 2000. http://www.usda.gov/cnpp/dietary_guidelines.htm

Aging

Campbell AJ, Buchner DM. Unstable disability and the fluctuations of frailty. Age and Ageng 1997; 26: 315–318.

Chapuy MC, Arlot ME, Duboeuf F, Brun J, Crouzet B, Arnaud S, Delmas PD, Meunier PJ. Vitamin D3 and calcium to prevent hip fractures in the elderly women. N Engl J Med. 1992 Dec 3; 327 (23): 1637–1642.

Fiatarone MA, O'Neill EF, Ryan ND, Clements KM, Solares GR, Nelson ME, Roberts SB, Kehayias JJ, Lipsitz LA, Evans WJ. Exercise training and nutritional supplementation for physical frailty in very elderly people. NEJM 1995; 330 (25): 1769–1775.

Glass TA, de Leon CM, Marattoli RA, Berkman LF. Population based study of social and productive activities as predictors of survival among elderly Americans. BMJ 1999; 319 (21): 478–483.

Grundy E. The epidemiology of aging. In: Textbook of Geriatric Medicine and Gerontology, 4th edn (JC Brocklehurst, RC Tallis, HM Fillit, eds), pp. 3–20. New York: Churchill Livingstone, 1992.

Khaw K-T. Healthy ageing. BMJ 1997; 315: 1090–1096. On-line full text: http://www.bmj.com/cgi/content/full/315/7115/1090

National Health and Medical Research Council. The Australian Dietary Guidelines for Older Adults. Canberra: Australian Government Publishing Service, 1999. On-line scientific background papers for each guideline. http://www.health.gov.au/nhmrc/publications/pdf/n23.pdf

Trichopoulou A, Kouris-Blazos A, Wahlqvist ML *et al.* Diet and overall survival in elderly people. BMJ 1995; 311: 1457–1460. On-line full text: http://www.bmj.com/cgi/content/full/311/7018/1457

Wahlqvist ML, Kouris-Blazos A. Requirements in maturity and ageing. In: Food and Nutrition: Australia and New Zealand (ML Wahlqvist, ed.). Sydney: Allen & Unwin, 2002. http://www.healthyeatingclub.com/bookstore/

8
Nutrition and the Brain

JD Fernstrom and MH Fernstrom

Key messages

- Brain chemistry and function are influenced by short-term and long-term changes in the diet.
- The blood–brain barrier is an important focal point for the nutrition of the brain: it is a selectively permeable barrier that promotes the uptake of water-soluble molecules via specific transporters (e.g. glucose, ketone bodies, amino acids, vitamins), excludes the uptake of other molecules, and allows the free diffusion of gases (e.g. oxygen, carbon dioxide) and other lipid-soluble molecules.
- Glucose is the principal energy substrate of the brain, although ketone bodies become major energy substrates during starvation.
- The dietary intake of carbohydrates, per se, does not influence the supply of hexoses to the brain.
- The dietary intake of protein and amino acids can influence the uptake of some amino acids into the brain, depending on the properties of amino acid transporters located at the blood–brain barrier.
- In the brain, amino acids are incorporated into proteins and functionally important small molecules, such as neurotransmitters. The production of these amino acid-derived small molecules is often surprisingly sensitive to the

supply of amino acid precursors from the circulation, and thus the diet.
- The brain does not use fatty acids directly as energy substrates, but does use them to construct a variety of complex lipid molecules that are incorporated into neuronal and glial cell membranes.
- Two fatty acids of functional importance to the brain are not synthesized in the brain or body of mammals (the essential fatty acids); certain brain functions thus depend on their adequate intake via the diet.
- Water-soluble vitamins gain access to the brain via blood–brain barrier (or blood–cerebrospinal fluid barrier) embedded transporters. Fat-soluble vitamins may also gain access to the brain by specialized transfer mechanisms that involve the macromolecules with which they circulate in the blood.
- Dietary deficiencies in certain water- and fat-soluble vitamins can produce functional deficits in the brain and retina of varying severity.
- The access of minerals to the brain, where studied, appears to involve the blood–brain barrier and special transport mechanisms; only prolonged deficiencies (for certain minerals) produce deficits in brain function.

8.1 Introduction

Until the 1960s, the brain was viewed as being 'protected' from both sudden and prolonged nutritional changes. This idea changed first with the realization that severe nutritional insults, such as malnutrition, could seriously retard normal brain development in the fetus and newborn. During the 1970s, a number of experimental findings emerged suggesting that in addition, fairly modest changes in the composition of the diet could directly influence the production of key

signaling molecules in the brain (the neurotransmitters), and thus brain functions.

A further factor that helped to change this early viewpoint of the brain's metabolic invulnerability was the elucidation by scientists of the true nature of the blood–brain barrier (BBB), a very old concept. Originally, the BBB was thought of as a 'barrier' between the blood and the brain, preventing environmental insults and metabolic changes in the body from disturbing the brain's chemistry and function. New work revealed that the BBB is not really a barrier at all, but instead an extensive set of transport carriers, located on the membranes of the cells that make up the capillaries of the brain, that promotes or restricts the entry of an endless number of molecules into brain, as well as their removal. Furthermore, in many cases transport carriers have been found to be 'plastic'; that is, the properties of specific carriers can change in relation to current demands for the nutrients they transport. A contemporary appreciation of how nutrition influences the brain thus requires an understanding of the nutrient transporters on capillary cells that modulate the flow of these molecules into and out of the brain.

This chapter will begin by providing an overview of the structure of the nervous system, and of the BBB. It will then consider how each of the nutrients in the diet finds its way into the brain, and whether vagaries in the diet can influence the uptake of nutrients into and ultimately their function within the brain.

8.2 General organization of the mammalian nervous system

The nervous system has two principal cell types, neurons and glia (Figure 8.1). Neurons are the cellular elements that provide information flow in the nervous system. They are organized into circuits that perform the various functions attributed to the nervous system. Neurons conduct electrical signals over short or long distances, depending on the circuit, and their anatomy bespeaks this function. Their cellular features are (a) one or more cellular extensions of variable length known as dendrites, which receive chemical and sometimes electrical signals from other neurons, (b) a cell body, which provides the normal housekeeping functions of cells, and passes electrical information received through dendrites across its surface membrane to the (c) axon, which conducts electrical signals away from the cell body to specialized endings, the nerve terminals. The nerve terminal contains special molecules, neurotransmitters, which are released by electrical signals arriving via the axon, which serve to modify the electrical activity of adjacent neurons. The nerve terminal, together with the adjacent neuron and the intracellular space between the two, is termed a synapse. The axon is the long conducting portion of the neuron, and depending on the circuit, can be short or extremely long. For example, a neuron in the cerebral cortex that controls a motor neuron that innervates a muscle in the toe must project an axon from an upper portion of the brain down into the lower reaches of the spinal cord, where it makes contact with the appropriate motor neuron. In a tall person, this axon could be 1 m in length; the axon of the motor neuron innervating the toe muscle could also be 1 m or more in length. This unusual cellular anatomy and function (maintenance and conduction of electrical impulses) suggests that neurons can have extraordinary metabolic needs.

Glial cells make up about 60% of the cellular mass of the brain, and provide (1) insulation and physical support and packing around neurons, (2) membranes (myelin sheaths) to insulate axons that insure privacy in the conduction of electrical impulses, and (3) metabolic support for dendrites, axons, nerve terminals and synapses. The glial cells found in peripheral nerve bundles serve the same functions.

At the organ level, the nervous system is divided into two parts, the central nervous system (CNS) and the peripheral nervous system (PNS) (Figure 8.2). The CNS consists of the brain (including the retina) and the spinal cord, and contains networks of neurons organized into circuits of functional importance (e.g. the regulation of blood pressure, the control of appetite, or the initiation and control of movement). The PNS consists of neurons that either serve to provide sensory information to the CNS (afferent neurons), or convey commands from the CNS to effector cells, such as muscle and gland cells (efferent neurons). The cell bodies of many sensory neurons lie outside the brain and spinal cord, while those of neurons conveying commands from the CNS lie within the brain or spinal cord. Hence, if the CNS provides a degree of metabolic organization and protection to the neurons and glia within it, such is not provided to peripheral neurons and/or their cellular processes. The structural organization of nerves and nerve bundles in the PNS, and their attendant glial cells, however, appears to provide some of the metabolic features enjoyed by neurons and glia within the CNS.

The following nutritional and metabolic discussion therefore focusses on the CNS, primarily the brain (since it has been easier to study). The presumption is, however, that what is found to be true for the brain will also be true for the spinal cord. Where evidence is available, relevant comments will also be made regarding nutrient and metabolic effects on peripheral nerves.

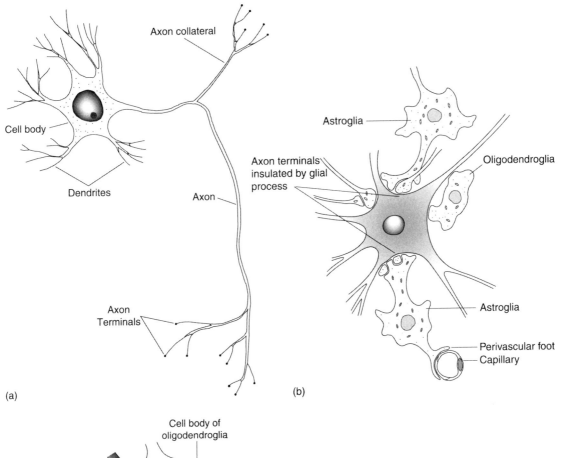

(a)

(b)

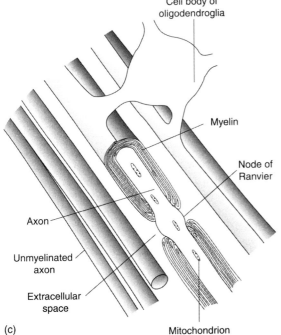

(c)

Figure 8.1 (a) Typical neuron; (b) glial cells and their relationships with brain neurons. Astroglia cells extend thin processes to surround regions where axon terminals make contact with neuronal surfaces (forming synapses), and separately to surround capllaries ("perivascular foot" in figure). Oligodendroglia cells can have relatively few processes, and provide physical packing and metabolic support around neurons; they can also have extensive processes, and form elaborate membranes around axons (myelin sheaths), as shown in (c). (c) Oligodendroglia wrapping axons with myelin. The three unmyelinated axons on the left lack myelin sheaths. The two axons on the right are myelinated by the same oligodendroglia cell (such cells can myelinate up to 50 axons). The myelin sheaths are connected by small cellular processes to the glial cell body. Outside the brain, the myelination of axons appears similar; glial cells performing this task are termed Schwann cells.

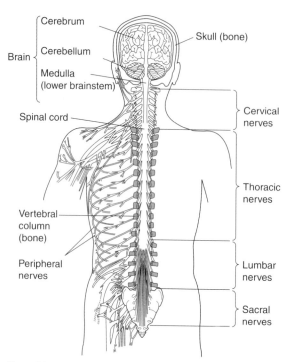

Figure 8.2 Gross structure of the human nervous system: brain, spinal cord and peripheral nerves.

8.3 The blood–brain barrier

A discussion of the BBB is central to any consideration of how food affects the brain (and other parts of the nervous system). This is because any solutes in blood must pass through this barrier to gain access to the brain extracellular fluid. Hence, the way in which the barrier handles blood-borne nutrients affects their availability to brain cells.

What do we mean by a blood–brain barrier? Historically, the concept arose a century ago with the observation that the intravenous administration to animals of certain dyes caused all tissues in the body, except for the brain, to be permeated by the dye. The brain, too, could become colored, but only when the dye was injected directly into the brain. Hence, the absence of color in the brain when the dye was administered into the blood did not result from some inability of brain cells to accumulate it, when they were exposed to it directly. Rather, some mechanism, a 'barrier', prevented the dye from penetrating from the blood into the brain.

With time, and much further experimentation, the blood–brain barrier was found to be a selective barrier to the penetration of solutes that are present in the circulation. It is now known to be located in the

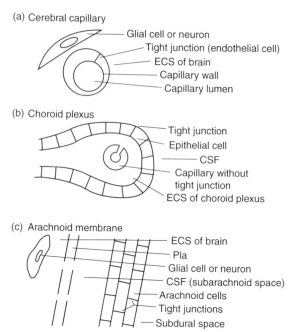

Figure 8.3 The physical nature of the blood–brain barrier. (a) The endothelial cells that form brain capillaries make tight junctions with each other, thereby preventing diffusion; capillary endothelial cells in other organs do not make tight junctions. (b) and (c) Capillaries that supply cerebral ventricles and choroid plexus are made up of endothelial cells *lacking* tight junctions. However, here the "barrier" is provided by tight junctions made by special epithelial and arachnoid cells, which prevent non-lipid molecules from entering the cerebrospinal fluid by simple diffusion. (From Spector, 1977.)

endothelial cells that make up the capillaries of the brain. Unlike capillaries elsewhere in the body, the endothelial cells of brain capillaries form tight junctions with each other, such that no fluid or solutes can pass into (or out of) brain without passing through these cells (Figure 8.3). Since this feature presents a continuous lipid barrier to solutes, as a first approximation, solutes in blood gain access to brain as a function of their lipid solubility. In fact, the ease of penetration of molecules into brain plots very reliably against their organic:aqueous partition coefficients: the greater the distribution into the organic phase, the greater the accessibility to brain by simple diffusion across cell membranes. However, many important exceptions exist, since most molecules of biological importance are water soluble, and thus do not readily diffuse into the brain. For example, the brain could not generate energy without a special, rapid means of acquiring glucose from the blood, since glucose is a water-soluble molecule. The same problem arises for other carbohydrates, as well as for amino acids, ketone bodies, vitamins and minerals. They are needed in the brain in amounts that could not be acquired rapidly enough if diffusion governed their rate of uptake into brain. The solution is that capillary endothelial cells have transport carriers for each of these (and other) nutrients, that greatly accelerate their uptake into the brain (relative to diffusion).

It should be noted as well that the brain does not have transport carriers for many water-soluble, biologically important compounds, for what seem to be very good reasons. Such molecules, when present in the blood, do not gain access to the brain. For example, certain neurotransmitters used by brain neurons are also used by peripheral neurons for the same purpose (e.g. norepinephrine, a neurotransmitter of the sympathetic nervous system). Significant concentrations of these molecules can sometimes occur in the blood, but they do not get into the brain, where they might indiscriminately modify brain functions. This protection occurs because they are water-soluble and brain capillary endothelial cells do not have transporters for them. Hence, viewed from this perspective, the BBB is a selectively permeable barrier, excluding some water-soluble molecules, promoting the uptake of other water-soluble molecules through carrier-mediated mechanisms, and further allowing the free penetration of gases (oxygen, carbon dioxide) and other lipid-soluble molecules. In addition, the BBB (capillary endothelial cells) appears to have transport carriers designed specifically to move molecules from the brain into the blood.

For completeness, it should be noted that not all parts of the CNS are protected by a BBB. Several small brain regions, known collectively as the circumventricular organs, receive their blood supplies from capillaries that do not have tight junctions. In such regions, neurons, nerve terminals and glial cells are exposed directly to all constituents of the blood. Compounds released by neurons and glia that would normally not penetrate the BBB are freely accessible to the blood in these areas. The absence of a BBB in these areas is presumably no accident. Indeed, it is thought that such areas lack a BBB because either they contain sensors for blood constituents that do not freely cross the barrier (e.g. the area postrema) or some of their neurons or glia release biologically important molecules into the circulation (e.g. nerve terminals in the median eminence, which release neurohormones into the blood that control the functions of the anterior pituitary gland).

These areas have been of some interest from a dietary perspective, as they have been argued to be gateways into the brain of amino acids that act as excitatory neurotransmitters. When consumed in excessive amounts in pure form, such amino acids (glutamic acid, aspartic acid, cysteine) have been reported to gain entry into brain via these areas, cause overexcitation of neurons and lead to their death. This issue is discussed further below.

A barrier known as the blood–cerebrospinal fluid (CSF) barrier is also found in a special region termed the choroid plexus. This special collection of blood vessels and brain ependymal cells lines a portion of the brain's ventricular system. It is the site of transport into (and out of) the brain of some nutritionally important molecules, and also is responsible for generating CSF. The blood–CSF barrier operates much like the BBB (Figure 8.3). It should also be noted that the retina (a portion of the CNS) is endowed with a blood–retinal barrier, the properties of which appear to be essentially identical to those of the BBB. Hence, as a first approximation, comments made in this chapter about the BBB also apply to the blood–retinal barrier.

Finally, the peripheral nerves lie outside the brain, and thus do not have a BBB to protect them. However, they do appear to have protection in the form of a blood–nerve barrier. Nerves running through the body are supplied by capillaries that have endothelial cells like those found in brain. That is, they have tight junctions between cells, restricting the passage of solutes. The properties of transport between blood and nerve, to the extent that they have been studied, have been found to be quite similar to those between blood and brain. The blood–nerve barrier does not appear to extend all the way to peripheral nerve terminals, however, which suggests that nerve endings are exposed to the circulation. This is most clearly evidenced by the occurrence in blood of neurotransmitters such as norepinephrine, which escape from peripheral nerve terminals located in the heart and other parts of the body, because no barrier surrounds terminal areas. It is also evident in the observation that when drugs such as 6-hydroxydopamine, which destroy norepinephrine nerve terminals in part by becoming concentrated in them, are given intravenously, they destroy peripheral, but not brain norepinephrine terminals. The peripheral norepinephrine nerve terminal lacks a barrier to circulating 6-hydroxydopamine; the brain norepinephrine terminal is protected by the BBB.

The BBB is discussed here because it figures prominently in the discussion that follows. The access of dietary nutrients to the brain occurs by way of the circulation. The BBB sits between the blood and the brain. The access of any nutrient to brain therefore depends to a considerable extent on the properties of the BBB (and blood–CSF barrier) and its transport systems for that nutrient.

8.4 Energy substrates

The brain uses glucose as its primary energy substrate. Because glucose is hydrophilic, and thus does not easily penetrate lipid membranes, its uptake into brain requires a transporter, which is located at the BBB. The properties of the transporter for glucose (actually, for hexoses: it mediates the uptake of any of several sugars, although in practice glucose is the principal passenger) can be described using simple Michelis–Menton kinetics. The carrier, which is saturable and competitive, non-concentrative and not insulin responsive, has a K_m for glucose of about 10 mM, somewhat higher than normal blood glucose levels (4–6 mM). This means that the carrier is about half-saturated at normal blood glucose concentrations. The V_{max} of the transporter for glucose is 1.4 μmol/min per gram of brain, or about 1200 g/day for the entire brain (a human brain weighs about 1400 g). The human brain normally consumes 15–20% of the body's oxygen consumption, which allows an estimation of glucose utilization by brain to be about 100 g/day. The carrier thus has a capacity for transporting glucose that is well in excess of that demanded daily by the brain. This fact presumably reflects the importance of glucose as the brain's primary fuel.

Once glucose has been transported across the BBB into the extracellular fluid, it is rapidly taken up into neurons by another glucose transporter, located on the cell membrane. This transporter has a glucose affinity some 30 times that of the BBB transporter. Within the cell, the glucose can then enter the glycolytic pathway. The initial enzyme, hexokinase, also has a very high affinity for glucose, and is therefore fully saturated at normal brain glucose concentrations (3–4 mM). Overall, then, each step in the glucose pipeline from the circulation to brain neurons is tuned to maximize glucose supply for energy production. It only fails when the blood glucose supply is abruptly curtailed (e.g. the rapid hypoglycemia that follows the accidental administration of too high a dose of insulin to a diabetic patient).

Blood glucose levels are normally regulated within bounds, except under unusual circumstances, such as starvation and diabetes. Hence, variations in the intake of carbohydrates, per se, are not thought to influence the uptake of glucose into the brain, or cerebral function. For example, consuming more or less sugar on any given day does not influence brain glucose uptake. The brain, however, monitors blood glucose concentrations, presumably to insure adequacy of supply, and uses behavior (food intake) as one mechanism for regulating blood glucose levels.

Blood glucose levels do not normally become low, but fall only under one extreme environmental circumstance, starvation. In starvation, when glucose supplies fall, the brain adds an additional energy source, ketone bodies. Ketone bodies are by-products of the breakdown of stored fat, and provide an extended supply of energy in the absence of food-derived energy. The brain will use ketone bodies whenever provided with them (i.e. whenever blood ketone body levels rise), and blood ketone body concentrations rise in starvation. Indeed, the brain participates in the mobilization of the body's fat stores, the key event that causes a cascade leading to increased blood ketone body concentrations. The BBB transporter for ketone bodies, required because ketone bodies are hydrophilic compounds that do not readily cross cell membranes, is induced during starvation, further promoting the flow of ketone bodies into brain. This transporter, like the glucose transporter, has a K_m that exceeds the concentrations of circulating ketone bodies that occur during starvation, and a V_{max} well in excess of energy demands. Ketone body delivery to brain will therefore never be limited by this transporter. During prolonged starvation, more than half of the energy used by the brain is derived from ketone bodies. Continued use of some glucose appears obligatory, and is supplied by way of hepatic gluconeogenesis.

The ingestion of certain foods can also induce the brain to use ketone bodies as an energy source. The chronic ingestion of very high-fat diets elevates blood ketone body concentrations, promoting their use by brain as an energy substrate. However, extremely high levels of fat intake are required to produce this effect, and such diets are found by most to be unpalatable. Hence, in practice, ketogenic diets are not sought after, and are hard to follow for extended periods.

Diet is therefore not thought normally to influence cerebral energy production via dietary fat manipulation of ketone body supply to brain (although it can).

High-fat diets are occasionally used clinically with success to treat intractable seizures, and the effect is linked to elevations in circulating ketone bodies. Although the mechanism of this effect is not understood, one hypothesis is that such diets somehow modify neuronal excitability to reduce seizure occurrence through the provision of this energy source to brain neurons.

As indicated earlier, blood glucose concentrations can fall abruptly, though not under physiological circumstances. An overdose of insulin administered by accident to a diabetic subject can cause a rapid, precipitous decline in blood glucose levels. The importance of maintaining blood glucose levels for the benefit of brain energy production quickly becomes evident, since confusion, delirium, seizures, coma and death occur as blood glucose concentrations drop below 50 mg/100 ml (2.5–3.0 mmoles/l). That such effects occur, and are most effectively and rapidly reversed by the infusion of glucose, suggests that there is no other compound present in the blood that can readily substitute for glucose as the primary energy source for the brain. When gradual, long-term declines in blood glucose are produced experimentally, the brain adapts by increasing the functioning of BBB transport carriers for glucose. The BBB hexose transporter is thus somewhat 'plastic'. Indeed, faced with chronic hyperglycemia, this hexose carrier can also reduce its ability to transport glucose into the brain.

The high rate of energy utilization by the brain is thought to reflect the fact that 10 billion or so neurons must generate and maintain electrochemical gradients across their cell membranes, which are used to produce neuronal impulses. This notion is supported by several types of evidence, and leads to the obvious prediction that when neuronal populations conduct more business, as they often do, glucose consumption rises. Conversely, when they conduct less, consumption falls. The mechanism for providing more glucose under conditions of increased neuronal firing involves increased blood flow to areas of enhanced neuronal activity. Glucose extraction increases simply because it is a flow-limited phenomenon. Such local mechanisms operate to ensure adequate cerebral supplies of glucose on a moment-to-moment basis. Their existence indirectly suggests that hunger and food intake,

if used by the brain as a mechanism for obtaining energy substrates, are relatively slow mechanisms for obtaining adequate cerebral energy supplies.

A final issue regarding brain energy substrates is ethanol, which supplies about 7 kcal/g when metabolized by the body (mainly in the liver and intestines). Is ethanol metabolized by the brain, and in the process, does it contribute to the brain's energy supply? Ethanol is lipid soluble, and thus readily penetrates into the brain as blood ethanol concentrations rise. However, the brain contains very little alcohol dehydrogenase (it may possibly be found in very small amounts in some neurons), and thus does not metabolize ethanol in appreciable amounts. Hence, the brain does not derive energy directly from local ethanol metabolism. This is probably not an accident, since the immediate product of ethanol metabolism, acetaldehyde, is toxic to the brain (indeed, acetaldehyde is not taken up into brain from the circulation). Ethanol consumption reduces glucose transport into and/or phosphorylation within the brain, and thus may actually limit the brain's energy supply. This action may contribute to its behavioral effects (CNS depression).

In sum, the dietary intake of carbohydrates does not appear to influence the availability of glucose or other hexoses to brain. Instead, blood glucose concentrations and cerebral blood flow are regulated, presumably to ensure the required supply to brain. In starvation, when glucose supply becomes severely limited, the body accelerates ketone body production, and the brain switches to these molecules as its primary energy source. While diets very high in fat can also lead to ketone body formation, and thus use by the brain, such diets are not typically consumed. Ethanol, an energy source in some parts of the body, is not an energy substrate in the brain.

8.5 Amino acids and protein

Neuronal and glial cells in the brain use all amino acids to produce proteins. In addition, they use certain amino acids for neurotransmission. The issue in relation to nutrition and the brain is the extent to which diet can influence the flow of amino acids into this organ, and thus their individual uses. Like other needed substrates, the path from diet to brain proceeds from their absorption by the gastrointestinal tract, through their insertion into the circulation, to their extraction by brain. As might be anticipated, this extraction process involves the BBB. The brain capillary endothelial cells that constitute the BBB contain on their cell surfaces a number of different transporters for amino

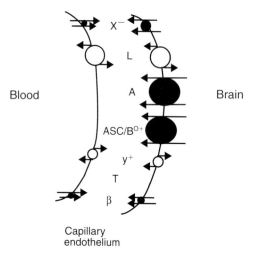

Figure 8.4 Blood–brain barrier amino acid transport carriers. Shaded Systems: Sodium dependent; unshaded systems: sodium independent. (Reproduced with permission from Smith and Stoll, 1998.)

acids. The properties of these transporters dictate how much of each amino acid enters and exits the brain.

Amino acids enter and exit the brain by one of several transport carriers. The choice of carrier relates to the size and charge of the amino acid side-chain. Currently, six carriers have been identified (Figure 8.4). The *first* is the large neutral amino acid carrier (L in the figure), which is a non-energy requiring, bidirectional transporter that is saturable and stereospecific. This carrier is shared by several amino acids (Table 8.1), including some that are precursors for neurotransmitters (phenylalanine, tyrosine, tryptophan, histidine). Because the carrier is almost saturated at normal plasma concentrations of these amino acids, it is competitive. Hence, changes in the plasma concentration of any one large, neutral amino acid will affect not only that amino acid's transport into brain, but also that of each of its transport competitors. Because glutamine is present in brain in extremely large concentrations (it is produced there for a variety of uses), this large neutral amino acid is thought to drive the uptake into the brain of the other large neutral amino acids, by serving as the principal amino acid that is

Table 8.1 Blood–brain barrier transport constants for brain uptake of neutral and basic amino acids, as measured by the *in situ* rat brain perfusion technique

Amino acid	Plasma concentration (μM)	κ_m (μM)	V_{max} (nmol/min/g)	κ_m (app) (μM)	Influx (nmol/min/g)
Neutral amino acids (system L)					
Phe	81	11	41	170	13.2
Trp	82	15	55	330	8.2[a]
Leu	175	29	59	500	14.5
Met	64	40	25	860	1.7
Ile	87	56	60	1210	4.0
Tyr	63	64	96	1420	4.1
His	95	100	61	2220	2.5
Val	181	210	49	4690	1.8
Thr	237	220	17	4860	0.8
Gln	485	880	43	19900	1.0
Basic amino acids (system y^+)					
Arg	117	56	24	302	6.7
Lys	245	70	22	279	10.3
Orn	98	109	26	718	3.1

[a]Estimated assuming ~70% of albumin-bound Trp contributes to brain uptake.
V_{max}: maximal saturable transport capacity; κ_m: half-saturation concentration in the absence of competitors; κ_m(app): 'apparent' κ_m under normal physiological conditions (i.e. in the presence of normal concentrations of plasma amino acids: κ_m(app) = $\kappa_m(1 + \Sigma(Ci/\kappa_m i))$; influx: unidirectional amino acid flux rate from plasma to brain. Apparent κ_m values *in vivo* are much greater than true κ_m because of transport saturation and competition. (Reproduced with permission from Smith and Stoll, 1998.)

counter-transported from brain to blood each time a large neutral amino acid is taken up into brain.

The *second* transporter is the basic amino acid carrier (y^+ in Figure 8.4), which is also non-energy requiring, bidirectional, saturable and stereospecific. It is responsible for transporting arginine, lysine and ornithine, and is competitive. The *third* transporter is the acidic amino acid carrier (X^- in Figure 8.4), transporting glutamic and aspartic acids. This carrier is energy requiring, although little uptake occurs from blood to brain. Instead, the major activity of this carrier is seen on the abluminal membrane (i.e. the membrane on the brain side) of capillary endothelial cells, such that most of the glutamate and aspartate transport is *from* the brain *to* the circulation. Indeed, balance studies of glutamate indicate that the brain is a net exporter of this amino acid, synthesizing much more than it needs. The *fourth* transporter is the small, neutral amino acid carrier (A in Figure 8.4), preferring amino acids with small, polar side-chains, also energy dependent, which transports primarily alanine, glycine, methionine and proline. This carrier is also located on abluminal side of the capillary endothelial cell, and like the X^- transporter, is thought to move amino acids primarily *from* brain *into* blood. The *fifth* carrier (ASC/B^{o+} in Figure 8.4) is also abluminal, and is specific to the small neutral amino acids alanine, serine and cysteine. Finally, the sixth carrier (β in Figure 8.4) is selective for taurine, and is energy requiring.

It is evident from the above discussion that the carriers oriented to move amino acids into the brain are those that transport mostly essential amino acids (the large, neutral and basic amino acids), while those oriented to move amino acids out of brain are those transporting non-essential amino acids (the acidic and small neutral amino acids). A small, net influx into the brain of the essential amino acids, notably tryptophan, tyrosine, phenylalanine, histidine and arginine, is no doubt required for the synthesis of the neurotransmitters from which they are derived (and are ultimately metabolized). The net efflux of the non-essential amino acids, notably aspartate, glutamate, glycine and cysteine, may serve as a means of removing amino acids that act *directly* as excitatory transmitters or cotransmitters in the brain. The brain carefully compartmentalizes these amino acids metabolically, as discussed below, because they excite (i.e. depolarize) neurons. A mechanism to remove these amino acids

from the brain may be a component of this compartmentalization design.

A better understanding of the fundamentally different manner in which the brain uses transport carriers to handle the essential amino acids that are neurotransmitter precursors, and the non-essential amino acids that are neurotransmitters, can be gained by studying an example of each. These examples also reveal important distinctions regarding the impact of the diet on amino acid transport into the brain. The examples are tryptophan, a large neutral amino acid, and glutamate, an acidic amino acid.

Tryptophan, a large neutral amino acid

Tryptophan is the precursor for the neurotransmitter serotonin (5-hydroxytryptamine). Serotonin neurons have their cell bodies in small regions (termed raphe nuclei) of the brainstem and midbrain, and project their axons extensively throughout the spinal cord and brain. This relatively small population of neurons (less than 1% of the total brain population) thus appears to communicate with most of the neurons in the CNS, and functions in neuronal circuitry that controls, for example, blood pressure, pituitary hormone secretion, sensory information processing (touch, pain, sound) and sleep.

Interest in this neurotransmitter in the present context derives from the fact that the concentration of tryptophan in the brain rapidly influences the rate of serotonin synthesis. This relationship holds because the enzyme that catalyzes the initial and rate-limiting step in serotonin synthesis (tryptophan hydroxylase; Figure 8.5) is relatively unsaturated with substrate at normal brain tryptophan concentrations. Hence, a rise in tryptophan concentration leads to an increase in serotonin synthesis as tryptophan hydroxylase becomes more saturated with substrate (causing the rate-limiting reaction to proceed more quickly). A fall in tryptophan concentration causes a reduction in serotonin synthesis as enzyme saturation declines (and the reaction proceeds more slowly).

Tryptophan concentrations in the brain are directly influenced by the tryptophan concentrations in plasma. Hence, a change in plasma tryptophan concentration can directly influence serotonin synthesis in brain neurons. However, because tryptophan is transported into brain by the competitive carrier for large neutral amino acids, tryptophan uptake and concentrations in brain, and thus serotonin synthesis, can *also* be modified by

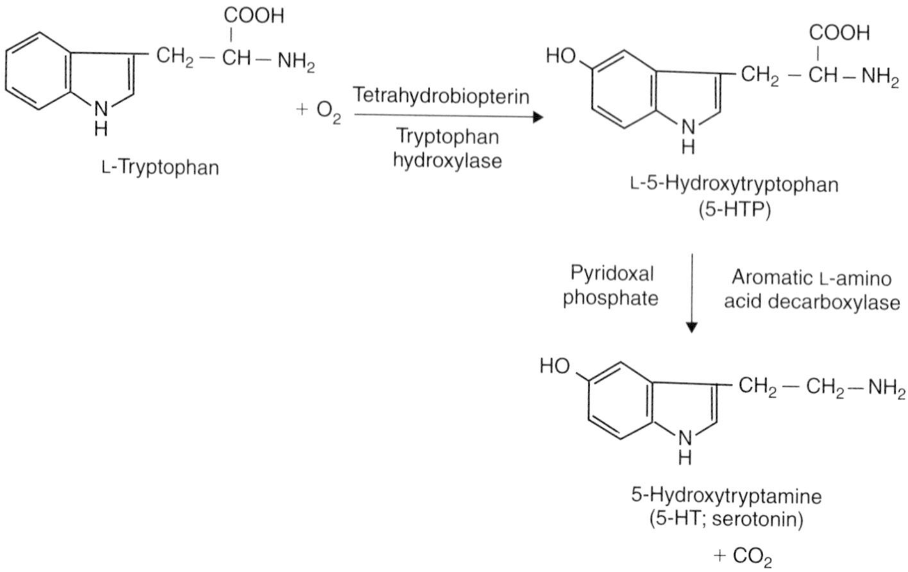

Figure 8.5 Pathway of serotonin synthesis from L-tryptophan. Serotonin is synthesized in two steps catalyzed by the enzymes tryptophan hydroxylase and aromatic L-amino acid decarboxylase. The cofactor for each reaction is also shown.

changing the plasma concentrations of *any* of its transport competitors. The plasma concentrations of most amino acids, including the large neutral amino acids, are readily influenced by food intake, thereby forming the final link between diet and serotonin synthesis in brain. But it is the competitive nature of the large neutral amino acid transporter that explains a seemingly confusing feature of how food intake modifies brain tryptophan concentrations and serotonin synthesis. When fasting animals ingest a meal of carbohydrates, plasma tryptophan increases within 1–2 h. This effect is paralleled by a like increase in brain tryptophan concentrations, and serotonin synthesis is accelerated. But when animals ingest a meal containing protein as well as carbohydrates, and plasma tryptophan rises even more than when carbohydrates are consumed alone, no rise in brain tryptophan concentration or serotonin synthesis occurs. The explanation for this effect involves tryptophan's competitors for transport at the BBB. When carbohydrates alone are consumed, not only does plasma tryptophan rise, but the plasma levels of most of its transport competitors fall, giving tryptophan a great advantage in competing for available transport sites into the brain. Brain tryptophan uptake and concentrations therefore increase. However, when a protein-containing meal is consumed, even though plasma tryptophan rises considerably, the

plasma concentrations of its many competitors not only fail to decline, but rise and by a proportionally *similar* amount to tryptophan. As a consequence, tryptophan experiences no change in its competitive standing for access to available transporters into brain, and brain tryptophan concentrations do not change. Hence, a key feature of the large neutral amino acid transporter, its competitive nature, explains the impact of meals containing or lacking protein on the production of a molecule important to normal brain function (serotonin).

The above example considers relatively rapid effects of food on tryptophan and serotonin. Longer term changes are also observed. For example, if rats are fed chronically with diets containing a protein naturally high in leucine content with normal amounts of tryptophan (sorghum), brain tryptophan and serotonin concentrations decline. This effect can be explained by an increase in the plasma leucine concentration (plasma concentrations of branched-chain amino acids reflect their content in the diet, because the liver cannot metabolize them), which competitively retards tryptophan transport into brain. In addition, when animals consume diets low in protein for extended periods, the plasma concentrations of all essential amino acids decline, including tryptophan and the other large, neutral amino acids. In this case, even

though the decline in plasma tryptophan may be proportionally similar to that of its transport competitors
(i.e. competition for the brain transporters does not
change), brain tryptophan and serotonin decline. The
most likely explanation for this effect is that the transport carriers, which are about 95% saturated when
normal amounts of protein are being consumed,
become much less saturated at low levels of protein
intake, because of the decline in the plasma concentrations of all large, neutral amino acids. At low carrier
saturation, competition ceases, and simple changes in
plasma tryptophan concentrations suffice to predict
brain tryptophan uptake and concentrations.

Other large, neutral amino acids serve as neurotransmitter precursors in substrate-driven pathways in
brain. Phenylalanine and tyrosine are substrates for the
synthesis of the catecholamines (dopamine, norepinephrine, epinephrine), and histidine is the precursor
of histamine. Like tryptophan, the brain concentrations of these amino acids are directly influenced by
their uptakes from the circulation, which in turn reflect
the plasma concentrations of all of the large, neutral
amino acids. For these transmitter precursors as well,
the influence of diet on their brain concentrations
reflects the impact the diet has on the plasma concentration of each amino acid in relation to those of
its competitors.

Glutamate, an acidic amino acid

The non-essential amino acid glutamate is used
directly as a transmitter by more than half of all nerve
terminals in brain. It is not known why there is such
extensive use of a single molecule of such great ubiquity in neuronal communications. Glutamate is an
excitatory neurotransmitter, which means that when
it is applied to neurons with appropriate glutamate
receptors on their surface, the neurons depolarize
(become electrically active). Within nerve terminals,
glutamate is packaged in small vesicles, where it resides
until it is released. Once released into the synapse, it
stimulates glutamate receptors on adjacent neurons,
and is then quickly cleared from the synapse. Glutamate
receptors fall into two broad categories, ionotropic and
metabotropic. Ionotropic receptors are linked to ion
channels and, when stimulated, directly alter transmembrane ion fluxes, thereby initiating depolarization.
Metabotropic receptors are linked to intracellular
second messengers and, when stimulated, modify signaling pathways (such as those initiated by adenylate

cyclase or protein kinases) that ultimately precipitate
changes in neuronal function. Because glutamate is so
ubiquitous as a transmitter in brain, it has been difficult to discern clearly the properties of the neuronal
circuits in which it operates, and the roles they play in
brain function. Nonetheless, glutamate neurons are
now actively studied, for example, for their involvement in learning and memory, in the control of
pituitary hormone secretion, and in blood pressure
control.

Because glutamate is an excitatory amino acid,
neurons with excitatory glutamate receptors on their
surface can become overexcited when exposed to high
concentrations of the amino acid, and die. The term
excitotoxicity was coined many years ago to describe
this effect. It led to the concern that perhaps because
glutamate is a major constituent of dietary proteins,
and also added to many foods as a flavoring agent, the
ingestion of food might cause the brain to become
flooded with glutamate, leading to widespread neurotoxicity. However, this possibility turns out not to be
the case. The principal reasons relates to the function
of the acidic amino acid transporter at the BBB
(X^- transporter in Figure 8.4). As noted earlier, this
transporter occurs primarily on the abluminal membrane of capillary endothelial cells. As a consequence,
the net transport of glutamate strongly favors transport out of the brain, not into it. Consequently, in this
case, the BBB really can be thought to function as
more than a 'barrier' regarding glutamate penetration.
This conclusion accords well with observations that
extremely large increases in plasma glutamate concentrations are required before signs of excitotoxicity
are evident in the brain (10–15-fold greater than would
ever be produced by food ingestion), increases that can
only be produced by administering extremely large
doses of free glutamate.

There is a second mechanism that protects brain
neurons from excessive exposure to glutamate, once
released by other neurons. It can also protect them
from glutamate that might accidentally penetrate into
brain from the blood. This mechanism involves the role
of glial cells in intracellular glutamate trafficking in
brain. In order for information flow in neuronal circuits to be rapid and accurate, neurotransmitters, once
released by nerve terminals, must quickly interact with
receptors on adjacent neurons, and then just as rapidly
be removed from the synapse (to reset it for the next
depolarization). For glutamate synapses, this process

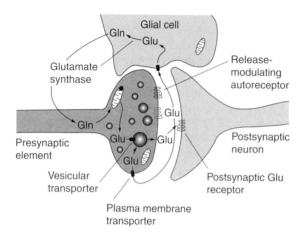

Figure 8.6 Glutamate synapse, showing glutamate and glutamine trafficking between neurons and glial cells in the brain. Glutamate, synthesized via metabolic pathways, is concentrated through a vesicular transporter into secretory granules. After release from the presynaptic terminal, glutamate can interact with receptors. Glutamate is then cleared from the synaptic region by the high-affinity plasma membrane transporters or by recycling through adjacent glia.

of neurotransmitter removal is accomplished primarily by local glial cells, which have energy-requiring, high-affinity glutamate transporters on their surface. Once inside the glial cell, the glutamate is quickly converted to glutamine (by glutamine synthetase) and released into the intercellular spaces, from which it is taken back up into neurons, reconverted to glutamate (by glutaminase) and stored for reuse (Figure 8.6). While the efficient removal of synaptic glutamate by glial cells functions primarily in glutamate–glutamine recycling between neurons and glia, it can also serve to remove from brain extracellular fluid glutamate molecules that may penetrate through the BBB.

Hence, overall, the BBB transporter for glutamate (and brain glial cell glutamate transporters as a backup system) prevents the glutamate ingested in food from entering the brain or influencing brain glutamate neurotransmission.

There are exceptions to this rule. One relates to the existence of several, small portions of the brain, termed the circumventricular organs, that lack a BBB. Presumably, this is not an accident of evolution, but serves to allow neurons in these regions to have access to blood constituents not permitted elsewhere in the brain (perhaps to allow sensing of particular molecules in blood) and their terminals to release molecules (e.g. neurohormones) into the circulation. It is possible that

these areas are exposed to circulating glutamate, for reasons not presently understood. However, the glial elements in these areas function as they do elsewhere in brain, and rapidly accumulate the glutamate that penetrates in from the circulation. As a consequence, the glial cells in these areas protect neural processes with glutamate receptors on their surfaces.

Protein

Amino acids are also used to synthesize protein in the brain, by mechanisms common to all cells in the body. Does dietary protein intake influence this process (as it does in liver, for example)? In adult animals, variations in dietary protein intake have no effects on brain protein synthesis. This includes the chronic ingestion of very low levels of dietary protein, and probably means that brain cells are quite efficient in reusing amino acids liberated during intracellular protein breakdown. Low levels of protein intake by neonatal and infant animals, however, are associated with below-normal rates of protein synthesis in brain. To date, one putative mechanism of this association, namely reduced uptake of essential amino acids into brain, and abnormally low brain concentrations of these amino acids, has not been proven.

Fatty acids and choline

Fatty Acids

Unlike other tissues in the body, the brain does not appear to use fatty acids directly as energy substrates. However, fatty acids are required by the brain on a continuing basis for the synthesis of the complex fat molecules that are used to construct neuronal and glial cell membranes. This process is extremely active in infant and growing animals, and it is also active in adults. The brain is thought to synthesize some fatty acids from smaller molecules, but uptake from the circulation is also considered to be an important, possibly the major source of most fatty acids found in the brain. (Indeed, the circulation is the ultimate source of all essential fatty acids in the brain.) In the blood, fatty acids circulate either as components of fat molecules or as non-esterified fatty acids. Some evidence suggests that lysophatidylcholine can be taken up into the brain, but non-esterified fatty acids presumably are the primary form in which fatty acids gain access to the brain. Indeed, uptake into the brain of both essential and non-essential fatty acids has repeatedly been demonstrated. The details of the uptake process are not presently understood, however, and fatty acid uptake presents certain conceptual problems. For example, the fact that fatty acids bind tightly to serum albumin suggests they might not be readily available for exchange with a transport carrier located at the BBB, and diffusion across capillary endothelial cell membranes may be limited, since fatty acids are almost completely ionized at physiological pH. At present, there is no generally accepted model of fatty acid transport to explain the available data for uptake into the brain and retina. Current hypotheses include multiple variants of the possibilities that fatty acids or albumin–fatty acid complexes bind to receptor sites on endothelial cells, and are moved across the membrane into the cell interior, either as the free fatty acid or as the complex, or that fatty acids diffuse in the non-ionized form across cell membranes.

Whatever the ultimate mechanism of transport proves to be, from the nutritional perspective, diet does influence essential fatty acid availability to brain, with potentially important functional consequences. In almost all mammals (cats are an exception), there are two long-chain fatty acids that cannot be synthesized, and thus are essential in the diet. These are the polyunsaturated fatty acids linoleic acid and α-linolenic acid. In the body (including the nervous system), linoleic acid is converted into arachadonic acid, a key precursor in the synthesis of prostaglandins and leukotrienes, families of important second messenger molecules. α-Linolenic acid is converted into docosahexanoic acid, a molecule found in very large amounts in the outer segments of rods and cones in retina, and in nerve terminal membranes in the brain (Figure 8.7). Docosahexanoic acid is thought to be a key component of phototransduction cells, and thus may be important in vision.

Inside the nervous system, linoleic and α-linolenic acid are incorporated into phospholipid molecules and inserted into cellular membranes. Typical phospholipids, which contain two fatty acid molecules, contain one saturated and one unsaturated fatty acid. In retinal rods and cones, where the docosahexanoic acid content is extremely high, both of the fatty acids in phospholipids can be unsaturated. Because they contain double bonds, essential fatty acids influence membrane fluidity and membrane-associated functions (e.g. the functionality of receptors, transporters and other membrane-embedded molecules). Arachidonic acid is a constituent of lipids in all cells, including those

n-3 Series

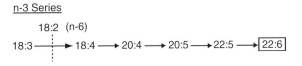

n-6 Series

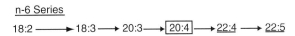

Figure 8.7 Pathway's of conversion of essential fatty acids to polyunsaturated fatty acids. The major pathways for synthesis of longer chain n-3 and n-6 fatty acids from linolenic (18:3) and linoleic (18:2) acids are shown. As indicated by the dotted line, high levels of linoleic acid block the desaturation of linolenic acid. In tissues, docosahexaenoic acid is the major n-3 fatty acid and arachidonic acid (20:4) is the major n-6 fatty acid. (From Connor *et al.* 1992.)

in the nervous system. It is released into the cytoplasm by phospholipase molecules that are activated by the occupancy of membrane receptors (of a variety of types). Once released, arachidonic acid is converted into prostaglandins and leukotrienes. These molecules influence cellular responses to second messenger molecules, such as cyclic adenosine monophosphate (cAMP), and are also released into the extracellular fluid, where they influence the functions of other cells. A dietary modification in essential fatty acid intake might therefore be expected to influence membrane functions in brain (and elsewhere), leading to alterations in brain function.

Thus far, the most illuminating studies linking the ingestion of an essential fatty acid to specific CNS functions have been those involving α-linolenic acid and its product, docosahexanoic acid. The outcome measure is vision. Unlike dietary amino acids, which can produce rapid changes in nervous system function (i.e. in hours), changes in the intake of α-linolenic acid require weeks to produce clear functional effects. In addition, such effects are produced by restricting intake (producing a deficiency), or by restoring the essential fatty acid to the diet of deficient animals (i.e. correcting a deficiency; no effects are seen by increasing intake in normal animals). Functional effects of restricting α-linolenic acid intake are typically seen when applied to animals during the late gestational and early postnatal periods, times when neurons are developing axonal and dendritic extensions, and forming nerve terminals and synapses, and glial cells are proliferating and developing their variety of membrane structures.

This also corresponds to the period when docosa-hexanoic acid is most actively accumulating in the CNS. While it may ultimately be shown that vagaries in essential fatty acid intake influence neuronal functions at other times of life, present evidence most strongly links essential fatty acid deficiency to the developmental period of the life cycle.

Studies of α-linolenic acid deficiency have been conducted in both rodents and primates, but the primate results are of greatest interest, because of the species proximity to humans. Female rhesus monkeys were fed a diet deficient in α-linolenic acid (but adequate in linoleic acid) throughout gestation, and the infants were fed an α-linolenic acid-deficient liquid diet from birth. Control animals were given diets containing adequate amounts of both α-linolenic and linoleic acids. At birth, biochemical determinations of blood and tissue samples affirmed that α-linolenic acid levels were greatly reduced in the offspring of the mothers fed the deficient diet, compared with those fed the adequate diet, and that this difference widened as the infants began to grow on their own. Moreover, brain and retinal docosahexaenoic acid levels were low at birth; this difference also widened as the infants aged. Measures of retinal function (non-invasive electrical recordings of retina activity, termed electroretinograms) in deficient animals were quite abnormal, and visual acuity was also found to be significantly below normal in α-linolenic acid-deficient infants (Figure 8.8). This effect persisted for at least 12 weeks postnatally. When animals were subsequently provided with diets containing adequate levels of α-linolenic acid, tissue

levels of docosahexaenoic acid rose rapidly (4–12 weeks), but abnormalities in the electroretinograms persisted. Hence, while the biochemical deficit was corrected by restoring α-linolenic acid adequacy, features of the functional effects persisted. The persistence of the functional deficit could indicate that a biochemical inadequacy during a critical period of development produced permanent effects on CNS function. Alternatively, it might simply mean that the functional deficit took longer to recover, once adequate α-linolenic acid levels were restored, than was examined in the study.

In humans, the development of the visual region of the cerebral cortex and the photoreceptors of the retina, as well as the accumulation of docosahexaenoic acid in the CNS, occur during the last trimester of pregnancy (gestation) and the early postnatal period. Some infants are born premature, however, removing them from the uterine environment during a significant portion of this important developmental period. For this reason, they may be deprived of the normal supply of α-linolenic and docosahexaenoic acids. In this case, visual development might be impaired, as it is in infant monkeys deprived of these fatty acids. Studies in premature infants, born at 7–8 months of gestation, suggested that this might be the case. The supplementation of a standard premature infant formula with α-linolenic acid, or α-linolenic acid and docosahexaenoic acids, was found to improve greatly functional indices of visual acuity at about 6 months after birth, suggesting effects at both the retinal and visual cortex levels. The formula containing both α-linolenic acid and docosahexaenoic acid produced the greatest benefit. Red blood cell membranes in premature infants fed the unsupplemented infant formula had very low levels of docosahexaenoic acid, compared with those in infants fed breast milk, considered the gold standard infant diet. These levels were notably increased by the addition of α-linolenic acid to the formula, although they remained below those in breast-fed infants. They rose even further with the additional inclusion of docosahexaenoic acid, to the point that they were no longer below those in breast-fed infants. (The red blood cell membrane is easily obtained in infants, and its fatty acid profile is used as an index of essential fatty acid adequacy in the diet.) Since it is known from animal studies that the addition of essential fatty acids to the diet of normal animals is without effect, but that such an addition to the diets of animals deficient in an essential fatty acid improves function, it may

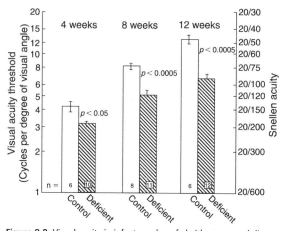

Figure 8.8 Visual acuity in infant monkeys fed either a normal diet or a diet deficient in α-linolenic acid. Reproduced with permission from Connor *et al.* (1992). © International Life Sciences Institute.

well be that the premature infants did indeed have a deficiency of α-linolenic acid and docosahexanoic acid, since vision improved with supplementation of the infant formula. Another interesting feature of this work was that the infants supplemented with docosahexanoic acid and α-linolenic acid showed a greater visual response that did those supplemented with α-linolenic acid alone. Breast milk contains docosahexanoic acid, while infants formulas do not. The finding may indicate that, like breast milk, infant formulas might be improved by the inclusion of this long-chain polyunsaturated fatty acid.

Choline

Choline occurs in the body as:

- a constitutent of lipid molecules (phosphatidylcholine, lysophophatidylcholine, sphingomyelin, choline plasmalogen) that are building blocks of cell membranes
- a source of methyl groups
- a precursor for the neurotransmitter acetylcholine.

Choline is not considered to be an essential nutrient, at least in humans, since the body can synthesize it. Moreover, deficiencies are rarely seen, since it is ubiquitous in the diet.

However, in recent decades, dietary choline has been a focus of interest in relation to brain function, because of the possibility that changes in choline intake could influence neuronal acetylcholine synthesis. Acetylcholine is a neurotransmitter in neurons in the brain and in the PNS. Indeed, ample evidence indicates that acetylcholine synthesis in and release by brain cholinergic neurons is influenced by neuronal choline availability, and that neuronal choline concentrations can be altered by dietary choline intake, in the form of either free choline or phosphatidylcholine. In addition, oral choline and phosphatidylcholine have found some application in human disease and brain functions thought to involve cholinergic neurons. For example, they have been used successfully to treat movement disorders such as tardive dyskinesia. Tardive dyskinesia is a drug-induced muscular disorder seen in schizophrenic patients. Cholinesterase inhibitors, which raise acetylcholine levels by inhibiting the transmitter's metabolism, have been used with success to reduce the uncontrollable muscle movements associated with antipsychotic treatment in these patients, and choline ingestion has also been found to produce some

beneficial effect. Choline and phosphatidylcholine, however, have proved to be of little value in controlling the muscle movements associated with Huntington's disease. Dietary choline and phosphatidylcholine supplements have also been studied as potential memory enhancers, based on the notion that acetylcholine neurons in the hippocampus have an important role in memory, and that enhancing acetylcholine levels might improve memory. (Memory is sometimes improved when acetylcholine levels are raised by administering a cholinesterase inhibitor.) Patients with Alzheimer's disease have been most studied and, in general, the disappointing outcome has been that neither choline nor phosphatidylcholine has offered much improvement in memory.

The production of choline deficiency in experimental animals (dietary choline deficiency in humans is rare) has been reported sometimes to reduce the brain content of choline, choline-containing lipids and acetylcholine. Since this has not been a uniform finding, it is not possible at present to state whether or not occasional occurrences of choline deficiency in humans would be expected to diminish the brain's content of choline-containing and/or choline-derived molecules.

8.6 Vitamins and minerals

Vitamins

Neurons and glia have the same functional demands for vitamins as do other cells in the body. Their access to the brain is thus an important consideration, particularly given the existence of the BBB. *Water-soluble vitamins* appear to be transported across the BBB and, in some cases, the blood–CSF barrier, usually (though not always) by non-energy-requiring carriers. After they are taken up into neurons and glial cells, most are rapidly converted into their biologically active derivatives, namely cofactors in enzyme-mediated reactions. Since cofactors are recycled, dietary deficiencies in one or another vitamin do not immediately lead to brain dysfunction, inasmuch as cofactor pools may take extended periods to become functionally compromised. *Fat-soluble vitamins* are hydrophobic (lipophilic), suggesting that their uptake into the CNS may involve simple diffusion across barrier endothelial cell membranes. The reality, however, is not so simple. The transport into and functions within the brain of micronutrients have not yet been studied to the same extent as has been the case for the macronutrients. However, available data do begin to provide some definition of these processes.

Water-soluble vitamins

Folic acid is transported into brain as methylenetetrahydrofolic acid, the major form of folic acid in the circulation. The transport site is located in the choroid plexus, at the blood–CSF barrier, and is about half-saturated at normal plasma concentrations of methylenetetrahydrofolate; little transport appears to occur at the BBB. CSF concentrations of methylenetetrahydrofolic acid are maintained at several times the circulating concentration, suggesting that transport is active (energy-requiring). The mechanism of transport of methylenetetrahydrofolate into neurons and glia from the CSF/extracellular fluid is not known, but is rapid. Once inside cells, folates are polyglutamated.

The brain appears to take up reduced folic acid, rather than folic acid itself, since it lacks the enzyme to reduce it (dihydrofolate reductase). Reduced folic acid (i.e. methylenetetrahydrofolate) is used by neurons and glia in transferring one carbon groups, such as in the conversion of serine to glycine or homocysteine to methionine. As methylenetetrahydrofolate is consumed in these reactions, folic acid is transported out of the brain into the circulation.

Considerable interest has been generated in the past decade regarding the consequences of folate deficiency to CNS development. The incidence of neural tube defects (NTDs, e.g. spina bifida, an abnormality in the formation of the spinal cord) has been found to be increased above the population mean in the children of women who are folate deficient during pregnancy. Moreover, the occurrence of this abnormality can be reduced by folic acid supplementation during pregnancy, beginning before conception. Initiating supplementation before conception is essential, since the basic design of the CNS is laid down during the first trimester. At present, the mechanisms by which folic acid deficiency leads to the improper formation of the spinal cord are unknown. Folate is important in single-carbon metabolism, contributing carbon atoms to purines, thymidine and amino acids. Methylation reactions involving folate may also be important in the formation and maintenance of neuronal and glial membrane lipids. A folate deficiency, by impeding DNA, protein and/or lipid synthesis, could also

conceivably influence neuronal and glial growth during critical points in neural tube development, leading to effects severe enough to induce NTDs. However, it is presently unknown which, if any, of these biochemical actions of folate might be involved in the production of NTDs.

Folate deficiency may also be linked to depression in adults. The clearest data supporting this connection come from findings in patients with megaloblastic anemia (i.e. non-psychiatric patients). Patients having a clear folate deficiency in the absence of vitamin B_{12} deficiency showed a very high incidence of depression. Other findings then indicated that depressed patients (who do not have anemia) have low plasma and red blood cell folate concentrations. Moreover, folate supplementation was found to improve mood in depressed patients. The mechanism(s) by which folate modifies mood might be related to the role of methylene tetrahydrofolate in methionine synthesis from homocysteine. It may thus help to maintain adequate methionine pools for *S*-adenosylmethionine synthesis. *S*-adenosylmethionine is a cofactor in methylation reactions in catecholamine synthesis and metabolism: catecholamines (dopamine, norepinephrine, epinephrine) are known to be important in maintaining mood, and *S*-adenosylmethionine ingestion is reputed to elevate mood. Folate has also been linked to the maintenance of adequate brain levels of tetrahydropterin, a cofactor in the synthesis of serotonin and catecholamines. It should be noted that although the above evidence suggests that a connection may exist between folate deficiency and abnormal mood, the connection is not widely accepted. Moreover, no mechanism for the effect has yet been convincingly demonstrated.

Ascorbic acid (vitamin C) is actively transported into the brain via the choroid plexus and the blood–CSF barrier, maintaining a concentration in the CSF that is four times circulating concentrations. Transport through the BBB does not occur; the absence of such transporters suggests that the BBB might retard the efflux of ascorbate from brain. The choroid plexus transporter is about half-saturated at normal blood ascorbate concentrations, such that increases in blood ascorbate do not produce large increments in brain concentrations. Moreover, the active transport mechanism insures that when plasma ascorbate falls, brain levels do not decline appreciably. Consequently, brain ascorbate concentrations show minimal fluctuations over a wide range of plasma ascorbate concentrations (indeed, brain ascorbate concentrations have been shown to vary only two-fold when plasma ascorbate concentrations were varied over a 100-fold range). Inside the CNS, ascorbate is actively transported into cells, although it is not known whether this uptake process is confined to neurons or glial cells, or occurs in both. Ascorbate is lost into the circulation at a rate of about 2% of the brain pool each hour, a loss thought to be caused by diffusion into the circulation, and by bulk flow of CSF returning to the circulation. The active transport mechanism readily compensates for this loss. Presumably because ascorbate is actively transported by the choroid plexus, and brain concentrations decline minimally at very low plasma concentrations, CNS signs are not notable in ascorbic acid deficiency states. To date, the only defined biochemical function of ascorbic acid in brain is to serve as a cofactor for dopamine β-hydroxylase, the enzyme that converts dopamine to norepinephrine (although ascorbate is thought by some to function as an antioxidant).

Thiamin (vitamin B_1) is taken up into brain by a transporter located at the BBB. It is non-energy requiring, and is about half-saturated at normal plasma thiamin concentrations. Small amounts of thiamin also gain entry via transport through the choroid plexus (blood–CSF barrier). Thiamin is then transported into neurons and glia, and phosphorylation effectively traps the molecule within the cell. In nervous tissue, thiamin functions as a cofactor for the pyruvate dehydrogenase complex, the α-ketoglutarate dehydrogenase complex, α-ketoacid decarboxylase and transketolase. It may also participate in nerve conduction. Severe thiamin deficiency in animals reduces thiamin pyrophosphate levels and the activities of thiamin-dependent reactions. It also produces difficulties in the coordinated control of muscle movement, suggestive of a compromise of vestibular function (e.g. unsteady gait, poor postural control and equilibrium). However, despite these biochemical–functional associations, the exact biochemical mechanism precipitating the functional deficits is unsettled. The functional deficits are rapidly corrected with thiamin treatment, suggesting that neurons have not been damaged or destroyed. Thiamin deficiency in humans (Wernicke's disease) produces similar deficits in the control of complex muscle movements, and also mental confusion. Korsakoff's syndrome, which occurs in almost all patients with Wernicke's disease, involves a loss of short-term memory as well as mental confusion. Severe thiamin deficiency in humans does appear to produce neuronal degeneration in certain brain regions. While the motor abnormalities can be corrected with thiamin treatment, the memory dysfunction is not improved.

Riboflavin enters brain via a saturable transport carrier, by a mechanism that has not been well described. It is probably located on capillary endothelial cells, although some transport appears to occur at the choroid plexus (blood–CSF barrier), and is about half-saturated at normal plasma riboflavin concentrations. The vitamin is readily transported into neurons and glia from the extracellular fluid, and trapped intracellularly by phosphorylation and subsequent conversion to flavin adenine dinucleotide and covalent linkage to functionally-active proteins (flavoproteins). In nervous tissue, these functional forms of riboflavin participate in numerous oxidation–reduction reactions that are key components of metabolic pathways for carbohydrates, amino acids and fats. A key enzyme in neurotransmitter metabolism, monoamine oxidase is a flavoprotein. The brain content of riboflavin and its derivatives is not notably altered in states of riboflavin deficiency or excess.

Pantothenic acid is transported into the brain by a saturable transport carrier located at the BBB. The carrier is almost completely unsaturated at normal plasma pantothenate concentrations; hence, increases in plasma levels would never be likely to saturate the transporter completely, and thereby limit transport. Neurons and glial cells take up pantothenic acid slowly by a mechanism of facilitated diffusion. Inside the cell, the vitamin becomes a component of coenzyme A, the coenzyme of acyl group transfer reactions. Relative to other tissues, the brain contains a high concentration of pantothenate, mostly in the form of coenzyme A. Brain coenzyme A concentrations do not become depleted in pantothenate deficiency states, indicating that the supply to brain of this vitamin is not the key factor governing coenzyme A concentrations in this organ.

Niacin (vitamin B_3) is transported into brain as niacinamide, primarily via the BBB (capillary endothelial cells), but possibly also to a small extent via the choroid plexus (blood–CSF barrier). Most niacin in brain is derived from the circulation, although the brain may be able to synthesize small amounts. Niacin is taken up into neurons and glia and rapidly converted to nicotinamide adenine dinucleotide (NAD). The half-life of NAD in the brain is considerably longer than in other tissues (e.g. seven to nine times that of liver). NAD and nicotinamide adenine dinucleotide phosphate (NADP) are involved in numerous oxidation–reduction reactions. Dietary niacin deficiency in the presence of a low intake of tryptophan causes pellagra in humans, a deficiency disease that includes changes in brain function such as mental depression and dementia, loss of motor coordination, and tremor. The mechanisms for these effects have not been identified.

Pyridoxine (vitamin B$_6$) is taken up into brain via a transport carrier that appears to be saturable; the details of the mechanism have not been well described. It is probably located on capillary endothelial cells, although some transport appears to occur at the blood–CSF barrier. The vitamin can be transported in any of its non-phosphorylated forms (pyridoxine, pyridoxal, pyridoxamine). Once within the brain extracellular fluid compartment, the vitamin is readily transported into neurons and glia, and phosphorylated (primarily to pyridoxal phosphate or pyridoxine phosphate). In neurons and glia, pyridoxal phosphate serves as a cofactor in a variety of reactions, including decarboxylation reactions, such as those mediated by aromatic L-amino acid decarboxylase (which converts dihydroxyphenylalanine to dopamine, and 5-hydroxy-tryptophan to serotonin) and glutamic acid decarboxylase [which converts glutamate to γ-amino butyric acid (GABA)], and transamination reactions, such as that mediated by GABA transaminase (which catabolizes GABA to glutamate and succinic semialdehyde). Dopamine, serotonin and GABA are neurotransmitters. In humans, pyridoxine deficiency is rare, because of its widespread occurrence in foodstuffs. However, where it has been identified, it has been associated with increased seizure activity, an effect that is dissipated with pyridoxine treatment. Production of pyridoxine deficiency in laboratory animals leads to reductions in pyridoxal phosphate levels in brain, and also in GABA concentrations. Reductions in GABA, an inhibitory transmitter, are known to be associated with increased seizure susceptibility, and electroencephalographic abnormalities have been recorded in deficient animals. Pyridoxine deficiency in rats also reduces serotonin concentrations in brain, almost certainly the result of diminished 5-hydroxytryptophan decarboxylation (a pyridoxal phosphate-dependent reaction).

Biotin is transported into the brain by a saturable, sodium-dependent (energy-requiring), carrier-mediated mechanism located at the BBB. Essentially no transport occurs at the blood–CSF barrier. The affinity of the transporter for biotin is such that the carrier would never become saturated. The biotin carrier shows sufficient transport activity to compensate for normal daily turnover of the vitamin. Biotin is a coenzyme for a variety of carboxylation reactions (e.g. pyruvate carboxylase).

Cobalamin (vitamin B$_{12}$) is thought to be transported into the brain by a carrier-mediated mechanism. Relatively little is known about this process or about the function of vitamin B$_{12}$ in the nervous system. However, vitamin B$_{12}$ deficiency has been known for over a century to be associated with neurological abnormalities. The neurological deficits are presumed to derive from the demyelinization of axons in spinal cord and brain that are seen in advanced deficiency cases. Left untreated, axonal degeneration eventually occurs. These effects can be reversed if vitamin B$_{12}$ treatment is provided early enough. Vitamin B$_{12}$ has been found to protect neurons from neurotoxin-induced damage, suggesting that it may be important in neuronal repair mechanisms, which may become compromised in deficiency states. Nervous system damage associated with vitamin B$_{12}$ deficiency can occur at any age.

Fat-soluble vitamins

Of the fat-soluble vitamins, *vitamin A* (retinol) has been the most studied in relation to CNS availability and function. The others have been much less well examined, although vitamin E is currently a compound of some interest, because of its function as an antioxidant. Vitamins D and K are not typically thought of as having the brain as a major focus of action, and thus little information is available regarding their involvement in brain function. Vitamin A therefore presently provides the best candidate to illustrate some of the complexities of fat-soluble vitamin flux and function in the CNS. Some of vitamin E's putative brain actions will also be mentioned.

The most noted role of vitamin A in the CNS is as a component of the photoreceptive pigment of the eye, rhodopsin. Rhodopsin is contained in the outer segments of the photoreceptor cells of the retina, which are in intimate proximity to retinal pigmented epithelium (RPE) cells. The RPE cells serve several functions. One is as the cellular analog to the ependymal cells of the brain that constitute the blood–CSF barrier. Another is as a participant in the maintenance of the rhodopsin pool in photoreceptor cells. The blood–retinal barrier function is served by the portion

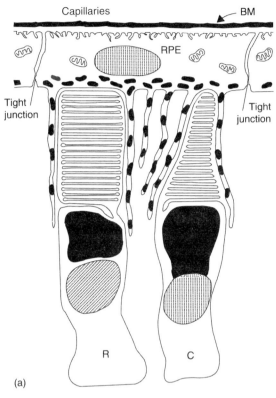

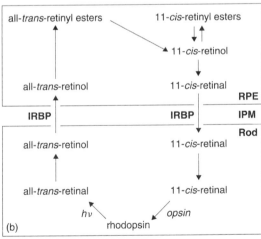

Figure 8.9 (a) Schematic drawing of the relation between the retinal pigment epithelial (RPE) cells and a rod (R) and a cone (C) in the retina. Villous processes containing pigment granules extend from the pigment epithelial cells and lie along the outer segments of both kinds of receptors. Adjacent RPE cells form close tight junctions, which serve to seal the extracellular space around the receptors from that found in the rest of the back of the eye. Some infoldings are found along the distal margin of the cell, and above those infoldings is a basement membrane (BM) and the interstitial space of the capillaries. (From Dowling, 1987.) (b) Retinoid cycle in the retina. IRBP, interstitial binding protein; IPM, interphotoreceptor matrix. (From Chader et al., 1998.)

of the RPE cell membrane exposed to retinal capillaries. The photoreceptor functions are handled by another portion of the RPE cell membrane, which lies on the opposite side of the tight junctions that are formed between RPE cells (Figure 8.9).

As the physical representation of the blood–retinal barrier, the RPE cells, joined by tight junctions, serve the same functions as the capillary endothelial cells of the BBB and the ependymal cells of the blood–CSF barriers, regarding the flow of nutrients and other molecules between blood and tissue. In this capacity, the RPE cells are also the passageway for vitamin A entry into the retina. In the blood, vitamin A (retinol, in the all-*trans* form) circulates bound to a protein complex consisting of retinol binding protein and transthyretin (prealbumin). This binding enables the blood to carry much more retinol than would otherwise be possible, since the vitamin is very hydrophobic. Protein binding also protects retinol from oxidation. Because retinal capillary endothelial cells do not have tight junctions, the retinol–carrier protein complex can readily penetrate into the immediate interstitial space. Here, it makes contact with the RPE cells, which have specific receptors for retinol binding protein. In a process that has not been completely characterized, once the receptor is occupied, retinol is released into the RPE cell. The retinol binding protein and transthyretin molecules are released back into the circulation. Inside the RPE cell, retinol is bound to a specific intracellular protein [cellular retinol binding protein (CRBP)] and ultimately esterified to a fatty acid. This latter molecule serves as the substrate for the conversion of retinol into the visually active form of the molecule, 11-*cis*-retinaldehyde, which will ultimately find its way into the photoreceptor and rhodopsin.

The RPE cell also participates in the maintenance of the rhodopsin pool in the photoreceptor cells, through its close proximity to these cells. RPE cells produce the active pigment molecule, 11-*cis*-retinaldehyde (11-*cis*-retinal in Figure 8.9b), and export it to photoreceptor cells. The 11-*cis*-retinaldehyde is produced from retinol entering the cell from the circulation, and from a very efficient mechanism for recycling the retinoid taken up from photoreceptor elements. This recycling process is not completely understood at the molecular level, but the general format is well described. Inside the photoreceptor, 11-*cis*-retinaldehyde is covalently bound to a protein, opsin, which resides in photoreceptor membranes. The 11-*cis*-retinaldehyde-opsin molecule is termed rhodopsin, and is the light-responsive pigment of the eye. When light strikes rhodopsin, the phototransduction process occurs as an isomerization of 11-*cis*-retinaldehyde to all-*trans*-retinaldehyde (all-*trans*-retinal in Figure 8.9b). Once this reaction has taken place, all-*trans*-retinaldehyde is hydrolyzed enzymically from opsin as all-*trans* retinol, and released from the photoreceptor into the extracellular space between the photoreceptor and the RPE cell. The opsin is retained in the photoreceptor and reactivated by binding with a new 11-*cis*-retinaldehyde molecule. In the interstitial space, the released all-*trans* retinol is bound to a carrier protein (IRBP in Figure 8.9b), which delivers it to the RPE cell membrane, from which it is transferred into the cell (this process has not yet been described at the molecular level). Inside the RPE cell, the all-*trans* retinol associates with CRBP and then is esterified to a fatty acid (all-*trans*-retinyl esters in Figure 8.9b).

The fatty acid-esterified form of all-*trans* retinol is enzymically converted to the 11-*cis*-retinaldehyde form, which is then exported into the interstitial space adjacent to the photoreceptors, where it again associates with a specific binding protein (IRBP in Figure 8.9b). It is delivered to the photoreceptor in this protein-bound form; the complex is presumed to bind to a receptor and release the 11-*cis*-retinaldehyde to the photoreceptor, where it can be covalently linked to opsin, thereby completing the cycle (Figure 8.9).

From the nutritional perspective, retinal cells clearly have a very refined system for managing and maintaining vitamin A pools. The molecule gains access to retina by a receptor specific for its transporter in blood, and is immediately sequestered within the RPE cell. Photoreceptor and RPE cells carefully recycle and conserve the vitamin. Hence, depletion of retinal vitamin A pools in relation to a dietary deficiency only occurs over an extended period. The ultimate appearance of a retinal deficiency develops functionally as 'night-blindness', resulting from the loss of rhodopsin. Extended vitamin A deficiency leads to a loss of photoreceptor elements, and eventually of the photoreceptor cells themselves. The cause of this cellular degeneration is not well understood.

Vitamin E is an antioxidant and free radical scavenger that (among other functions) protects fatty acids in cellular membranes. It is transported in blood bound associated with lipoproteins. The mechanism of its transfer into nervous tissue is presently unknown, but the vitamin generally transfers rapidly between lipoproteins and cellular membranes. Dietary vitamin E deficiency is extremely rare in humans. It occurs in association with certain abnormalities of vitamin E transport and fat absorption, and sometimes in individuals with protein–calorie malnutrition. The neurological manifestations are peripheral nerve degeneration, spinocerebellar ataxia and retinopathy.

Vitamin E has been *proposed* to play a role in a number of diseases of the CNS that have been linked to oxidative damage. One example is Parkinson's disease, a disorder of movement control induced by the degeneration of certain populations of brain neurons. Evidence of oxidative damage is present in the brains of parkinsonian patients, although controlled clinical trials of vitamin E supplementation have proved to be of no benefit in retarding the disease's progression. Such negative findings question the likelihood of a vitamin E link to the etiology of the degenerative changes. A second example is Alzheimer's disease (a form of senile dementia), which is associated with a progressive, generalized, ultimately catastrophic degeneration of the brain. Several types of oxidative damage have been found in the brains of Alzheimer's patients, although it is unclear whether this damage is cause or effect. The observation from a well-designed clinical trial that vitamin E supplementation can slow the progression of Alzheimer's disease in affected humans suggests that the oxidative damage may be causative in the disease. However, such findings do not indicate whether vagaries in vitamin E intake over an extended period are a cause of the disease.

Minerals

All of the essential minerals are important for cellular functions in brain, as they are elsewhere in the body. These are sodium, potassium, calcium, magnesium, iron, copper, zinc, manganese, cobalt and molybdenum. While most function as cofactors in enzymic reactions, sodium and potassium are key ions in electrical conduction in neuronal membranes, calcium functions as a second messenger within neurons, and magnesium functions at certain ligand-gated ion channels on neurons [e.g. the N-methyl-D-aspartate (NMDA) glutamate receptor]. The diet normally provides more than adequate amounts of almost all minerals, except possibly for calcium, iron, magnesium and zinc. The permeability of the BBB to most metals is quite low, generally much lower than in other organs. Indeed, as a point of reference, the brain extracts

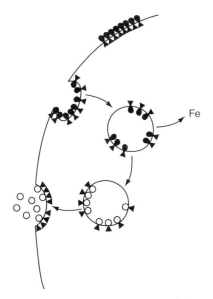

Figure 8.10 Iron-transferrin uptake across the cellular membrane. ●: iron-bound transferrin; ▲: receptors; ○: iron-free transferrin. (From Smith, 1990.)

20–30% of the glucose in blood in a single capillary transit, but less than 0.3% of any metal is normally extracted. The mechanisms of transport into brain for most metals are unknown. However, some details regarding the transport and/or functions of iron, calcium and copper are available.

Iron circulates bound to a protein, transferrin. More than 90% of plasma iron is bound to transferrin. Iron uptake into brain occurs at the BBB, although some also appears to take place across the blood–CSF barrier (choroid plexus). Iron transport occurs by a transferrin receptor-mediated endocytosis of the iron–transferrin complex by capillary endothelial cells (Figure 8.10). Iron dissociates from transferrin inside the endothelial cell; the iron is delivered into the brain interstitial fluid, while the transferrin is returned to the circulation. Brain iron associates with ferretin and is stored intracellularly. The bulk of the iron–ferretin stores in brain reside in glial cells (oligodendrocytes and microglia), and are laid down early in postnatal life. Marked regional differences in iron and ferretin concentrations occur in the brain, with levels in some areas being as high as those in the liver. This distribution, however, does not correlate with the density of transferrin receptors in brain capillaries, and it is presently unknown how or why the unequal distribution of iron develops. Numerous

enzymes in brain are iron requiring, including several hydroxylases that mediate rate-limiting reactions in the production of neurotransmitters (tryptophan hydroxylase, phenylalanine hydroxylase, tyrosine hydroxylase) and a key enzyme in the metabolism of the monoamine neurotransmitters (monoamine oxidase).

Iron deficiency can cause impairments in attention and cognition in children. Similar effects are seen in animals. In rats made iron deficient, despite increases in the efficiency of iron uptake by the brain, brain iron concentrations decline, with newborn and infant animals showing more rapid declines than older animals. Iron repletion in the brain occurs (slowly) in infant and adult rats with iron supplementation, but not in animals depleted at birth. While outside the brain the activities of many iron-dependent enzymes are depressed by iron deficiency, inside the brain their activities are unaffected. The activitites of the hydroxylase enzymes are not reduced by severe iron restriction, nor are the rates of production of the neurotransmitters derived from them (serotonin for tryptophan hydroxylase; dopamine, norepinephrine and epinephrine from phenylalanine and tyrosine hydroxylases). However, a reduction in dopamine receptors (D_2 subtype) does occur, and coincides with aberrations in dopamine-dependent behaviors in rats. The inability of brain iron stores to recover in rats made iron deficient as newborns coincides with a persistence of dopamine receptor-linked behavioral deficits, despite normal repletion of iron stores elsewhere in the body. Restoration of normal behavior with iron supplementation, along with brain iron stores, is seen in animals made iron deficient at other ages.

Iron deficiency also interferes with myelinization. Since marked glial proliferation and myelin formation occur early in infancy, iron deficiency during this period could compromise the optimal development of neuronal communications (e.g. glial cells provide insulation for axons and synapses). This effect could account for some of the behavioral deficits associated with neonatal iron deficiency. If brain function is permanently affected by the occurrence of iron deficiency shortly after birth, this vulnerability should be an issue of great concern in those parts of the world where iron deficiency in infancy is an endemic problem.

Calcium is transported into the CNS via a saturable, probably active transport mechanism located in the choroid plexus (the blood–CSF barrier). At normal plasma calcium concentrations (calcium circulates mostly in the free form, i.e. unbound to a blood protein), it operates at near saturation, presumably enabling brain calcium levels to remain relatively constant in the face of increases in plasma calcium. Unlike intestinal calcium transport, transport into the brain is not vitamin D sensitive. Some calcium is taken up into the brain via the brain capillary system (i.e. across the BBB), but this fraction is less than 40% of total calcium uptake each day. This transport mechanism has not been defined. The active transport of calcium at the blood–CSF barrier would presumably enable brain calcium levels to be maintained at or near normal levels in the face of dietary calcium deficits. Since calcium concentrations in the circulation are also regulated, under most circumstances, this process would also be expected to help maintain brain calcium uptake and levels in the face of vagaries in calcium intake. Deficiencies in brain calcium should thus be a relatively rare occurrence.

Copper functions as a cofactor for numerous enzymes, including dopamine β-hydroxylase, which mediates the reaction converting dopamine to norepinephrine. Dietary copper deficiency in humans is fairly rare, but experimentally induced in animals, lowers copper concentrations throughout the body, including the brain, and blocks the conversion of dopamine to norepinephrine in brain neurons. This enzyme block also occurs in peripheral sympathetic nerves and the adrenal gland, which synthesize norepinephrine and epinephrine. The mechanism of copper transport into the brain is unknown, but capillary endothelial cells have a copper-ATPase that could function as a transporter. One hypothesis is that copper transported into the endothelial cells is then directly transferred into astrocytes (through 'end-feet' that surround brain capillaries) and subsequently provided to neurons through astrocytic processes that impinge on neurons. In this manner, copper availability to neurons could be metered, since excess copper is neurotoxic. Copper deficiency occurs as an X-linked genetic disease of copper transport in Menkes disease, in which tissue and brain copper levels become extremely low, and produce neurodegeneration. Children with Menkes' disease die at a very young age.

8.7 Perspectives on the future

The brain is influenced by the availability to it of many of the nutrients it needs, and not simply in relation to chronic, dietary deficiencies. Indeed, the brain depends from minute to minute on its supply of glucose, and this nutrient is therefore carefully regulated in blood (i.e. not directly dependent on the vagaries of dietary supply). Moreover, in the absence of an adequate glucose supply, the body turns to an alternate energy source, ketone bodies, which are supplied through body fat deposits. Variations in amino acid supply to the brain do not influence protein synthesis, but hour-to-hour variations in the plasma concentrations of certain amino acids, such as follow a meal, can directly influence their conversion to neurotransmitter derivatives, and thus presumably brain functions. Variations in the dietary intake of essential fatty acids also impact on brain and retinal composition, and on function (vision). These effects, however, take weeks to develop, and developing animals are most susceptible. Variations in micronutrient intake tend not to influence brain uptake and functions on a short-term basis. The manner in which they are supplied to, sequestered in and used by the brain indicates that considerable buffering exists between brain pools and dietary supply. Such seems to be the case for water-soluble and fat-soluble vitamins, and for minerals.

It is clear why glucose supply to brain needs to be supplied without interruption (cutting off glucose supply has an immediate, drastically negative impact on the brain), and why so many nutrient pools should be buffered from metabolic and dietary vagaries. It is thus somewhat surprising that the transmitter products of some amino acids are so vulnerable to diet-induced variations. Perhaps some function is served by this rapid diet–brain link, such as the monitoring of protein intake, but no real answer has yet been identified.

In contrast to the impact on brain chemistry and function of dietary vagaries in nutrient intake in relation to normal food sources, relatively little is known about the effects on the nervous system of consuming excessive amounts of most nutrients. The issue of potential toxicities of excessive nutrient intake gains importance with the current and growing practice of ingesting 'megadose' amounts of individual nutrients for perceived medical and physiological benefits, but this discussion remains for the future when, hopefully, the knowledge base will have expanded.

Further reading

Chader GJ, Pepperberg DR, Crouch R, Wiggert B. Retinoids and the retinal pigment epithelium. In: The Retinal Pigment Epithelium:

Function and Disease (Marmor MF, Wolfensberger TJ, eds.), New York: Oxford Univeristy Press, 1998, pp. 135–151.

Connor WE, Neuringer M, Reisbick S, Essential fatty acids: The importance of n-3 fatty acids in the retina and brain. Nutrition Reviews 50(4): 21–29, 1992.

Davson H, Zlokovic B, Rakic L, Segal MB, eds., An Introduction to the Blood–Brain Barrier. Boca Raton, FL: CRC Press, 1993.

Deutsch AY, Roth RH, Neurotransmitters. In: Fundamental Neuroscience (Zigmond MJ, Bloom FE, Landis SC, Roberts JL, Squire LR, eds), San Diego, CA: Academic Press, 1999, pp. 193–234.

Dowling JE, The Retina: An Approachable Part of the Brain, Cambridge, MA: Belknap Press of Harvard University Press, 1987.

Fernstrom JD, Fernstrom MH. Diet, monoamine neurotransmitters and appetite control. In: Nutrition and Brain, Nestlé Nutrition Workshop Series Clinical and Performance Program, Vol 5 (Fernstrom JD, Uauy R, Arroyo P, eds), pp 117–134. Basel: Karger, 2001.

Fernstrom JD, Garattini S, eds., International Symposium on Glutamate. J Nutr 2000; 130 (4S): 891S–1079S.

Innis SM. The 1993 Borden Award Lecture. Fatty acid requirements of the newborn. Can J Physiol Pharmacol 1994; 72: 1483–1492.

Smith QR, Stoll J, Blood–Brain Barrier Amino Acid Transport, in: Introduction to the Blood–Brain Barrier (PartridgeWM, ed). New York, Cambridge University Press, 1998, pp. 188–197.

Smith QR, Regulation of metal uptake and distribution within brain, in: Nutrition and the Brain, Volume 8 (Wurtman RJ, Wurtman JJ, eds). New York: Raven Press, 1990, pp. 25–74.

Spector, R., Vitamin homeostasis in the central nervous system. New Engl J Med 1977; 296: 1393–1398.

Spector R., Micronutrient homeostasis in the mammalian brain and cerebrospinal fluid. J Neurochem 1989; 53: 1667–1774.

Zigmond MJ, Bloom FE, Landis SC, Roberts JL, Squire LR, eds., Fundamental Neuroscience. New York: Academic Press, 1999.

9
The Sensory Systems: Taste, Smell, Chemesthesis and Vision

CM Delahunty and TAB Sanders

Key messages

- Taste, smell and chemesthesis are the three distinct sensory modalities that contribute to flavor perception.
- Cross-modal sensory interactions are observed when two or more perceptible components of a food system are studied together. The halo effect refers to how learning places greater reliance on one sensory modality over another. Flavor perception is influenced by the dominant senses and by changing food properties.
- Flavor can be defined as the integrated response to stimulation of all the chemical senses and it is of key importance for food acceptance. The chemical senses alter significantly across the lifespan; this in turn may change flavor perceptions and influence nutritional status.

- The visual system consists of the outer eye, the inner eye including the lens, the vitreous body and the retina, which is connected to the optic nerve.
- Retinol, docosahexaenoic acid and taurine are key nutrients in the visual process.
- The lens is susceptible to oxidative damage; antioxidant protection falls with increasing age and may be involved in the etiology of cataract and age-related maculopathy. It remains to be determined whether dietary antioxidants alter the pathogenesis or progression of cataract and age-related maculopathy

9.1 Introduction to taste, smell and chemesthesis

Taste, olfaction and chemesthesis (the common chemical sense) are the sensory modalities that respond to chemical stimuli in the foods that we eat. Collectively, these sensory modalities are referred to as the chemical senses. The chemical senses function as 'gatekeepers' to the body, evaluating and distinguishing the foods that are acceptable for consumption from those that should be rejected. Food intake and nutritional status are strongly related, and it is for this reason that the function and selectivity of the chemical senses is an essential component of nutritional science.

In normal eating, all food enters the body through the mouth. From the time of birth, we select what is beneficial to eat and reject that which will cause ill-health.

The chemical senses have evolved to aid this decision-making process. In present life, the protective role of chemical sensation is primarily that to detect microbiologically spoiled foods or tainted foods, as few roam the countryside hunting, gathering and sampling unusual 'food'. Within the range of food selected as palatable, subtle differences in taste or smell can have dramatic influences on preferences, ultimately determining repeated intake and potential nutrition. Individual preferences are determined by genetics and the impact of environment and experience from early life.

The taste, smell and chemesthesis sensory systems have independent physiology and will be considered separately in this chapter. However, during consumption, these distinct sensory modalities interact to provide flavor, and few consumers make any distinction. In fact, flavor is often referred to as a combination of all sensations relevant to food acceptability, including taste, smell, warmth or cold, touch, texture, pain and even visual sensations. Therefore, in remaining parts of this chapter it will be necessary to consider the perception of the senses together, particularly with regard to the understanding of sensory preferences.

9.2 The taste system

Unlike vision, hearing or olfaction, taste is a proximal sense, meaning that the primary stimulus for taste must make contact with the taste receptors. Therefore, the process of tasting begins in the oral cavity, and primarily on the tongue. Taste receptors are stimulated by contact with liquid compounds, creating perceptions that endow distinctive taste qualities such as sweet, salty, sour and bitter to these compounds.

Anatomy of the taste system

Taste receptors, located primarily on the tongue and soft palate, are termed taste buds. Each taste bud is a cluster of between 30 and 50 specialized epithelial cells. Taste bud cells end in hair-like cilia called microvilli, which make contact with the fluid environment in the mouth through a taste pore at the top of the taste bud. Taste-stimulating compounds are believed to bind to these microvilli, initiating taste transduction. Taste buds, of which there are about 6000 in total, are located within small, but visible, structures known as papillae (Figure 9.1). There are four types: fungiform papillae located at the tip and sides of the tongue, foliate papillae which appear as a series of folds along the sides of the tongue; circumvallate papillae which are found at the back of the tongue, and filliform papillae which cover

the entire surface of the tongue and give the tongue a rough appearance. All papillae, apart from the filliform type, contain taste buds. Filliform papillae grip food on the tongue and play a role in mouthfeel. Stimulation of the back or sides of the tongue produces a broad range of taste sensations. The soft palate, root of the tongue and upper part of the throat are also sensitive to tastes. Taste papillae are supplied by a number of nerves. The chorda tympani nerve conducts signals from the front and sides of the tongue, and from the fungiform papillae in particular. The glossopharangeal nerve conducts signals from the back of the tongue. The vagus nerve conducts signals from taste receptors in the mouth and larynx. The sense of taste is robust by comparison with other sensory modalities, and this may be partly explained by the fact that different nerves innervate the tongue. It would therefore be difficult to knock out all taste areas through trauma.

Taste transduction involves complex chemical events occurring within the taste cell. Organic molecules such as sweet and bitter tastants interact with membrane-bound protein receptors. These in turn activate a second protein complex, called G-protein, which releases a subunit. The subunit activates enzyme systems within the cell that affect calcium deposits and membrane permeability to various ions such as sodium, potassium and calcium. The membrane conductance changes lead to transmission of the nerve signal at synaptic terminals via release packets of chemical neurotransmitters, which stimulate the next cell in the sequence.

Each taste cell has a lifespan of about 1 week. New cells differentiate from the surrounding epithelium and during their lifetime migrate towards the center of the bud, where they eventually die. Differences in cell type within the taste bud represent differences in age and development. As a person ages, replacement of taste cells may slow, and this may have adverse effects on taste function.

Taste coding

The taste neurons branch before entering the taste papillae, and branch again inside the taste bud. Therefore a single nerve fiber may innervate more than one papilla and a large number of taste buds. Two theories have been proposed to explain taste coding, or how we can distinguish different taste qualities. The first is across-fiber pattern coding. The principle is that a taste compound stimulates many fibers, but not all to the same extent, and that the pattern of stimulation across

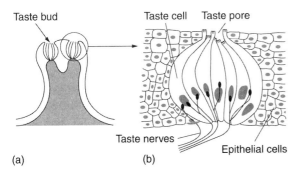

Figure 9.1 (a) Cross-section of a fungiform papilla showing the location of taste buds. (b) Cross-section of a taste bud, showing the taste pore where the taste enters, the taste cells and the taste nerve fibers.

fibers is used to recognize, or code, the stimulus quality. The alternative theory is that of specificity coding, which assumes that some neurons respond best to specific compounds. However, results show that both mechanisms operate together. The firing of specific neurons may identify, for example, compound group or type, and then more subtle qualities of a compound can be determined by the pattern of firing across large groups of neurons.

Taste quality

It is most widely recognized that there are four basic taste qualities, referred to as sweet, salty, sour and bitter. A fifth taste, 'umami', has been accepted more recently, particularly in Japan and other cultures where it is most familiar and most easily perceived. There have been attempts to define, or classify, the stimuli for specific taste qualities. Such a definition might explain an evolutionary basis for quality discrimination that is linked to the nutritional value of foods. Sweet taste is typical of sugars and other carbohydrates, although many artificial sweeteners are not carbohydrate. Salt taste is typical of salts of alkali metals and halogens, although again not without exception. Sour taste is very closely linked to the pH of a substance. Most bitter substances are organic compounds having biological activity, and many of them are poisonous. Thus, bitter taste seems to be a poison detector. Umami is used to describe the taste of monosodium glutamate (MSG) and ribosides, such as salts of 5'-ionosine monophosphate (IMP) and 5'-guanine monophosphate (GMP). Europeans and Americans generally describe the umami taste as 'brothy', 'savory' or 'meaty', and are not certain whether it is a distinct taste quality or due to a mouth-filling sensation and interaction with other tactile sensory modalities. Some compounds have a predominant taste: sodium chloride (NaCl) is predominantly salty, hydrochloric acid (HCl) is predominantly sour, sucrose predominantly sweet and quinine predominantly bitter. However, most compounds have more than one taste quality. For example, potassium chloride (KCl) has substantial salty and bitter tastes, and sodium nitrate ($NaNO_3$) tastes of salty, sour and bitter.

Taste thresholds

Two types of taste threshold measurement can be considered. Absolute thresholds refer to the minimum concentration of a substance or compound that can be detected. Differential thresholds refer to the just noticeable difference between two levels of concentration above the absolute threshold (i.e. suprathreshold). At absolute threshold, a taste sensation may not have any discernable quality, but as its concentration in solution increases, quality becomes more defined. The taste quality of a compound may also change as concentration continues to increase. For example, NaCl tastes sweet at very low concentrations, and salt solutions below the concentration of saliva may give rise to bitter tastes. In general, intensity of perception increases with increases in the physical concentration of a compound. Psychometric taste functions relating concentration to response are sigmoidally shaped, with an initial flat portion where response at levels below threshold hover around a baseline or background noise level, an accelerating function as threshold is surpassed, and a decelerating function that eventually becomes flat as receptor sites are filled, or as the maximum number of sensitive nerves respond at or near their maximum frequency (Figure 9.2). Sigmoidal shaped psychometric functions can also represent olfactory and chemesthesis stimuli, and will be referred to again later in this chapter. The duration of taste sensation is also an important quality consideration and could be considered as a type of threshold. Long-lasting tastes are generally referred to as aftertastes, and most often have negative association with preference.

It was believed that different taste sensations were located exclusively on different areas of the tongue. This 'map' of the tongue was not accurate as a range of tastes can be detected on all parts. However, it is true that not all regions of the tongue are equally sensitive

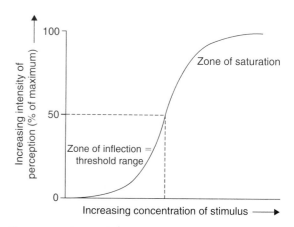

Figure 9.2 Psychometric function of increasing intensity of perception of a taste stimulus with increasing concentration of the stimulus in solution.

to all chemical stimuli: for sweet taste, the threshold is lowest at the front; for sour taste, the rear sides are most sensitive; for salt taste, the front and sides are most sensitive; and for bitter taste, the front of the tongue and the soft palate are most sensitive. This localization of taste sensitivity may aid in identification of food, manipulation of the food bolus, or removal of selected portions of the bolus that have an unacceptable taste quality. However, this spatial ability also creates an obstacle to the development of substitute sweeteners and salts, as these generally have more than one taste quality, and differ in the part of the tongue that they stimulate to the pure tastes of sucrose and NaCl, which they seek to replace.

Widespread individual differences in taste sensitivity are observed for most compounds, especially for bitter compounds, intensive sweeteners and multiquality salts. For some compounds, the range in sensitivity across a population can be several orders of magnitude. There is a genetically inherited difference in sensitivity to the bitter compound 6-*n*-propylthiouracil (PROP). Individuals may be classified into one of three PROP sensitivity status, termed non-tasters, medium tasters and super tasters. Anatomical differences have also been observed between groups with different PROP taste status, as papillae and taste bud numbers are correlated with taster status. PROP status has also been related to sensitivity to other taste compounds, to mouthfeel and to chemical irritant sensitivity. However, these relationships are tentative and high thresholds for one compound do not predict high thresholds for all compounds.

Taste mixtures

The taste qualities of mixed compounds are perceived separately, and no taste quality results from a mixture that is not present in the individual constituents of the mixture. Also, sapid compounds in the mixture cannot mutually suppress one another to produce a tasteless mixture. Consumers often assume that sweet and sour are opposite in taste quality. However, if that were the case, a mixture of these taste qualities would have no taste. In fact, when acetic acid and sucrose are mixed, the resultant solution tastes both sweet and sour. Mutual suppression can raise the threshold of each mixed compound, and if one compound is stronger than the other, it will dominate and may mask the weaker taste entirely. A solution of quinine and sucrose is less sweet than an equimolar concentration of sucrose tasted alone. Similarly, the mixture is less bitter than equimolar

quinine. In general, this inhibitory criterion applies to mixtures of all four basic taste qualities, and is referred to as mixture suppression. Since the majority of foods contain more than one taste compound, mixture suppression is important for determining a balanced sensation and providing overall appeal. For example, in fruit juices, the unpleasant sourness of acids can be partially masked by the pleasant sweetness from sugars. However, it is difficult to characterize taste mixture interactions without also considering the sequential effects of adaptation, a concept that will be dealt with later in this chapter. PROP taste status can also manifest itself in taste mixture sensitivity, as people who are not sensitive to PROP will not show some mixture suppression effects on other flavors, particularly when bitterness is present in the mixture. Therefore, the relative intensity of other flavors may be enhanced.

The sense of taste also demonstrates integrative, or additive, effects across the taste qualities. Solutions of taste compounds, regardless of quality, cannot be perceived when diluted below threshold (Table 9.1). However, when two solutions of different taste quality that

Table 9.1 Absolute taste thresholds for common taste compounds

Compound	Threshold[a] (molar concentration)[b]
Bitter	
Urea	0.015
Caffeine	0.0005
Quinine HCl	0.000014
Sour	
HCl	0.00016
Acetic acid	0.00011
Citric acid	0.00007
Salt	
NaCl	0.001
KCl	0.0064
Sweet	
Glucose	0.0073
Sucrose	0.00065
Apartame	0.00002
Umami	
Monosodium glutamate	0.0005

[a] Thresholds are based on compounds' major taste quality, although several have additional tastes.
[b] Molar concentration represents the number of grams of solute divided by its molecular weight, per liter of solution.

are diluted to 50% below absolute threshold are mixed, the mixture can be perceived. This additive effect has been demonstrated for up to 24 solutions of varied quality diluted to 1/24th of their absolute threshold.

9.3 The olfactory system

As for taste, the primary stimuli for smell must also make contact with the olfactory receptors. However, the stimuli for smell are airborne compounds of volatile substances. The odor stimulating compounds create perceptions that are endowed with distinctive smells. The olfactory system is both an external sensory system and an internal sensory system, as it responds to odor (sensed orthonasally) and aroma (sensed retronasally from volatile compounds released in the oral cavity during consumption). The largest contribution to the diversity of food flavors comes from volatile compounds sensed by the olfactory system, and much of what we commonly refer to as 'taste' is incorrectly localized smell detection. The significant contribution of smell to flavor can easily be demonstrated if you pinch your nose shut while eating, effectively blocking air circulation through the nasal passages. Familiar foods will not be recognized and it is even possible to confuse apples with onions if tasting blind.

Anatomy of the olfactory system

The receptors for odor are olfactory cells. These cells are long, narrow, column-shaped cells, each less than 1 μm in diameter. Olfactory cells are true nerve cells. There are between 6 and 10 million olfactory cells in the human nose. These are located within the olfactory epithelium, a region of tissue of around 5 cm^2 in area, located high in the upper part of each of two nasal cavities (Figure 9.3). A layer of mucus coats the olfactory epithelium. This mucus provides protection for the sensitive olfactory cells, and also regulates transport of olfactory stimuli to the receptors aiding in smell quality determination. The olfactory receptors have very fine fibers (cilia), which project into the mucous layer where they contact the stimulus. The cilia serve to enlarge the surface area of the cell enormously so that it is about the same size as the total skin area for humans. Extending from the other end of the olfactory cells are nerve fibers, which pass through the cribriform plate of the skull into the olfactory bulb and connect at a junction called the glomerulus, then further connect with other

parts of the brain by olfactory tracts. Therefore, olfactory receptors both receive and conduct stimuli.

During inspiration, or when air refluxes retronasally from the mouth carrying aroma during eating, it is directed into the nasal cavity below the level of the olfactory epithelium. At the interface of the air with the mucous layer covering the olfactory receptors, there is an opportunity for chemically selective processes to take place. Compounds first partition from the air into the mucous medium and therefore for any compound to have smell potential it must be soluble in the olfactory mucosa. These compounds may then bind to other compounds called olfactory receptor proteins, of which there are many hundreds of different types. Compounds eventually stimulate the cilia, and by some poorly understood biochemical process provoke the olfactory neural activity. The more vigorous the inhalation, the more of the olfactory epithelium is bathed by the odorant and the greater the stimulation. Olfactory receptors transmit signals directly to the olfactory bulb in the brain, where signals are then processed before being sent to the olfactory cortex and to the orbitofrontal cortex. In addition, olfactory nerves project to many different sites in the brain, some of them closely associated with emotion and memory.

Smell coding

Olfactory receptors respond to many hundreds of different odor-active compounds, giving rise to thousands of different odor qualities. To account for this

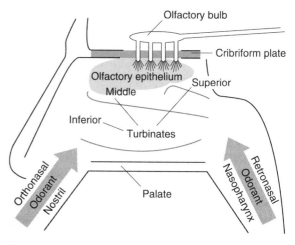

Figure 9.3 Human nasal cavity, illustrating the olfactory receptors, the olfactory epithelium and the different means of entry for volatile compounds.

incredible discriminative ability it is likely that smell is coded by a pattern of response across many receptors. The ability of the system to form a pattern is facilitated by differential movement of potential odorants through the olfactory mucosa. Some volatile compounds are strongly attracted to the mucosa, so they flow slowly through it, and are potentially deposited close to its surface. Others are more weakly attracted to the mucosa and so flow more rapidly and stimulate receptors more uniformly throughout the mucosa. Each compound creates a different pattern of receptor stimulation because of differences in how each is deposited on the receptor surface, termed a regional sensitivity effect. In addition, the stimulus causes fairly widespread and diffuse activity in the olfactory bulb. Areas of the nervous system higher than the olfactory bulb may be important to intrepret the complex neural activity, and the orbitofrontal cortex has been implicated. The amount of neural activity increases with increases in the concentration of a given odorant and it is also possible that different odorants, owing to specific differences in molecular properties, produce specific and distinctive spatial and temporal patterns of activity.

Smell quality

The sense of smell is capable of distinguishing and recognizing a wide range of qualities. However, researchers have yet to identify a relationship between a compound's smell and a physical property that causes that smell. Compounds that are structurally very different from one another can smell the same, whereas compounds almost identical in structure can have very different smell quality. In addition, many smells that we perceive as unitary are in fact complex mixtures of many volatile compounds. For example, the smell of coffee contains over 800 volatile compounds, although only 20 or 30 of these have odor activity. Adding to complexity, different individuals may describe the same sensation in different ways, although fixed terminologies and objective descriptive analysis techniques are now used to overcome this problem. However, terminology systems work better on a product-by-product basis (e.g. there are agreed terminologies for wine, beer and other product categories) than across product categories.

There have been many attempts to classify odor quality, and researchers have searched for primary odors believing that their discovery will elucidate odor quality as did the discovery of the primary colors. The stereochemical theory proposes seven primary odors (camphoraceous, musky, floral, minty, ethereal, pungent and putrid). This theory proposes that all compounds with similar odor quality have similar geometric structures that fit specific olfactory receptor sites. However, this theory is not widely accepted, as there is no evidence of clear and distinct receptor sites, and some compounds of similar quality have different structures. Odorants can be classified according to common structural features, such as aldehydes, alcohols, esters or ketones. Odors can also be classified according to physicochemical features such as carbon chain length, or the number and polarity of side-groups. These properties determine the volatility and the mucus solubility of the odorant. In addition, the three-dimensional structure of the compound may determine what olfactory receptor protein the compound is capable of interacting with, and thus the nature of the neuron activity that it will elicit.

Smell thresholds

There are several million olfactory receptor cells on each side of the nose, and these are highly ciliated, with six to 12 cilia per cell. The cilia greatly increase the surface area of exposure. In the olfactory bulb, a relatively large number of olfactory cells converge on a single glomerular cell, which in turn proceeds directly to the higher cortical regions. Therefore, there is neural convergence from the cilia to the olfactory cells, and again from the olfactory cells to the olfactory bulb. This general funneling of olfactory information makes the olfactory system extremely sensitive. As for taste, absolute and differential thresholds can be determined for smell. Olfaction has far lower absolute thresholds to concentration than does taste, and may be 10 000 times more sensitive. In contrast, the sense of smell has a poor ability to discriminate intensity levels, and differential thresholds are high relative to other sensory modalities (in the region of 15–25% concentration change is required before a difference can be detected). Odor thresholds are not related only to the concentration of compound. Odor activity is also related to physical and chemical properties described earlier. The absolute odor thresholds for some common odor compounds are presented in Table 9.2. Methyl mercaptan, which has the objectionable smell of rotten cabbage, can be detected at extremely low concentrations. Methyl salicylate, the smell of wintergreen, has a relatively high threshold, whereas water, which is also volatile, is odorless.

Table 9.2 Absolute odor thresholds for common odor compounds

Compound	Smell quality	Threshold (mg/l of air)
Methyl salicylate	Wintergreen	0.100
Amyl acetate	Banana	0.039
Butyric acid	Rancid butter	0.009
Pyridine	Burnt, smokey	0.0074
Safrol	Sassafras (woody–floral)	0.005
Ethyl acetate	Pineapple	0.0036
Benzaldehyde	Almond	0.003
Hydrogen sulfide	Rotten eggs	0.00018
Courmarin	Haylike, nutlike	0.00002
Citral	Lemon	0.000003
Methyl mercaptan	Rotten cabbage	0.0000002

Odor thresholds can vary significantly, both within and between people, and some people with an otherwise normal sense of smell are unable to detect families of similar smelling compounds. This condition is termed specific anosmia, and can be defined as a smell threshold more than two standard deviations above the population mean. Specific anosmias identified include that to androstenone, a component of boar taint; cineole, a terpene found in many herbs, diacetyl, which is a butter-like smell important for dairy flavor; and trimethyl amine, a fish spoilage taint. Thresholds for odor may also be affected by an interaction of gender and hormonal variation in an individual. It has been reported that the absolute threshold for exaltolide (cyclopentadecanolide), a musk-like synthetic lactone odorant used as a fixative in perfume, varies significantly in the human female according to the stage of her reproductive or menstrual cycle. Similar differences might be expected for foods odors.

Smell mixtures

As for taste, the sense of smell also shows mixture interactions. In fact, it is smell mixtures, and not single odorants, that are encountered in almost every instance of everyday life. It may be for this reason that the sense of smell is limited in identifying individual odors even in the simplest of mixtures, and in deciding whether a stimulus is a single odorant or a mixture. There are several basic principles that hold in general: odors of different quality tend to mask or suppress one another, or may remain distinct, whereas odors of similar quality tend to blend to produce a third unitary odor quality. The extent to which these interactions occur depends on the compounds that are mixed, and can

be influenced by chemical interaction between compounds, or by interaction or filtering at the olfactory receptor sites. The perception of the mixture is also determined by the odor thresholds of the compounds that are mixed, their concentration response functions, and their potential to cause adaptation (adaptation will be discussed in more detail later in this chapter). In general, odor mixtures bear a strong resemblance in character to the quality characteristics of the individual components, and obtaining a wholly new odor as a function of mixing is rare. However, in very complex mixtures, such as those that are typical of cheese or wine, often odors of dissimilar quality can be found. In cheese, for example Cheddar, subtle fruity character is provided by fatty acid esters. However, this character complements the dairy characteristics of the cheese because of the inherent complexity of a blend of up to 30 compounds, which are above threshold. In fact, the majority of natural odors are mixtures of many chemical components, and none of the individual components of the mixture can produce the complexity of mixed odor on its own. It is this complexity and fine balance of natural odors that has made it difficult for flavor companies to reproduce accurately the character of natural flavors in manufactured foods.

9.4 Chemesthesis

Chemesthesis is the term used to describe the sensory system responsible for detecting chemical irritants. Detection is more general than that of taste and smell, and takes place primarily in the eyes, nose and mouth. The perception is closely related to the somatosensory characteristics of pain and temperature change, and provokes a strong behavioral response. The primary function of chemesthesis is to protect the body from noxious chemical stimuli; however, this high-influence sense has also been exploited to great effect commercially. The fizzy tingle of carbon dioxide so desired in soft drinks, the cooling sensation of menthol in mint sweets or toothpastes, and the burning sensation of chili in curry or salsa are perhaps the best examples of how chemical irritation can provide additional character that is very much desired.

Anatomy of chemesthesis

The general chemical responsiveness to irritation is mediated by nerve fibers in the trigeminal (fifth cranial)

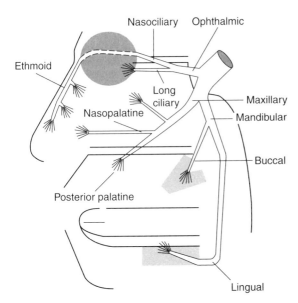

Figure 9.4 Diagram of the branches of the trigeminal nerves that innervate the nasal and oral cavities. A person is bilaterally symmetrical with two of each of the branches illustrated.

nerves, which innervate the mucosae and skin of the mouth, nose and eyes (Figure 9.4). The trigeminal nerves have three main branches: ophthalmic, maxillary and mandibular. The chorda tympani and glossopharyngeal nerves, which serve taste reception, may also convey information about chemical irritation. All of the areas served by the trigeminal nerves are sensitive to chemical irritants. Tears caused when cutting onions readily demonstrate sensitivity in the eye, whereas the pungency of mustard demonstrates sensitivity in the nose. Chemical irritant sensitivity is by no means less important than that of taste or odor, and as already mentioned can have a strong influence on food acceptability.

Chemesthesis quality

The anatomical requirement to enable perception of different irritant qualities appears to be present, and there seems to be variety in the quality of irritative experiences. However, these differences could arise from intensity differences or additional taste or odor qualities. Examples of sensations arising from chemesthesis include the fizzy tingle of carbon dioxide, the burn of hot peppers, the cooling of menthol, the nasal pungency of mustard and horseradish, the oral pungency of spices such as ginger, cumin and black pepper, and the bite of raw onions and garlic. However, each of these substances has additional qualities that stimulate other

parts of the chemesthesis anatomy, or that stimulate olfaction and taste. Mustard, onions and garlic also have lachrymatory effects (tearing), not to mention strong odor. Menthol has a number of sensory properties that include cooling, warming, odor and other sensory effects depending on isomeric conformation, concentration and temporal parameters of exposure.

A majority of compounds, including those that stimulate common odors and tastes, have some degree of irritation. For example, completely anosmic individuals can detect many odor compounds, presumably from the ability of odorants to stimulate the trigeminal nerve branches in the nasal cavity. The trigeminal nerves also signal tactile, thermal and pain sensations, and therefore the distinction between a true chemical sense and a tactile sense becomes blurred.

Chemesthesis thresholds

Psychophysical principles (absolute thresholds, differential thresholds, sigmoidal concentration–response functions) can again be applied to understanding the relationship between concentration and the perception of chemical irritant stimuli. However, such relationships are often difficult to study because irritant stimuli, and in particular capsaicin burn, cause desensitization following stimulation, which can be long lasting. Upon first stimulation with capsaicin, a warm, burning and painful sensation is perceived. This is termed sensitization. However, repeated stimulation with the same concentration of capsaicin can be without effect as the receptors become desensitized. The quantity of irritant compound consumed is also important. Irritation from chili continues to build to higher levels if stimulation proceeds in rapid sequences without allowing sufficient time for the senses to recover. The absolute threshold of capsaicin, the active irritant in chili pepper, has been measured at below 1 ppm. In pure form, capsaicin causes a warm or burning sensation, with little or no apparent taste or smell. Piperine, black pepper, is around 100 times less potent. The rate of increase in perceived intensity as a function of concentration for common chemical irritants is often high relative to those for tastants and odorants. The relationship between the concentration of carbon dioxide, which provides the fizziness in soft drinks, and perceived fizziness is greater than 1:2. This response to stimulus is much greater than that typical of other sensory modalities, apart from electric shock. The long-lasting nature of irritant stimulus is an important aspect of both quality and threshold of perception. Stimulation with capsaicin or piperine with concentrations above threshold may last for 10 min or longer.

In addition, individual thresholds may change depending on regularity of exposure. People who regularly consume chili peppers, or spices derived from chili pepper, show chronic desensitization. Often reported 'addiction' to spicy food may have a physiological basis, as desensitization by capsaicin is thought to be due to depletion of substance P, a neurotransmitter in the somatic pain system. Substance P has been linked to the functioning of endorphins, which have the effect of improving mood or giving a feeling of high. Irritant stimulation also has a strong cognitive component, as it results in strong defensive mechanisms in the body, including sweating, tearing and salivary flow.

9.5 Role of saliva

Saliva plays an important role in taste function. It contains substances that modulate taste response and acts as a carrier for sapid compounds to the taste buds. Saliva contains a weak solution of NaCl, and ionic constituents of chlorides, phosphates, sulfates and carbonates, as well as other organic components, proteins, enzymes and carbon dioxide. It is capable of buffering acids, and the salivary proteins and mucopolysaccharides give it its slippery and coating properties, which are essential for lubrication of the mouth. The importance of saliva lubrication is most noticeable when it is lost following strong astringent sensation. However, saliva is not necessary for taste response as extensive rinsing of the tongue with deionized water does not inhibit the taste response, but actually sharpens it owing to release from adaptation and, for example, the absolute threshold for NaCl is decreased significantly. Saliva is also very important as a solvent that is mixed with food by mastication, aiding food breakdown and bolus preparation. The structural deformation and mixing of food has a significant influence on the release and availability of flavor-active compounds, both sapid and volatile, for sensory stimulation. With regard to chemesthesis, there is strong correlation between increased oral chemical irritation and increased salivary flow rate. There are differences between individuals in both salivary flow rate and composition, and this can have significant impact on the potential of food compounds to stimulate the sensory systems.

Astringency is a sensation that does not result from stimulation of the chemical senses per se, although it is caused by chemical stimuli. Astringency sensations are largely tactile, and are experienced as a dry and rough mouth, and a drawing, puckering or tightening sensation in the cheeks and muscles of the face. It is believed that tannins or acids binding to salivary proteins and inhibiting their lubricating function cause the dominant astringent sensations. People with a low salivary flow rate have prolonged astringency responses, and those with less salivary protein have higher astringency responses.

9.6 Adaptation

Adaptation can be defined as the decrement in intensity or sensitivity to a compound under constant stimulation by this compound. Adaptation results in a higher threshold or a reduced perception of intensity. It is an important operating characteristic of the chemical sensory systems that enables perception of change: the status quo is rarely of interest. We use adaptation constantly to adjust to our changing environment by becoming unresponsive to stimuli that are stable in space and time. An obvious example of adaptation in everyday life is as follows. Consider entering an active kitchen, filled with the odor of food. After a short time there you will no longer notice the odor, which upon entering you could perceive strongly. If you leave the kitchen for a time and then return, the odor will be perceived as strongly as before. What is experienced in this example is a feature of all adaptation. Threshold will increase following periods of constant stimulation, and ratings of perceived intensity will decrease over time, and may even approach a judgment of 'no sensation'. If the stimulus is removed, then sensitivity returns. The fact that we cannot taste our own saliva, although it contains NaCl and other potentially sapid compounds, is another everyday example of necessary adaptation. Similarly, our odor world is continually filled, so that usually we are at least partially odor adapted.

Adaptation also has a role to play in the perception of mixtures. For example, the sweetness of sucrose and the bitterness of quinine are each partially suppressed when presented in a mixture. However, following adaptation to sucrose, the bitterness of the quinine–sucrose mixture will be perceived at a higher intensity, comparable to that of an equimolar unmixed quinine solution.

The opposite occurs following adaptation to quinine. Wine has dominant sweet and sour tastes. If wine is consumed with a salad dressed with a vinegar base (which is essentially sour), it will appear sweet to taste. If the same wine is consumed with dessert (which is essentially sweet), it will appear sour to taste. Similar principles hold for odor mixtures. Adaptation to one component of an odor mixture can make another stand out. Returning to wine, differential adaptation may explain why wine character appears to change with time of exposure.

Compounds of the same quality tend to cross-adapt. For example, after adapting to NaCl, the salty taste of other salts is perceived to be less intense, and other taste qualities are unaffected. Adaptation to sucrose reduces sensitivity to other sweet compounds and, similarly, adaptation to one odorant may affect the threshold of another odorant.

9.7 Cross-modal sensory interactions

Cross-modal sensory interactions are often observed when two or more perceptible components of a food system are studied together. It is important to identify the nature of these interactions as they may influence consumers' perceptions and preferences in unexpected ways. The factors that cause apparent cross-modal sensory interaction are not always the same. Sensory differences can be caused by interactions between the components of the food before introduction to the senses. For example, differences in temperature can change the vapor pressure and partition coefficients of volatile compounds and therefore their release from a solute. Differences in viscosity (perceived as texture) can also influence partition and availability of compounds for perception. Changing fat content or salt content also influences the physical chemistry of a food matrix dramatically, changing its flavor significantly. Sensory interactions are also determined by a halo effect which is due to learning to place greater reliance on one sensory modality over another to make behavioral decisions. This effect is most obvious by the dominance, or bias, of the visual sense over the taste or olfactory sense when familiar color and flavor combinations are confused, or when the color intensity is varied beyond expectation (e.g. imagine a dark beverage with no taste). This type of bias can be modified by directing attention to specific characteristics of the

product, or those of most interest. A true cross-modal sensory interaction is one where the function of one sense (e.g. threshold measures, concentration–response functions) is changed by stimulation of another sense. Some examples of all three interactions that influence sensory perception will be given here.

Interactions between the chemical senses of taste and smell have received much attention. Consumers often do not make any distinction between taste and smell, and most often refer to the combined sensation as 'taste'. Therefore, incorrect localization is often misinterpreted as representing interaction. There is very little specific interaction between taste and odor. However, when taste compounds and odor compounds that have complementary character are presented together, the intensity of perception of the combination is stronger than when either is presented alone. It has been shown that a below-threshold tastant can be combined with a below-threshold odorant to provide a flavor stimulus above threshold. In addition, sucrose is perceived as sweeter when presented with fruit character odor compounds, but not when presented with peanut butter odor. These types of interaction are dependent on the characteristics of the compounds or substances combined, and whether there is any pattern or rule is not yet clear. Recent experiments conducted with a sucrose and mint-based chewing gum showed that intensity ratings for mint decreased as sucrose was lost from the gum, although mint release was unchanged (measured using real-time mass spectrometry). The intensity of mint perception increased if sucrose was introduced to the mouth. These results may demonstrate an inability to localize the perception of taste and aroma, or may be related to attention mechanisms.

Interactions between chemesthesis and both odor and taste have been demonstrated. These interactions are truly cross-modal, as they are manifest as suppression effects that can be measured using psychophysical functions. When odor molecules and irritant molecules are mixed they produce mutual suppression, in a similar way to when odors alone are mixed. As most odorants have irritant effect in addition to their odor quality, suppression may be a common occurrence. If a person had reduced sensitivity to irritation, then the balance of aromatic flavor they perceive may be changed. Capsaicin desensitization has partial inhibitory effects on sweetness, sourness and bitterness perception, but not on saltiness. However, when capsaicin is presented mixed with these tastants, inhibitory effects are not found. This is probably because the capsaicin has not had sufficient time to cause desensitization before the tastants are perceived. There is less evidence to show how tastes can influence the burn of capsaicin, although studies suggest that sweet, sour and salt will reduce the intensity of burn, with sweet working best. Fat, or fat content, may also reduce burn as capsaicin is highly lipophilic, and fat may remove excess capsaicin that is available for perception. Irritation of various types can also improve preferences significantly. Soft drinks, or sodas, are not particularly pleasant without the fizziness provided by carbon dioxide, and are in fact sweeter to taste.

Interactions between the somatory senses, the visual senses and the chemical senses are also common. An intense sweet taste increases the perception of viscosity, although this is observed as a halo effect. The change in perception caused by sweetness identity may be due to prior association between high levels of sugars and high viscosity. Thresholds for the four basic tastes, and for most odorants, are higher in solid foods, foams and gels than in water. However, this interaction is most influenced by physicochemical interactions occurring in the food matrix, rather than effects on the sensory receptors. This influence is particularly so for odor.

Color has a strong influence on flavor perception. It influences absolute threshold measures, differential threshold measures, discrimination and even the ability of beverages to quench thirst. Darker colored foods and beverages are rated as having more intense flavor. Uncolored foods receive lower odor quality ratings, and incorrect identification is common when familiar flavor and color combinations are confused. These interactions also demonstrate halo effects.

Temperature changes influence the intensity of perception for all of the chemical sense modalities. Thresholds for taste compounds are lowest between 22 and 32°C. The effect of temperature can be represented by a U-shaped curve. In practical terms, salted foods taste more salty when they are heated or cooled to the 22–32°C range. Similarly, sweet-tasting foods will be most sweet in the 22–32°C range. A good cook knows to adjust seasoning to the temperature at which the food will be served. Temperature also influences chemical irritation perception. The most obvious example is that of the temporary, but significant, relief from chili burn given by a cold drink.

9.8 Flavor preferences

Flavor can be defined as the integrated response to stimulation of all of the chemical senses in combination. It is most logical to refer to flavor when attempting to relate chemical sense perceptions to preferences, as regular consumers, whose preferences are of most interest, do not normally distinguish between taste, smell and chemesthesis when they respond to food during consumption. Some authors stretch the scope of flavor definition even wider, by including texture, temperature and even visual sensations. However, to do so in this chapter would depart from the principles of chemical stimulation already discussed and enter the realm of food structure, where the psychophysical principle differs somewhat. In the sections of this chapter to follow flavor will be defined as above, but relevant consideration will be paid to texture and other food properties.

In developed society, the significance of food has changed from providing basic nutritional needs to providing protocols that define a person, their cultural identity and social standing. Flavor could now be called the social sense, because we tend to eat with other people when possible, sharing flavor experiences as we eat. However, when we do share flavor experience, labels are usually prefaced with pleasant or unpleasant remarks. Comments such as 'this soup is too salty', or 'I really like the taste of this sauce' are typical. These labels determine which foods we choose to eat and which we avoid.

With regard to chemical sensation, there is a strong relationship between the sensory perception and hedonic response to food. As the sensory intensity of a given stimulus increases, for example the sweetness of sugar, its hedonic tone becomes increasingly pleasant, reaches a maximum (ideal point) and then decreases in pleasantness to the point of neutral hedonic tone. Further increases in concentration become unpleasant (Figure 9.5). This inverted U-shaped curve is typical of the hedonic response to most chemical stimuli. However, there are many factors that influence an individual person's perception of a food's flavor. These include how much has already been eaten, what has already been eaten and how long ago, past experiences with different foods, genetic make-up, nutritional state and, with reference to the preceding paragraph, the culture and personal company that have most influence on a person. Such factors will not negate the relationship between sensory perception and hedonic response described

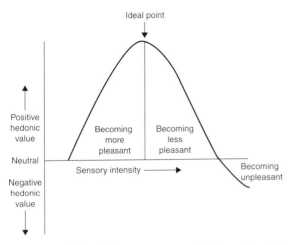

Figure 9.5 Relationship between sensory intensity and hedonic response.

above, but they may alter the shape of psychophysical concentration–response curves, hedonic response curves, or both.

Our reaction to a flavor stimulus may be positive when we first taste it, but this positive response may become negative after we have eaten for a while. This change in response can be due to changes in internal state, or satiety, signaling the body to stop eating. However, other factors may also be involved. Consider ordering a dark chocolate pudding, with intense chocolate flavor, at a café. At first, you may feel that the piece you have received is rather small; however, you will be doing well to finish it all off, even if you are quite hungry. This latter response is more likely to do with flavor fatigue, or sensory specific satiety, than a signal from inside the body. This response to strongly flavored foods is common. Sensory-specific satiety is also manifest if the same food is presented repeatedly over time to an individual, and can result in reduced intake. This may explain why humans characteristically seek variety in their diet, at least to a point.

People in certain cultures develop preferences for certain foods that are typically associated with that culture. Consider the differences between Asian and European cuisines. However, there is little evidence to suggest that peoples of different cultures have different sensitivity to flavors. In addition, children, who often avoid unfamiliar foods because of their flavor, come to prefer these foods if repeatedly exposed to them. People also learn to like and to appreciate bitter-tasting foods and beverages such as alcoholic beverages and

coffee. People who perform blind preference tests among a range of products within type more often than not choose the product with which they are most familiar or the one that they themselves consume. Evidence suggests that even subtle flavor preferences are learned and are strongly related to past experience with food. However, flavor preferences are not fixed when one reaches a particular point in life; they continuously change as experience increases.

Food preferences also demonstrate evolutionary design, instinctive response and adaptive value. At birth, infants prefer sweet taste, which indicates the presence of sugar, an important source of energy. They also tend to dislike bitter taste, which indicates substances that might cause sickness. These responses remain strong throughout life, and only change through experience as referred to above. Salt is liked at low concentrations but disliked at high concentrations, which makes sense as high intake might disrupt the body's careful osmotic balance. However, rats deprived of salt, a necessary component of their diets, have been shown to compensate and develop a specific hunger for sodium. Food preferences can also be affected by a single pairing of a food with sickness. This response is termed conditioned flavor aversion. There is good evolutionary justification for this extreme response, as sickness was most likely caused by poisoning, and conditioned flavor aversion prevents us from making the same mistake again.

There are well-documented differences between individuals in ability to taste PROP, and this difference has a genetic cause. Significant individual differences in thresholds to other sapid and odor compounds have also been shown. There are also documented differences in saliva composition and flow rate, mastication behavior and the quantities of sapid and volatile compounds that individuals can release from their food during eating. With these differences in mind, it may be that some foods may taste differently to different people, and that these differences can be genetic. These differences may explain differences in individual food preferences, particularly within cultures.

Memory for taste and smell is especially durable when compared with that for visual stimuli. Recollection, particularly for smell, is linked to an emotional component that aids the sensory systems in their role as gatekeeper. Long-term memory, often subconscious, enables humans to form associations between tastes and smells and foods that are good and bad to consume, and between tastes and smells and a particular place or occasion. A celebratory meal in a good restaurant will be recalled with more satisfaction than a meal eaten alone or when feeling low. These emotional factors can have a large influence on preferences. It is important to recognize that these emotions are closely associated with sensory memory, and recent evidence suggests that sensory memory for some tastes and smells is stronger than for others, perhaps referring to physiological need in the past. For example, memory for sweet taste and flavors associated with fats is relatively short term, whereas that for bitterness is longer term. This difference in memory for tastes may have implications for food intake.

9.9 Changing function of the chemical senses across the lifespan

When examining the changing function of the chemical senses across the lifespan, it is difficult to distinguish sensitivity from hedonic response. As discussed in Section 9.8, it is preferences, or hedonic response to stimuli, rather than the stimuli themselves, that determine behavior towards food and relate best to food intake. To recap: the performance of the chemical senses is responsible for determining initial preferences, and may determine how easily new preferences can be learned during life; and the chemical senses constantly maintain their gatekeeping function, screening stimuli to check that they meet preferred criteria, sourcing those that provide positive feelings, and rejecting those associated with unhappy experiences or ill health.

There are several stages of life, from early infancy, through childhood, adolescence, adulthood, middle-age and elderly to the oldest old. Food preferences and food intake change across the lifespan. Nutritional requirements also change. Malnutrition, manifest in undereating, overeating or insufficient nutrient intake, is widespread among almost all age groups or life stages. When considering the contribution of the chemical senses to food choice and intake, one should approach the subject from two perspectives. The first is to seek knowledge of how chemical sensitivity and hedonic response change across the lifespan, and ultimately to determine relationships between these factors and eating behavior that can be exploited in age-appropriate new product development. The other perspective is to understand how society and the food industry are currently contributing to incorrect dietary habits and dietary

guidance strategy through a lack of understanding of changing sensory function and its significance in helping to regulate optimum dietary intake, and to use this knowledge to restrict flavors that cause indulgence and promote flavors that signal nutritive value.

Newborn infants can discriminate between basic tastes. They demonstrate this by responding with positive facial expressions to sweet taste, and with negative facial expressions to sour and bitter tastes. They are indifferent to salty taste, probably because they are relatively insensitive to it. However, a preference for salt emerges at around 4 months of age owing to taste system development. Innate taste preferences remain strong throughout the lifetime, but may be modified by experience, and it is unclear how changes are related to changing sensitivity. For example, salt taste preference can be modified in infants as young as 6 months of age through experience. Children maintain a strong preference for sweet taste, certainly up to 5 years of age, but sweet taste preferences tend to decline between adolescence and adulthood.

The human olfactory system is anatomically complete before birth, and perception of odors via the amniotic fluid and early in infancy may play a role in later responses and preferences to odor stimuli. Studies have shown that newborns can smell and can discriminate between different odors, although they do not demonstrate typical preferences initially. Infants may like smells that are offputting to adults, such as those of fecal odors; however, these infants soon learn to develop preferences that are more in keeping with their peers, and by the age of 3 years tend to match those of adults. This and other evidence suggests that lifelong preferences and aversions for odors, as well as other strong emotional associations with odors, are formed during infancy and childhood. Preferences for the flavors of fat also appear to be learned, as children may associate specific flavors with high energy density. Children's preferences for fat are correlated with the body mass index (BMI) of their parents. This suggests a possible genetic link, but may equally be due to the dietary habits these parents give their children. Given the evidence presented, the variety of the diet in later life may be compromised by flavor preferences or food experiences learned during infancy and in early childhood. This relationship highlights a need to introduce a variety of flavors linked to positive nutritional value early in life. Relatively little is known about changes in sensitivity or hedonic response to chemesthesis that accompany the change from infancy to adolescence and adulthood. Given the impact of chemical irritation on hedonic response, research work is now needed.

Nutritional disorders may begin during childhood, but are more commonly initiated during the transition from adolesence to adulthood, and are established as adulthood progresses. Studies have been conducted to determine whether sensitivity and preferences for sweet taste, the flavor of fat and prevalence of obesity are related. No causal relationship has been found, although obese people tend to prefer foods high in sugar and fat and select fat-rich taste stimuli in sensory tests. Additional factors such as income, socioeconomic status, and the availability of sugars and fats are related to intake. People with the eating disorder anorexia nervosa seem to have dissociated taste responsiveness and eating patterns. Their taste preferences for sweet and fat do not differ from those of other people, but they use them to aid food avoidance rather than selection. Although not conclusive, these studies may demonstrate that it is not sensitivity per se that is important, but how we have learned to use our sensory system as a guide to consumption.

In the elderly, and in particularly in the oldest old, a new sensory requirement emerges. Older people lose chemical sense function, in parallel with the loss of other biological functions. This loss is greatest to olfactory function, which is manifest as higher absolute odor thresholds, less ability to perceive differences between suprathreshold odor intensity levels, and decreased ability to identify odors. Anatomically, decrement can be seen by morphological change to the olfactory bulb. Taste function remains relatively intact. Thresholds for salt and bitter taste may increase, whereas sweet and sour thresholds show little change. There are also some intensity decrements to chemesthesis function, although little is known for certain. In general, adaptation proceeds more slowly, recovery from adaptation is more lengthy and cross-adaptation is more severe in the elderly compared with the young. In addition, interactions within and between sensory modalities may be affected by a changed contribution of specific compounds or modalities to perception owing to differential loss of function. For example, as smell declines at a faster rate, foods that are bitter but have pleasant odor may be experienced as just plain bitter by an older person with poor odor ability. There are also effects of aging on saliva flow and composition. This change influences the ability to break down food,

inhibits mixing, retards flavor release and makes swallowing difficult.

Loss of sensory function with aging may cause older people to lose interest in food and food-related activities such as cooking or dining out, leading to reduced energy intakes and a reduction in essential nutrient consumption. In addition, the motivation that sensory-specific satiety gives to seek variety may be reduced, leading to consumption of a monotonous diet, which can also lead to reduced intake of specific essential nutrients. Losses in the ability to sense saltiness can create problems in elderly hypertensive populations, as they are likely to put more salt in their food. However, the impact that an age-related change in sensory function has on food preferences and food intake is unclear as no study has demonstrated a causal relationship between sensory impairment, diminished hedonic response and altered food intake in the same group of elderly people.

In all age groups, the perception of food in the mouth signals an innate biological response termed the cephalic phase response. This response stimulates saliva flow, and gastric and pancreatic secretions, preparing the gastrointestinal tract for foods that are about to be ingested so that these may be processed efficiently by the digestive system. The extent to which cephalic phase responses change over the lifespan, and the importance of these responses to long-term nutritional status, has yet to be determined. Changes in nutritional status, resulting from physiological disturbances that affect nutrient or energy balance, from normal fluctuations in energy status associated with hunger and satiety (sensory-specific satiety was discussed previously) or from modifications in diet (e.g. resulting in specific hunger for salt) can influence sensitivity and hedonic response, although these changes are generally short term. Extreme cases of nutrient deficiency or toxicity can influence the function of the chemical senses. This effect has been observed for vitamins A, B_6 and B_{12}, and for the trace metals zinc and copper. For example, zinc deficiency has been associated with histological changes in taste buds as well as degeneration and loss of taste papillae. Vitamin A deficiency results in gradual, but reversible, loss of taste, although zinc may again be involved as it plays an important role in transporting vitamin A from the liver. Diabetes results in a general reduction in taste sensitivity, and losses in ability to sense sweetness may cause diabetics to add more sugar to their food. This can create additional nutritional problems, particularly in the elderly who develop late-onset diabetes and find it difficult to manage their diet. Although not directly related to nutrition per se, poor oral and dental health influences sensory function, and can also cause dietary restriction if mechanical difficulties or pain are associated with the eating of some food types. Medications that are taken for chronic illness also contribute significantly to sensory loss, particularly in the elderly. The average older person in the USA takes 3.7 different medications at a time.

9.10 Introduction to the visual system

The visual system is our main portal with the outside world and consists of specialized tissues that are vulnerable to nutritional insults. For example, vitamin A deficiency results in night blindness and xerophthalmia. Thiamin deficiency can result in ophthalmoplegia (paralysis of movement of the eye). The eye is also susceptible to damage by toxic material in food and drink. For example, the consumption of methanol results in the formation of formic acid in the body, which damages the retina and can cause blindness; cyanide toxicity can damage the optic nerves and cause amblyopia (dimness of vision without obvious defect or change in the eye). The outer tissues of the eye are susceptible to damage and infection if the production of tears and mucus are affected. The lens of the eye is at risk of developing opacities if the proteins from which it is made become oxidatively damaged. The extremely high oxygen tension within the retina and the high level of exposure of the eye to ionizing radiation make this tissue susceptible to oxidative damage. To protect against damage mediated by free radicals, the eye has a number of protective system to mop up free radicals. With increasing age the effectiveness of this system decreases and two major causes of blindness, cataracts and age-related macular degeneration, are consequences. This chapter describes the physiology of the visual system and the role played by specific nutrients in the system, and considers the evidence that modification of diet can influence visual function and the risk of the major degenerative diseases in the eye.

9.11 Outline of the physiology of the visual system

The visual system consists of the outer eye, the inner eye including the lens and vitreous body, and the retina, which is connected to the optic nerve. The outer surfaces of the eye are susceptible to damage and infection and heat. In this respect, vitamin A plays a crucial role in maintaining the normal differentiation of epithelial cells which facilitate mucus production by goblet cells needed to lubricate the outer surfaces of the eye. The iris regulates the amount of light entering the eye, and the lens, which is mounted between two ciliary muscles, is able to focus the image on the retina (Figure 9.6). The fundus of the eye includes the retina, macula, fovea, optic disk and retinal vessels. The retina acts as a transducer converting radiant energy into molecular events in the photoreceptors. The retina consists of two types of photoreceptor cells: rods, which are sensitive to low-intensity black and white vision (scotopic), and cones, which are sensitive to color (photopic vision). Both types of cell are connected synaptically to a variety of bipolar cells. These in turn connect with ganglion cells, the axons of which form the optic nerve and lead to the lateral geniculate bodies and then to the cerebral cortex, where visual images are processed. A variety of optical and spatial filters enables the visual system to discard information. The mobility of each eye is controlled by six extraocular muscles and promoted by a virtually frictionless and largely shock-proof environment. The ball-and-socket complex is kept lubricated by an active lachrymal

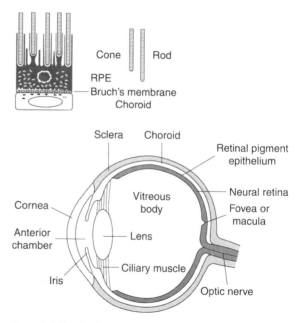

Figure 9.6 The visual system.

system, which also insures the maintenance of an optimal optical quality of the exposed cornea.

The amount of light entering the eye is controlled by the iris and the lens is a glycoprotein that focusses light on the retina. The lens aids in the refraction of light, but the primary refractive structure in the eye is the cornea. The lens can flex to aid focus and vision of close objects (accommodation). The lens also helps to filter out dangerous ultraviolet (UV) light from the retina. The optic disk, which is also called the blind spot, is the part of the retina where there are no photoceptors. It is where all of the axons of the ganglion cells exit the retina to form the optic nerve. The arteries and vessels also converge at the disk in a central area called the optic cup. The macula is an oval area lateral to the disk used for central vision and has an orange tinge when viewed via an ophthalmoscope, owing to the accumulation of carotenoid pigments such as zeaxanthin and lutein. These pigments may serve as scavengers of singlet oxygen O$^{\cdot}$ and protect the retina from oxidative damage, but they also reduce the effects of chromatic aberration by absorbing blue and violet rays for which the eye is myopic. The fovea is a small depression in the macula composed almost entirely of cones. Contrast, fine detail and color are dependent on data from the foveal cones, whereas movement is best detected by the more peripherol rod-dense regions of the retina. The proportion of rods and cones in the eye varies markedly between species; cones are dominant in humans. Color vision is facilitated by the iodopsins with differing sensitivity to varying wavelengths; these are referred to as cones with red, blue and green sensitivities. The signals from each retina are projected partly on both sides of the brain, therefore permitting the operation of stereoscopic vision. However, the visual signals are deciphered in the visual cortex, with the signals from the left eye being interpreted in the right cerebral cortex and those of the right eye in the left. Consequently, damage to the cerebral cortex results in visual loss in the contralateral eye. There appear to be critical windows of development of the visual processing system. Stimulation of the visual cortex during early life seems to increase the number of synaptic connections that are made. For example, in kittens, if one eye is sutured at birth development of the contralateral visual cortex is impaired. Evidence that this occurs in humans comes from the study of children born with congenital cataracts who have impaired visual processing which can be ameliorated by early removal of the cataract.

9.12 Role of the retina in signal transduction and the specific roles of retinol, docosahexaenoic acid and taurine in the visual process

In rods the light-responsive pigment is termed rhodopsin (visual purple) and is a complex between 11-*cis*-retinal and opsin (in cones there are similar pigments that bind with 11-*cis*-retinal but they are called iodopsins). 11-*cis*-Retinal is formed in the retina from 11-*cis*-retinol, which in turn is derived from all-*trans*-retinol. The *cis*-configuration allows the retinal to fit into a cleft in the opsin protein and the purple color can be ascribed to resonance of the conjugated double-bond system of 11-*cis*-retinal. When a photon interacts with rhodopsin, the configuration of 11-*cis*-retinal changes to 11-*trans*-retinal. The *cis*–*trans* isomerization causes the retinal to disassociate from opsin (bleaching of the pigment) and results in the release of energy and membrane depolarization, which is transmitted via bipolar cells to the optic nerve. The activated rhodopsin repeatedly contacts molecules of the heterotrimeric G-protein, catalyzing the exchange of guanosine diphosphate (GDP) for guanosine triphosphate (GTP), producing the active form, Gα-GTP. Two of the Gα-GTP subunits bind to two inhibitory subunits of phosphodiesterase, which then catalyzes the hydrolysis of cyclic GMP (cGMP). The consequent reduction in cytoplasmic concentration of cGMP leads to closure of the cyclic nucleotide gated channels and blockage of the inwards flux of Na$^+$ and Ca^{2+} (thereby reducing the circulating electrical current). The molecular mechanisms involved in the visual process are complex and beyond the scope of this chapter, but reviews dedicated to this subject are given in the Further reading list. 11-*cis*-Retinal is regenerated within the retina but is strongly dependent on a continued supply in plasma. This is why night blindness (nyctalopia) is one of the earliest signs of vitamin A deficiency disease.

The n-3 polyunsaturated fatty acid (PUFA) docosahexaenoic acid (DHA, 22:6n-3) is found in high concentrations in cells of the retina. It appears to perform an important physiological function in the eye of both higher and lower animals. This function does not appear to be dependent on conversion to secondary metabolites such as prostaglandins. The reflecting layer in the eye of sand trout (*Cyonscion arenarius*) consists almost entirely of tridocosahexaenoin, in the form of lipid spherules, which has a high refractive index.

In all mammalian species DHA is concentrated in the phospholipids of the retina, especially in the rod outer segment where DHA, which is mainly present in the sn-2 position, accounts for about half of the total fatty acids. Elongated homologs of DHA, notably 22:6n-3, have been found in retinal phosphatidyl cholines. The rod outer segment consists of a series of disk-like membranes. Rhodopsin is imbedded within and spans these disk membranes. The disk membrane needs to be flexible to accommodate the dynamics of rhodopsin behavior. Studies of model membranes have shown that phosphatidyl cholines containing DHA have an unexpectedly high melting point. DHA is believed to exist in a helical conformation in the membrane. It has been argued that this may produce greater flexibility and compressibility and, therefore, lower resistance to conformational changes in rhodopsin. The high DHA content may also increase the permeability of the disk to ions involved in neural signaling.

Taurine (ethaneaminosulfonic acid) is also found in high concentrations in the retina and is believed to act as a membrane-stabilizing component because of its ability to form a zwitterion (an ion that has both positive and negative charges on the same group of atoms; taurine has the capacity to transfer a proton from the sulfate group to the amino group). Taurine can be synthesized in humans from cysteine. However, its rate of synthesis may not be commensurate with needs in the newborn infant and preformed taurine may be required in the diet of the human infant. Taurine deficiency was first shown to cause retinal degenerations in kittens. However, in cats there is an obligatory loss of taurine in bile as they are unable to synthesize glycocholic acid and must conjugate bile acids with taurine. Visual function in rhesus monkey infants raised from birth until 6 or 12 months of age on a taurine-free soy protein-based human infant formula has been compared with a control group that received the same formula supplemented with taurine. An additional group received taurine-free formula until 6 months and then the supplemented diet from 6 until 12 months. The densities of rhodopsin, measured in the near periphery after a white bleach, and of cone pigment, measured in the macula after a red bleach, were significantly reduced in the taurine-deprived monkeys at 6 months, but not at 12 months. The retinae of 6-month-old taurine-deprived infants showed degenerative morphological changes in photoreceptors, particularly in cones in the foveal region. Therefore,

most breast milk substitutes are fortified to contain taurine at the same level as that found in human breast milk. The main dietary sources of taurine are meat and seafood, and these determine the level of taurine in breast milk. This explains why in human breast milk taurine concentration is lower in vegetarians than in meat eaters.

9.13 Evidence for a specific requirement for docosahexaenoic acid in the visual process

The electroretinogram is used as an index of visual function. It represents depolarization/repolarisation reactions following light stimulation. Studies have shown that the electroretinogram amplitude is reduced in rats fed a source of n-6 PUFA only (ethyl linoleate) compared with those also fed a source of n-3 PUFA (ethyl linolenate). Other studies have confirmed that the proportion of dietary n-6:n-3 PUFA affects the visual process. The amplitude of the electroretinogram a-wave was reduced in young rats reared on a diet with a high linoleic acid (LA, 18:2n-6):α-linolenic acid (ALA, 18:3n-3) ratio, compared with controls reared on a diet with a low LA:ALA ratio. This effect was most evident in young animals, and any effect of the dietary LA:ALA ratio on visual function decreased with age. It is difficult to deplete the retina of DHA in adult life, which would suggest that DHA is avidly conserved by the retina. Monkeys born to a mother fed a diet in which the fat was provided by safflower oil, then reared on an artificial formula containing the same source of dietary fat, were found to exhibit differences in the electroretinogram recordings compared with animals fed soybean oil. There was a decrease in the amplitude of the a-wave and an increased latency in response to light stimulation. This can be interpreted as meaning that the response of the photoreceptors and the propagation of the signal were slower in the deprived animals. Again, the differences between groups diminished with increasing age. The animals exhibited marked reductions in the proportion of DHA in retinal and cerebral cortex phospholipids and its replacement with 22:5n-6, a derivative of the n-6 PUFA arachidonic acid. The biochemical changes were shown to be reversible by supplementing the diet with fish oil but, surprisingly, the electroretinogram recordings did not recover. This could be interpreted as meaning that an inadequate supply of DHA during a vulnerable phase of development leads to irreversible damage. Impaired visual-evoked potential measurement has been reported in preterm infants fed formula containing LA (18:2n-6) but virtually no ALA (18:3n-3). This did not occur in infants fed breast milk or formula containing DHA. It has been argued that the conversion of ALA to DHA may be limited in humans, particularly when the intake of linoleic acid is high. Consequently, DHA may be required in the diet for normal visual development. Several randomized controlled trials have assessed the impact of supplementing preterm and term infants with formula containing DHA. A systematic review of these trials suggests that supplementation of preterm infants with formula containing DHA results in a transient improvement in visual function. However, the benefits of including DHA in term formula are equivocal. While claims have been made in relation to the benefits of DHA on visual function and reading ability, data do not currently exist to support the claims.

9.14 Specific problems associated with the visual process

The lens is susceptible to oxidative damage owing to its exposure to ionizing radiation. The retina is susceptible to oxidative damage because of its high oxygen tension, and high concentrations of DHA and retinal make it vulnerable to lipid peroxidation. Age-related increases in the rise of fluorescent material in both the lens and the retina are believed to result from oxidative changes. Retinal degeneration in rats induced by oxidants or constant light exposure leads to a selective loss of DHA from the rod outer segment. To counteract the vulnerability to lipid peroxidation, the retina contains a variety of membrane-stabilizing substances such as vitamin E and taurine, as well as enzymes involved in protection from free radicals. Retinopathy of prematurity is a common problem and can result from exposure to hyperbaric oxygen in early life, such as when preterm infants are kept in incubators. Attempts to prevent retinopathy of prematurity with additional vitamin E did not significantly lower the overall incidence of retinopathy. However, a meta-analysis of the randomized controlled trials suggested that vitamin E may reduce the risk of threshold (stage 3+) retinopathy of prematurity by half.

Hypertension and type II diabetes mellitus are two conditions that are common in old age and can result in damage to the eye. Hypertension can result in the rupture of small vessels in the retina (retinal hemorrhage), leading to damage to the retina. In diabetes mellitus there may be associated hypertension and lipid infiltrates may affect the retina. Diabetic retinopathy is a progressive disease that destroys capillaries in the eye by depositing abnormal material along the walls of the microcirculation of the retina. Blurred vision and often blindness follow. The longer a person has diabetes the greater their chances of developing diabetic retinopathy. Neovascularization, a proliferative growth of abnormal blood vessels, is particularly harmful. This latter process can be controlled by laser coagulation of the vessels. Glycosylation reactions that result as a consequence of high blood glucose concentrations can also cause damage to the basement membranes in the retina. Good control of blood pressure and blood glucose in patients with type II diabetes mellitus has been shown to decrease the risk of visual complications.

Antioxidant protection falls with increasing age and may be involved in the etiology of cataracts and age-related maculopathy, which are major causes of visual loss in old age. The third major cause of blindness in older people is glaucoma (increased pressure within the eyeball, causing gradual loss of sight through damage to the optic nerve). There is little evidence that diet influences the risk of glaucoma, but there is some evidence that it does influence the risk of cataract and age-related maculopathy.

9.15 Cataract

Cataract is the term used to describe lens opacity and is a major cause of reversible blindness worldwide. Cataract has often been presented as a terminal condition. First, there is yellowing of the lens, which then becomes presbyopic (loss of accommodation that normally develops in the eye in middle age, which is a result of a loss of elasticity in the lens and can be corrected by reading glasses). Then the pupil size is decreased, reducing the amount of light entering the eye, and there is degeneration of the retina leading to loss of visual acuity (Figure 9.7). The incidence of cataract increases with age, but is modified by environmental and genetic factors.

The incidence of cataract is high among the elderly population of developed countries, but occurs at a younger age in some less economically developed

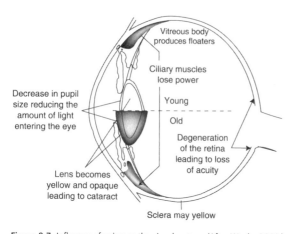

Figure 9.7 Influence of aging on the visual system. (After Weale, 2000.)

countries such as India. In the Beaver Dam Eye Study in the USA, the overall incidence of cataract was 27% over a 5 year period in subjects aged 43 to >75 years at age of recruitment. Cataract can be subdivided into nuclear, cortical and subcapsular cataract, the former being more prevalent. Cortical cataract, which is characterized by streaks, clefts and wedges seen with a slit lamp in the lenticular cortex, is more frequent among black people. In contrast, nuclear cataract, which involves opacities in the nucleus, occurs frequently among those born in the Indian subcontinent. Posterior subcapsular caratact, a condensation located near the visual axis intersecting the posterior lenticular pole, is a most disabling form of cataract that can result from systemic causes such as diabetes and ingestion of steroids. Cataract occurs when the protein making up the lens undergoes post-translational changes. Some of these changes may be due to wear and tear, while others may be due to environmental influences such as heat shock, cross-linking and glycosylation of proteins. It has been suggested that the high incidence of nuclear cataract and presbyopia among people born in the Indian subcontinent is related to average environmental temperature. It has also been suggested that diarrhea in childhood may predispose to nuclear cataract. α-Crystallin may act as a chaperone, protecting proteins from heat shock and other causes of denaturation. The age-related decline in this protein might therefore be related to the risk of cataract. If this is correct then it is the loss of the protection rather than degradation that increases the vulnerability of the lens to cataract.

Cortical changes entail the rupture of cell membranes and free radical damage. There is some evidence that cortical cataract is more strongly related to light exposure than nuclear cataract. Free radicals such as the hydroxy radical OH· can cause changes in protein conformation. However, these disorganizational effects are retarded by scavengers of free radicals. Consequently, vitamins and minerals (selenium, zinc, copper and manganese) involved in free-radical scavenging mechanisms may have a role to play in influencing the etiology of cataract. Reduced glutathione appears to play a particularly important role in maintaining the clarity of the lens. There is an age-related decline in lenticular glutathione content with age, which is associated with an increased incidence of cataract.

Several risk factors for cataract have been established from prospective cohort studies in developed countries. Exposure to sunlight appears to promote both cortical and posterior subscapsular lesions and to protect from nuclear cataract. Smoking may promote nuclear cataract. Individuals with glucose-6-phosphate dehydrogenase deficiency, which is needed to maintain glutathione in a reduced state, have an increased risk of cataract. Case–control studies in developed countries suggest that multivitamin intake protects from nuclear cataract. Furthermore, several prospective studies show lower rates of self-reported cataracts among those who took mulitvitamin supplements or who were long-term users of vitamin C. Low educational attainment is a risk factor for all types of cataract and this may be an important confounder in the dietary studies in developed countries. There have been few randomized controlled trials on the effect of diet on the prevention of cataract.

In a nutritionally deprived area of China, multivitamin or riboflavin and niacin supplements resulted in a lower prevalence of nuclear cataracts among subjects aged 65–74 years. However, a combination of selenium, vitamin E and β-carotene was not effective. An analysis of the cataract incidence in the Alpha Tocopherol Betacarotene Trial did not find any effect of these nutrients. These findings suggest that lipid soluble antioxidants are not important in the etiology of nuclear cataract. The finding that riboflavin and niacin helped to prevent nuclear cataract is consistent with their physiological role in maintaining adequate production of reduced glutathione. Several large randomized controlled trials are currently underway which should be able to ascertain whether vitamin and/or mineral supplementation is of benefit in delaying the onset of caratact, but it will be several years until any firm conclusions can be drawn.

9.16 Age-related macular degeneration

Age-related macular degeneration (ARMD) is now recognized as the most common cause of registered blindness in Western society and it is evident that the prevalence is rising because of the aging of the population. Although it rarely results in total blindness, it involves a failure of central vision, manifest by a greatly reduced ability to perceive fine detail and contrast. Reading becomes impossible and tasks such as watching television become difficult and unenjoyable. ARMD occurs in two main forms, wet and dry. The former involves retinal hemorrhages, which can be partly controlled by laser coagulation of the leaky vessels. The lesions identified as causing loss of central vision are subretinal neovascularization, detachment of the retinal pigment epithelium and geographical atrophy of the retinal pigment epithelium. These are widely believed to occur in response to deposition of abnormal material (drusen) within Bruch's membrane. Neither cause nor cure is known, but several risk factors have been identified. Eye color (low ocular melanin, e.g. blue eyes) is a risk factor. Exposure to sunlight and smoking are among the controllable factors shown to be associated with risk. Loss of DHA from the retina may be involved in the causation of ARMD. However a case–control study in patients with overt drusen demonstrated that plasma and erythrocyte phospholipids DHA and eicosapentaenoic acid (EPA) levels were similar to those in controls. This suggests that dietary DHA is not important in the etiology of ARMD.

Some case–control studies have suggested that people who eat a diet rich in antioxidant vitamins (carotenoids, vitamins E and C) or minerals (selenium, zinc) may be at less risk from the disease. Some prospective studies show that the intake of specific carotenoids, lutein and zeaxanthin, is associated with a decreased risk of ARMD. However, in the Alpha-Tocopherol Beta-carotene Trial supplementation with α-tocopherol or β-carotene, or both, was not found to influence the incidence of ARMD. One trial suggested that a combination of zinc and lutein may decrease the risk of developing ARMD, but results from further trials are awaited before any firm conclusion can be drawn. Caution should be exercised regarding carotenoid supplements because high intakes of canthoxanthin can lead to the formation of crystalline deposits in the retina. Canthoxanthin was at one time sold as a health-food supplement to change skin color, but has now been withdrawn because of concern that it may have adverse effects on vision.

9.17 Epidemic optic nerve neuropathy

Optic nerve neuropathy can occur in both thiamin and vitamin B_{12} deficiency. Formerly, optic nerve neuropathy was associated with heavy tobacco consumption and a poor diet (termed tobacco amblyopia). Vitamin B_{12} is involved in the detoxification of cyanide which is produced from tobacco smoke. Cyanide-induced neuropathy is also associated with cassava use in Nigeria. From late 1991 an epidemic of optic nerve neuropathy occurred in Cuba affecting some 51 000 people in a country with a population of 11 million. This disorder was associated with weight loss, cigar smoking, heavy alcohol intake and the increased use of cassava by the Cuban population. The epidemic dramatically was resolved by the administration of multivitamin supplements. To this day the exact cause of the epidemic remains uncertain, but a plausible explanation is that the vitamin B_{12} intake of the Cuban diet deteriorated following the withdrawal of economic support from the former USSR. This, together with the increased cultivation and consumption of cassava, heavy cigar smoking and high alcohol intake, precipitated an outbreak of optic nerve neuropathy.

9.18 Perspectives on the future

Earlier in this chapter it was stated that the primary function of the chemical senses is to detect foods that would be bad for the body and should be rejected, and to identify foods that the body needs for survival and that therefore should be consumed. Nevertheless 'what is bad for the body' can be interpreted as flavors that we dislike for whatever personal reasons, and 'what is good for the body' can be interpreted as flavors that we like for whatever personal reasons. The factors determining personal likes and dislikes for flavors are influenced by genetics, age, nutrition and health status, but most importantly by experience. In addition, individual nutritional status is determined by individual likes and dislikes, and by the quantity of liked foods that are consumed.

The aim of nutritional sciences is to improve dietary quality. Most focus to date has been directed at improving the nutritional quality of foods, by the provision of nutritionally enhanced foods and the recommendation of ideal eating habits. Little regard has been paid to 'tastes' or 'taste' preferences. To address this, efforts should now be made to develop dietary strategies that take account of the chemosensory properties of food. Unacceptable flavor, or flavor that does not match individual likes or expectations, is an obstacle to compliance with a recommended change in diet, particularly now that consumers are becoming more affluent and more discerning. The potential nutritional value of functional ingredients may be compromised because they have tastes that do not meet acceptable criteria. For example, phytochemicals, linked with cancer prevention, have a bitter taste for which there is an innate dislike. Sugar, salt and fat, substitutes do not taste the same as the substances that they seek to replace as their taste is not pure.

However, the hedonics of taste is arguably malleable through experience. As many bitter-tasting compounds are associated with foods that have high nutritive benefit, e.g. fruits and vegetables, hedonic responses to these bitter tastes needs to be adjusted. Conversely, macronutrients, such as sugar, salt and fat are generally most liked. As these are linked with chronic disease when consumed in excessive quantities, hedonic response to these flavors needs to be adjusted to reduce consumption. More research attention should be aimed at linking changes in chemosensory function and food preferences with diet selection and intake under real-life situations. To facilitate this, more work is needed to understand the role of olfaction and chemical irritation in diet selection and food preferences, to complement that already carried out on taste. More research with real food products is needed, which has greater ecological validity than working with pure tastants or odorants in solution. Nutritional scientists should also recognize the technological challenges facing the food manufacturing industry, as they seek to produce acceptable foods that contain new ingredients and formulations that differ markedly from tradition. In addition, dietary intervention strategies should consider the relationships between sensory likes and dislikes, and demographic, economic and sociocultural factors. It is important to consider sensory requirements and dietary needs in parallel, but at different stages in life. What is the contribution of sensory variety in infancy to lifelong variety-seeking behavior, and do breast-fed and formula-fed infants have different hedonic potential? Although preference studies may

show that older consumers are satisfied with foods currently available, these foods should be improved to compensate for specific sensory losses, which will with time lead to reaquaintance with an increased sensory variety. Given the strong link between sensory properties and digestive response, this compensation may have unforeseen benefits. However, it is important to recognize that the older population is very heterogeneous, and individual preferences are likely to differ significantly. Responsible nutritional intervention and functional food use may also reduce the need for widespread pharmaceutical use as old age progresses. This will have the added benefit of delaying the adverse effects of medicines on the ability to taste and smell, which may contribute to continued good eating habits.

Therefore, rather than attempting to play down the importance of the chemical senses to food intake, by demonstrating that price or, say, availability is a more significant determinant, it is time to understand better the development of food preferences with positive nutrition in mind and to exploit sensory properties to increase the intake of foods with high nutritive value. Future research should direct product development for individual nutrition needs, rather than consider sensory quality as part of market positioning after a product has already been produced, which is currently the norm.

Within the context of nutrition and the visual system, it is apparent that there are roles for specific nutrients in the functioning of the eye. Vitamin A plays a crucial role in the visual system by maintaining the outer surfaces of the eye and participating in the tranduction of light into electrical signals within the retina as rhodopsins and iodopsins. The conformational changes that occur upon light stimulation in rhodopsin, which is embedded in the photoreceptor membrane, appear to be facilitated by the presence of DHA in the membrane phospholipids. Nevertheless, the true nature of the role of dietary DHA in vision, especially throughout the different stages of life, has yet to be established. Taurine also appears to play an important role as a membrane stabilizer in the eye, but its exact role remains uncertain. Deficiencies of thiamin and vitamin B_{12} can result in optic nerve neuropathy. Hypertension and diabetes mellitus if untreated can result in damage to the retina and in the case of the latter can result in diabetic cataract. In developing countries, the incidence of nuclear cataract is high. Risk of cataract may be increased by malnutrition in childhood, which occurs as a consequence of repeated attacks of diarrhea. There is some evidence from China that niacin and riboflavin supplements decrease the risk of nuclear cataracts. In developing countries, the risk of cataract may be decreased by high intakes of vitamin C. Randomized controlled trials are required to confirm the role of vitamin C in cataract. ARMD is a major cause of blindness in the developed world and there is some evidence that an increased intake of zinc and lutein may be associated with decreased risk. Again, the results of large-scale randomized controlled trials are required to answer this question in the next few years.

Further reading

Finger TE, Silver WL, Restrepo D. The Neurobiology of Taste and Smell, 2nd edn. New York: Wiley-Liss, 2000.

Getchell TV, Bartoshuk LM, Doty RL, Snow JB. Smell and Taste in Health and Disease. New York: Raven Press, 1991.

Lawless HT, Heymann H. Sensory Evaluation of Foods, Principles and Practices. London: Chapman & Hall, 1998.

Pugh EN, Jr, Nikonov S, Lamb TD. Molecular mechanisms of vertebrate photoreceptor light adaptation. Curr Opin Neurobiol 1999; 9: 410–418.

Weale RA. The eye and senescence. In: The Oxford Textbook of Geriatric Medicine (J Grimley Evans ed.), pp. 863–873. Oxford: Oxford University Press, 2000.

10
The Gastrointestinal Tract

M Mañas, E Martínez de Victoria, A Gil, M Yago and J Mathers

Key messages

- The four basic processes that constitute the functions of the gastrointestinal tract are motility, secretion, digestion and absorption.
- The pancreas is a mixed gland containing both endocrine and exocrine portions. These two parts of the pancreas have a level of interaction.
- The most important digestive function of the liver is the secretion of bile, but it also plays a role in lipid, protein and carbohydrate metabolism, as well as the excretion of bile pigments and the storage of several vitamins and minerals, and the processing of hormones, drugs and toxins.

- The intestinal epithelium is a complex system of multiple cell types that maintain precise interrelationships. The regulatory mechanisms involved with developmental processes are at organism, cellular and molecular levels.
- The primary function of the large bowel is in salvage of energy via bacterial fermentation of food residues, but it also plays a role in the absorption of water and electrolytes, lipid metabolism, the synthesis of certain vitamins, essential amino acids, and the metabolism and absorption of phytochemicals.

10.1 Introduction

The overall function of the gastrointestinal system is to process ingested foods into molecular forms that can be transferred, along with salts and water, from the external environment to the internal environment of the body. The digestive processes are largely determined by the composition of food ingested. This fact determines the importance of the food and thus the diet, in most aspects of the physiology of the gastrointestinal system, including its regulation.

10.2 Structure and function of the gastrointestinal system

The structure of the gastrointestinal system (Figure 10.1) includes the gastrointestinal tract and the accessory glands (salivary, exocrine pancreas and liver). The structure of the gastrointestinal tract varies greatly from region to region, but there are common features in the overall organization of the tissue.

The layered structure of the wall of the gastrointestinal tract (Figure 10.2) includes, from the inside to the outside:

- *mucosa*: consists of an epithelium, the lamina propria and the muscularis mucosae
- *submucosa*: consists largely of loose connective tissue with collagen and elastin fibers. Some submucosal glands are present in some regions. In this layer there is a dense network of nerve cells highly interconnected called the submucosal plexus (Meissner's plexus)
- *muscularis externa*: consists of two substantial layers of smooth-muscle cells, an inner circular layer and an outer longitudinal layer. Between these layers there is another prominent network of highly interconnected nerve cells called the myenteric plexus (Auerbach's plexus). Both submucosal and myenteric plexuses (intramural plexuses) constitute, with the other neurons, the enteric nervous system. This innervation constitutes the intrinsic innervation (Figure 10.3)

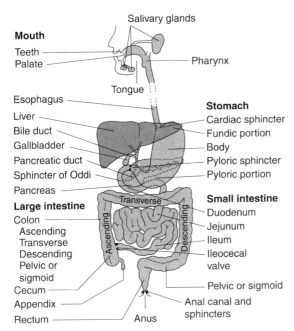

Figure 10.1 Structure of the gastrointestinal system, including the gastrointestinal tract and accessory glands (salivary, exocrine pancreas and liver).

- *serosa*: the outer most layer consists mainly of connective tissue and mesothelial cells.

The gastrointestinal system receives innervations from neurons of the autonomic nervous system, both sympathetic and parasympathetic. This constitutes the extrinsic innervation.

Both types of innervation are important for the regulation of the different functions of the gastrointestinal tract, mainly related to motility and secretion (exocrine and endocrine).

The oral cavity (or mouth) is the first portion of the gastrointestinal tract and is bounded by the lips (anteriorly), the fauces (posteriorly), the cheek (laterally), the palate (superiorly) and a muscular floor (inferiorly). The next structure is the pharynx, which is the common opening of both the digestive and the respiratory systems. The pharynx can be divided into three regions: the nasopharynx, the oropharynx and the laryngopharynx. The first includes the uvula, while the second extends from the uvula to the epiglottis and communicates with the oral cavity through the fauces. The laryngopharynx extends from the tip of the epiglottis to the glottis and esophagus.

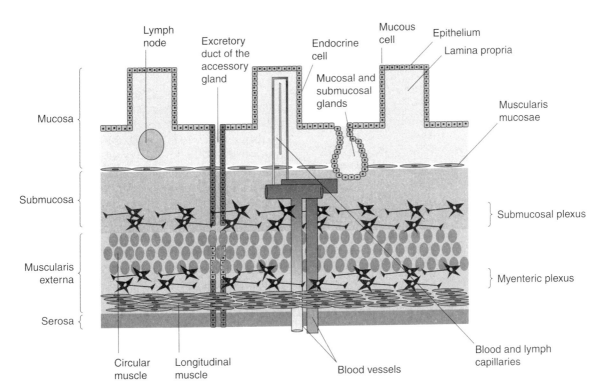

Figure 10.2 Layered structure of the gastrointestinal tract.

accumulating effects of years of poor eating habits can increase the risk of many health conditions as one grows older; yet, it is never too late to change!

Compression of morbidity

The accumulating effects of years of poor eating habits can increase the risk of many health conditions as one grows older. The good news is, however, that food habits may be amenable to modification. In other words, we can adopt lifestyle habits such as regular exercise and healthy eating that will slow functional decline and compositional changes within the limits set by genetics. It is possible to compress morbidity into the last few years of life (i.e. increase health span potential) if we take care of lifestyle and environmental factors throughout life, even once we reach old age. For example, an exercise intervention study in mid-life has been shown to compress morbidity (measured with disability score) towards the end of life. Several of the health problems and bodily changes experienced by older adults that have been attributed to the normal aging process are increasingly being recognized as linked to lifestyle or environmental factors. For example, decline in LBM and increases in body fat which tend to occur as people grow older cannot be entirely attributed to the aging process per se. A major contributor to these changes is the increasingly sedentary nature of people's lifestyles as they grow older in Western countries. Social and physical inactivity and inadequate nutrient and phytochemical intakes are now thought to be instrumental in trying to compress morbidity towards the end of life, and in maintaining or increasing physiological and nutritional reserves.

Physiological reserves, frailty and prevention strategies

Many bodily functions remain relatively unaffected until about 75 years of age when, on average, they start to decrease more noticeably. Nutritionally related health problems are often compounded in later life by reduced physiological reserves of many organs and functions. This applies to both reduced metabolic tissues (e.g. insulin resistance or reduced insulin response to a meal load or a greater glycemic response to the same food) and organ tissues (e.g. reduced cardiac reserve means that an added salt load may tip someone into heart failure, whereas otherwise it would not). While a younger person will be able to consume an inadequate diet with no foreseeable consequences, an elderly person is more likely to experience problems

because of diminished physiological function. Many studies have shown significant reductions in different body functions with age. These may not be inevitable, however. For example, what used to be regarded as a decline in brain function at about the age of 70 may not be seen until much later, raising the possibility that biological age in some body functions may be occurring at a later and later chronological age. Measures of physiological and nutritional reserves may be important indicators of health in older adults. Prevention of associated health problems may be possible if physiological and nutritional reserve levels are known.

Frailty

Avoidance of frailty is one of the major challenges facing older people and their carers. Frailty among older people has been defined as 'a condition or syndrome which results from a multi-system reduction in reserve capacity to the extent that a number of physiological systems are close to, or past, the threshold of symptomatic clinical failure. As a consequence the frail person is at an increased risk of disability and death from minor external stresses' (Campbell and Buchner, 1997). As the number of chronic conditions increases with age they contribute to disability and frailty, which in turn reduce a person's level of independence, sometimes resulting in institutionalization. Falls, incontinence and confusion are regarded as clinical consequences of frailty, and a number of risk factors is associated with each of these conditions. The risk of falling is increased as muscle strength and flexibility decline, and if balance and reaction time are impaired. Urinary incontinence is also a risk factor for falls among elderly people. Dehydration and PEM are two nutritional factors that can contribute to the confusion often experienced by elderly adults. Urinary incontinence often results in elderly people restricting their fluid intake in an effort to control their incontinence or reduce their frequency of urination. Studies are underway in relation to its prevention and management, and there is great interest in the extent to which it is reversible.

Prevention strategies

The major prevention strategies that elderly individuals can take to increase their physiological and nutritional reserves include:

- consuming a wide variety of foods
- engaging in physical activity, as this maintains lean muscle and bone mass, thus increasing nutritional

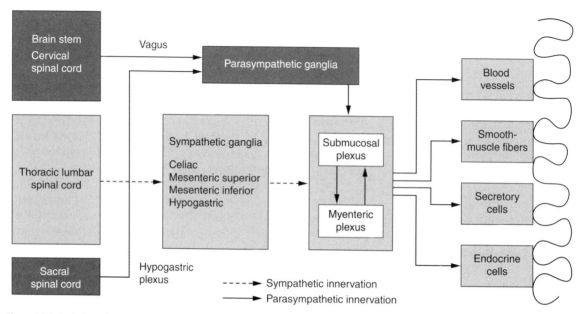

Figure 10.3 Intrinsic and extrinsic innervation of the gastrointestinal tract.

The esophagus is a segment of the gastrointestinal tract, 25 cm in length, that extends between the pharynx and stomach. It lies in the mediastinum, anterior to the vertebrae and posterior to the trachea. It passes through the esophageal hiatus (opening) of the diaphragm and ends at the cardiac opening of the stomach. The esophagus has two sphincters, the upper esophageal sphincter between the pharynx and esophagus, and the lower esophageal sphincter between the esophagus and stomach, near the cardiac opening. Both sphincters regulate the movement of the ingested meal into and out of the esophagus.

The stomach is an enlarged segment of the gastrointestinal tract in the left superior portion of the abdomen. The upper opening from the esophagus is the gastroesophageal or cardiac opening. The region near this opening is called the cardiac region. In the left and upper parts of the cardiac region is the fundus. The body, the largest portion of the stomach, turns to the right, creating a greater curvature and a lesser curvature. The lower opening of the stomach which communicates with the proximal segment of the small intestine (duodenal bulb) is the pylorus (or pyloric opening). The pylorus is surrounded by a thick ring of smooth muscle, the pyloric sphincter.

The small intestine is a long tube that consists of three portions: the duodenum, the jejunum and the ileum. The large intestine includes the cecum (most proximal), colon (ascending, transverse and descending), rectum and anal

canal. The longitudinal layer of smooth muscle of the large intestine is incomplete and forms three bands called teniae coli. The contraction of teniae coli causes pouches called haustra along the length of the colon.

The function of the gastrointestinal tract includes four general processes: motility, secretion, digestion and absorption (Figure 10.4).

- *Motility*: includes contractions of the smooth muscle of the gastrointestinal tract wall to mix the luminal contents with the various secretions and move them through the tract from mouth to anus. The components of motility are: chewing, swallowing, gastric motility, gastric emptying, small and large intestinal motility, gallbladder contraction and defecation.
- *Secretion*: the wall of the gastrointestinal tract and the accessory glands produce several secretions that contribute to the breakdown of food into small molecules. These secretions consist of saliva, pancreatic juice and bile secreted by accessory glands (salivary, pancreas and liver respectively), and gastric and intestinal juices secreted by the glands lining the wall of the stomach and the small and large intestine.
- *Digestion*: most food is ingested as large particles containing macromolecules, such as proteins and polysaccharides, which are unable to cross the wall of the gastrointestinal tract. Before the ingested food can be absorbed, therefore, it must be broken down and dissolved. These processes of breakdown and

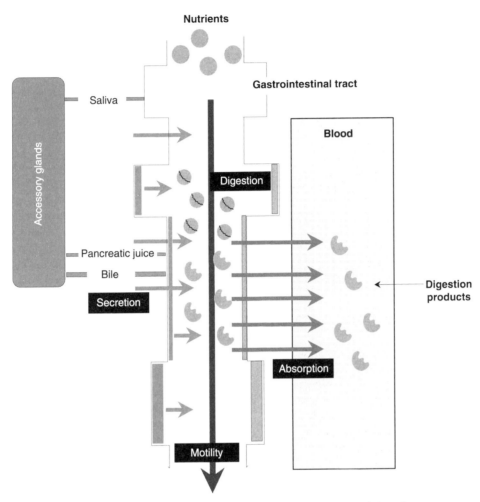

Figure 10.4 The four general functions of the gastrointestinal tract: motility, secretion, digestion and absorption.

dissolution of the food involve both gastrointestinal motility and secretion, and are termed mechanical and chemical digestion.

- *Absorption*: the molecules produced by digestion then move from the lumen of the gastrointestinal tract across a layer of epithelial cells and enter the blood or the lymph (internal environment).

These are the four basic processes that, with the mechanisms controlling them, constitute the functions of the gastrointestinal system.

10.3 Motility

Chewing can be carried out voluntarily, but thereafter the process is almost entirely under reflex control.

Chewing serves to lubricate the food by mixing it with saliva, to start the starch digestion with ptyalin (α-amylase) and to subdivide the food.

Swallowing is a rigidly ordered reflex that results in the propulsion of food from the mouth to the stomach. The swallowing center in the medulla and lower pons controls this reflex. There are three phases: oral, pharyngeal and esophageal. The last phase is carried out by the motor activity of the esophagus.

Gastric motility serves the following major functions:

- to allow the stomach to serve as a reservoir for the large volume of food that may be ingested at a single meal
- to fragment food into smaller particles and mix the luminal contents with gastric juice to begin digestion

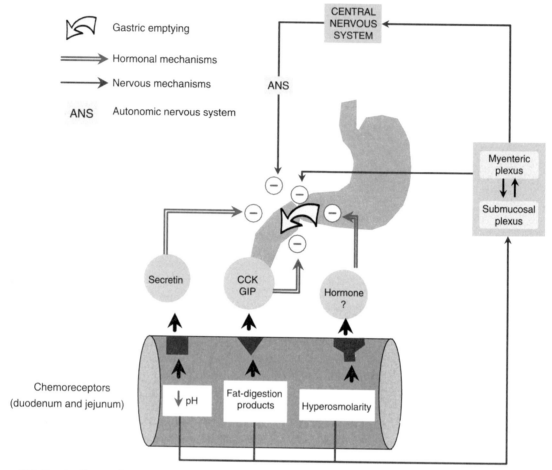

Figure 10.5 Neural and hormonal mechanisms involved in the regulation of gastric emptying. CCK: cholecystokinin; GIP: gastric inhibitory polypeptide.

- to empty gastric contents into the duodenum at a controlled rate. This last function is closely regulated by several mechanisms so that the chyme is not delivered to the duodenum too rapidly.

The mixing and mechanical fragmentation of the luminal contents and gastric emptying are carried out by peristaltic waves that begin in the pacemaker zone in the middle of the body of the stomach and travel towards the pylorus and through the gastroduodenal junction. The gastroduodenal junction (pyloric sphincter) allows the carefully regulated emptying of gastric contents to the duodenum for optimal digestion and absorption of nutrients.

Gastric emptying is regulated by both neural and hormonal mechanisms. The signals come from duodenal and jejunal receptors that sense acidity, osmotic pressure and fat content (Figure 10.5).

If the pH of chyme is less than 3.5, the rate of gastric emptying is reduced by neural mechanisms (vagal reflex) and through the release of secretin, an intestinal hormone that inhibits the antral contractions and stimulates the contraction of the pyloric sphincter.

The chyme emptying into the duodenal bulb is usually hypertonic and becomes more hypertonic in the duodenum because of the action of digestive enzymes. The hypertonic duodenal contents slow gastric emptying. The luminal hypertonic solution releases an unidentified humoral factor (hormone) that diminishes the rate of gastric emptying. A neural component may also be involved. The presence of fat-digestion products (mainly fatty acids and 2-mono-glycerides) dramatically decreases the rate of gastric emptying owing to an increase in the contractility of the pyloric sphincter. This inhibition of gastric emptying is mediated by both hormonal and neural mechanisms. The effect of unsaturated and long-chain (>14 carbons) fatty acids is greater than that of saturated and medium short-chain fatty acids. Cholecystokinin (CCK) is an intestinal hormone released by the presence of fatty acids and other fat-digestion products. The net effect of CCK is to slow the rate of gastric emptying. Other gastrointestinal hormones such as gastric inhibitory polypeptide (GIP, also termed glucose-dependent insulinotropic peptide) and peptide tyrosine-tyrosine (PYY) are involved in the delayed inhibition of gastric emptying by the presence of fatty acids in the ileum ('ileal brake').

Finally, the presence of proteins and peptides in the stomach also slows gastric emptying via the release of gastrin. This gastric hormone has a net effect of diminishing gastric emptying. Further inhibition is achieved by the presence of tryptophan, other amino acids and peptides in the duodenum, probably via CCK release.

Motility of the small intestine

The movements of the small intestine can be classified in two major patterns: segmentation that occurs in the postprandial period and the migrating motor complex (MMC) seen during fasting. The postprandial motility involves alternating contractions of the intestine, which mixes the chyme with digestive secretions, bringing fresh chyme into contact with the mucosal surface for absorption. The interdigestive period consists of bursts of intense electrical and contractile activity separated by longer quiescent periods. This pattern appears to be propagated from the stomach to the terminal ileum. The MMCs sweep the small intestine clean, emptying its contents into the cecum. The mechanisms that regulate the MMCs are both neural (vagal) and hormonal (motilin).

Motility of the colon

There are two major types of movement: segmentation (haustration), with a mixing function, and segmental propulsion, which allows the luminal contents to move in the distal direction.

Control of the contractile activities of the gastrointestinal tract involves the central nervous system (long reflexes), the intrinsic plexuses of gut (short

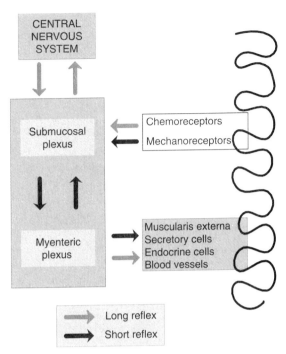

Figure 10.6 Neural control of the motility of the gastrointestinal tract.

reflexes) (Figure 10.6), humoral factors (e.g. gastrin, CCK, secretin) and electrical coupling among the smooth-muscle cells.

10.4 Secretion

Salivary secretion

Salivary secretion is produced by the three major salivary glands (parotids, submandibular and sublingual) and other minor glands in the oral mucosa. Saliva lubricates food for swallowing, facilitates speaking and begins the digestion of starch. The functional unit of the salivary gland is the acinus (secretory end-piece). The composition of saliva includes inorganic (salts) and organic (amylase, mucoproteins) components. The primary control of salivary secretion is exerted by the autonomic nervous system, which regulates several gland effectors including acinar cells, blood vessels, ductular cells and myoepithelial cells.

Gastric secretions

The major secretions of the stomach are hydrochloric acid (HCl), pepsinogens, intrinsic factor and mucus.

These components arise from the many secretory glands in the wall of the gastric mucosa. These glands have different cellular types: mucous neck cells (which secrete mucus), parietal or oxyntic cells (which secrete HCl and intrinsic factor) and chief or peptic cells (which secrete pepsinogens). The regulation of gastric secretion is carried out by neural and humoral mechanisms. There are three phases in the regulation process: cephalic, gastric and intestinal. The first is elicited by sight, smell and taste of food. The second is brought about by the presence of food in the stomach. The last phase is elicited by the presence of chyme in the duodenum.

In the past few years it has been recognized that *Helicobacter pylori*, a Gram-negative microaerophilic, flagellated, urease-producing rod found in the gastric mucosa, is related to the development of peptic ulcer disease. The studies suggest that *H. pylori* can induce mucosal damage via both direct and indirect mechanisms. The direct mechanisms imply the production by the microorganisms of urease, lipopolysaccharides and cytotoxins that induce mucosal inflammation. The indirect mechanisms include the release of gastrin and somatostatin. The importance of *H. pylori* infection of the gastric mucosa has led to the development of treatments for both gastritis and duodenal ulcers with anti-*H. pylori* regimens such as antacids and antibiotics.

Intestinal secretions

The mucosa of all segments of the gastrointestinal tract elaborates secretions that contain mucus, electrolytes and water.

Exocrine pancreatic secretion and bile secretion are covered in Sections 10.8 and 10.10, respectively.

10.5 Digestion and absorption

Digestion and absorption of carbohydrates

The major source of carbohydrates in the diet is starch. The starch is hydrolyzed by salivary and pancreatic α-amylase. The further digestion of the oligosaccharides is accomplished by enzymes in the brush-border membrane of the epithelium of the duodenum and jejunum. The major brush-border oligosaccharidases are lactase, sucrase, α-dextrinase and glucoamylase. The end-products of the disaccharidases are glucose, galactose and fructose. Several mechanisms transport these products across the

intestinal mucosa to the blood, including Na^+-dependent and Na^+-independent active transport.

Digestion and absorption of proteins

The process of digestion of dietary protein begins in the stomach. In the gastric lumen the pepsinogens secreted by the chief cells are activated by hydrogen ions to pepsins which hydrolyze the proteins to amino acids and small peptides. In the duodenum and small intestine, the proteases secreted by the pancreas (trypsin, chymotrypsin and carboxypeptidase) play a major role in protein digestion. The brush border of the small intestine contains a number of peptidases. They reduce the peptides produced by pancreatic enzymes to oligopeptides and amino acids. The principal products of protein digestion are small peptides and amino acids. These products are transported across the intestinal mucosa via specific amino acid and oligopeptide transport systems.

Digestion and absorption of lipids

The digestion of dietary fat is carried out by lipolytic enzymes of the exocrine pancreas (lipase and colipase), and requires the presence of biliary phospholipid and bile salts. The absorption of lipids needs the formation of micelles with bile lecithin, bile salt and products of the fat digestion. Inside the intestinal epithelial cell the lipids are reprocessed and the 2-monoglycerides are re-esterified, lysophospholipids are reconverted to phospholipids and most of the cholesterol is re-esterified. The reprocessed lipids, along with those that are synthesized *de novo,* combine with proteins to form chylomicrons that enter the bloodstream at the thoracic vena cava, via the lymphatics draining the gut.

Absorption of water and electrolytes

Water movement into or out of the lumen of the gastrointestinal tract is passive. The water moves across the cell plasma membrane or in between cells via the paracellular pathways composed of tight junctions and lateral intercellular spaces between epithelial cells. Water molecules follow the osmotic gradients created by electrolyte movement. Electrolytes are transported by both passive and active processes, and these ionic movements control water absorption and secretion.

Net intestinal fluid transport depends on the balance between intestinal water absorption and secretion. The

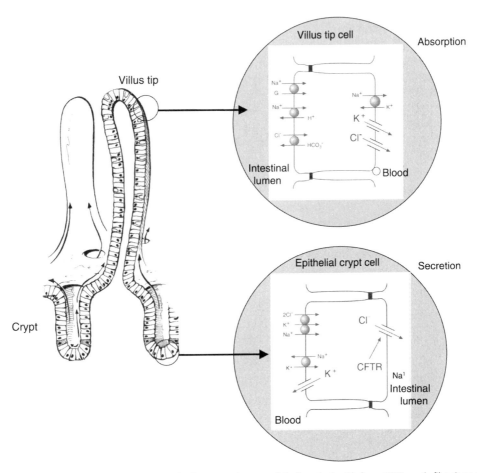

Figure 10.7 Transport mechanisms in the enterocytes of villus tips and crypts of the intestinal epithelium. CFTR: cystic fibrosis transmembrane conductance regulator.

processes are localized to specific regions of the intestinal epithelium. The cells of the villus tip are differentiated so as to promote fluid and solute absorption, whereas those in the crypt region promote fluid and solute secretion. Figure 10.7 shows the transport mechanisms in the enterocytes of both regions (villus tip and crypts).

Na^+ entry into the epithelial cell from the intestinal lumen is passive. This occurs via two mechanisms. One is a Na^+/H^+ antiporter protein, which exchanges one sodium ion (in) and one proton (out). The second is the Na^+/glucose cotransporter, which mediates the coupled entry of Na^+ and glucose into the epithelial cell against a concentration gradient. The presence of

glucose in the intestinal lumen enhances Na^+ absorption, which is the basis for the use of glucose in rehydratation solutions during diarrhea. The absorption of other sugars (galactose) and some neutral and acidic amino acids uses a similar mechanism.

Cl^- is absorbed following different pathways. Some Cl^- is absorbed across a paracellular path, and some through a cellular pathway composed of an apical Cl^-/HCO_3^- antiporter and possibly using an unidentified basolateral Cl^- selective channel or a K^+/Cl^- cotransporter. There is a linkage between H^+ and HCO_3^- via carbonic acid and carbonic anhydrase that provides a degree of coupling between the entry of Na^+ and Cl^-.

K^+ is passively absorbed in the small intestine (jejunum and ileum) when its luminal concentration rises because of the absorption of water.

10.6 Water balance in the gastrointestinal tract

The water balance in the gastrointestinal tract depends on the inputs and output of water to and from the gastrointestinal lumen. The water inputs can be exogenous or endogenous. Average oral (i.e. exogenous) intake of water is about 2 liters per day. The major components of the endogenous inputs are: saliva (1.5 liters), gastric juice (2.5 liters), bile (0.5 liter), pancreatic juice (1.5 liters) and intestinal secretions (in normal state 1 liter). Thus, the final daily water volume load in the duodenal lumen is 8–10 liters. Most of the fluid is absorbed by the small intestine, and about 1–1.5 liters reach the colon, which continues to absorb water, reducing fecal water volume to about 100 ml/day (Figure 10.8).

The maximum absorptive capacity of the colon is only about 4 l/day, so if volumes of fluid greater than this enter the small intestine, diarrhea will ensue despite normal colonic function. The normal intestinal secretion is about 1 l/day but can be as much as

20 l/day. This striking difference between the absorptive and secretory capacity of the small intestine and colon means that large-volume diarrhea is most often caused by small intestinal dysfunction.

Diarrhea

Diarrhea is a problem of intestinal water and electrolyte balance. It results when excess water and electrolytes are actively transported into the lumen (secretory diarrhea) or when water is retained in the lumen by osmotically active agents (osmotic diarrhea). Another major contributor to diarrhea is gastrointestinal motility. The rate of transit through the gut determines the time available for intestinal absorption of water and very rapid transit can result in diarrhea.

Vomiting

Vomiting is a reflex behavior controlled and coordinated by the vomiting center in the medulla, and involving the somatic and autonomic nervous systems, the oropharynx, the gastrointestinal tract and the skeletal muscles of the thorax and abdomen. It is the expulsion of gastric (or sometimes gastric and duodenal) contents from the gastrointestinal tract via the mouth. This can result from irritation (e.g. overdistension or overexcitation) of both chemoreceptors and mechanoreceptors anywhere along the gastrointestinal. It is usually preceded by nausea and retching.

The events of the vomiting reflex are independent of the initiating stimulus and include:

1. a wave of reverse peristalsis that sweeps from the middle of the small intestine to the duodenum
2. relaxation of the pylorus and stomach
3. forced inspiration against a closed glottis
4. increase in the abdominal pressure owing to diaphragm and abdominal muscle contraction
5. relaxation of the lower esophageal sphincter and entry of gastric contents into the esophagus
6. forward movement of the hyoid bone and larynx, closure by approximation of the vocal chords and closure of the glottis
7. projection of gastrointestinal contents into the pharynx and mouth.

Several physiological changes accompany vomiting, including hypersalivation, tachycardia, inhibition of gastric acid secretion and sometime defecation.

Certain chemicals, called emetics, can elicit vomiting. Their action is mediated by stimulating receptors

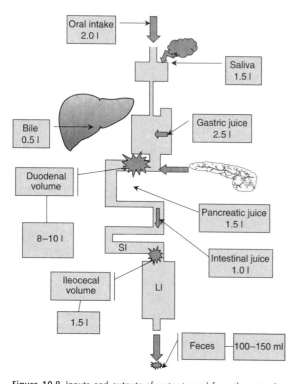

Figure 10.8 Inputs and outputs of water to and from the gastrointestinal lumen in a healthy adult. SG: salivary glands; SI: small intestine; LI: large intestine.

in the stomach, or more commonly in the duodenum, or by acting in the central nervous system on the chemoreceptor trigger zone near the area postrema in the floor of the fourth ventricle (brainstem).

10.7 The exocrine pancreas

Anatomy and histology of the pancreas

The human pancreas is a pink, soft, elongated organ weighing less than 100 g and lying posterior to the greater curvature of the stomach. It consists of a head, located within the duodenal loop, a body and a tail. The latter extends towards the spleen, onto which it has morphological relations. The pancreas is a mixed gland, containing both exocrine and endocrine portions (Figure 10.9). The major structural components responsible for the exocrine function of the pancreas are the acinar units (acini) and the duct system, accounting for about 86% of the gland mass. The acini, the enzyme-secreting units of the exocrine pancreas, are round or oval structures composed of epithelial cells (acinar cells) bordering a common luminal space where enzymes are delivered. The acini form lobules that are separated by thin septa. The tiny ducts that drain the acini are called intercalated ducts. Within a lobule, a number of intercalated ducts empty into somewhat larger intralobular ducts. All of the intralobular ducts of a particular lobule then drain into a single extralobular duct; this duct in turn empties into still larger ducts. These larger ducts ultimately converge to form two ducts that drain the secretions into the small intes-tine. The main duct is called the pancreatic duct (duct of Wirsung), which joins the common bile duct form-ing the hepatopancreatic ampulla (ampulla of Vater). The ampulla opens on an elevation of the duodenal mucosa known as the major duodenal papilla. The smaller of the two ducts, the accessory duct (duct of Santorini) leads from the pancreas and empties into the duodenum at the apex of the lesser duodenal papilla.

The endocrine portion of the pancreas is composed of cells organized into clusters called islets of Langer-hans, which secrete the hormones insulin, glucagon, somatostatin and pancreatic polypeptide. Insulin and glucagon play a major role in the regulation of macronutrient metabolism. The main functions of these hormones are dealt with in other chapters. The functional interactions between the endocrine and exocrine pancreas are discussed in Section 10.9.

The pancreas is innervated by the vagus and sym-pathetic nerves. The vagal fibers innervate both exocrine and endocrine cells, while the sympathetic nerves innervate the endocrine cells.

Composition of the pancreatic juice

The exocrine secretion of the pancreas is important in the digestion of foodstuffs. It is made up of an aqueous component and an enzyme component.

The aqueous component of pancreatic juice

This is secreted by the epithelial cells lining the pancreatic ducts, and is composed of water, sodium, potassium, bicarbonate and chloride (Figure 10.10).

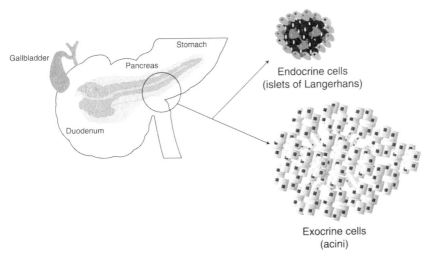

Endocrine cells
(islets of Langerhans)

Exocrine cells
(acini)

Figure 10.9 Endocrine and exocrine portions of the pancreas.

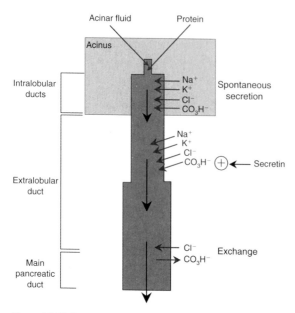

Figure 10.10 Composition and secretion of the aqueous component of pancreatic juice.

Bicarbonate and chloride are the major anions contained in pancreatic juice. The bicarbonate concentration increases and chloride concentration decreases reciprocally with the rate of secretion.

The primary pancreatic fluid is hypertonic to plasma. Pancreatic duct cells are water permeable, and as this primary secretion flows through the ducts water moves into the duct and makes the pancreatic juice isotonic to plasma.

The function of the pancreatic bicarbonate is to neutralize gastric acid entering the duodenum, creating the optimum pH for action of digestive enzymes in the small intestine.

The hormone secretin is the primary stimulant for bicarbonate secretion. The fluid secreted under secretin stimulation has a higher bicarbonate concentration than that secreted under resting conditions (spontaneous secretion).

Since the function of pancreatic bicarbonate is to neutralize duodenal acidity it is logical that the acidity of the chyme entering the duodenum stimulates the release of secretin.

The enzyme component of pancreatic juice

The acinar cells secrete the enzyme component of the pancreatic juice. The enzyme component in pancreatic

Table 10.1 Enzymes produced in pancreatic juice and the substrate they digest

Enzyme	Substrate
Amylase	Starches (polysaccharides)
Lipase	Trigycerides
Phospholipase A_2	Phospholipids
Carboxypeptidase	Proteins (exopeptidase)
Trypsin	Proteins (endopentidase)
Chymotrypsin	Proteins (endopeptidase)
Elastase	Elastin and fibrous proteins
Ribonuclease	Ribonucleic acids
Deoxyribonuclease	Deoxyribonucleic acids

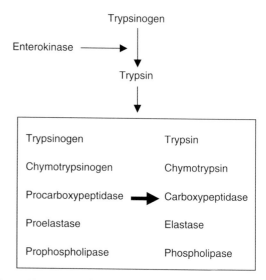

Figure 10.11 Process for converting inactive proteolytic enzymes to their active form.

juice includes enzymes for digesting carbohydrates, proteins, fats and nucleic acids (Table 10.1).

The proteases and phospholipases (enzymes that degrade phospholipids) are secreted in the form of zymogen granules; zymogens are inactive precursors of the proteolytic enzymes. In the duodenum inactive pancreatic zymogens are converted to their active form. Enterokinase, an enzyme embedded in the membrane of duodenum epithelial cells, converts the trypsinogen (inactive proteolityc zymogen) to trypsin (Figure 10.11).

The trypsin then activates the other pancreatic zymogens by removing specific peptides from them. A protein present in the pancreatic juice, trypsin inhibitor,

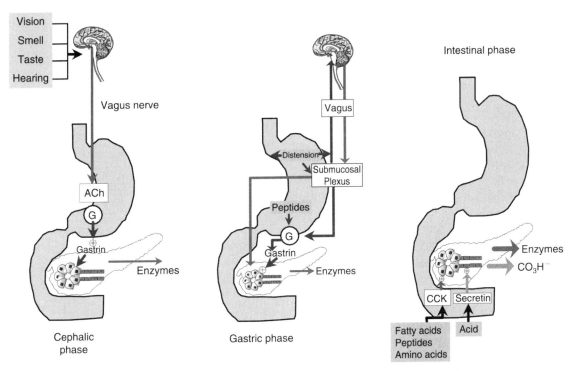

Figure 10.12 Neural and hormonal reflexes regulating pancreatic exocrine secretion. ACh: acetylcholine; CCK: cholecystokinin.

prevents the activation of inactive enzymes inside the pancreas. If the pancreatic duct is blocked the concentration of endogenous trypsin can rise, and when the concentration of trypsin inhibitor becomes insufficient the pancreas begins to autodigest (acute pancreatitis).

The major pancreatic proteolytic enzymes are trypsin, chymotrypsin, elastase and carboxypeptidase.

The non-proteolytic enzymes are released by the pancreas in their active form. The most important are:

- amylase: carbohydrate-digesting enzyme that degrades starch molecules into oligosaccharides
- ribonuclease and deoxyribonuclease: nucleic acid-digesting enzymes
- lipase: degrades triglycerides into fatty acids and glycerol.

The presence of fat and amino acids in the duodenum is the stimulus for the release of the intestinal hormone CCK. This hormone is the most potent stimulus of secretion of the enzymic component of the pancreatic juice.

The nutrients of the diet initiate, via CCK release, the enzymic secretion involved in their own digestion.

Regulation of the pancreatic exocrine secretion

Neural and hormonal reflexes regulate pancreatic exocrine secretion (Figure 10.12). The secretion of pancreatic juice is released during three phases.

- **Cephalic phase**: the taste and the smell of food lead to increased pancreatic secretion via the parasympathetic nerves to the pancreas. The vagal impulses stimulate the secretion of the enzyme component of the pancreatic juice.
- **Gastric phase**: the distenstion of the stomach by food transmits impulses via vagus afferents to the brain, then efferent activity via the vagus nerves to the pancreas, increasing the enzyme secretion of the pancreas.

  During these two phases, vagal impulses, distension of the stomach and the presence of amino acids and peptides in the stomach evoke release of the hormone gastrin, which also stimulates pancreatic secretion. Vagotomy reduces pancreatic exocrine secretion.
- **Intestinal phase**: the acidity of the chyme emptied into the duodenum stimulates the release of secretin. This

hormone causes the ductular epithelial cells to secrete a solution high in bicarbonate and, in doing so, increases the pancreatic flow. Secretin produces a large volume of pancreatic juice with low protein concentration.

CCK is released into the blood by fatty acids and polypeptides in the chyme and stimulates the secretion of digestive enzymes by the acinar cells. CCK potentiates the pancreatic stimulatory effects of secretin and vice versa. Secretin and CCK are released in the mucosa of the duodenum and upper jejunum by enteroendocrine cells and pass into the capillaries and thus into the systemic circulation.

10.8 Diet and exocrine pancreatic function

Adaptation of the exocrine pancreas to diet

The pancreas is very sensitive to a variety of physiological and pathological stimuli, the most important of which are nutritional in origin. Severe alterations in the diet leading to a state of malnutrition are associated with the occurrence of pancreatic injury. This section will focus on the functional changes that may occur when nutritional components in the diet are altered within non-pathological limits.

Pancreatic adaptation, a phenomenon first noted by Pavlov in the early twentieth century, refers to the ability of the pancreas to modify the volume and composition of its exocrine secretion according to the levels of nutritional substrates available in the diet. Most of the information in this scientific area has been obtained from studies on rats.

With an adequate dietary protein supply, the content and synthesis of the major digestive enzymes (proteases, amylase and lipase) change proportionally to the amount of their respective substrates (protein, carbohydrate and fat) in the diet. This adaptation would optimize the digestion and utilization of such substrates.

In response to high-protein diets, the trypsinogen and chymotrypsinogen content and synthesis increase. The quality of dietary protein also affects this adaptation. Increasing the intake of high-quality proteins such as casein or fish protein increases chymotrypsinogen, whereas low-quality proteins such as gelatin or zein do not.

High-carbohydrate diets increase the pancreatic amylase content and synthesis. This effect occurs as the level of dietary carbohydrate increases at the expense of dietary fat or protein, which implies a primary response to the amount of carbohydrate.

The intake of high-fat diets stimulates the content and synthesis of pancreatic lipase, independently of whether the amount of dietary fat increases at the expense of protein or carbohydrate. Although lipase adapts to increasing dietary fat levels, there may be a threshold of fat content below which there is little adaptation and above which there is significant adaptation. Colipase may adapt to increasing dietary fat levels, but the response seems to be weaker than that of lipase. Considerable controversy exists over the effects of the type of fat (degree of saturation or major chain length) on the adaptation of pancreatic enzymes.

There have been few studies of pancreatic adaptation to the diet in humans, and the literature available is controversial. Studies in premature infants suggest that adaptive responses occur in humans in a manner similar to that observed in experimental animals. In contrast, altering the quantity of carbohydrate, protein or fat in the diet of adult volunteers for 10 or 15 days failed to induce any changes in the ratios among the enzymes secreted. In humans adapted for 30 days to diets containing either olive oil (rich in oleic acid, a monounsaturated fatty acid) or sunflower oil (rich in linoleic acid, a polyunsaturated fatty acid) as the main source of dietary fat, no differences in the activity of proteases, amylase, lipase and colipase measured in duodenal contents were apparent after the administration of a liquid meal.

Is pancreatic adaptation mediated by specific hormones?

Several studies have demonstrated that stimulation with individual hormones results in marked changes in the rate of synthesis of different sets of exocrine proteins (Table 10.2). CCK increases dramatically the synthesis and tissue level of proteases, so it has been proposed as the mediator of pancreatic adaptation to dietary protein. This action is exerted through the negative feedback regulation of CCK release. Figure 10.13 is a schematic diagram of the feedback mechanism.

Secretin and/or GIP are believed to mediate pancreatic adaptation to lipid in the diet. Both are produced by cells of the upper intestine and their release is stimulated, among other factors, by the hydrolytic products of fat. Moreover, the administration of either secretin or glucose-dependent insulinotropic peptide has proved to augment the synthesis and content of lipase and colipase in pancreatic acinar cells.

A role for insulin in the adaptation of the pancreas to high-carbohydrate diets has been proposed.

The type of dietary fat affects the circulating levels of hormones involved in the control of pancreatic secretion, as shown in a study conducted in humans. They were fed for 30 days on diets containing either olive or sunflower oil as the main source of dietary fat, and plasma CCK levels were higher in the olive oil group than in the sunflower oil group. Also, greater plasma PYY and pancreatic polypeptide (PP) concentrations were found in the subjects who received the olive oil diet. Similar results have been found in dogs adapted for 6 months to diets rich in either of the two same fats. The higher concentrations of inhibiting hormones such as PP and PYY in response to an olive oil diet can explain, at least in part, why long-term adaptation to olive oil leads in this species to an attenuation of pancreatic response to food compared with the typical one in the animals fed sunflower oil.

Regulation of pancreatic gene expression by diet

Gene expression in the pancreas seems to be regulated at multiple levels. Theoretically, diet can alter the expression of genes encoding specific pancreatic enzymes through mechanisms involving the gene (transcription), its mRNA (processing, extranuclear

Table 10.2 Hormonal mediators of pancreatic adaptation to increased nutritional substrates

Substrate	Hormone	(Pro)enzyme synthesis and tissue content
Protein	CCK	↑ Trypsinogen and chymotrypsinogen
Triglyceride	Secretin, GIP	↑ Lipase
Starch	Insulin?	↑ Amylase

CCK: cholecystokinin; GIP: gastric inhibitory peptide.

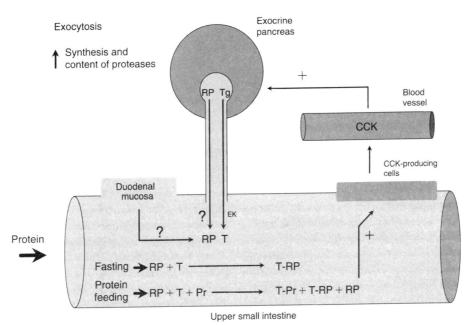

Figure 10.13 Negative feedback regulation of exocrine pancreatic secretion by proteases in the rat. Two different peptides may be involved in this mechanism. One is secreted by the exocrine pancreas and the other by the duodenal mucosa. They both are protease sensitive and stimulate cholecystokinin (CCK) release from the corresponding endocrine cells in the gut epithelium. They are represented by RP (releasing peptide) in the diagram. Under conditions of protein fasting, RP becomes complexed with trypsin (T) in the intestinal lumen. In this form, RP is not capable of stimulating CCK release. When abundant protein is present, this interacts with trypsin (T), leading to substrate competition for the binding with RP. Consequently, the amount of free RP increases progressively, which enhances the release of CCK into the blood circulation. CCK stimulation of acinar cells not only evokes exocytosis of pancreatic enzymes but also regulates selectively gene expression, increasing the synthesis of proteases. Tg: trypsinogen; EK: enterokinase; Pr: protein.

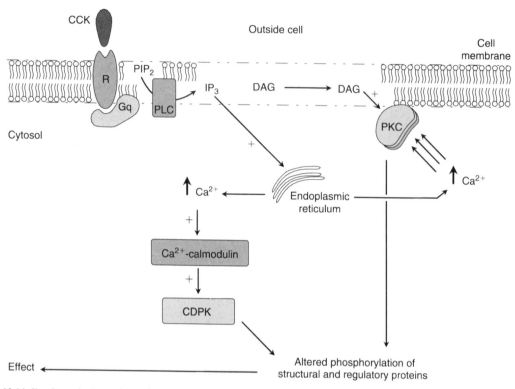

Figure 10.14 Signal transduction pathway triggered by cholecystokinin (CCK) in the pancreatic acinar cell. Binding of CCK to its specific receptor (R) activates the Gq class of heterotrimeric G proteins (Gq). The activated Gq then stimulates the activity of phospholipase C (PLC) to hydrolyze the membrane phospholipid phosphatidylinositol 4,5-bisphosphate (PIP$_2$). This cleavage releases inositol 1,4,5-trisphosphate (IP$_3$) and diacylglycerol (DAG). IP$_3$ binds to specific Ca^{2+} channels in the endoplasmic reticulum membrane causing Ca^{2+} to be released. The rise in cytosolic Ca^{2+} favors the formation of the complex Ca^{2+} calmodulin, which in turn activates a number of calmodulin-dependent protein kinases (CDPK). In the presence of enhanced Ca^{2+}, protein kinase C (PKC) (which in unstimulated conditions is in the cytosol) also binds Ca^{2+}, and this causes PKC to migrate to the inner surface of the plasma membrane, where it can be activated by the DAG produced by hydrolysis of PIP$_2$. All PKCs and CDPKs phophorylate key intracellular enzymes, leading to either activation or inactivation of downstream regulatory proteins and producing the cellular response.

transport or cytoplasmic stability) and its translation into protein.

Modifications in the synthesis and content of a particular enzyme following dietary changes in animals are clearly associated with changes in the corresponding mRNA level, thus suggesting a transcriptional change. In contrast, studies using administration of hormonal mediators show that the effects on enzyme synthesis depend on the infusion period. Single periods of hormone stimulation modify the efficiency of mRNA translation into protein, whereas repeated periods of stimulation (up to 7 days) lead to changes in mRNA levels. It seems that sequential phases of biological response should be expected depending on the integration of several mechanisms activated over different periods. This illustrates the importance of the duration of the adaptation period to a dietary change.

So, how do hormones exert these effects? CCK, secretin and GIP are peptide hormones which interact with specific receptors on the plasma membrane of the pancreatic acinar cell. Their cellular effects are associated with activation of separate intracellular messenger pathways. The action of CCK (Figure 10.14) results in the hydrolysis of membrane phospholipids known as phosphoinositides and the consequent generation of inositol 1,4,5-trisphosphate (IP$_3$) and diacylglycerol. IP$_3$ mobilizes cellular calcium (Ca^{2+}) and this ultimately leads to activation of a calmodulin-dependent protein kinase, diacylglycerol activates protein kinase C (PKC). Secretin and glucose-dependent insulinotropic peptide evoke increases in the level of cyclic adenosine monophosphate (cAMP), which activates cAMP-dependent protein kinase (Figure 10.15).

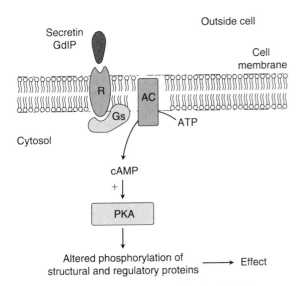

Figure 10.15 The cyclic adenosine monophosphate (cAMP) messenger system. After interacting with specific receptors on the plasma membrane, the cellular effects of secretin and gastric inhibitory polypeptide (GIP) are mediated by trimeric G-protein activation (Gs type), which activates the membrane enzyme adenylyl cyclase (AC). The activated AC, the catalytic site for which is located on the cytosolic surface of the plasma membrane, catalyzes the conversion of some cytosolic adenosine triphosphate (ATP) molecules to cAMP, which then diffuses throughout the cell to bind and activate the cAMP-dependent protein kinase, also termed protein kinase A (PKA). Similarly to the kinases involved in the CCK pathway, PKA phosphorylates other proteins and the change in the activity of these proteins brings about the response of the cell. Although all of these kinases operate in a similar manner, they are distinct from one another and have their own specific substrates.

Application of calcium ionophores, which produces an increase in intracellular Ca^{2+} levels similar to that observed with CCK stimulation, results specifically in increases in the synthesis of pancreatic proteases, the same effect observed after CCK infusion or after adaptation to high-protein diets. Forskolin, a drug that enhances cAMP levels, causes an increase in pancreatic lipase and colipase synthesis similar to that produced by secretin and glucose-dependent insulinotropic peptide or by intake of high-fat diets. The mechanism by which activation of second messenger pathways and their associated protein kinases regulate gene expression in the exocrine pancreas has been demonstrated to involve the induction of primary response genes (PRGs, also called immediate–early genes). These genes encode regulatory proteins that control the expression of late response genes (LRGs). Thus, an initial transcription factor (a protein that directly affects gene expression) activated in the signal transduction

pathway causes the synthesis of a different transcription factor which, in turn, causes the synthesis of additional proteins. In pancreatic acinar cells CCK has been shown to induce the expression of PRGs by increasing their nuclear transcription, and this response occurs at 60 min after the application of the hormone. The role of second messengers has also been established: increases in intracellular Ca^{2+} or cAMP and direct activation of protein kinase C induces, especially when combined, the expression of PRGs to levels comparable to those observed with CCK stimulation. However, the role of these PRGs in linking second messenger pathways to activation of LRGs has not been determined in this tissue. Figure 10.16 proposes a model to explain the relationships between the transduction pathways and the control of gene expression in the pancreas.

Effect of pancreatic insufficiency on nutrition

It is clear from the previous sections that various nutritional factors can affect exocrine pancreatic function. Conversely, pathological modifications of this function lead to an altered nutritional state.

The pancreas has a reserve capacity that is many times the physiological requirement. Steatorrhea and creatorrhea (excessive amounts of fat and protein, respectively, in the feces) occur only when the secretion of pancreatic lipase and trypsin is reduced to less than 10% of normal. Patients with severe and chronic pancreatic insufficiency are at high risk for developing different forms of malabsorption, the common end-stage of which is protein–energy malnutrition. Apart from defective absorption of the three major nutrients, there may be other nutritional disorders:

- deficiencies of fat-soluble vitamins (in patients with pancreatic steatorrhea)
- in healthy subjects, a zinc-binding compound of pancreatic origin facilitates intestinal zinc absorption. In chronic pancreatitis, clinically significant malabsorption of zinc may ensue
- vitamin B_{12} deficiency: certain proteins of saliva and gastric juice (R proteins) are able to bind vitamin B_{12}, forming a complex that is not available for absorption. In normal conditions, pancreatic proteases degrade these proteins, releasing the vitamin. In pancreatic insufficiency due to deficiency of proteases, the amount of vitamin B_{12} absorbed can decrease markedly.

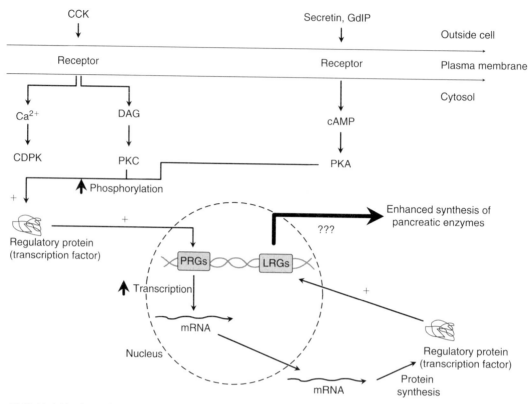

Figure 10.16 Model for the regulation of pancreatic gene expression by hormones and their intracellular messengers. CCK: cholecystokinin; DAG: diacylglycerol; CDPK: calmodulin-dependent protein kinase; PKC: protein kinase C; GIP: gastric inhibitory polypeptide; PKA: protein kinase A; PRGs: primary response genes; LRGs: late response genes.

10.9 Interactions between the endocrine and exocrine pancreas

Acute effects of the islet hormones on the secretory activity of the exocrine pancreas

The pancreas is usually regarded as two separate systems. However, several observations support the idea that marked interactions must occur between the endocrine and exocrine parts.

- The endocrine cells, arranged into the islets of Langerhans, are in close contact with the acinar tissue.
- An islet–acinar portal blood system has been demonstrated.
- Abnormal secretory responses to secretagogues exist in human diabetes.
- Exocrine pancreatic insufficiency often results in pancreatic endocrine changes.

The concept of the pancreas being an integrated organ seems reasonable when one considers that the exocrine portion secretes enzymes and bicarbonate, which affect digestion and absorption of nutrients, whereas the endocrine part releases hormones that regulate the metabolism and disposal of breakdown products of food within the body.

Insulin

For different reasons, the effects of insulin on interdigestive or stimulated exocrine pancreatic secretion (quantity and quality) are difficult to study in conscious animals. *In vitro* secretory effects have been examined more extensively. Specific insulin receptors exist on acini prepared from different species. Apart from the effects of insulin on the regulation of the synthesis of some pancreatic enzymes as indicated earlier, there is evidence that insulin may exert short-term actions on the exocrine pancreas by potentiating the secretory responses to hormones (CCK) and neurotransmitters (acetylcholine). This positive effect requires the intact pancreas for its expression, which may partly explain the derangement of exocrine pancreatic function in diabetes.

Glucagon

In vivo studies have been conducted on the actions of glucagon on exocrine pancreatic secretion in different species. Although little effect is seen in the resting (unstimulated) pancreas, exogenous administration of glucagon has been demonstrated to inhibit exocrine pancreatic secretion induced by a meal or by application of secretin and/or CCK. *In vitro*, glucagon can elicit differential effects on the exocrine pancreas depending on the concentration, the animal species and the type of preparation. When administered alone or combined with CCK, acetylcholine or secretin, glucagon can result in either an inhibition or a potentiation of the secretory responses. In general, these responses decrease gradually with increasing doses of the islet hormone.

Somatostatin

The effects of somatostatin on exocrine pancreatic secretion have been investigated in many studies and yet major discrepancies are apparent. The available data indicate that, *in vivo*, somatostatin administration inhibits both resting and stimulated pancreatic enzyme secretion, whereas the effects on water and bicarbonate secretion are less well defined. *In vitro* studies show that somatostatin is able to act directly on the acinar cells (specific receptors have been found in both intact acinar cells and subcellular organelles) to evoke either a decrease, an increase or no change in exocrine pancreatic secretion. This depends to a great extent on the concentration of the islet hormone.

Pancreatic polypeptide

PP, another islet hormone, is released into the blood in response to the ingestion of a meal, and has been consistently shown to inhibit both basal and stimulated exocrine pancreatic secretion in different species. Moreover, these effects are produced at concentrations of PP assayed in plasma after a normal meal. For a long time, little was known concerning the mechanism for the inhibitory actions of PP. Several investigators failed to reproduce in isolated acini the observed *in vivo* effects of PP. The strongest hypotheses supported an indirect role for this peptide in the regulation of pancreatic secretion. Recently, PP receptors have been found on acinar and duct cells, which means that a great advance in the understanding of the effects of this peptide is expected very soon.

In conclusion, morphological evidence coupled with functional studies indicate that the islet hormones

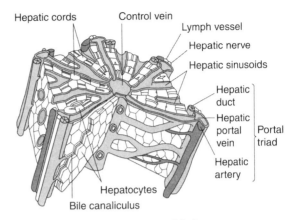

Figure 10.17 Histology and anatomy of the liver.

insulin, glucagon, somatostatin and PP are involved in the regulation of exocrine pancreatic secretion. Much of this regulation is likely to be exerted at a local level. The precise mechanisms for the interaction between the islet hormones and secretagogues is not yet fully established, and confirmation of a true physiological role of the islet hormones in this area is awaited.

10.10 Physiology of bile secretion and enterohepatic circulation

The liver of all vertebrates produces and secretes bile. This digestive secretion is elaborated from transport processes in the hepatocyte and is modified along the bile canaliculus and ducts. Finally, it is stored in the gallbladder, from which it is released into the common hepatic duct and duodenum after a meal.

The liver cells (hepatocytes) are arranged in many functional units called lobules. The lobules are sheets of hepatocytes organized around a central vein (Figure 10.17). Instead of capillaries the liver has large spaces called sinusoids. The sinusoids receive blood containing absorbed nutrients from the hepatic portal vein. The hepatic arterial blood supply to the liver brings oxygen to the liver cells.

Branches of both the hepatic portal vein and the hepatic artery carry blood into the liver sinusoids, where nutrients and oxygen are taken up by the hepatocytes. The liver secretes back into the blood products synthesized by the hepatocytes and nutrients needed by other cells. Blood from both origins leaves the liver in the hepatic vein.

Functions of the liver

The most important digestive function of the liver is the secretion of bile, which is essential for lipid digestion in the intestine. Bile is secreted continuously into specialized ducts, called bile canaliculi, located within each lobule of the liver. These canaliculi empty into bile ducts at the periphery of the lobules. The bile ducts merge and form the right and left hepatic ducts, which unite to form a single common hepatic duct. The common hepatic duct is joined by the cystic duct from the gallbladder to form the common bile duct, which empties into the duodenum.

Surrounding the common bile duct at the point where it enters the duodenum is the sphincter of Oddi. When the sphincter is closed the dilute bile secreted by the liver passes into the gallbladder and becomes concentrated until it is needed in the small intestine.

After the beginning of a meal, the sphincter of Oddi relaxes and the gallbladder contracts, discharging concentrated bile into duodenum. The signal for gallbladder contraction is the intestinal hormone CCK. The presence of fat and amino acids in the duodenum is the stimulus for the release of CCK, a hormone that also causes relaxation of the sphincter of Oddi.

Apart from bile secretion the liver has other important functions.

- *Lipid metabolism*: the hepatocytes synthesize lipoprotein and cholesterol, store some tryglicerides and use cholesterol to synthesize bile acids.
- *Carbohydrate metabolism*: the liver is one of the major sites of glycogen storage in the body. This occurs after carbohydrate containing meals and is stimulated by insulin. When blood glucose is low, glycogen is broken down to glucose (glycogenolysis) and the glucose is released into the bloodstream. Under these conditions the liver also synthesizes glucose from amino acids and lactic acid (gluconeogenesis).
- *Protein metabolism*: hepatocytes deaminate amino acids to form ammonia (NH_3), which is converted into a much less toxic product, urea. The latter is excreted in urine. The liver synthesizes all the major plasma proteins (albumin, globulin, apoproteins, fibrinogen and prothrombin).
- *Excretion of bile pigments*: bile pigments are derived from the heme portion of hemoglobin in aged erythrocytes. The most important is bilirubin, which is absorbed by the liver from the blood and actively secreted into the bile. After entering the intestinal tract bilirubin is metabolized by bacteria and eliminated in feces.
- *Storage*: the liver stores some vitamins (A, D, E, K and B_{12}) and minerals (iron and copper), and participates in the activation of vitamin D.
- *Processing of hormones, drugs and toxins*: the liver converts these substances to inactive forms in the hepatocytes for subsequent excretion in bile or urine.

Role and composition of the bile

Bile is a mixture of substances synthesized by the liver. It has several components: bile acids, cholesterol, phospholipids (lecithin), bile pigments, and small amounts of other metabolic end-products, bicarbonate ions and other salts and trace elements. Bile acids are synthesized from cholesterol and before they are secreted are conjugated with the amino acids glycine or taurine. Conjugated bile acids are called bile salts. Bile salts emulsify lipids in the lumen of the small intestine to form micelles, increasing the surface area available to lipolytic enzymes. Micelles transport the products of lipid digestion to the brush-border surface of the epithelial cells, helping the absorption of lipids.

Cholesterol is made soluble in bile by bile acids and lecithin.

The epithelial cells lining the ducts secrete a bicarbonate solution, similar to that produced by the pancreas, which contributes to the volume of bile leaving the liver. This salt solution neutralizes acid in the duodenum.

Bile secretion

The hepatocytes produce a primary secretion isotonic to plasma that contains the substances that carry out the main digestive functions (bile acids, cholesterol and lecithin). The bicarbonate-rich fluid secreted by the epithelial cells of the ducts modifies the primary secretion of the liver (Figure 10.18).

Fraction of bile secreted by the hepatocytes

Bile acids, phospholipids, cholesterol, bile pigments and proteins are the most important substances secreted by the hepatocytes into the bile. Bile acids synthesized from cholesterol by the liver are called primary bile acids (cholic acid and chenodeoxycholic acid). The bacteria of the small intestine dehydroxylate primary bile acids to form secondary bile acids (deoxycholic acid and lithocholic acid).

Before they are secreted, bile acids are conjugated with the amino acids glycine or taurine to make them

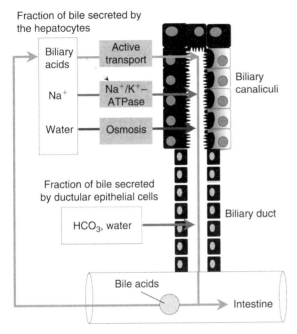

Fraction of bile secreted by the hepatocytes

Figure 10.18 Process of bile secretion in the hepatocytes of the liver.

more water soluble. Bacteria in the intestine deconjugate bile salts into bile acids, which are absorbed in the ileum and return to the liver, where they are converted into bile salts again and secreted along with newly synthesized bile acids. The uptake of bile acids by the liver stimulates bile salts release. This process is known as the enterohepatic recirculation of bile salts (Figure 10.19).

Hepatocytes secrete phospholipids, especially lecithin, which help to solubilize fat, cholesterol and bile pigments in the small intestine. The synthesis of bile acids from cholesterol and the excretion of cholesterol and bile acids in feces comprise one of the mechanisms to maintain cholesterol homeostasis. Hepatocytes remove bilirubin from the bloodstream, attached to glucuronic molecules. The resultant conjugated bilirubin is secreted into the bile.

Fraction of bile secreted by ductular epithelial cells.

These cells secrete a bicarbonate-rich salt solution that accounts for about half of the total bile volume. The

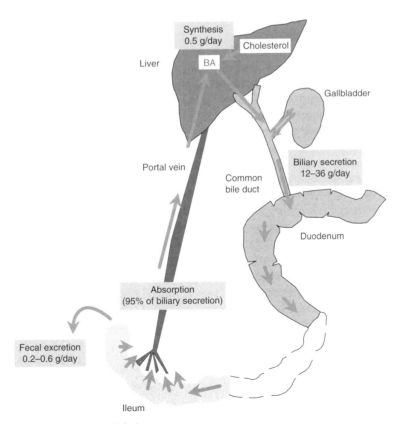

Figure 10.19 Enterohepatic circulation of bile acids (BA).

concentration of HCO_3 is greater than in the plasma and helps to neutralize the intestinal acid. This secretion is stimulated by secretin in response to the presence of acid in the duodenum.

Bile concentration and storage in the gallbladder

Between meals the sphincter of Oddi is closed and the dilute bile secreted by the liver passes through the cystic duct into the gallbladder and becomes concentrated. The gallbladder mucosa absorbs water and ions (Na^+, Cl^-, HCO_3^-) and can concentrate bile salts by 10-fold. The active transport of Na^+ into the interstitial space produces an elevated osmolarity in this region and the osmotic flow of water across the epithelium; HCO_3^- and Cl^- are transported to the interstitial space to preserve electroneutrality.

Regulation of bile secretion

Several factors increase the production or release of bile (Figure 10.20):

- The rate of return of the bile acids to the liver via portal blood affects the rate of secretion of bile acids. Bile acids stimulate bile production and secretion; there is a linear relationship between the secretion rate of bile acids and bile flow. Bile acids increase bile flow because they provide an osmotic driving force for filtration of water and electrolytes (choleretic effect).

- During a meal CCK is released into the blood by fatty acids and polypeptides in the chyme. This causes contraction of the gallbladder and release of concentrated bile. CCK also relaxes the sphincter of Oddi, allowing bile flow, rich in bile salts, into the duodenum. These bile salts return via the enterohepatic circulation to the liver, further stimulating bile acid secretion and bile flow. CCK also directly stimulates the primary secretion by the liver.

- Parasympathetic impulses along the vagus nerve (cephalic influences) also cause contraction of the gallbladder.

- The acidity of the chyme emptying to the duodenum stimulates the release of secretin. This hormone causes the ductular epithelial cells to secrete a solution high in bicarbonate and in doing so increases the bile flow.

10.11 Adaptation of the biliary response to the diet

There is abundant information on adaptation of the pancreatic exocrine secretion in response to the composition of the diet. The physiological significance of this adaptation would be to optimize the digestion and

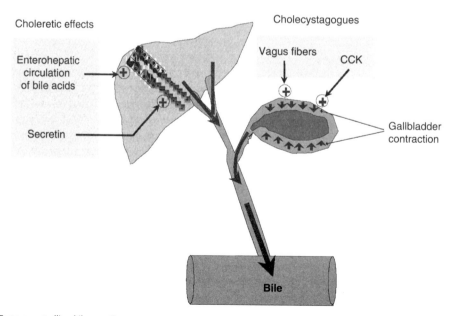

Figure 10.20 Factors controlling bile secretion.

utilization of macronutrients. Reports about the role of major dietary components in bile secretion are relatively scarce, in spite of the fact that this secretion is essential for lipid digestion.

Bile salts are synthesized and secreted by the liver, stored and concentrated in the gallbladder and delivered into duodenum in response to a meal. Postprandial gallbladder contraction and sphincter of Oddi relaxation are mainly regulated by CCK. This hormone is released into blood by the products of macronutrient digestion. Changing the composition of macronutrients in the diet may evoke different plasma levels of CCK and thus modify the bile flow, the supply of bile salts into the duodenum, the enterohepatic circulation, the hepatic synthesis of bile acids and the amount excreted into the bile.

In healthy subjects, higher CCK release in response to food has been associated with stronger gallbladder emptying. There is a positive linear relationship between CCK release and gallbladder contraction. Meals differing in either the type or the amount of fat, protein or carbohydrates may be effective in stimulating CCK release and biliary secretion to varying degrees.

In addition, decreased postprandial gallbladder emptying has been suggested to play a major role in the development of gallstones in humans; therefore, dietary factors may be important in the pathogenesis of gallbladder stasis.

Major dietary components, cholecystokinin release and gallbladder contraction

Carbohydrates

Carbohydrates seem to have no influence upon bile secretion when they constitute the standard proportion of the diet. Institution of a 95% carbohydrate diet reduces gallbladder emptying and diminishes bile salt pool size and bile acid secretion. Fat is the stronger stimulant for the release of CCK. Diets very rich in carbohydrates and with an adequate protein supply are very low in fat, and these diets has been shown to be especially ineffective in the stimulation of CCK secretion and gallbladder contraction.

Protein

Several studies have shown that the amount and type of dietary protein influences biliary secretion. High-protein diets have been shown to increase bile acid secretion and the presence of bile salts in the lumen of the small intestine, and have been shown to stimulate plasma CCK secretion. The effect of low-protein diets on the postprandial emptying of the gallbladder has also been examined. A 3 day low-protein/low-fat diet increased fasting gall-bladder volume and significantly decreased fasting plasma CCK levels in humans. This suggests that CCK secretion regulates fasting gallbladder volume and that basal CCK release depends on diet composition. This diminished gallbladder stimulation affects bile flow and bile acid secretion in resting conditions and in response to food. The quality of the dietary protein also affects CCK release. Animal studies have demonstrated this, although more human studies in this area are necessary before the relationship between the biliary response to a meal and protein quality is fully understood. Intravenous infusion of amino acid solutions appears to have different effects on gallbladder contraction and CCK secretion depending on the amino acid composition. Tryptophan and phenylalanine seem to be the most potent stimulants to CCK secretion and gallbladder contraction in humans.

Fat

The amount and type of dietary fat ingested also affect biliary secretion. In general, when the amount of fat ingested increases, the biliary response shows a marked rise in bile acid concentration and output. It has been suggested that this response is an adaptation process ensuring adequate fat digestion. In humans, CCK release and gallbladder contraction after a meal depend mainly on fat intake. Low-fat diets and fat-free diets decrease gallbladder emptying and CCK levels compared with a normal mixed diet. High-fat diets produce the opposite results. Some studies suggest that meals high in long-chain triacylglycerols (LCT) produce a postprandial increase in plasma CCK concentration, while meals containing medium-chain triacylglycerols (MCT) inhibit CCK release. The type of dietary fat also affects gallbladder emptying. Oleic acid, the major fatty acid in olive oil, is one of the most potent stimulators of CCK release known.

10.12 Growth, development and differentiation of the gastrointestinal tract

The intestinal epithelium is a complex equilibrium system of multiple cell types undergoing continual renewal while maintaining precise interrelationships.

The crypt–villous axis is composed of a dynamic cell population in perpetual change from a crypt proliferative and undifferentiated stage to a mature villous stage. The migration of crypt cells is accompanied by cellular differentiation, which leads to morphological and functional changes.

The regulatory mechanisms involved with developmental processes are at organism, cellular and molecular levels. At the organism level there is an expanded array of hormones and dietary effects that modulate the ontogeny of the intestine. The adult phenotype of the small intestine is established via a series of developmental transitions resulting from the interaction of visceral endoderm and mesoderm.

During development and in the adult epithelium, cellular phenotypes are defined by the expression of specific sets of genes in individual cells. These genes are mainly regulated at the transcriptional level, although some genes may be regulated after initiation of the transcription during translation or even by late modifications of synthesized proteins in the endoplasmic reticulum and Golgi system. The particular set of genes expressed in a single cell type has recently been referred to as the 'transcriptome'. Intestinal epithelial cell transcriptomes shift in well-orchestrated patterns during the development, differentiation and adaptive processes of the intestinal mucosa. In addition to this intrinsic gene program, intestinal epithelial cells respond to extrinsic signals including nutrients and other dietary components by producing various molecules. Using different experimental approaches, recent studies have further characterized intestinal epithelial-cell biology and provided evidence of their polyvalent nature and important role in gut homeostasis.

Ontogeny of digestive and absorptive functions in humans

By the time of birth, all mammals must be able to digest all the nutritional components of their mother's milk. Lactose is the primary carbohydrate in the diet of the infant until the time of weaning. Lactase, sucrase and maltase activities appear between 8 and 9 weeks of gestational age in the jejunum. The greatest increase in lactase activity occurs during the third trimester, while at 20 weeks sucrase and maltase activities are already 50–75% of those found in term infants and adults. The appearance of lactase coincides with the appearance of microvilli. Unlike other species in which lactase activity declines at weaning, in the human it is maintained well beyond the weaning period especially in Caucasians. However, a decline occurs between 3 and 5 years of life. Sucrase and maltase activities are maintained throughout life.

Glucoamylase is the most important enzyme for digestion of complex carbohydrates. This enzyme is detectable by 20 weeks of gestational age and the greatest increase occurs between the period of fetal development and early postnatal development. Its activity in infants less than 1 year old is comparable to that of adolescents.

Alkaline phosphatase is detectable by 7 weeks of gestation but levels in newborns are substantially less than in adults.

As for sucrase and maltase, most brush-border peptidases appear to mature more rapidly in humans than in rats. γ-Glutamyl transpeptidase (γ-GT) activity increases more than two-fold between 13 and 20 weeks of gestational age, and its activity is higher in fetuses than in infants and adults. Aminopeptidase activity appears at 8 weeks of gestation, and adult values are attained by 14 weeks. Oligoaminopeptidase, dipeptidylaminopeptidase IV and carboxypeptidase increase in activity from 8 to 22 weeks of gestational age and are present in infants. Lysosomal enzymes undergo little ontogenic change in the human.

Longitudinal distribution of the various enzymes along the small intestine often varies with the stage of development. Lactase and sucrase show a proximodistal gradient through adulthood, and glucoamylase and γ-GT activities are fairly uniform throughout the small intestine.

Active transport of glucose is demonstrable by 10 weeks of life in the jejunum and by 12 weeks in the ileum. *In vivo* data suggest that little change occurs between 30 weeks and term. A high-affinity, low-capacity Na/glucose cotransport system along the length of the small intestine and a low-affinity, high-capacity system in the proximal intestine have been found in human fetuses. Glucose absorptive capacity seems to increase as a function of age from fetal life to adulthood.

Amino acid transport can also be demonstrated by 12 weeks of gestational age. Amino acid uptake is accomplished by sodium-dependent and -independent transport mechanisms. The Na$^-$ dependent pathways include the NBB and Phe systems for neutral amino acids, the X^{ag} system for acidic amino acids, and the imino system for proline and hydroxyproline. The Na-independent pathways include the L system for neutral amino acids and the y^+ system for basic amino acids. The NBB system, which transports leucine, is demonstrable in the entire small intestine of both infants and adults.

Macromolecules are also capable of crossing the small intestinal mucosa. The pathway of macromolecular uptake in the human is unclear, although endocytic and pinocytic processes can occur. The ability of the human intestinal mucosa to take up macromolecules is increased in infancy and during episodes of intestinal injury, such as diarrhea and malnutrition. The intestinal closure is enhanced in breast-fed infants compared with those fed formula.

Calcium absorptive capacity in preterm infants is greater than 50% of adult levels. In agreement with the needs of the growing infant, iron absorption is more efficient in infants than in adults, although iron bioavailability is fairly dependent on dietary components, namely the presence of lactoferrin in human milk.

By 8–11 weeks of gestational age, gastrin, secretin, motilin, GIP, enteroglucagon, somatostatin, vasoactive intestinal polypeptide (VIP), gastrin and CCK are demonstrable. The concentration of these peptides increases throughout gestation and reaches adult levels between 31 and 40 weeks of gestational age. Gastrin, secretin, motilin and GIP are localized to the duodenum and jejunum, whereas enteroglucagon, neurotensin, somatostatin and VIP are distributed throughout the small intestine.

Hormonal and dietary regulation of ontogenic changes in the small intestine

Administration of exogenous glucocorticoids during the first or second postnatal week causes precocious maturation of intestinal structure and function. In the absence of glucocorticoids, there is a dramatic reduction in the rate of maturation. Glucocorticoids cause intestinal maturation by transcriptional changes, but hormones may also have post-translational effects on proteins of the microvillous membrane as a result of their capacity to alter membrane fluidity and glycosylation patterns. Glucocorticoids are capable of eliciting terminal maturation of the human intestine in a manner analogous to their effects in the rat. These hormones increase lactase activity *in vitro*. In addition, retrospective and prospective studies have shown that prenatal corticosteroid treatment is associated with a significantly reduced incidence of necrotizing enterocolitis in preterm infants.

Thyroxine (T_4) is a reasonable candidate for mediating the ontogeny of enzyme changes in the human small intestine, and total and free serum T_4 increase during the latter half of gestation. Insulin levels increase just before ontogenic changes in disaccharidase activities. For example, in the human, amniotic fluid insulin directly reflects fetal insulin output, and the concentration increases during the last trimester. The rise in insulin precedes the prenatal increase in lactase activity that occurs in the third trimester.

Other hormones and substances have been proposed to play a role in the regulation of intestinal mucosal ontogeny. Many of them are known growth factors, but their direct effects on intestinal maturation are largely unknown.

In preterm infants, the provision of small amounts of milk enterally within the first week of life shortens the time it takes for infants to be able to tolerate all nutrients. Early introduction of feeding also appears to enhance the development of a more mature small intestinal motility pattern and improve enteral feeding tolerance. In addition, water feeding is not as effective as formula feeding in stimulating the release of gastrointestinal peptides in the premature infant.

Epithelial growth and differentiation

The small intestinal epithelium originates from stem cells that give rise to four different cell lineages:

- absorptive enterocytes
- mucus-producing goblet cells
- enteroendocrine cells
- Paneth cells.

The first three cell types migrate towards the villi, whereas Paneth cells migrate downward to the crypt base. The intestinal epithelial cells form intimate contacts with T-lymphocytes, which in turn may regulate epithelial cell growth and barrier function. The intestinal epithelium provides unique opportunities for the study of cell differentiation and apoptosis. The gut epithelium along the crypt–villus axis is dynamic, with an equilibrium between crypt cell production and the senescence and exfoliation of differentiated cells. Regulation of normal intestinal epithelial growth is thought to be dependent on mesenchymal–epithelial interactions as well as interactions with extracellular matrix proteins. Mesenchymal fibroblasts secrete growth factors that influence intestinal epithelial cell migration, proliferation and differentiation. As mature epithelial cells are produced, they express a variety of intestine-specific gene products involved in digestive, absorptive, cell migratory and cell protection functions.

Proteinase-activated receptors (PARs) are a family of G-coupled receptors for serine protease. PAR-2 has been recently found to be expressed in the villi and crypt region of the rat small intestine and in the basolateral and apical membrane of the rat enterocytes. Trypsin at physiological concentrations activates PAR-2, which triggers the release of inositol triphosphate, arachidonic acid, and prostaglandin E_2 and F_{1a}. Therefore, luminal trypsin may serve as a signaling protein for enterocyte activation via PAR-2.

PKC is involved in cell growth and differentiation in various cell types. PKC-α expression is increased in Caco-2 spontaneous cell differentiation, although levels of other kinases remain unchanged in postconfluent cells. Concurrently, expression of PKC-α-regulated cyclin-dependent kinase inhibitor p21^{waf1} increases in differentiated cells. Therefore, the PKC-α and p21^{waf1} cascade could direct a signal that influences the differentiation status of intestinal epithelial cells. Paneth cells play a role in secretion and protection against microflora. Paneth cell allocation occurs early during epithelial cytodifferentiation and crypt formation, and leads to the production of marker proteins such as phospholipase A_2 (PLA$_2$), cryptidins and lysozyme.

Transforming growth factor-α (TGF-α) and TGF-β, as well as epidermal growth factor (EGF) and hepatocyte growth factor (HGF), are potent multifunctional growth factors that appear to play critical roles in the intestine under normal development and during injury. Using immunohistochemistry, TGF-β_1 has been localized to the smooth-muscle cells of the muscularis propria in the human fetal intestine. In untreated adult rats TGF-α expression has been also demonstrated in the epithelial cells at the villous tip and TGF-β expression in epithelial cells in the upper crypt. TGF-α and TGF-β may accelerate wound healing in the intestine. Polyamines and ornithine decarboxylase-dependent cations have been demonstrated to be crucial for the migration of epithelial cells into regions of damaged tissue to promote early mucosal repair. Insulin-like growth factor (IGF) peptides are known to stimulate gastrointestinal growth

in normal adult rats and IGF-1 has been shown selectively to stimulate intestinal growth in developing rats.

Brush-border hydrolases

Lactase and sucrase isomaltase

The developmental expression of lactase and sucrase–isomaltase (SI) enzyme activity correlates with the change in diet at the time of weaning from predominantly lactose-containing milk to non-lactose-containing foods. The expression of the two enzymes appears to be largely genetically determined and transcriptionally regulated. However, the profiles are markedly different, with lactase mRNA appearing before SI mRNA, peaking earlier and then rapidly declining. SI mRNA peaks later and is maintained at 70% of its peak value thereafter. A second major determinant of enzyme activity is the stability of the proteins, with lactase having a longer half-life than SI.

There is strong support for additional independent transcription factors to allow for the differential regulation of these two genes. Further support for differential regulation is provided by the observation that increased cAMP levels increase lactase biosynthesis and mRNA levels but inhibit SI synthesis. Transgenic mouse experiments show that the patterns of SI gene expression are regulated by multiple functional *cis*-acting DNA elements. There are at least three groups of transcriptional factors involved in SI promoter activation, including hepatocyte nuclear factor 1 (HNF-1), Cdx proteins and nuclear proteins that interact with a GATA binding site. There is little correlation of SI transcription with the expression of these transcription factors, which is apparently due to the differential expression of coactivator proteins that thereby modulate the activation of the SI promoter.

Each of the intestinal epithelial cell lineages contains the necessary components for SI expression, and normal enterocyte-specific expression probably involves a repression mechanism in the goblet, enteroendocrine and Paneth cell lineages.

Peptidases

γ-GT catalyzes the transfer of glutamic acid from a donor molecule such as glutathione to an acceptor molecule such as a peptide. The mouse γ-GT gene is unique since it has seven different promoters and contains six 5$'$-exons. The combination of different promoter usage along with alternative splicing generates tissue-specific mRNAs from this single gene.

Enterokinase is a hydrolase that activates latent hydrolytic enzymes in the intestinal lumen by proteolytic cleavage of the proenzymes. The cloning of the bovine enterokinase has revealed a complex protease with multiple domains. Its amino acid sequence suggests that the enterokinase is activated by an unidentified protease and therefore is not the first enzyme of the intestinal digestive hydrolase cascade. The regulation of the expression of the enterokinase gene is largely unknown.

Dipeptidyl peptidase IV (DP-IV), a brush-border hydrolase, is identical to the T-cell activation molecule CD26. It is a member of the prolyl oligopeptidase family of serine proteases that plays an important role in the hydrolysis of proline-rich peptides. Differential expression of DP-IV is seen along the vertical axis, with high levels of expression in the villous cells and lower levels in the crypt cells and horizontal axis.

Alkaline phosphatase

Intestinal alkaline phosphatase (IAP) is a brush-border enzyme that is secreted into the serum and lumen and undergoes extensive postnatal developmental regulation of expression. The adult rat intestine expresses two IAP mRNAs, IAP-I and IAP-II, which have about 70% nucleotide sequence identity with complete divergence at the carboxy-terminus.

Transporters

The sodium-dependent glucose cotransporter (SGLT1) and seven facilitative glucose transporters (GLUT1–GLUT7) have been cloned. SGLT1, GLUT2 and GLUT5 are expressed in the small intestine. SGLT1 is located in the apical membrane of the enterocytes, GLUT2 is anchored to the basolateral membrane and GLUT5 appears to function as an intestinal fructose transporter.

The Na-dependent uptake of bile is also developmentally regulated, with a marked increase at weaning. This cotransporter is regulated at the transcriptional level at the time of weaning, with changes in the apparent molecular weight of the protein after weaning.

Regulatory peptides

Pituitary adenylate cyclase-activating peptide (PACAP) is a neuropeptide that exists in two functional forms, and is a member of a group of regulatory peptides that includes secretin, glucagons, GIP, growth hormone-releasing factor and VIP. PACAP receptors have tissue-specific affinity for both PACAP and VIP. PACAP nerves exist within the myenteric plexus, deep muscular plexus and submucosal plexus in the canine terminal ileum. In addition, PACAP receptors are present in deep muscular plexus and circular muscular fibers.

Uroguanylin and guanylin are endogenous proteins that regulate intestinal chloride secretion by binding to guanylate cyclase C, and guanylin also has been shown to be involved in duodenal bicarbonate secretion. Uroguanylin is expressed throughout the intestinal tract and also in the kidney. This gene is predominantly expressed in the villous. Guanilyn, however, is localized to the distal small intestine and proximal colon, and is expressed in both the crypt and villus.

Intestinal cytoprotection

Cyclooxygenases

Two cyclooxygenase (Cox) isoforms, Cox-1 and Cox-2, catalyze the synthesis of prostaglandins. Cox-1 is expressed constitutively in most mammalian tissues, and prostaglandins produced by Cox-1 are thought to play a major role in the maintenance of gastrointestinal homeostasis, including gastric cytoprotection and blood flow. Cox-2 is induced in monocytes and macrophages by proinflammatory cytokines, mitogens, serum and endotoxin. Prostaglandins synthesized by Cox-2 mediate the inflammatory response. Cox-2 is expressed at very low levels in the intestinal epithelium, but at high levels in human colon cancers and adenomas and in spontaneous adenomas in mice that carry a mutant *APC* gene. In the normal colonic epithelium there is no significant Cox-2 expression, but in ulcerative colitis and Crohn's disease Cox-2 is expressed in epithelial cells in upper crypts and on the surface, but not in the lower crypts.

The area of Cox-1 expression in the small and large intestine corresponds to the area of epithelial proliferation in the crypt. As the epithelial cell migrates up out of the crypt and onto the villus it differentiates and stops expressing Cox-1.

Trefoil peptides

Trefoil peptides contain a unique motif with six cysteine residues and three intrachain disulfide bonds, resulting in a three-loop structure. They are expressed highly in gastrointestinal mucosa and are resistant to protease digestion in the lumen, probably owing to their unusual trefoil domain. Known members of the trefoil peptide family include pS2, spasmolitic peptide (SP) and intestinal trefoil factor (ITF), all cloned from several species. The stomach secretes pS2, the stomach and duodenum secrete spasmolitic peptide, and the small and large intestine secretes ITF. Although the exact function of these proteins has not yet been determined, they are found in high levels at the edges of healing ulcers and are believed to be involved in protective function of the mucosal barrier.

Mucins

Mucins are a key component of the protective gel layer that coats the mucosal surface. Whether secretory or membrane bound, mucins contain diverse, highly O-glycosylated repeat amino acid residues. Mucin expression is known to be both cell type and tissue specific as different mucins have been localized to specific regions of the gastrointestinal tract. Mucin precursors for mucins, MUC2–MUC6, have been identified from the stomach to the small and large intestine, MUC3 from the small intestine, MUC4 from the large intestine, and both MUC5AC and MUC6 from the stomach. Litle is known about the specific function of individual MUCs, but the site-specific expression of these molecules suggests that the composition of MUC5AC and MUC6 is beneficial in protecting the stomach from acid-induced damage.

Human MUC2 is expressed almost exclusively in goblet cells and may be abnormally expressed in colon cancer. The gene for human MUC2 maps to chromosome 11p15 and analysis of the locus reveals two regulatory elements, an enhancer and an inhibitor, upstream from the MUC2 translation start site. MUC1 protein expression has been located to microvilli on the luminal surface of the epithelial cell in the intestine.

Regulation of intestinal gene expression mediated by nutrients

Traditionally it has been assumed that gene expression in higher eukaryotes was not directly influenced by food components but by the action of hormones, growth factors and cytokines. However, it is now known that diet is a powerful means to modify the cellular environment of the gastrointestinal tract. Dietary regulation of the genes expressed by the epithelium confers three fundamental advantages for mammals. It enables the epithelium to adapt to the luminal environment better to digest and absorb nutrients; it provides the means whereby breast milk can influence the development of the gastrointestinal tract and, when the proteins expressed by the epithelium act on the immune system,

it constitutes a signaling mechanism from the intestinal lumen to the body's defenses. Each of these mechanisms is amenable to manipulation for therapeutic purposes. Major nutrients (e.g. glucose and fatty acids) as well as minor nutrients (e.g. vitamins A and D, and minerals, iron, zinc and copper) influence the expression of a number of genes directly or in a concerted action with hormones.

The regulation of genes by nutrients requires that some enzymes, transporters and membrane receptors interact with the particular nutrient, giving rise to a series of cellular events leading to modulation of the transcriptional or translational gene processes.

There is some evidence of the direct control of a number of genes by amino acids. The expression of the neutral amino acid A system is proportional to the extracellular amino acid concentrations. In addition, the charge level of specific tRNA is a determining factor in the regulation of protein synthesis. Moreover, some genes coding for ribosomal proteins are tightly regulated by the availability of exogenous amino acids. Glutamine has been demonstrated to reduce cellular death due to thermal shock; hsp70 and hsp72 genes are expressed in the presence of glutamine by intestinal cells.

In addition to EGF, insulin and other growth factors and nutrients, human milk contains some nutrients that influence gene expression. Lactoferrin, a protein involved in iron bioavailability, is a proliferative factor for lymphocytes, embryonic fibroblasts and human intestinal HT-29 cells. It also increases sucrase and alkaline phosphatase activities in intestinal cells. These data suggest that lactoferrin may affect intestinal growth and differentiation, probably by internalization of the lactoferrin-receptor complex.

Soluble nucleotides are present in milk from various mammals, contributing up to 20% of the non-protein nitrogen. Although nucleotide deficiency has not been related to any particular disease, dietary nucleotides are reportedly beneficial for infants since they positively influence lipid metabolism, immunity, and tissue growth, development and repair. Nucleotides are naturally present in all foods of animal and vegetable origin as free nucleotides and nucleic acids. Concentrations of RNA and DNA in foods depend mainly on their cell density, whereas the content of free nucleotides is species specific. Thus, meat, fish and seeds have a high content of nucleic acids, and milk, eggs and fruits have lower levels. Milk has a specific free-nucleotide profile for each species. The nucleotide content of colostrum is qualitatively similar but quantitatively distinct in human and ruminants. In general, total colostrum nucleotide content increases immediately after parturition, reaches maximum levels from 24 to 48 after birth, and decreases thereafter with advancing lactation. Dietary nucleotides appear to modulate lipoprotein and fatty acid metabolism in early human life, and affect the growth, development and repair of the small intestine and liver in experimental animals. Moreover, dietary nucleotides modify the intestinal ecology of newborn infants, enhancing the growth of bifidobacteria and limiting that of enterobacteria, and have a role in the maintenance of the immune response both in animals and in human neonates.

Erythrocytes, lymphocytes, enterocytes and glial cells have a common characteristic: their ability to synthesize nucleotides by the *de novo* pathway is very low. Thus, an external supply of nucleosides seems to be needed for optimal functioning. Several investigations support the hypothesis that the enterocyte is not fully capable of developing the *de novo* purine synthesis and that this metabolic pathway may be inactive unless it is induced by a purine-deficient diet. The purine salvage pathway, as measured by the activity of its rate-limiting enzyme hypoxanthine-guanine phosphoribosyl transferase (HGPRT), is highest in the small intestine relative to liver and colon; moreover, a purine-free diet lowers HGPRT activity.

A number of studies have demonstrated that dietary nucleotides in part regulate gene expression in the intestine (Figure 10.21). Intestinal mRNA levels of the enzymes HGPRT and adenine phosphoribosyl transfera (APRT) decline in response to nucleotide restriction in the diet. Nuclear 'run-on' assays in nuclei isolated both from the small intestine and from an intestinal epithelial cell line (IEC-18) demonstrated that dietary-nucleotide restriction significantly altered the transcription rate. A 35 base-pair region (HCRE) in the promoter of the HPGRT gene has been identified as the element necessary for this response, and the protein that interacts with this region has been identified and purified.

Glucose, fructose, sucrose, galactose and glycerol increase the expression of lactase in rat jejunum homogenates. Long-chain fatty acids decrease lactase expression, whereas high-starch diets increase its expression. In mice, the expression of the sodium/glucose cotransporter SGLT1 is increased by dietary carbohydrates and the effect is apparent only in the

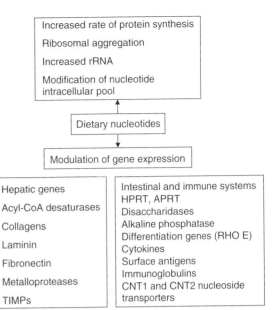

Figure 10.21 Modulation of gene expression by dietary nucleotides. TIMPs: tissue inhibitor of metalloproteases; HPRT: hypoxanthine phosphoribosyl transferase; APRT: aderine phosphoribosyl transferase; CNT: concentrative nucleoside transporter

crypts. In addition, high-fructose diets increase the expression of GLUT5.

Dietary fat plays a key role in the regulation of gene expression in many tissues (Figure 10.22). Several transcription factors, including peroxisome proliferator receptors (PPARs), HNF4, nuclear factor KB (NFκB) and steroid response binding protein type c (SREBP1c), have been shown to be modulated by exogenous polyunsaturated fatty acids or their metabolites, namely eicosanoids.

Vitamins D and A acts as true hormones, and their action on the expression of many genes occurs via binding to nuclear receptors in many organs, including the intestine (Figure 10.23). In addition, it is well known that metals can influence the regulation of some genes. The post-transcriptional regulation of ferritin and transferrin receptor by dietary iron levels is well recognized.

10.13 The large bowel

Until the 1980s, the large bowel was a relatively neglected organ, once described as a 'sophisticated way of producing manure' which, unfortunately, was inclined to go wrong, resulting in common diseases and

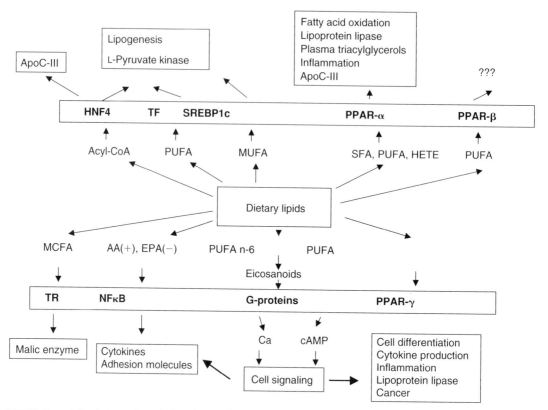

Figure 10.22 Transcription factors and metabolic pathways affected by dietary lipids. AA: arachidonic acid; ApoC-III: apoprotein C-III; EPA: eicosapentanoic acid; HETE: hydroxides of trienoic acids; HNF-4: hepatic nuclear factor-4; MCFA: medium-chain fatty acids; NFKB: nuclear factor KB; PPAR: peroxisome proliferator receptor; PUFA: polyunsaturated fatty acids; SFA: saturated fatty acids; SREBP: sterol response element binding protein; TF: tyroxine factor.

disorders such as constipation, ulcerative colitis and colorectal cancer. Fortunately, recent investigations on the etiology, prevention and treatment of these diseases and disorders have illuminated the structure and function of the large bowel. From a nutritional perspective, recognition that the primary function of this organ is salvage of energy via bacterial fermentation of food residues has revolutionized understanding of this area of the body. The human body contains about 10^{14} cells, of which only one-tenth are human cells. The remainder are bacterial cells, most of which are found in the colon where they dominate metabolic processes.

Structure

The large bowel forms the last 1.5 m of the intestine and is divided into the appendix, cecum, transverse colon, descending colon, sigmoid colon and rectum. It is about 6 cm in diameter, becoming narrower towards the rectum. With the exception of the rectum

(the final 12 cm of the intestine), the large bowel has a complex mesentery supplying blood from the superior and inferior mesenteric arteries. Blood drained from the colon reaches the liver via the portal vein. As with the more proximal regions of the intestine, the large bowel has two layers of muscle, an outer longitudinal layer and an inner circular layer, which work together to sequester and move digesta along the tract. Although food residues travel through the small bowel in just a few hours, digesta may be retained in the large bowel for 2–4 days or longer. The colon has a sacculated appearance composed of pouches known as haustra. These are formed by the organization of the outer longitudinal smooth-muscle layer into three bands called the taeniae coli (which are shorter than the other longitudinal muscles) and by segmental thickening of the inner circular smooth muscles.

The parasympathetic vagus nerve innervates the ascending colon and most of the transverse colon, with

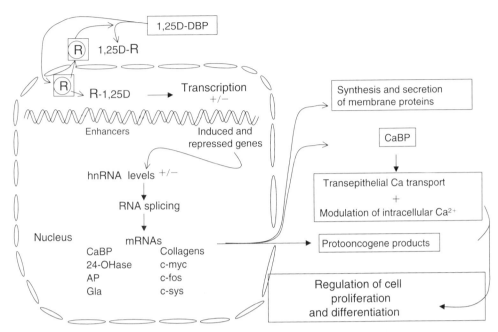

Figure 10.23 Regulation of gene expression mediated by vitamin D. AP: alkaline phosphatase; 24-OHase: 24-calciferol hydroxylase.

the pelvic nerves innervating the more distal regions. There are also connections to the colon from the lower thoracic and upper lumbar segments of the spinal cord via noradrenergic sympathetic nerves.

The mucosa of the colon consists of a single layer of columnar epithelial cells which are derived from stem cells located at or near the base of the crypts. Unlike the small bowel, there are no villi, so that the inner surface of the colon is relatively flat, which may have contributed to the misapprehension that this organ is unimportant in digestion and absorption. There is a higher density of goblet cells than in the small intestine, producing mucus that both protects the colonic surface and coats the increasingly more solid feces as it is propelled through the large bowel. The water content of the gut contents decreases from about 85% in the cecum to 77% in the sigmoid colon. Immune protection extends into the large intestine with the presence of gut-associated lymphoid tissue (GALT) in nodules within the mucosa and extending into the submucosa.

Functions of the large bowel

Energy salvage

Many animal species have evolved a symbiotic relationship with microorganisms which allows them to extract energy from food materials that otherwise would be indigestible by the animal's enzymes. This is best exemplified by mammalian herbivores, which may obtain up to three-quarters of their energy as the by-products of anaerobic fermentation in specialized sacs before the gastric stomach (e.g. in ruminants) or in a massively enlarged large bowel (e.g. in equids, members of the horse family). In each case, commensal bacteria (and sometimes other microorganisms such as protozoa and fungi) proliferate by fermenting plant matter in specialized regions of the intestine that do not secrete digestive enzymes. The energy-containing end-products of this fermentation, principally short-chain fatty acids (SCFAs), are absorbed readily and metabolized. For those animals in which fermentation precedes the gastric stomach or where there is ingestion of feces (best described for lagomorphs such as the rabbit) the bacterial biomass is also an important source of nutrients.

In humans consuming Westernized diets, the equivalent of 50–60 g dry weight of food residues and endogenous material dissolved and suspended in approximately 1–1.5 litres of fluid flow into the cecum from the ileum every day. For those eating low-fat diets with lots of plant foods rich in carbohydrates which are poorly, or not at all, digested in the small bowel

Table 10.3 Examples of major bacterial species found in the human colon and their fermentation end-products

Bacterial species	Major end-products
Bacteroides	Acetate, propionate and succinate
Eubacteria	Acetate, butyrate and lactate
Bifidobacteria	Acetate and lactate
Lactobacilli	Lactate
Ruminococci	Acetate
Methanobrevibacter	Methane

(e.g. non-starch polysaccharides and resistant starch), considerably more carbohydrate and other energy-containing food components escape into the colon. In a world with an increasing proportion of obese people, loss of this potential energy would not be a problem but, throughout human history, shortage of food has been much more common. Therefore, the ability to salvage as much energy as possible from food will have been an evolutionary advantage and may have made the difference between survival and death. This energy salvage is achieved by bacterial fermentation of carbohydrates and, to a lesser extent, proteins. Bacterial cells make up at least 50% by weight of colonic contents, where they are present at concentrations of about 10^{10}–10^{11} cells/g wet matter. There are several hundreds of bacterial species (see Table 10.3 for examples) and this great diversity, together with the inability to grow some of the organisms in pure culture, has proved a big challenge for conventional bacteriology. However, the application of modern molecular biological techniques, including the use of 16S-rRNA probes, offers considerable promise as a means of characterizing the colonic microflora.

The virtual absence of oxygen in the anaerobic conditions in the lumen of the large bowel means that the bacterial inhabitants cannot oxidize organic matter using the Krebs cycle and oxidative phosphorylation. Instead, reduced dinucleotides, generated via the glycolytic pathway, are converted to their oxidized counterparts via metabolism of pyruvate to SCFAs. In this way, most of the energy present in the intractable carbohydrates escaping small bowel digestion is absorbed across the colonic epithelial cells as the SCFAs acetate, propionate and butyrate. SCFA absorption is largely by transcellular mechanisms, including carrier-mediated transport and non-ionic diffusion. Only a very small proportion, usually much less than 5%, of SCFA production is lost in the feces. The principal

gaseous end-products of large bowel fermentation are carbon dioxide, hydrogen and methane, with everyone generating carbon dioxide and hydrogen, but only 30–40% of people producing significant quantities of methane. These gases are released in the flatus (about 500 ml/day) or absorbed and excreted via the lungs.

It appears as if the colonic microflora prefer to ferment carbohydrates, switching to proteins and other nitrogenous substrates only in the more distal large bowel when accessible carbohydrates become exhausted. Degradation of the 10–12 g of nitrogenous compounds entering the colon from the small bowel daily yields a range of quantitatively minor end-products, including branched-chain and longer chain SCFAs, ammonia, hydrogen sulfide, indole, skatole and volatile amines. However, several of these compounds are implicated in colonic diseases; for example, hydrogen sulfide is believed to contribute to the etiology or recurrence of ulcerative colitis, while ammonia and sulfide may play a part in damaging colonocytes leading to colorectal cancer.

Absorption of water and electrolytes

Daily fecal output is highly variable, but is in the order of 100–150 g stool containing about 25 g dry matter. This means that the large bowel absorbs approximately 1 liter of water every day. Water is absorbed down an osmotic gradient, mainly from the proximal colon, following the absorption of sodium and chloride ions and of SCFAs. Sodium uptake is driven by an active process powered by a Na^+/K^+-ATPase pump situated on the basolateral membrane of the colonocyte. Chloride ions are absorbed passively in exchange for bicarbonate ions. Water absorption is under both neural (via the enteric nerve plexus) and hormonal control. Aldosterone, angiotensin and the glucocorticoids stimulate water absorption, while the antidiuretic hormone, vasopressin, decreases water absorption. An unpleasant side-effect of treatment with some antibiotics can be the development of diarrhea as a result of suppression of colonic bacteria and subsequent reduction in SCFA production.

Lipid metabolism

The most extensively studied aspect of lipid metabolism in the colon is the bacterial transformation of the up to 5% of bile salts that are not absorbed in the ileum. Bile salts are deconjugated (removal of glycine and taurine residues) and, depending on the pH of the digesta (which ranges from about 5.5 in the cecum to 6.5 in the distal colon), the primary bile acids may be converted to secondary bile acids by dehydroxylation. The latter are more lipid soluble, and are absorbed by passive diffusion (probably about 50 mg/day) and returned to the liver. Most of the cholesterol entering the colon is excreted as such in feces, but some is metabolized to the relatively insoluble derivatives coprostanol and coprostanone, which are not absorbed. The anaerobic nature of the colonic lumen does not allow the oxidation of long-chain fatty acids, which explains why diseases causing fat malabsorption in the small intestine result in greatly increased excretion of fat in the feces (stearorrhea). However, in the colon, unsaturated fatty acids may be biohydrogenated using the reducing power (H_2) generated as a by-product of carbohydrate fermentation.

Synthesis of vitamins and essential amino acids

Although it has been known for more than 50 years that the bacteria in the large bowel synthesize a wide range of vitamins, in particular, several of the B vitamins and vitamin K, there is rather poor understanding of the nutritional significance of this synthesis. In part this is due to the considerable technical difficulty in making quantitative measurements of vitamin absorption from the human colon. The presence of menaquinones (bacterially derived forms of vitamin K) in human blood and tissues attests to uptake of these substances from the human gut, but there is only modest experimental evidence for the frequently cited assertion that about half of vitamin K needs can be obtained by colonic synthesis. The observation that low intakes of folate are associated with an increased risk of colorectal cancer and the accumulating evidence that low folate status can compromise the integrity of the genome are stimulating interest in factors (dietary or otherwise) that may modulate folate synthesis in the large intestine. It is possible that bacterially synthesized folate could be absorbed and utilized by colonocytes (affording protection against colorectal cancer) with or without an impact on folate status elsewhere in the body.

In the same way that colonic bacteria synthesize vitamins for their own use, they synthesize amino acids including the essential amino acids. Some of the nitrogen required for this synthesis is derived from urea circulating in the bloodstream, which diffuses readily into the bowel where it is hydrolyzed by the gut microflora to ammonia. It has been proposed that intestinally synthesized amino acids may make a significant contribution to the amino acid needs of children and adults on very low protein intakes. However, quantifying this contribution remains a tough challenge. The factors that lead to effective salvage by the colon of nitrogen as amino acids are unknown, but may include adequate supplies of ammonia and carbohydrate to stimulate colonic bacterial proliferation. Even if the colonic bacteria can be encouraged to produce extra essential amino acids it is not clear how those amino acids are transferred from the bacteria to, and taken up by, colonocytes. This is an important research area with potentially profound implications for the understanding of colonic physiology and for the derivation of human protein and amino acid needs.

Metabolism and absorption of phytochemicals

The strong epidemiological evidence that those consuming diets rich in vegetables and fruits have a lower risk of developing several common non-communicable diseases, including cardiovascular disease and cancer, has stimulated research on components of these plant foods that may be protective. There is particular interest in the non-nutrient secondary metabolites of plants described collectively as phytochemicals or phytoprotectants, which have bioactivity when consumed by humans. To be effective in protecting human cells against oxidative damage, for example, these compounds must be released from the plant tissue, absorbed across the intestinal mucosa and transported in sufficient concentrations to their site of action. Disruption of plant cells by cooking may help to release phytochemicals, but for uncooked foods degradation of plant cell walls and release of their phytochemical contents will be aided greatly by bacterial fermentation in the colon. Phytochemicals are chemically diverse, but a large proportion is found naturally as glycosides. In many cases, these must be converted to the aglycone derivatives (a process that is accomplished readily by colonic bacteria) before they can be absorbed. Bacterial metabolism is also believed to be responsible for the production of the active derivatives of some phytochemicals. Among the best known are enterolactone and enterodiol, which are estrogen-like compounds derived by bacterial degradation of the plant lignans matairesinol and secoisolariciresinol, respectively.

Manipulation of the large bowel to enhance or protect health

An unpleasant side-effect of treatment with some antibiotics can be the development of diarrhea as a result of suppression of colonic bacteria and subsequent reduction in SCFA production. This is one of the most frequent, albeit unwanted, illustrations of the ease with which the colonic flora can be manipulated. The recognition that the balance of microflora within the large bowel may influence health has stimulated attempts to manipulate the flora in health-promoting ways using two main approaches.

Probiotics

A probiotic is a live microbial food ingredient that is beneficial to health. The concept is quite straightforward. All one needs is a 'gut-friendly' bacterium that is both demonstrably safe and beneficial to health and that can be consumed in an attractive food product. Several probiotic products (mostly fermented milk-based products) are on the market in Japan, Europe and elsewhere. Some potential probiotic species may help to overcome pathogenic bacteria such as *Clostridium difficile,* which can become dominant if the endogenous flora is disturbed, such as by the use of broad-spectrum antibiotics. Other potential probiotics are intended to improve immune defences, for example by direct interaction with the GALT or the production of 'protective' end-products such as butyrate. However, in practice, it has proved difficult to identify microbes that produce demonstrable benefits to human health *in vivo,* and the development of delivery systems (foods) that have both a good shelf-life and ensure that an appropriate and effective dose of bacteria reaches the large bowel (or other site of activity) remains a challenge. It is possible using genetic engineering to tailor the potential benefit of probiotic organisms. For example, a food-grade *Lactococcus lactis* was engineered to secrete the anti-inflammatory cytokine interleukin-10 and was as effective as conventional steroid drugs in the treatment of inflammatory bowel disease in mice. Whether such approaches are developed as far as food products will depend on the public's acceptance or otherwise of genetically modified food ingredients and the demonstration that such products are safe and effective for human use.

Prebiotics

Prebiotics are food ingredients that stimulate selectively the growth and activity of bifidobacteria and lactobacteria in the gut and thereby benefit health. Given the difficulty of delivering enough 'gut-friendly' bacteria in foods in the form of probiotics, an alternative approach is to augment the numbers of the desired bacteria in the large bowel by supplying them with substrates that give them a competitive advantage. All prebiotics developed to date are relatively small carbohydrates (degree of polymerization 2–60) which are essentially indigestible by mammalian enzymes and so are delivered in digesta to the colon. There is good evidence that some of these oligosaccharides can produce significant shifts in the balance of bacterial species in the human colon, but how they do so is not yet certain. For example, consumption of 15 g/day of the probiotic oligofructose for 15 days increased bifidobacteria, and decreased bacteroides, clostridia and fusobacteria in the feces (Gibson *et al.,* 1995). Because many of them are present in commonly used foods such as onions and some cereal products, it is probable that such carbohydrates are safe in the amounts likely to be eaten. However, research to obtain sound evidence for the effectiveness of probiotics in protecting or enhancing health is in its early stages.

10.14 Perspectives on the future

Recently, the hypothesis has emerged that digestive end-products and/or their metabolic derivatives may regulate pancreatic gene expression directly and independently of hormone stimulation. The quantity, type (mainly degree of unsaturation) and duration of the fat ingested affect the final response. The role of fatty acids in the control of gene expression is now at an early stage of understanding, and whether this mechanism is related to pancreatic adaptation to dietary fat is unknown and will have to be defined by additional research.

Current information on developmental gene expression in the intestine as well as the dietary regulation of genes expressed in the developing intestinal epithelium is limited to only a handful of genes, which are primarily highly expressed genes involved in differentiated cellular functions. However, in the future expression patterns of transcriptional regulatory factors and signaling proteins involved in the regulation of intestinal transcriptomes will enable the assessment of the entire transcriptome of each cell type of the intestinal mucosa.

Further reading

Gibson GR, Beatty ER, Wang X, Cummings JH. Selective stimulation of bifidobacteria in the human colon by oligofructose and inulin. *Gastroenterology* 1995; **108**: 975–982.

Jackson AA. Salvage of urea-nitrogen and protein requirements. *Proc Nutr Soc* 1995; **54:** 535–547.

Macfarlane GT, Gibson GR. Microbiological aspects of the production of short-chain fatty acids in the large bowel. In: *Physiological and Clinical Aspects of Short-chain Fatty Acids.* (JH Cummings, JL Rombeau, T Sakata, eds), pp. 87–105. Cambridge: Cambridge University Press, 1995.

Sandford PA. *Digestive System Physiology,* 2nd edn. London: Edward Arnold, 1992.

Smith ME, Morton DG. *The Digestive System.* Edinburgh: Churchill Livingstone, 2001.

Steidler L, Hans W, Schotte L *et al.* Treatment of murine colitis by *Lactococcus lactis* secreting interleukin-10. *Science* 2000; **289**: 1352–1355.

11
The Cardiovascular System

G Riccardi, A Rivellese and C Williams

Key messages

- Raised plasma low-density lipoprotein (LDL) cholesterol, raised triacylglycerol (TAG), raised blood pressure and reduced levels of high-density lipoprotein (HDL) cholesterol are established independent risk factors for cardiovascular disease (CVD).
- Raised levels of the clotting factors (factor VII, fibrinogen and von Willebrand factor) and of the fibrinolytic system (tissue plasminogen activator and plasminogen activator inhibitor-1) have been shown to be independent risk factors for CVD.
- Diabetes and obesity are associated with an increased risk of CVD due in part to elevated glucose levels and the blood lipoprotein abnormalities that occur in insulin resistance.
- There is general agreement that a reduced intake of saturated fat is essential to decrease LDL cholesterol levels and related cardiovascular risk. Replacing saturated fat with monounsaturated or n-6 polyunsaturated fatty acids (PUFA) induces a similar decrease in LDL cholesterol.
- Among the different types of fatty acids, long-chain n-3 fatty acids have the most relevant hypotriacylglycerolemic effect. Modest intakes of long-chain n-3 PUFA significantly reduce the risk of CVD without affecting plasma lipid levels.
- Carbohydrate increases plasma TAG, but dietary fiber counteracts this negative effect.
- Beside *trans*-fatty acids, which have a clear negative effect on HDL cholesterol, the influences of dietary components on this parameter are not yet well defined.
- A combination diet that includes increased fruit and vegetables, reduced salt and reduced total and saturated fat intakes has a more powerful effect on blood pressure than a single-nutrient intervention.

11.1 Introduction

Epidemiological research in the 1950s began to show quite clearly that diseases of the vascular system, particularly coronary heart disease and stroke, have a strong root in lifestyle factors. As our knowledge of epidemiological predictors of heart disease, now referred to as risk factors, grew, so too did our understanding of how specific nutrients can influence their manifestation. The present chapter aims to provide the reader with an overview of this large and complex topic. The first part of the chapter examines pathophysiological aspects of the cardiovascular system, while the second part examines the roles of specific nutrients in modifying the risk factors for cardiovascular disease (CVD).

Section 11.2 discusses the physiological factors involved in maintaining a healthy vascular system and which, by definition, lead to morbidity and mortality when they operate outside the norms of physiology. Section 11.3 examines the pathology of CVD and the concept of risk factors, and Section 11.4 describes the manner in which each of the factors involved in vascular function contributes to risk of disease. Subsequent sections examine the role of individual dietary components on CVD. The key areas of metabolism that need to be considered when studying nutrition and the cardiovascular system are plasma lipids, blood pressure, endothelial function, the hemostatic and fibrinolytic pathways, and insulin sensitivity.

11.2 Factors involved in a healthy vascular system

Lipids [cholesterol, triacylglycerol (TAG) and phospholipids] are transported in blood plasma as lipoprotein particles, consisting of a neutral lipid core (TAG and esterified cholesterol) surrounded by a coating of the more hydrophilic phospholipids and free cholesterol (Figure 11.1). The lipoproteins present in plasma are of varying density and size according to the relative amounts of lipid and protein present in the particle (Table 11.1). Cholesterol is carried in the smaller, denser particles, low-density lipoprotein (LDL) and high-density lipoprotein (HDL) cholesterol. TAG is carried in the larger, less dense particles, very low-density lipoprotein (VLDL) and chylomicrons. Because raised levels of LDL cholesterol and TAG, and reduced levels of HDL cholesterol, have been identified as risk factors for cardiovascular disease, an understanding of their normal metabolism is important to appreciate the way in which diet and other lifestyle factors can influence the circulating concentrations of these lipoprotein particles.

Low-density lipoprotein metabolism

LDL particles are largely formed within the circulation from VLDL particles secreted by the liver (Figure 11.2). Through the action of lipoprotein lipase (LPL, an enzyme present in muscle and adipose tissue), TAG is progressively removed from the VLDL particle. The fatty acids that are released by the action of the lipase are taken up and used as an energy substrate by tissues (especially skeletal and cardiac muscles), or are stored within adipose tissue. This progressive removal of triacylglycerol from the core of the VLDL particle leads to the formation of a smaller, more cholesterol-rich particle, sometimes referred to as intermediate-density

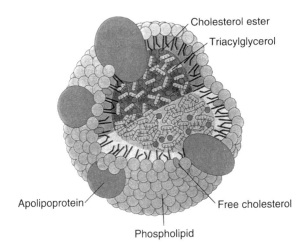

Figure 11.1 Diagrammatic representation of a typical lipoprotein particle showing the major lipid and protein components.

Table 11.1 Characteristics of the major lipoprotein classes

Fraction	Diameter (nm)	Site of synthesis	Function of major lipids	Major apolipoproteins	Composition (% by weight)			
					Protein	TAG	TC	PL
Chylomicron	80–1000	Gut	Transport of dietary fat	B48, A1, A2, C	1	90	5	4
VLDL	30–80	Gut, liver	Transport of endogenous fat from liver	B100, C	10	65	13	13
LDL	20–22	Capillaries of peripheral tissue, liver	Transport of cholesterol to peripheral tissues	B100	20	10	45	23
HDL	9–15	Gut, liver	Removal of cholesterol from peripheral tissues to liver	A1, A2, C	50	2	18	30

TAG: triacylglycerol; TC: total cholesterol; PL: phospholipid; VLDL: very low-density lipoprotein; LDL: low-density lipoprotein; HDL: high-density lipoprotein. The proportions shown are approximate only and vary within each major class.

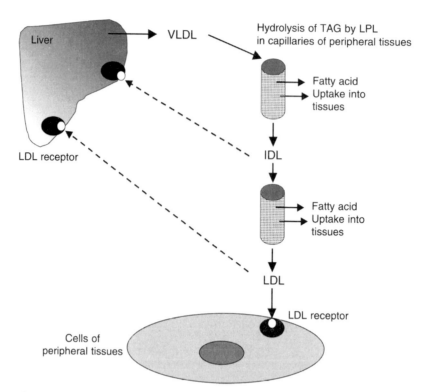

Figure 11.2 Pathway of low-density lipoprotein (LDL) metabolism from production of very low-density lipoprotein (VLDL) particles in liver, their hydrolysis by lipoprotein lipase (LPL) in capillaries of peripheral tissues with progressive removal of triacylglycerol (TAG) to form intermediate-density lipoprotein (IDL) and then LDL. LDL is removed from circulation via LDL receptors on all cell membranes, with the highest density of receptors found in the liver.

lipoprotein (IDL). IDL may be removed from the circulation by the liver or, by the further action of LPL, may be converted to LDL cholesterol. The essential function of LDL is the transport of cholesterol to peripheral tissues for the formation of cell membranes and synthesis of steroid hormones. LDL formed from VLDL and IDL is taken up by specific receptors (LDL or apoB/E receptors) present on all cell membranes. When the levels of cholesterol within cells are high, the LDL receptors are reduced in number (down-regulated) to prevent excessive uptake of cholesterol. Under such circumstances, LDL particles remain within the circulation. It is clear from this that the major factors that will determine the concentration of LDL in the circulation are:

- the rate of formation of VLDL and its conversion to LDL in the circulation
- the density of the LDL receptor on cell membranes.

Since half of the body's LDL receptors are present in the liver, it follows that hepatic LDL receptor density is a major determinant of circulating LDL concentrations.

The majority of cholesterol carried by LDL is endogenously synthesized in the liver. The rate-limiting enzyme in cholesterol biosynthesis, 3-hydroxy-3-methylglutamyl-coenzyme A (HMG-CoA) reductase, can be regulated to a very significant extent by a family of drugs known as statins, as well as by dietary fats. Another route to the lowering of blood cholesterol is the plant sterols, which are not capable of being incorporated into micellar lipid and thus create a pool of unabsorbed lipid in the distal gut in which some ingested cholesterol becomes trapped. Equally, gut sequestration of bile acids by dietary fiber disrupts the enterohepatic recirculation of bile acids back to the liver and thus requires a greater diversion of hepatic cholesterol to bile acids. This reduces the flow of hepatic free cholesterol to LDL cholesterol for export to plasma.

High-density lipoprotein metabolism

Precursor HDL particles are formed in the small intestine and the liver, and consist of small amounts of cholesterol and phospholipid complexed with a transport

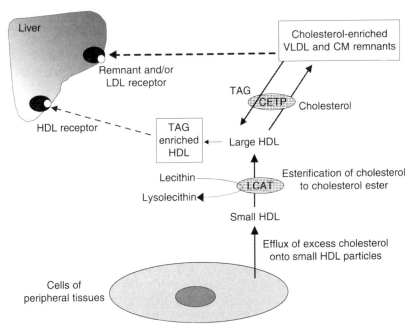

Figure 11.3 Major steps in reverse cholesterol transport. Small high-density lipoprotein (HDL) receives free cholesterol secreted by peripheral cells. By the action of lecithin cholesterol acyl transferase (LCAT), free cholesterol is esterified on HDL to form the large HDL particle. HDL returns cholesterol to the liver, either directly via uptake on HDL receptors, or indirectly via transfer of cholesterol onto very low-density lipoprotein (VLDL) and chylomicron (CM) remnant particles in exchange for triacylglycerol (TAG). The latter step is catalyzed by cholesterol ester transfer protein (CETP), a circulating enzyme associated with lipoprotein particles. Cholesterol-enriched VLDL and CM remnants are taken up by remnant receptors or by the low-density lipoprotein (LDL) receptor on the liver.

protein, apolipoprotein A1(apo A1). HDL particles play a central role in reverse cholesterol transport (Figure 11.3), whereby cholesterol is transported back from peripheral tissues to liver for oxidation and removal. Although peripheral cells can synthesize cholesterol, they are unable to oxidize the cholesterol molecule. Excess cholesterol is therefore removed from cells and transported to the liver for oxidation and excretion via reverse cholesterol transport. This is one of the prime functions of the HDL particle. Cells secrete excess cholesterol in the free unesterified form. This is initially taken up by the precursor HDL particle. By the action of lecithin cholesterol acyl transferase (LCAT), a fatty acid (usually linoleic acid) is removed from lecithin and transferred to cholesterol on HDL, forming the more stable and hydrophobic cholesterol ester, which migrates to the hydrophobic HDL core. HDL, now enriched with cholesterol ester, can be removed directly by the liver through the action of a putative receptor that has not yet been isolated. However, an alternative and more active pathway appears to be the transfer of cholesterol ester from HDL onto the

TAG-rich particles, VLDL and CMs. In return, TAG is transferred onto the HDL particles. The reciprocal transfer of cholesterol ester and TAG between HDL and TAG-rich particles is catalyzed by the action of cholesterol ester transfer protein (CETP). The cholesterol ester that is transferred onto VLDL and chylomicron particles is rapidly removed by the liver when these particles are take up by hepatic receptors. Because the remnants of VLDL and chylomicron particles are removed by the liver via high-throughput remnant receptors as well as by the LDL receptor, this mechanism provides a very efficient means of returning excess cholesterol to the liver for excretion. Therefore, in simple terms, the HDL particle uses the TAG-rich particles as vehicles for transferring the excess cholesterol removed from cells back to the liver for conversion to bile acids.

Very low-density lipoprotein and chylomicron metabolism

For convenience it is useful to consider the metabolism of chylomicron particles as the exogenous pathway and of VLDL particles as the endogenous pathway,

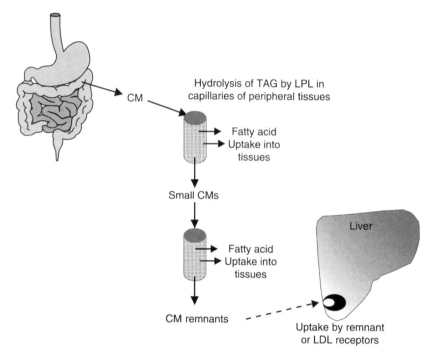

Figure 11.4 Outline of the exogenous pathway of triacylglycerol (TAG) metabolism. Chylomicron (CM) particles are formed in the enterocyte following the digestion and absorption of dietary fat and are secreted for 4–8 h after a fat-containing meal. The particles are hydrolyzed by lipoprotein lipase (LPL, present on the capillary lining of blood vessels supplying adipose tissue, skeletal muscle and heart), with removal of TAG and eventual removal of smaller delipidated particles (remnants) via specific remnant receptors or by the low-density lipoprotein (LDL) receptor.

although in essence they form part of a continuous common transport system for TAG-rich lipoproteins.

Exogenous pathway

Dietary TAG is hydrolyzed in the small intestine to form free fatty acids and monoacyl glycerol. Once absorbed across the brush-border membrane of the enterocyte, monoacylglycerol and free fatty acids are re-esterified to form TAG. The mature chylomicron particle is formed when TAG combines with cholesterol and the transport protein apo B-48 in the endoplasmic reticulum. A surface coating of phospholipid and free cholesterol increases the water solubility of the particles, which are then secreted into the lacteals and, via the lymphatic system, enter the blood circulation via the thoracic duct. It is clear from this account that dietary fat, unlike other digested nutrients, does not enter the circulation via the portal vein and liver, but bypasses the liver and enters directly from the gut. This means that dietary TAG can be directly taken up from the circulating chylomicron particles into adipose tissue, skeletal and cardiac muscle (Figure 11.4). These tissues possess LPL. Following a fat-containing meal the amount of LPL on adipose tissue capillary endothelial cell membranes is increased (by the action of insulin). This activates the enzyme and allows hydrolysis of TAG on chylomicron particles. The particles become progressively smaller as TAG is gradually removed. Eventually the action of lipoprotein lipase on chylomicrons is terminated and the smaller particles, known as chylomicron remnants, are removed by the liver via the remnant or the LDL receptors. Whereas this is the pathway followed by most dietary fatty acids, the medium-chain and short-chain fatty acids ($\leqslant$ C12:0) pass directly to the liver in the portal vein rather than being absorbed via the lymphatic system. This is a consequence of their higher water solubility and, thus, the complex pathway for water-insoluble fatty acids is not needed. It follows that these fatty acids do not contribute to the increase in blood TAG (postprandial lipemia) that occurs following ingestion of a fat-containing meal.

Endogenous pathway

The endogenous pathway of TAG metabolism involves the hepatic synthesis, secretion and subsequent metabolism of the VLDL particles. VLDL synthesis is stimulated in the liver by increased availability of free fatty acids (FFA). Increased FFA delivery to the liver occurs either in the fed state when large amounts of FFA are being released from circulating chylomicrons, or in the fasted state, when there is breakdown of stored TAG from adipose tissue. The FFA are delivered to the liver and through the action of insulin are re-esterified to TAG. As in the enterocyte, the TAG combines with cholesterol and a specific apolipoprotein (in this case apo B-100), together with a surface coating of phospholipid and cholesterol ester, to form the mature VLDL particles. The secretion of VLDL is regulated by insulin, being inhibited by high levels of insulin and stimulated when insulin levels begin to fall. Therefore, following a meal, increased secretion of VLDL tends to occur 2–3 h after meal consumption when insulin levels are beginning to fall.

In the fasted state most of the circulating TAG-rich particles are VLDL. In the fed state after a fat-containing meal, chylomicrons begin to enter the circulation within 30 min and reach their highest concentration 2–4 h after the meal. During this time, VLDL secretion tends to be low owing to the high circulating insulin concentrations. However, as insulin falls the secretion of VLDL particles from the liver increases and these particles become the dominant postprandial TAG-rich particle in the late postprandial stage after a meal. VLDL metabolism is very similar to that outlined for chylomicrons above. VLDL particles are hydrolyzed by LPL. Hydrolysis of TAG and uptake of FFA into tissues proceeds in the same way as for chylomicrons, but VLDL appear to be a better substrate for skeletal muscle lipase than for adipose tissue. Partial removal of TAG results in the formation of the VLDL remnant (also known as IDL); complete removal leads to the formation of circulating LDL as outlined in the section above (Figure 11.2).

Blood pressure

Blood pressure is the force that causes blood to flow through the arteries and capillaries, and finally via the veins back to the heart. Blood pressure is maintained by regulation of cardiac output and peripheral resistance at the arterioles, postcapillary venules and heart. Blood pressure is regulated by central as well as peripheral neuronal mechanisms, by capillary fluid shifts and by central and local hormone secretions. The kidney also contributes to maintenance of blood pressure by regulating blood volume. The autonomic nervous system is the most rapidly responding regulator of blood pressure and receives continuous information from the baroreceptors (pressure-sensitive nerve endings) situated in the carotid sinus and the aortic arch. This information is relayed to the vasomotor center in the brainstem. A decrease in blood pressure causes activation of the sympathetic nervous system, resulting in increased contractility of the heart (via β-adrenoceptors) and vasoconstriction of both the arterial and venous side of the circulation (via α-adrenoceptors). The capillary fluid shift mechanism refers to the exchange of fluid that occurs across the capillary membrane between the blood and the interstitial fluid. This fluid movement is controlled by the capillary blood pressure, the interstitial fluid pressure and the colloid osmotic pressure of the plasma. Hormonal mechanisms operate in various ways to maintain blood pressure, including vasoconstriction, vasodilatation and alteration of blood volume. The principal hormones involved in raising blood pressure are epinephrine and norepinephrine, secreted from the adrenal medulla in response to sympathetic nervous system stimulation. They increase cardiac output and cause vasoconstriction and act very rapidly. Renin release from the kidney increases in states such as hypotension owing to both sympathetic nerve stimulation of the kidneys and a reduction in glomerular filtration. This renin stimulates the conversion of angiotensinogen to angiotensin, both in the circulation and in vascular tissue. Plasma angiotensin is converted in the lung to angiotensin II, which is a potent vasoconstrictor. In addition, angiotensin II stimulates the production of aldosterone from the adrenal cortex, which decreases urinary fluid and electrolyte (sodium) loss from the body. The kidneys help to regulate the blood pressure by increasing or decreasing the blood volume via alterations in water and sodium reabsorption in the kidney tubules, and also by the renin–angiotensin system, and are consequently the most important organs for long-term blood pressure regulation.

The vascular endothelium

Damage to the vascular endothelium appears to be the unifying pathophysiological event through which the adverse effects of raised circulating blood lipids, glucose, homocysteine and thrombotic factors result in atherosclerosis and thrombosis. The vascular endothelium should be considered as an organ regulating vascular tone through its response to, and production of, vasodilator and vasoconstrictor substances. It regulates the balance between thrombosis and fibrinolysis, and platelet aggregation, through the production of prostacyclin and other bioactive substances. The adhesion of monocytes to the endothelium is mediated in part through the presence of adhesion molecules [intercellular adhesion molecule-1 (ICAM-1), vascular cell adhesion molecule (VCAM)] on the surface of the endothelial cell. The key regulatory component of the endothelial cell is nitric oxide (NO), the production of which is central to all of the above functions. NO is formed from L-arginine by nitric oxide synthase. NO is a vasodilator, it inhibits platelet aggregation and smooth muscle cell proliferation and reduces adhesion of monocytes to the endothelium. When there is impaired endothelial function, the vasodilatory response to standard drugs is impaired; this is now used as a dynamic *in vivo* measure of endothelial dysfunction. Other meaures of endothelial dysfunction include measurement of circulating proteins that are derived from the endothelium [e.g. endothelin, von Willebrand factor (vWf), ICAM-1, VCAM and plasminogen activator inhibitor-1 (PAI-1)].

The hemostatic system

The hemostatic system coordinates a finely regulated series of reactions that occur at the surface of damaged blood vessels to reduce or terminate bleeding following tissue injury. Cessation of bleeding occurs via three overlapping pathways. First, there is adhesion and aggregation of blood platelets at the site of injury. Secondly, there is conversion of soluble protein fibrinogen to its insoluble product, the fibrin fibril, by activation of the clotting pathway and generation of the clotting enzyme, thrombin, which in turn triggers platelet activation and aggregation. Finally, the fibrin fibrils cross-link with the aid of factor XIII (FXIII), thereby 'wringing' the clot of plasma and increasing its firmness by retraction. The cessation of clot formation is achieved via activation of another pathway, the fibrinolytic pathway, which prevents excessive clot formation in response to activation of the clotting cascade.

The following sections outline the major steps involved in coagulation, platelet aggregation and fibrinolysis.

Coagulation (clotting) pathway

As shown in outline in Figure 11.5, this pathway comprises two separate activation pathways (the intrinsic and extrinsic pathways), which feed into the final common pathway leading to thrombin generation and fibrin production. Although the pathways are activated separately there are many cross-reactions between them that provide autoregulation.

- **The extrinsic and final common pathways.** The main trigger of coagulation is a protein called tissue factor, which is exposed on the blood vessel wall when there is injury. Cellular tissue factor then initiates coagulation through interactions with a circulating clotting protein called factor VII (FVII). Once FVII binds to accessible tissue factor it undergoes a single cleavage which converts it to its active enzyme, FVIIa (the 'a' suffix indicates the activated state). Cleavage is performed either by autoactivation (by FVIIa already present and bound to tissue factor) or by activated factor IX (FIXa) or activated factor X (FXa). Coagulation occurs when the initial stimulus is sufficient to cause conversion of activity in the pathway from a basal or steady state to a 'cascade' of activation. As amplification occurs at each step of the pathway, one molecule of FVIIa–tissue factor complex is responsible for many thousands of molecules of thrombin generated from prothrombin. Thus, in secondary hemostasis, FVIIa–tissue factor activates FIX and FX. Plasma FIXa, with its cofactor vWf (VIIIa), also activates FX. Plasma FXa, with its cofactor factor Va, then cleaves prothrombin to thrombin.

- **The intrinsic pathway and the contact system.** The four proteins of the contact system are factor XII (FXII), factor XI (FXI), prekallikrein (PK) and high molecular weight kininogen (HMK). The proteins play major roles in coagulation, with their activation at negatively charged surfaces leading to formation of FXIIa and FXIa. Likely activators of the intrinsic pathway include collagen (like tissue factor, collagen is exposed on blood-vessel walls on tissue damage), heparans and FFA. Surface-bound FXIa then activates FIX, and FIXa will activate FVII and FX. *In vitro* studies show long-chain saturated fatty acids such as stearate (C18) to be potent activators of the intrinsic system, while unsaturated fatty acids such as oleate are ineffective.

Platelets

Platelets are formed from the megakaryocytes of the bone marrow, each of which releases about 4000 platelets on maturation. On stimulation, platelets

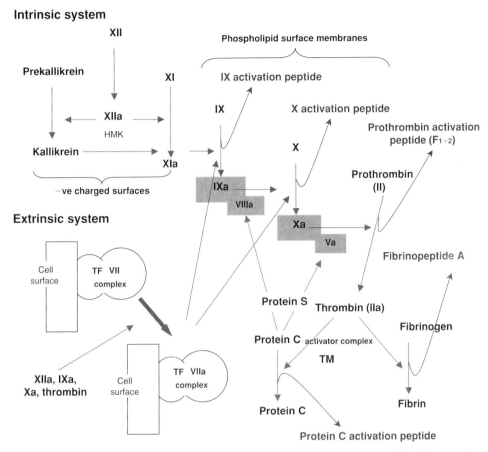

Intrinsic system

XII

Prekallikrein

XI

XIIa

HMK

Kallikrein

XIa

−ve charged surfaces

Phospholipid surface membranes

IX activation peptide

IX

X activation peptide

X

Prothrombin activation peptide (F_{1+2})

IXa

VIIIa

Xa

Va

Prothrombin (II)

Extrinsic system

Cell surface

TF VII complex

Fibrinopeptide A

XIIa, IXa, Xa, thrombin

Cell surface

TF VIIa complex

Protein S   Thrombin (IIa)

Protein C activator complex

TM

Fibrinogen

Protein C

Fibrin

Protein C activation peptide

Figure 11.5 Outline of the intrinsic and extrinsic pathways of coagulation. Exposure of blood to negatively charged non-membranous surfaces activates the intrinsic pathway. The extrinsic pathway is activated when blood comes into contact with cell membranes, exposing tissue factor (TF). The sequence of protein activations are dependent on phospholipids and take place on cell membrane surfaces. HMK: high molecular weight kininogen; TM: thrombomodulin. 'a' denotes the enzyme product of the inactive precursor protein.

form aggregates as a result of exposure, on their surface membranes, of binding sites that allow adjacent platelets to adhere to one another. The exposure of 'sticky' binding sites on the platelet comes about as the result of activation of platelet receptors by aggregating factors (thrombin, collagen), clotting factors (vWf, fibrinogen) and inhibitors. Running through the platelet is an open canalicular system of invaginated plasma membrane, thus increasing the effective platelet surface area many-fold. In the platelet interior are dense granules packed with adenosine diphosphate (ADP) and serotonin. Other granules (α-granules) contain many compounds, including platelet derived growth factor (PDGF), fibrinogen, vWf and factor V. Adhesion of platelets to the endothelium triggers intracellular signals which result in release of active compounds

(e.g. ADP) that release the contents of the granules, promote striking shape change and favor aggregation. For example, collagen binding and binding of thrombin to its platelet receptors trigger platelet synthesis of prostaglandins from membrane arachidonic acid. The product, thromboxane A_2, initiates the release reaction, thereby encouraging aggregation of activated platelets. With sustained activation, a plug of aggregated platelets incorporating fibrin and entrapped red and white blood cells results in the formation of a clot or thrombus.

Fibrinolytic pathway

The fibrinolytic pathway operates as a feedback system to prevent excessive activation of fibrinogen and regulate the extent of clot formation. The main regulatory

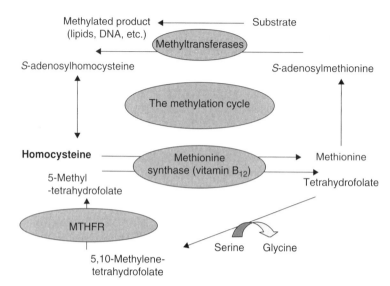

Figure 11.6 Outline of the role of homocysteine in the remethylation pathway. The vitamin B_{12}-dependent enzyme methionine synthase catalyzes the methylation of homocysteine to methionine. Conversion of methionine to S-adenosylmethionine and its subsequent demethylation to S-adenosylhomocysteine generate methyl groups essential to the synthesis of phsopholipids, DNA, etc. Further methylation of homocysteine required to sustain the remethylation pathway is through the action of methylene tetrahydrofolate reductase (MTHFR), which generates the methyl donor 5-methyltetrahydrofolate from 5,10-methylene tetrahydrolfolate. The latter is in turn dependent on the dietary supply of folic acid.

steps lead to the conversion of inactive plasminogen to the active enzyme, plasmin, which activates the breakdown of fibrin. Plasminogen activation is achieved by a number of different plasminogen activators, the most important of which is tissue plasminogen activator (tPA), the release of which from vascular endothelial cells is stimulated by a variety of agents. When a fibrin clot is evolving, tPA and plasminogen bind sequentially to fibrin, thereby providing the conditions for rapid generation of plasmin. By the lytic action of plasmin, a complex array of fibrin and fibrinogen degradation products is generated and clot formation terminated. An important regulatory component of this complex system is PAI-1, activation of which prevents conversion of plasminogen to plasmin, thereby reducing fibrinolysis.

Homocysteine

Homocysteine is a sulfur-containing amino acid found in all cells, where it plays a role in the generation of methyl groups, required for a range of essential functions, particularly in DNA synthesis. Its relevance with respect to the functioning of the cardiovascular system, is that elevated levels of homocysteine appear to cause damage to the vascular endothelium and may play a primary role in initiating the damage that leads to atherosclerosis.

Homocysteine is an intermediate in one-carbon metabolism, lying between two connected metabolic cycles (remethylation and trans-sulfuration). In the remethylation reaction (Figure 11.6), homocysteine accepts a methyl group from methyl tetrahydrofolate to form methionine. Methionine, in turn, is converted to S-adenosylmethionine (SAM), which is the main donor of methyl groups in the synthesis of DNA, proteins and phospholipids. The micronutrients folic acid and vitamin B_{12} play an important part in this cycle, folate as a component part of methyl tetrahydrofolate, and vitamin B_{12} as a cofactor for the enzyme methionine synthase, the enzyme that catalyzes the remethylation step. Another enzyme, methylene tetrahydrofolate reductase (MTHFR), plays an important role by supplying methyl tetrahydrofolate for the remethylation step.

Insulin sensitivity

Insulin is a metabolic hormone secreted by the β-cells of the pancreas in response to food ingestion. The main stimulus for insulin release is the increase in blood glucose that occurs within a few minutes of ingesting a carbohydrate-containing meal. Insulin has a wide variety of actions on cellular glucose metabolism (see Chapter 5), but its main effects are to decrease blood glucose following a meal, thereby maintaining circulating glucose concentrations within narrow normal limits (4–10 mmol/l). However, insulin also has important effects on lipid metabolism, and through its actions in stimulating hydrolysis of circulating TAGs, and uptake of the released FFAs into adipose tissue, skeletal and cardiac muscle, this hormone plays a central role in maintaining plasma TAG concentrations within normal limits during the fasted and postprandial state (0.5–4 mmol/l).

11.3 Pathogenesis of cardiovascular disease

Atherogenesis is a very complex and slowly progressive process involving several pathophysiological systems, on which both genetic and environmental factors act. This process occurs in the intima and media of large and medium-sized arteries and leads to the formation of focal lesions (plaques), which might be complicated by intraplaque hemorrhage, rupture and overimposed thrombosis that causes ischemia in the region supplied by the artery.

In the twentieth century, two major hypotheses – the thrombogenic and the lipidic – were postulated for the origin of CVD. The two theories can be unified into a single multifactorial theory involving one common step represented by endothelial dysfunction. This widely accepted theory is generally called the response to injury hypothesis and its main steps are summarized in Figure 11.7. Different risk factors (hyperlipidemia, LDL oxidation, hypertension, etc.) induce endothelial injury, leading to compensatory responses that alter the normal homeostatic functions of the endothelium. This is particularly so at certain areas of the coronary tree such as the branching points. In particular, a variety of forms of injury increase the permeability of the endothelium to lipids and proteins, and increase the adhesion to monocytes and platelets. This in turn induces the endothelium to have procoagulant instead of anticoagulant properties and to form vasoactive molecules, such as cytokines and growth factors, which promote the migration and internalization of monocytes and proliferation of vascular smooth-muscle cells. These, together with increased lipid accumulation and

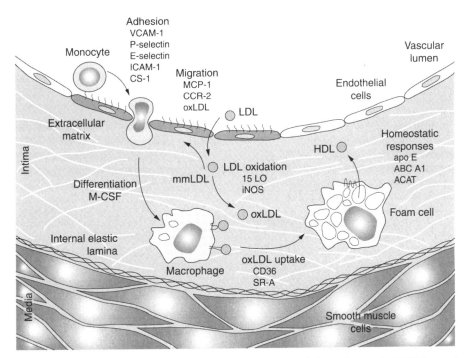

Figure 11.7 The response to injury hypothesis. LDL: low-density lipoprotein; HDL: high-density lipoprotein; VCAM-1: vascular cell adhesion molecule-1; ICAM-1: intercellular adhesion molecule-1; CS-1: connecting segment-1; MCP-1: monocyte chemoattractant protein-1; CCR-2: chemokine receptor-2; M-CSF: macrophage-chemokine stimulating factor; 15 LO: 15 lipoxygenase; iNOS: inducible nitric oxide synthatase; apoE: apolipoprotein E; MMLDL: minimally modified LDL: ABC A1: ATP binding cassette A1; ACAT: acylcholesterol acyltransferase; SR-A: scavenger receptor A. Reproduced from Glass and Witztum (2001) with permission of Elsevier Science.

Table 11.2 Risk factors for cardiovascular diseases

Untreatable	Potentially treatable
Men	Cigarette smoking
Age >45 years for men, after menopause for women	Dyslipidemia: increased cholesterol, triacylglycerol, low-density and very low-density lipoproteins levels, decreased high-density lipoprotein levels
Genetic traits	Oxidability of low-density lipoproteins
	Obesity, especially central obesity
Psychosocial	Hypertension
Low socio-economic class	Hyperglycemia, diabetes and thematabolic syndrome
Stressful situations	Prothrombotic factors
Coronary-prone behaviour patterns, type A behavior	High homocysteine levels

increased connective tissue synthesis, lead to the formation of atheromas. If the atherogenic process continues, there will be cycles of accumulation and activation of mononuclear cells, migration and proliferation of smooth-muscle cells with cell necrosis and formation of fibrous tissue, which eventually lead to the formation of advanced lesions, the fibrous atheromas. Fibroatheromas grow slowly and can induce arterial stenosis, but often represent an unstable lesion that can be complicated by intraplaque hemorrhage and rupture. Plaque rupture is followed by blood entry into the plaque core from the lumen, with activation of platelets and the coagulation cascade. This leads to the formation of a thrombus, which can cause acute ischemia. The primary cause of arterial thrombosis involves tissue factors, which are present in normal adventitia and atherosclerotic plaques and which, as mentioned in the previous sections, are able to initiate the extrinsic clotting cascade. The general hypercoagulable or prothrombotic state of subjects with atherosclerosis is of great importance in the final stages leading to myocardial infarction or stroke. As a consequence, these individuals have increased plasma levels of clotting factors (fibrinogen, factor VII, vWf), enhanced platelet reactivity and reduced fibrinolysis.

When the arterial lumen is significantly narrowed or closed following the progressive increase in arterial stenosis or, more frequently, the formation of thrombus, atherosclerosis becomes clinically manifest: depending on the arteries involved in this process, the individual will suffer from myocardial or cerebral infarction, peripheral vascular disease or mesenteric ischemia. The progression of the atherosclerotic lesions throughout life is highly variable, partly because of the presence and severity of different cardiovascular risk factors.

Cardiovascular risk factors

The term cardiovascular risk factor is used to identify factors predicting an increased likelihood of developing CVD. Many of these factors have been identified (Table 11.2); some of these factors are modifiable (lifestyle, e.g. diet, exercise and smoking), while others are not (gender, age and genetic traits). The following section will focus on the main cardiovascular risk factors and their normal physiology and metabolism. Section 11.5 will consider the extent to which specific nutrients influence the functioning of these risk factors.

11.4 Risk factors for cardiovascular disease

Plasma cholesterol and cardiovascular disease risk

Increased plasma cholesterol levels, particularly LDL cholesterol, are undoubtedly one of the most important risk factors for CVD. This is true not only for very high cholesterol levels, such as those occurring in genetically determined lipid disorders (familial hypercholesterolemia, familial combined hyperlipidemia, type III hyperlipidemia), but also in a large majority of people (about half the adult population in high-risk countries) with only moderately high plasma cholesterol levels. Familial hypercholesterolemia is a rare genetic condition caused by a defect in the gene that codes for the LDL receptor. Homozygous individuals have no LDL receptors, while heterozygotes have half the normal number of LDL receptors. Because the hepatic LDL receptors are reduced in number or absent, these individuals cannot regulate their circulating LDL levels and develop extremely high plasma LDL cholesterol concentrations at a very young age. However, in most individuals raised levels of LDL cholesterol are determined by an interaction between genetically transmitted, but relatively minor, metabolic abnormalities (often multiple genes are involved) and lifestyle-related factors (polygenic or common hypercholesterolemia). All the cross-sectional and prospective studies on this topic have clearly shown that the association between plasma total cholesterol levels and coronary heart disease (CHD) mortality is very strong, is independent of other risk factors, and is characterized by increased risk with increasing plasma cholesterol concentrations, starting even at 'low' cholesterol levels. The causal relationship with atherosclerosis has also been proven by the fact that interventions that reduce total and LDL cholesterol have significantly reduced total and CHD mortality.

Although the concentration of LDL in the circulation is important in determining its uptake into the endothelium, other factors, including the oxidative modification of LDL in the arterial wall, appear to be just as important. LDL particles are taken up by macrophages, especially after being oxidized or otherwise modified, and may be then deposited in the arterial intima, thus leading to the formation of atheroma. Thus, oxidation and other modifications of LDL seem to play an important role within the pathogenic mechanisms of atherosclerosis. The dietary relevance of oxidized LDL is clear, since the capacity of LDL to resist oxidation is dependent on the type of fatty acids present and the antioxidant content of the particle.

High-density lipoprotein cholesterol and cardiovascular disease risk

The inverse association between HDL cholesterol levels and incidence of CVD has so far been confirmed by many cross-sectional and prospective studies. Low HDL levels are now considered a strong risk factor for CVD and the LDL:HDL cholesterol ratio a much stronger predictor of risk than an elevated LDL cholesterol level alone. However, it should be stated that low HDL levels often occur along with moderately raised plasma TAG and, indeed, a low HDL level may be a marker for the presence of the metabolic syndrome or syndrome X. This is a syndrome that is characterized by a collection of abnormalities, including raised blood glucose, raised TAG, low HDL, an increased proportion of small, dense LDL and raised blood pressure. The underlying cause of the abnormalities

appears to be insulin resistance, whereby increased secretion of insulin fails to return circulating glucose and TAG to normal concentrations owing to resistance to the actions of insulin in peripheral cells and the liver (see Chapter 16).

A clear identification of the mechanisms through which HDL protect from CVD is lacking, although it is clear from the account of the role of HDL in maintaining normal reverse cholesterol transport (Section 11.2) that reduced circulating levels of HDL will have severely compromised the ability to maintain cellular and circulating cholesterol homeostasis. In particular, there will be reduced ability to remove excess cholesterol from cells. This will lead to accumulation of cholesterol in peripheral cells, leading to down-regulation of LDL receptors on cell membranes, thereby reducing the rate of uptake of LDL from the circulation. There is also evidence that HDL acts as an antioxidant and protects LDL from oxidation.

Plasma triacylglycerol and cardiovascular disease risk

Many studies have shown an association between high levels of plasma TAG and CVD. However, what has been disputed over the years is whether hypertriacylglycerolemia represents a risk factor independent of other factors that are often associated with it (obesity, hyperglycemia, low HDL cholesterol levels, hypertension, abnormalities in coagulation factors). The role of TAGs as an independent risk factor seems more consistent in people with diabetes. Moreover, in cross-sectional and prospective studies, higher levels of TAGs and chylomicron remnants in the postprandial period have been found to be associated with higher risk of CHD. Recently published intervention trials have clearly shown that hypertriacylglycerolemia is indeed an important modifiable risk factor. There are a number of mechanisms by which elevated plasma TAG may lead to an increased risk of CVD. Some studies have shown that chylomicron and VLDL remnants that are enriched with cholesterol can be taken up by monocytes in a similar manner to LDL and form the characteristic foam cell of the atherosclerotic lesion. However, elevated TAG levels have also been shown to lead to adverse changes in LDL and HDL cholesterol via excessive transfer of TAG onto the HDL and LDL particles via the CETP-catalyzed reaction (Figure 11.3). When LDL and HDL acquire large amounts of TAG from the

TAG-rich lipoproteins, the TAG undergoes hydrolysis by the hepatic lipase. Removal of TAG from LDL and HDL leads to the formation of small, dense LDL and HDL particles. Small, dense HDL particles are rapidly catabolized by the liver, leading to reductions in circulating HDL concentrations. Conversely, small dense LDL is poorly recognized by the normal LDL receptor and remains in the circulation longer than normal. Because of its smaller size and longer half-life, small, dense LDL is more able to penetrate the endothelium and contribute to atherogenesis.

Many studies have shown raised levels of TAG, small, dense LDL and lowered levels of HDL in type II diabetes and in subjects with insulin resistance. These abnormalities in lipoprotein concentration and composition are likely to be the one of the main causes of the greater risk of CVD that is associated with these conditions. The atherogenic consequences of raised plasma TAG therefore include: direct atherogenic effects of chylomicron and VLDL remnant particles, reduced levels of HDL and raised levels of the atherogenic small, dense LDL. In addition to these atherogenic actions, raised TAG, particularly in the postprandial state, may be prothrombotic since it has been shown to lead to the activation of factor VII, part of the extrinsic pathway of blood clotting.

Blood pressure and cardiovascular disease risk

High blood pressure is a reversible risk factor for CVD for which a strong causal relationship has clearly been found. The positive relationship between both systolic and diastolic blood pressure and CVD are found not only among hypertensive individuals but also among those considered to be normotensive. Studies have suggested that even small reductions in blood pressure can have large beneficial effects on the risk of CVD. The relation of blood pressure to CVD risk is important with respect to potential preventive nutritional strategies, since high blood pressure is one of the 'deadly quartet' of obesity, hyperlipidemia, hypertension and hyperinsulinemia, that make up the metabolic syndrome or syndrome X. This syndrome has repeatedly been linked with modern lifestyles characterized by high levels of stress, inappropriate diets and lack of exercise. The well-known roles of ions such as sodium, potassium, calcium, magnesium and chloride in regulating blood volume, vascular tone and membrane ion-channel activity also indicate the potential role of micronutrients as well as macronutrients in blood-pressure regulation.

Endothelial dysfunction and cardiovascular disease risk

Because endothelial dysfunction is an important early step in atherogenesis, measurement of endothelial function *in vivo* is being studied as a means of risk assessment. Some of the early studies indicate that these new measurements may prove useful in identifying subjects at risk of CVD, but it is not yet known whether they will prove to be more valuable than the conventional risk factors such as serum cholesterol and blood pressure which are currently used.

Homocysteine and cardiovascular disease risk

Very high homocysteine levels, due to inborn errors of the metabolism of this amino acid, cause severe atherosclerosis with clinical manifestations at a very early age. However, the importance of more moderately raised levels of homocysteine as a risk factor for CVD remains uncertain. Although retrospective epidemiological studies have suggested a strong association between raised homocysteine and CVD risk, recent prospective studies suggest that the risk may be smaller. The issue is important for the dietary prevention of CVD since moderate hyperhomocysteinemia is due in part to inadequate dietary intake of folic acid and vitamins B_6 and B_{12}. The adverse effects of low folate intakes appear to be particularly important for those individuals (30% of most populations) who carry a variant form of the MTHFR enzyme and who demonstrate elevated homocysteine levels. The exact mechanism by which elevated homocysteine levels may cause vascular disease are uncertain but may involve disruption of normal endothelial physiology. The endothelial dysfunction leads to multiple biological effects as described above, including abnormal vasoconstriction, platelet aggregation, monocyte adhesion and procoagulation.

Coagulation, platelets and fibrinolytic factors and cardiovascular disease risk

Prospective epidemiological studies have shown that raised concentrations of specific clotting and fibrinolytic factors are predictive of CHD. Plasma FVIIc has been found to be a marker of risk of fatal, but not non-fatal, CVD. Many studies have found plasma fibrinogen concentration to be a strongly positive predictor of CHD, and vWf has also been shown to be an independent risk factor in a number of studies. Elevated levels of these clotting factors in people at risk of CVD are believed to reflect a prothrombotic state that could contribute to their increased risk. In the fibrinolytic system, both tPA and PAI-1 are positive risk factors for CHD. Both are believed to be markers of hypofibrinolysis.

Although the platelet plays a central role in thrombosis, and platelet hyperactivation is believed to be one of the mechanisms involved in inducing a prothrombotic state, platelet hyperreactivity is not established as a strong risk factor, largely because of difficulties in carrying out measurements of platelet aggregability *in vitro*.

11.5 Dietary components and their effect on plasma lipids

Cholesterol levels

The effects of different dietary components on plasma cholesterol levels have been studied for many years, so a large body of data exists in the literature on the effect of different types of dietary fatty acids on plasma cholesterol (Table 11.3). However, many of these studies, especially the older ones, have only taken into account the effects of diet on total plasma cholesterol, without differentiating between the cholesterol present in LDL and that present in HDL. This is of fundamental importance, as indicated in the previous section, since the two lipoproteins have opposite effects on CVD.

Saturated fatty acids

Epidemiological studies have consistently shown that the intake of saturated fatty acids is directly correlated with plasma cholesterol levels and with mortality from coronary artery disease. All the intervention studies performed on humans since the early 1950s have shown that saturated fatty acids are the key dietary factor responsible for increased plasma cholesterol, and that this effect is largely due to increased LDL cholesterol. Although the increase in LDL cholesterol during high saturated fat diets is greater in subjects with higher baseline cholesterol levels, it is still of significance even in normocholesterolemic individuals.

Recently there has been increased emphasis on the possible difference between the individual saturated fatty acids and plasma cholesterol fractions. Among the saturated fatty acids, the most hypercholesterolemic are

Table 11.3 Effects of different dietary components on low-density lipoprotein (LDL) cholesterol

Nutrients	Effect on LDL cholesterol
Saturated fatty acids	↑↑
Trans-fatty acids	↑↑
Dietary cholesterol	↑
Plant sterols	↓
MUFA	↓
n-6 PUFA	↓
n-3 PUFA	↑
Soy protein	↓
Carbohydrate	−
Fiber	↓↓
Alcohol	−

↑: increase; ↓: decrease; −: no effect.
MUFA: monounsaturated fatty acid; PUFA: polyunsaturated fatty acid.

C14:0 (myristic acid) and C16:0 (palmitic acid), while stearic acid (C18:0) appears to be neutral, or even hypocholesterolemic. However, this evidence is based on a limited number of studies and requires further research before conclusions can be drawn and recommendations made. The ability of saturated fatty acids to raise LDL cholesterol levels appears to be due to the effect of these fatty acids in regulating the expression of the LDL receptor on hepatic cell membranes. When levels of these fatty acids in hepatic cell membranes is high there is down-regulation of the LDL receptor protein and thus a reduced rate of removal of LDL from the circulation.

Unsaturated fatty acids

In the past 30 years, many intervention studies have been performed to investigate the possible hypocholesterolemic effect of the unsaturated fatty acids [monounsaturated fatty acids (MUFA) and n-6 polyunsaturated fatty acids (PUFA)]. From the results of these studies some definite conclusions can be drawn. Both MUFA and PUFA are able to reduce total and, in particular, LDL cholesterol. It is now possible to derive equations that predict the hypocholesterolemic effect of MUFA or n-6 PUFA. According to these equations, if 10% of the dietary energy derived from SFA were replaced by MUFA or n-6 PUFA, LDL cholesterol would decrease by 0.39 mmol/l (15 mg/dl) and by 0.42 mmol/l (18 mg/dl), respectively. Therefore, the effects of MUFA and PUFA on LDL cholesterol are quite similar.

In relation to the effects of long-chain n-3 PUFA on LDL cholesterol, a review of all the controlled studies performed clearly showed that doses of approximately 3 g/day of n-3 PUFA given as supplements increase LDL cholesterol by 5–10%, especially in hypertriacyl-glycerolemic patients. These responses have also been reported in healthy people and may be more common in certain susceptible genotypes. These reported LDL-raising effects of n-3 PUFA have been observed with fish oil supplements but not with fish. Nevertheless, whether intakes of the long-chain n-3 PUFA are increased via fish or fish oils, pronounced cardiovascular benefits of modest increases in intakes of long-chain n-3 PUFA have been observed in secondary prevention trials. Two recent studies have shown that intakes of approximately 1 g/day of long-chain n-3 PUFA reduce the rate of cardiovascular mortality by 30–45%. In both studies there were very limited effects on plasma lipid levels and the decreased risk of cardiovascular mortality was probably due to the beneficial influence of n-3 PUFA on thrombosis or on cardiac arrhythmias.

Unlike saturated fatty acids, which cause down-regulation of the LDL receptor and reduced rates of LDL removal from the circulation, unsaturated fatty acids increase the expression of the LDL receptor protein, causing a greater rate of removal of LDL from the circulation. In this respect, unsaturated fatty acids act like the statin drugs which lower LDL cholesterol through their actions on genes that regulate hepatic lipid metabolism. These drugs reduce rates of hepatic cholesterol synthesis and increase rates of LDL removal from the circulation by up-regulation of the LDL receptor.

Trans-fatty acids

Trans-unsaturated fatty acids are produced in the rumen during ruminant fermentation and are therefore found in meat and dairy products. They are also produced commercially in large quantities by partial hydrogenation of vegetable oil in the preparation of shortening and margarine.

All the metabolic studies on trans-fatty acids have clearly shown that they significantly increase LDL cholesterol levels (replacing 10% of dietary energy derived from oleic acid with trans-fatty acids induces an average LDL cholesterol increase of about 0.37 mmol/l) and, contrary to what happens with saturated fatty acids, trans-fatty acids also reduce HDL cholesterol levels. These two opposite effects imply an increase in the LDL:HDL cholesterol ratio (Table 11.3), with major

effects increasing the risk of CHD, as reported by both cross-sectional and prospective studies.

Dietary cholesterol

Prospective studies have shown a positive significant correlation between cholesterol intake and CHD mortality, which is partly independent of plasma cholesterol levels. Several intervention studies on humans have evaluated the effects of dietary cholesterol on lipid metabolism, and the most consistent results on LDL levels can be summarized as follows.

There is great variability among individuals. Some people are able to reduce their endogenous cholesterol synthesis in response to an increase in cholesterol intake, without changing their levels of LDL cholesterol (the 'compensators'). Others do not have this ability and their plasma cholesterol levels increase after a cholesterol-rich diet (the 'non-compensators'). Unfortunately, there are no simple markers, clinical or otherwise, that allow these two types of individuals to be differentiated. Moreover, for very high levels of dietary cholesterol (>850–1000 mg/day), the ability of compensators to maintain normal plasma cholesterol levels may be overcome.

In practice, high levels of dietary cholesterol are generally associated with high levels of saturated fat and often the more powerful effect of the latter is dominant. The increase in LDL cholesterol in response to a diet high in cholesterol is usually more consistent in high-risk individuals, such as hyperlipidemic and diabetic patients.

Carbohydrates and dietary fiber

Carbohydrates do not have a direct and independent effect on LDL cholesterol and, therefore, it can be said that they are 'neutral' in this respect. However, foods rich in carbohydrates represent one of the easiest ways to replace saturated fats and are thus very important for practical reasons. On the other hand, dietary fiber, which is naturally present particularly in carbohydrate-rich foods, has a direct hypocholesterolemic effect. In fact, the studies performed either with diets naturally rich in fiber, especially soluble fiber, or with different types of fiber added to foods (guar, psyllium, oats, etc.) have consistently shown that dietary fiber per se, independently of other dietary changes, is able to reduce LDL cholesterol. This effect is present in healthy people, patients with hyperlipidemia and those with diabetes, and is still more evident in patients with both hyperlipidemia and diabetes.

Proteins

In the context of dietary proteins and lipid metabolism, a brief mention of soy protein is merited. A meta-analysis on this topic has indicated that soy protein is effective in lowering LDL cholesterol in hypercholesterolemic subjects, while this effect is much more variable in those with normal lipid values.

Dietary composition and plasma triacylglycerol levels

Fatty acids

Among the fatty acids, the most important relevant hypotriacylglycerolemic effect is observed with the long-chain n-3 fatty acids. In fact, supplementation with long-chain n-3 fatty acids (even by as little as 2–3 g/day) can reduce TAG levels by 25–30% in both normolipidemic and hyperlipidemic individuals. The precursor n-3 fatty acid (α-linolenic acid, present in some plants and oils) has not been observed to alter plasma TAG levels, except when very high intake levels (>40 g/day) have been used; recent studies have supported the view that α-linolenic acid may not have comparable TAG-lowering effects to the long-chain n-3 PUFA. Long-chain n-3 fatty acids have also been reported to reduce the postprandial lipemic response, with a reduction particularly in chylomicron and chylomicron remnants. The effects of the other fatty acids on postprandial lipemia are less well defined. Chronic and acute ingestion of food enriched with saturated fat produces enhanced postprandial lipemia in comparison with MUFA and n-6 PUFA. Only a few studies have compared these two types of fatty acid (MUFA versus n-6 PUFA) on postprandial lipemia, and their results are variable.

Carbohydrates

The majority of intervention studies that have examined the effect of high-carbohydrate, low-fat diets on plasma TAG levels have shown that such diets lead to an elevation of plasma TAG. This is accompanied by a fall in plasma HDL levels and an increase in the percentage of LDL as small, dense particles. It is important to note that whereas the majority of studies have recorded these effects, not all have done so. It is also important to note that these effects occur with diets varying in the ratio of simple to complex carbohydrates. These potentially adverse effects of high-carbohydrate, low-fat diets have led many eminent nutritionists to advocate a more vigorous pursuit of

Table 11.4 Effects of different dietary components on plasma triacylglycerol (TAG)

	Fasting TAG	Postprandial TAG
Saturated fatty acids	–	↑
MUFA	↓	?
n-6 PUFA	↓	?
n-3 PUFA	↓↓	↓
Carbohydrate	↑	?
Fiber	– or ↓	?
Alcohol	↑	↑

↑: increase; ↓: decrease; – : no effect; ?: no sound data.
MUFA: monounsaturated fatty acid; PUFA: polyunsaturated fatty acid.

Table 11.5 Effects of different dietary components on high-density lipoprotein (HDL) cholesterol

Nutrients	Effect on HDL cholesterol
Saturated fatty acids	↑
Dietary cholesterol	– or ↑
MUFA	–
Trans-fatty acids	↓
n-6 PUFA	↓
n-3 PUFA	–
Carbohydrate	– or ↓
Fiber	–
Alcohol	↑

↑: increase; ↓: decrease; –: no effect.
MUFA: monounsaturated fatty acid; PUFA: polyunsaturated fatty acid.

changing the composition of the dietary fat, while paying less attention to changing total fat level. However, the potential adverse effects of low-fat, high-carbohydrate diets should be seen in the wider context of public health nutrition strategies to reduce CVD. An increase in physical activity, a reduction in body-fat content and increased intake of long-chain n-3 PUFA will all lead to reduced TAG levels and increased HDL levels, thus overcoming the effect observed in narrow, single-factor intervention studies. No doubt, this area will be one to watch for the future. The data on dietary effects on TAG are summarized in Table 11.4.

Diet and high-density lipoprotein cholesterol levels

In comparison with effects of diet on LDL cholesterol, less is known of the influence of dietary components on HDL cholesterol, since little attention has been paid to this powerful cardiovascular risk factor until recently (Table 11.5).

Fatty acids

Saturated fatty acids, considered as a group or as individual fatty acids, do not reduce HDL cholesterol and most studies show that saturated fats increase this cholesterol fraction. However, these data have to be seen in the context of the very deleterious effects of saturated fatty acids on LDL cholesterol. In contrast, *trans*-fatty acids have a combined negative effect on both LDL and HDL cholesterol, since they increase the former and reduce the latter.

MUFA and n-6 PUFA have almost comparable effects on HDL cholesterol, based on studies in which moderate amounts of PUFA have been used (<10% of total energy intake). In fact, with higher levels of PUFA in the diet (>10%, an amount no longer recommended because of a putative effect on carcinogenesis and gallstones), reductions in HDL cholesterol have been observed. Finally, n-3 fatty acids, both long and short chain, do not seem to have significant and relevant effects on HDL cholesterol levels.

Carbohydrate and fiber

In contrast to what happens with plasma TAG levels, the effects of dietary carbohydrate on HDL cholesterol levels are quite variable. However, in general, the isocaloric replacement of dietary fat with carbohydrate leads to a reduction in HDL. This probably depends on the type of carbohydrate (carbohydrate with high glycemic index versus carbohydrate with low glycemic index). In support of this observation, a prospective study in a middle-aged population has recently shown that the only independent determinant of lower HDL cholesterol levels is the higher glycemic index of foods consumed. In this context, dietary fiber does not seem to influence HDL cholesterol directly, but only indirectly through its effect on the glycemic index of the foods.

Alcohol and plasma lipids

The effects of alcohol on plasma lipids are quite contradictory. On the one hand, alcohol increases plasma TAG levels (a negative effect). On the other, it increases HDL cholesterol levels (a positive effect). The latter effect seems to be one of the possible mechanisms accounting, at least in part, for the protective effect of moderate alcohol consumption on the risk of CHD that has been shown in many epidemiological studies.

Therefore, taking into account the energy intake deriving from alcohol and its possible influence on hypertriacylglycerolemia and overweight, a moderate

Table 11.6 Nutritional recommendations for the treatment of hyperlipidemia

Saturated fat	<7% of total calories
Monounsaturated fat	15–20% of total calories
Polyunsaturated fat	≤10% of total calories
Total fat	30–35% of total calories
Cholesterol	<200 mg/day
Carbohydrate	50–60% of total calories
Fiber	30 g/day
Protein	≈15% of total calories
Total calories[a]	Balanced between energy intake and expenditure to maintain body weight/prevent weight gain

National Cholesterol Education Programme (NCEP), Adult Panel Treatment III. The National Heart, Lung and Blood Institute.

[a] Daily energy expenditure should include at least moderate physical activity, contributing approximately 200 kcal/day.

consumption of alcohol (two or three drinks/day) may have beneficial effects by means of the increased HDL levels that it causes.

Nutritional recommendations for the treatment of hyperlipidemia are summarized in Table 11.6.

11.6 Diet and blood pressure

Hypertension is one of the major cardiovascular risk factors, and many intervention studies have clearly shown that reducing blood pressure leads to a significant reduction in the incidence of CHD, congestive heart failure, stroke and renal disease, as well as mortality rate.

The prevalence of hypertension in Western countries is very high, with about 50–60% of individuals above 55 years being classified as hypertensive (systolic/ diastolic blood pressure > 140/90). Although genetic factors play a significant role in determining who will become hypertensive, lifestyle factors contribute strongly to the high prevalence of hypertension. This section will focus on the possible role of micronutrients and macronutrients on blood pressure regulation.

Dietary macronutrient composition and blood pressure

Fat, particularly the type of fat rather than the total amount consumed, seems to be the most important macronutrient in relation to blood pressure regulation. All of the available evidence (cross-sectional studies and controlled clinical trials) fails to support any relationship between average total fat intake and average blood pressure. However, there is evidence that n-3 PUFA and MUFA have some influence on blood pressure. Supplementation with n-3 fatty acids reduces blood pressure in hypertensive subjects but not in normotensive ones. For significant effects to occur, doses above 3.3 g/day are needed, and this intake can only be achieved through n-3 fatty acid supplementation.

Data on MUFA are somewhat contradictory, as some show a blood pressure reduction in both hypertensive and normotensive individuals, and others no effect. However, a recent multicenter intervention trial has shown a significant reduction of systolic and diastolic blood pressure (an average of 3 mmHg) in healthy normotensive people when moderate amounts of saturated fat were replaced with monounsaturated fat.

There are various possible explanations for the blood pressure-modulating effects induced by the different types of fat: the incorporation of unsaturated fat into lipid cell membranes increases the membrane permeability, thereby stimulating sodium and cation transport, Increased synthesis of related prostaglandins, with a possible influence on factors such as arterial vasodilatation, electrolyte balance and renal renin secretion, may also play a role.

Findings of a relationship between other macronutrients (carbohydrate, dietary fiber, protein) and blood pressure are inconsistent.

Alcohol and blood pressure

All of the available evidence shows that there is a significant direct relationship between alcohol intake and blood pressure, with an increase especially for intakes above three or four drinks per day. As a reduction in alcohol intake improves blood pressure, the recommendation for the management of hypertension is to limit daily alcohol intake to no more than 30 ml for men and 15 ml for women.

Minerals and blood pressure

Sodium intake

Epidemiological studies have shown a positive association between dietary salt intake, blood-pressure levels and the prevalence of hypertension. Most intervention trials indicate that a reduction in salt intake significantly reduces both systolic and diastolic blood pressure. This effect is more evident in hypertensive, diabetic, obese and elderly subjects, and in certain populations such as African–Americans, while it is less evident in normotensive people. Some studies in normotensive people failed to find a significant reduction in diastolic blood pressure, but it is important to remember that the response to salt intake reduction is highly variable among individuals and this different response may be modulated by genetic factors. Considering all the available evidence, the recommendations are to reduce sodium intake to no more than 100 mmol/day (approximately 6 g of sodium chloride or 2.4 g/day of sodium).

Potassium intake

Epidemiological studies show an inverse correlation between blood-pressure levels and potassium intake. Almost all of the intervention trials performed have shown a significant reduction in systolic and diastolic blood pressure with potassium supplementation. Again, as for salt, this effect is more evident in hypertensive than in normotensive people and in studies where participants were accustomed to high salt intake. Potassium may act on blood-pressure regulation through its natriuretic effect or its possible effect on vascular smooth-muscle cells.

Calcium intake

Calcium supplementation has not been shown to have a significant effect on blood-pressure reduction in subjects with adequate calcium intake.

Multiple dietary changes and recommendations

Since a variety of macronutrients and micronutrients is involved in the regulation of blood pressure, it is likely that a 'combination diet' that includes changes in overall dietary habits could have a more powerful effect on blood pressure than the modulation of individual dietary constituents. This hypothesis has been established by the DASH Study (Dietary Approaches to Stop Hypertension), where a diet rich in fruit and vegetables (to increase potassium and fiber intake), low in saturated and total fat, and rich in low-fat dairy products (to increase calcium intake) was able to decrease significantly systolic and diastolic blood pressure, compared with a 'Western' diet, in both normotensive and mildly hypertensive individuals. It has been shown that if these combined diets also include a reduction in salt intake, systolic and diastolic blood pressure can be reduced even further.

11.7 Effects of dietary factors on coagulation and fibrinolysis

While it is probable that diet interacts with both coagulation and fibrinolysis, the exact nature of this is not yet completely understood. Much of the information in relation to the effect of dietary factors on coagulation and fibrinolysis derives from animal studies and epidemiological observations. To date, few properly controlled human dietary intervention studies have examined the effect of dietary components on hemostasis. Many of the human studies provide conflicting results. These divergent results probably reflect the fact that many studies have used different biochemical indices to measure coagulation and fibrinolysis. In addition, the assays used to measure coagulation and fibrinolysis are rather crude and it is unlikely that they reflect the true state *in vivo*. For example, platelet aggregation is often measured in platelet-rich plasma, but *in vivo* platelet aggregation is a very complex process that represents the interaction of the platelet with several other components of the blood and the vascular endothelium. The effect of dietary fat on coagulation and fibrinolysis has been widely studied, but there is little consistent information in relation to the effects of other nutrients and non-nutritive food components. Dietary intervention studies show that dietary fatty acids have a minimal effect on plasma fibrinogen levels. It has been shown that very high intake of saturated fat, particularly stearic acid, induces a modest increase in plasma fibrinogen concentrations, but the biological significance of this effect is questionable. Epidemiological studies have shown a negative relationship between plasma fibrinogen and n-3 PUFA intake. Several intervention studies investigated the potential effects of increasing dietary n-3 PUFA in lowering fibrinogen levels, but the results have been inconsistent.

In contrast, several epidemiological and human intervention studies have shown a consistent effect of dietary fat on coagulation factor VII. The level and activity of factor VII are affected by the amount of dietary fat consumed. It is reduced by low-fat diets and increased when high-fat diets are consumed. Factor VII activity is also related to postprandial lipid metabolism, whereby it is activated during the postprandial state following the ingestion of a meal containing fat. This effect is probably related to the presence of greater levels of TAG-rich lipoproteins (chylomicrons and VLDL), which provide a surface capable of activating the protein. Dietary fatty acid composition may also affect factor VII activity. Although short-term experiments show little effect, there is evidence from longer human dietary intervention studies that habitual high intakes of saturated fat increase factor VII, compared with monounsaturated fat. There is considerable variability in terms of how studies have measured factor VII, and not all assays reflect the true state *in vivo*. Factor VII assays can measure the amount of the protein or the activation status; the latter is probably more relevant since it is only the active proportion of factor VII that contributes to coagulation.

Fibrinolysis is influenced by dietary factors, and in particular by dietary fat. tPA is a major initiator of fibrinolysis in the normal circulation. It binds to the fibrin in a clot and promotes the generation of plasmin, which promotes clot dissolution. tPA activity is increased by a low-fat, high-fiber diet. In general, dietary fat composition does not have a major influence on tPA activity. Conversely, dietary fat composition has important effects on PAI-1. PAI-1 is increased by a high intake of n-3 PUFA and decreased when the diet is rich in oleic acid. PAI-1 activity is also increased by dietary carbohydrate intake, moreso if the carbohydrate-rich foods have a high glycemic index.

Platelets are important contributors to both coagulation and fibrinolysis. Platelet procoagulant activity, also called platelet factor 3, is closely related to platelet aggregation. Dietary fatty acid composition can have significant effects on platelet membrane fatty acid composition. For example, n-3 PUFA supplementation will lead to a significant increase in platelet phospholipid eicosapenatoic and docosahexaenoic acids levels. There is no doubt that altered platelet membrane fatty acid composition affects the activation of coagulation and fibrinolysis, nevertheless the exact nature of this is not fully understood. However, there is some evidence that saturated fatty acids promote a prothrombotic state. Again, the true nature of this effect is unknown because it is very difficult to measure platelet activity *ex vivo* in a manner that accurately reflects the *in vivo* situation.

11.8 Homocysteine

Homocysteine is a central metabolic intermediate in the metabolism of sulfur-containing amino acids. Homocysteine, which is formed as a result of the breakdown of dietary methionine, can be converted to either methionine (by the remethylation pathway) or cysteine (by the trans-sulfuration pathway) (Figure 11.6). These pathways are dependent on up to four B-vitamins: folate, vitamin B_{12}, vitamin B_6 and riboflavin. In recent years, evidence has been accumulating implicating elevated plasma homocysteine (hyperhomocysteinemia) as an independent risk factor for occlusive CVD.

The causes of hyperhomocysteinemia are both nutritional and genetic. In the extreme, patients with rare inborn errors of metabolism that impair trans-sulfuration (cystathionine β-synthetase deficiency) have profoundly elevated homocysteine in plasma and urine (homocysteinuria), and develop occlusive vascular disease in early adulthood or even childhood. Although such inborn errors are extremely rare, genetically inherited functional variants of the enzymes involved in homocysteine metabolism are commonly found in the general population, and are associated with mild to moderate elevations in homocysteine. However, the most common cause of elevated homocysteine is low status of one or more of the B-vitamins associated with its metabolism.

Vitamin therapy with folic acid, alone or in combination with vitamins B_6 and B_{12}, and dietary supplementation with cereal products fortified with these vitamins, can significantly lower plasma homocysteine levels. As a consequence of the introduction of a mandatory folic acid fortification policy in the USA, plasma homocysteine levels in the population have declined considerably in recent years.

Although, as yet, there is no conclusive evidence to show that lowering homocysteine reduces vascular disease, the case for homocysteine being implicated in CVD is very plausible and ongoing intervention trials will provide important information in this respect. Thus, from a public health viewpoint, it is important to identify modifiable factors, such as low or suboptimal status of the relevant B-vitamins, which may be particularly important in preventing homocysteine accumulation in the face of genetic predisposition to elevated plasma homocysteine levels.

11.9 Diet and antioxidant function

As a by-product of oxygen metabolism and transport, the cells of human body produce oxidants – reactive oxygen species (ROS) – that damage biological macromolecules such as DNA, proteins, lipids and carbohydrates. However, cells also contain complex defense systems against the actions of ROS, comprising different antioxidants, some of endogenous origin (superoxide dismutases to remove the superoxide anion, enzymes for removing hydrogen peroxide and organic peroxides, such as glutathione peroxidase), and some derive from the diet (e.g. vitamins C and E, β-carotene). In general, there is a balance between oxidant production and antioxidant defense: the imbalance between the two induces 'oxidative stress', which is now considered to be a very important process in the development of atherosclerosis. Oxidized LDL, more than native LDL, is involved in several steps of atherosclerosis, such as endothelial injury, monocyte chemotaxis, perturbation of vascular tone, growth factor synthesis and antibody formation. Moreover, aside from LDL oxidation, oxidative stress could be important in the development of atherosclerosis through other mechanisms, such as activation or repression of gene expression, apoptosis and cell death. Lipoprotein oxidation, in particular the susceptibility of LDL to oxidation, may be influenced also by the type of the diet, in particular by the type of fats. The few studies performed on this topic have shown that a diet rich in n-6 polyunsaturated fat increases *ex vivo* LDL oxidation in comparison to monounsaturated fat, which is more stable and, therefore, less liable to be oxidized. The few data on the effect of n-3 polyunsaturated fat on LDL oxidation are very discordant, as some of them show no effect, and others increased or even decreased *ex vivo* susceptibility of LDL to oxidation. It should be stated that, although the role of LDL oxidation in the pathogenesis of atherosclerosis is well accepted, there is much debate as to the physiological relevance of *ex vivo* measurements of LDL oxidation and its use as a risk for CVD.

If oxidative stress is so important, the supply of antioxidants through the diet, as well as the choice of nutrients capable of reducing oxidation, could be crucial in the prevention of CVD. The antioxidant hypothesis proposes that antioxidant vitamins may slow the progression of atherosclerosis by blocking the oxidative modification of LDL cholesterol and thus decreasing its uptake into the arterial lumen. The most important dietary antioxidants are vitamins C and E and β-carotene (provitamin A). All of these vitamins are able to reduce oxidation of LDL *in vitro,* but their effectiveness in preventing CVD is yet unresolved. Most observational epidemiological studies support a

Table 11.7 Primary Prevention Trials of dietary antioxidants

	ATCB (1994)	Physicians' Health Study (1996)	CARET (1996)
No. of participants	29 133	22 071	18 134
Follow-up (years)	5–8	12	4
Intervention	β-carotene 20 mg, vitamin E 50 mg	β-carotene 50 mg every other day	β-carotene 20 mg, vitamin A 2500 U
Mortality	+2% vitamin E +8% β-carotene	+0.1%	17%
Cardiovascular mortality		+0.9%	+17%
Myocardial infarction		−4%	

Modified from: Kris-Etherton PM, Shaomey Y. Individual fatty acid effects on plasma lipids and lipoproteins: human studies. Am J Clin Nutr 1997; 65 (Suppl): 1628s–1644s.
ATCB: Alpha Tocopherol Beta-Carotene Cancer Prevention Study; CARET: Beta-Carotene and Retinol Efficacy Trial.

cardioprotective effect of carotenoids and vitamin E, whereas the relationship between vitamin C intake and the risk of heart disease is weak and inconsistent. However, intervention studies with vitamin E and β-carotene, at least those in primary prevention, have failed to show a significant benefit of these vitamins taken as a dietary supplement for the prevention of CHD (Table 11.7).

11.10 Insulin sensitivity

Diet composition and insulin sensitivity

The effects of insulin on lipid, carbohydrate and protein metabolism depend not only on insulin concentrations at the level of the target organ, but also on the cells' ability to transmit insulin signaling (insulin sensitivity). Impaired insulin sensitivity not only is associated with type II diabetes but also facilitates the occurrence of metabolic abnormalities and CVD risk factors that, in turn, predispose to ischemic cardiovascular disease (the metabolic syndrome). Weight reduction represents the most effective means to improve insulin sensitivity in overweight individuals. Even a modest weight reduction (4.5 kg) is able to improve significantly insulin's action in relation to glucose, lipid and protein metabolism.

Insulin sensitivity can be influenced not only by total energy intake, but also by dietary composition. In this respect, of great interest are the specific effects of the quality of dietary fat, as there is considerable evidence in experimental animals that the increased amounts of saturated fat in the diet may lead to insulin resistance.

In humans, there is indirect evidence for the same effect: a higher saturated fat intake is associated with impaired insulin action. However, intervention studies on changes in dietary fat quality and insulin sensitivity in humans have so far been inconclusive, perhaps because of the short duration of the study period and the inadequate sample size.

Human studies have also attempted to evaluate the relationship between total fat intake and insulin sensitivity. Many epidemiological studies, both cross-sectional and prospective, are now available showing that fat intake is correlated with both plasma insulin values (positively) and insulin sensitivity (negatively). These correlations are largely mediated by body weight, which may explain why in these studies saturated and unsaturated fats (which have identical energy content) show similar relationships with insulin sensitivity. If the effect of total fat intake on body weight is properly accounted for, the relationship between dietary fat and insulin sensitivity becomes less consistent.

A more appropriate study design to evaluate the effect of total fat intake on insulin sensitivity independently of all possible confounders is the intervention trial. Few such studies are available in the literature, but these studies are consistent in showing that when total fat intake is increased from 20% to 40% no major effect is observed on insulin sensitivity. Only more extreme experimental conditions, such as when fat intake varies from almost 0% to as much as 55%, may be able to modify insulin sensitivity. Undoubtedly, the impact of dietary fat composition on insulin function will differ between healthy subjects and diabetics. A large, multicenter intervention study undertaken in healthy individuals given either a high saturated fat or a high monounsaturated fat diet for 3 months showed that a high monounsaturated fat diet significantly improved insulin sensitivity compared with a high saturated fat diet. However, this beneficial effect of monounsaturated fat disappears in individuals whose total fat intake is high (35–40% of total energy).

By and large, there are insufficient data available to draw any firm conclusions as to whether and how insulin sensitivity may be influenced by the glycemic index of diets, alcohol and micronutrient intakes.

Nutritional influence on fasting and postprandial blood glucose levels

Although closely related, fasting and postprandial blood glucose levels are regulated by mechanisms that are, to some extent, different. While postprandial blood glucose concentrations depend largely on meal composition, fasting values are only minimally influenced by the amount and/or rate of glucose absorption during the previous meal, and reflect the rate of glucose production in the liver by means of two key processes, glycogenolysis and gluconeogenesis, which are regulated by insulin secretion and insulin sensitivity.

Diabetes is a disease that results from either a failure in insulin secretion (type I or juvenile-onset diabetes) or a failure in the sensitivity to insulin (type II or insulin-resistant diabetes). Although both types of diabetes increase the risk of CVD, less severe forms of insulin resistance, which manifest as disturbed lipid metabolism in the absence of overt hyperglycemia, are present in a significant proportion of middle-aged adults in developed countries and also confer increased cardiovascular risk.

11.11 Perspectives on the future

Lipids, genetics and cardiovascular disease

A great deal of the advances in our understanding of the role of lipids in the pathophysiology of cardiovascular disease has arisen from the study of rare mutations such as those of genes coding for proteins involved in the LDL receptor pathway. However, as pointed out in Chapter 2, more commonly genetic variation plays a significant role in determining individual responsiveness to diet. Numerous apolipoproteins (e.g. apoE, apoA1,2, apoC1,2,3, apoB-48, apoB-100), enzymes (e.g.

LPL, CETP, HMG-CoA reductase), receptors (e.g. LDL receptor, remnant receptor) and transcription factors (e.g. PPAR-α, PPAR-γ, SREBP) are involved in lipid and lipoprotein metabolism. It is likely that polymorphisms in these and other regulatory proteins will prove to be responsible for modifying both the risk of CVD and interindividual responsiveness to dietary components that can modify CVD risk.

The most widely studied polymorphism is that of the apoE gene, which produces three main isoforms: E_2, E_3 and E_4. The prevalence of these alleles varies between populations, but is generally in the region of 14% (E_2), 60% (E_3) and 26% (E_4). The apoE isoforms represent examples of single nucleotide polymorphisms (SNPs) which, in the case of E_4, involves an arginine for cysteine substitution at residue 112, whereas E_2 involves a cysteine for arginine substitution at residue 158. Some 2% of the population are homozygous for E_2 and display markedly delayed chylomicron clearance, while 14% are heterozygous and show much less effect on chylomicron clearance. In contrast, the E_4 allele is associated with an increased risk of CVD, higher LDL cholesterol and greater than average responsiveness in terms of LDL cholesterol to dietary saturated fat but not statin therapy. Given the number of potential SNPs in the large number of proteins involved in lipid and lipoprotein metabolism that could confer variability in dietary responsiveness, it is clear that the big challenge for the future will be in exploiting the forthcoming explosion of data in this area, arising from the application of technology for high-throughput genomic analysis and the advances in the understanding of the huge array of data that will arrive through bioinformatics. It is probable that this will lead to the ability to predict an individual's responsiveness to a particular dietary change and thereby provide customized dietary advice based on their particular gene profile. There are enormous social and economic benefits to accurately titrating the proper effective diet to an individual's needs. While this might be true of all diseases, the high social and economic cost of diseases of the cardiovascular system will put CVD in the front line of this technology.

Bioactive microcomponents in foods and their effects on cardiovascular disease risk factors: role of gene expression screening

Recognition of the potential cardioprotective effects of many nutrient and non-nutrient components of foods

Table 11.8 Dietary components with known or putative cardioprotective effects

Component	Effect
Known effects	
Long-chain n-3 PUFA	Prevention of secondary cardiovascular disease
PUFA, MUFA	LDL cholesterol reduction
Plant sterols	LDL cholesterol reduction
Dietary fiber	LDL cholesterol lowering effect
Putative effects	
Soy protein and soy isoflavones, CLA	Reduction of LDL and increase in HDL cholesterol
Milk peptides	Reduction of blood pressure
Isoflavones, long-chain n-3 PUFA, CLA	Reduction endothelial inflammation
PUFA, MUFA	Reduction of platelet aggregation
Carotenoids, vitamin E, flavonoids, e.g. reservatrol	Reduction of susceptibility of LDL to oxidation
Quercetin	Reduction of platelet aggregation

PUFA: polyunsaturated fatty acid; MUFA: monounsaturated fatty acid; CLA: conjugated linoleic acid; LDL: low-density Lipoprotein; HDL: high-density lipoprotein.

in recent years (Table 11.8) has led to the introduction of the concept of 'functional foods' (or nutraceuticals): foods in which normal levels of these bioactive compounds are increased, either through their enrichment at source [e.g. increased levels of conjugated linoleic acid (CLA) in milk] or through their addition during the manufacturing process (e.g. plant sterols in spreads and margarines). The dietary compounds for which cardioprotective effects have been suggested are exceedingly diverse and include possible blood pressure-lowering peptides in milk, cholesterol-lowering effects of soy proteins and plant isoflavones, antioxidant effects of flavonoids found in wine and tea, and platelet antiaggregating effects of quercetin found in onions (see Chapter 14). Not all of the studies conducted in human volunteers have provided conclusive or convincing findings, but considerable research effort is currently being applied and is likely to reveal that at least some of the compounds have potential application for the prevention of CVD. Already it is clear from secondary

prevention trials that modest amounts of eicosapentaenoic and docosahexaenoic acid have powerful cardioprotective effects that could be harnessed via their enrichment in the diet. There has been considerable research into the effects of CLA on risk factors for atherosclerosis. CLA is a mix of conjugated isomers of all-*cis* C18:2n-6 and the different isomers have different and sometimes divergent effects. Whereas CLA is the focus of present attention, there are almost certainly likely to be other conjugated isomers of very biologically active fatty acids such as arachidonic, eicosapentaenoic or docosahexaenoic acids that may prove to be even more potent than the parent compounds.

One of the factors that has limited the development of this exciting area is the cost and complexity of conducting intervention trials in human volunteers. Compromise of cost over study design means that many trials are too small to demonstrate statistically significant findings. However, the availability of high-throughput microarray technology (genomics) and proteomics, applied to cell-culture models, will enable putative bioactive compounds to be screened for their ability to influence the expression of target genes. This will allow nutritional trials to be limited to compounds already shown to influence key pathways in relevant cell systems.

Further reading

Glass CK, Witztum JL. Atherosclerosis: the road ahead. Cell 2001; 104(4): 503–516.

Hermansen K. Diet, blood pressure and hypertension. Br J Nutr 2000; 83 (Suppl 1): s113–s119.

Hornstra G, Barth CA, Galli C. Functional food science and the cardiovascular system. Br J Nutr 1998 (Suppl 1): s113–s146.

Kris-Etherton PM, Shaomey Y. Individual fatty acid effects on plasma lipids and lipoproteins: human studies. Am J Clin Nutr 1997; 65 (Suppl): 1628s–1644s.

NHLBI. Third Report of the Expert Panel on Detection Evaluation and Treatment of High Blood Cholesterol in Adults. National Cholesterol Education, 2001.

Riccardi G, Rivellese AA. Dietary treatment of the metabolic syndrome: the optimal diet. Br J Nutr 2000; 83 (Suppl 1): s143–s148.

Zaman AG, Halft G, Worthly SG, Badimon JJ. The role of plaque rupture and thrombosis in coronary artery diseases. Athero≠sclerosis 2000; 149: 251–266.

12
The Skeletal System

JM Pettifor, A Prentice and P Cleaton-Jones

Key messages

- Bone plays important supportive and protective functions for the body, and its constituent cells are in close relationship with those of the bone marrow, from which they are derived.
- Bone is a dynamic tissue, which is continually being resorbed and replaced (the process of remodeling). The rate of remodeling is influenced by a number of different factors, including circulating hormones such as sex steroids and parathyroid hormone. Bone formation and resorption can be measured by various different biochemical assays, which may be of use in assessing bone and mineral metabolism.
- Bone mass can be accurately measured by several techniques, including dual-energy X-ray absorptiometry (DXA) and computed tomography. Each method has its advantages and disadvantages, which may complicate the interpretation of the results.
- Peak bone mass, which is reached in early adulthood, is influenced by different factors, including heredity,

gender, nutrition, hormonal status and lifestyle patterns. Peak bone mass may influence the prevalence of fragility fractures occurring in later life.
- Important metabolic bone diseases include osteomalacia/rickets and osteoporosis. The former is common in infants, young children and the elderly in a number of developing and developed countries owing to vitamin D deficiency, while the latter is becoming an increasingly severe problem in the aging population of developed countries.
- Several nutritional factors play permissive roles in ensuring optimal bone health. Among the most important of these are vitamin D and calcium, but many other nutrients, singly or in combination, may influence bone and mineral homeostasis.
- The nutritional factors influencing tooth development and dental caries are less well understood, but it appears that genetic factors combine with nutritional patterns to influence caries prevalence.

12.1 Introduction

Rickets and osteoporosis are two diseases of bone which have major impacts on the state of health and quality of life of young and old, respectively, in both developing and industrialized countries. Nutritional factors play important roles in determining the prevalence of these two diseases. This chapter sets the scene for the reader by providing an overview of the structure and physiology of bone, and of the factors that determine bone and teeth growth and development. The physiological changes that occur during pregnancy and lactation and with aging are discussed and the factors that may influence these changes are

described. This chapter should be read in conjunction with other chapters in other books in this series.

12.2 Bone architecture and physiology

The skeletal system plays a number of important physiological roles, thus its integrity must be maintained for the normal function of the human body. These physiological functions include:

- **support** for the body: in this role the skeleton is responsible for posture, for allowing normal joint movement and muscle activity through providing the levers on which muscles act, and for withstanding functional load bearing

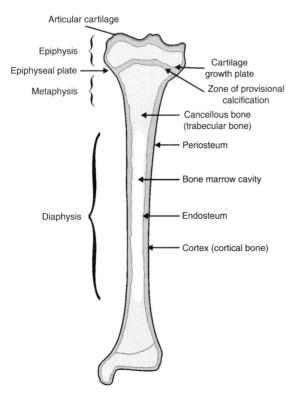

Figure 12.1 Schematic representation of a long bone with the important anatomical areas labeled.

Box 12.1 Composition of bone

Mineral (calcium hydroxyapatite)	50–70% or ~ 1000 g
Organic matrix	20–30%
Water	5–10%
Lipids	3%

bone such as the femur or tibia and highlights the various anatomical regions of the bone.

Bone composition

Unlike most other tissues, which are composed mainly of cells, bone is mainly composed of an extracellular matrix. The cells that maintain this matrix are relatively sparse, being present only on the various surfaces of the calcified matrix and scattered within the matrix that makes up cortical bone. Bone thus consists of a non-cellular calcified matrix and the cells that maintain this matrix. As shown in Box 12.1, mineral is the major constituent of bone.

Bone matrix

The matrix is made up of both **collagenous** and **non-collagenous** proteins, with type I collagen making up 90% of total bone protein (Box 12.2). The fibrous nature of collagen provides elasticity and flexibility to bone as well as the scaffolding on which mineralization can occur. The collagen fibers are oriented in directions influenced by the stresses and strains experienced by the developing bone through weight bearing, and the attachments of muscles, tendons and ligaments. Type I collagen is a triple-helical molecule containing two identical α_1 (I) chains and an α_2 (I) chain. These chains are rich in lysine and proline, which undergo post-translational modifications including hydroxylation of lysyl and prolyl residues (which requires vitamin C), glycosylation of lysyl and hydroxylysyl residues, and the formation of intramolecular and intermolecular covalent cross-links (Figure 12.2). These post-translational modifications are important in ensuring the linkage of the collagen molecules into fibrils, thus increasing the strength of the collagen network. The collagen molecules are linked end-to-end and side-to-side in a staggered pattern, resulting in gaps between the molecules, where mineral deposition occurs. Measurement of these various collagen cross-links has been used successfully to assess the rate of bone resorption in the clinical situation.

- **protection** of organs, such as the brain and lungs
- **providing a reservoir** of calcium
- **acting as a buffer** to maintain normal acid–base balance
- through its close relationship with bone marrow, **maintaining a normal hemopoietic and immune system**.

Bone may be divided into compact (cortical) bone which provides mainly the supporting and protective functions of bone and makes up approximately 85% of bone tissue, and trabecular, cancellous or spongy bone, which is composed of thin calcified trabeculae enclosing the hemopoietic bone marrow and adipose tissue and comprises only 15% of the skeleton. Trabecular bone is considered to be physiologically more active than cortical bone because of its larger surface area. The internal trabecular structure of bones such as that found in the vertebral bodies and femoral neck plays an important supportive role, preventing collapse or fracture. Figure 12.1 schematically depicts a long

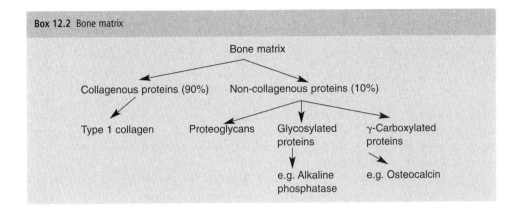

Box 12.2 Bone matrix

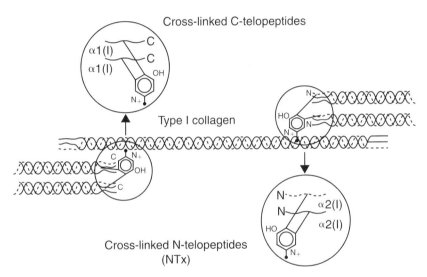

Cross-linked C-telopeptides

Type I collagen

Cross-linked N-telopeptides
(NTx)

Figure 12.2 Schematic diagram of type I collagen, highlighting its linkages with other fibers. (Reproduced from Calvo *et al.*, 1996 with permission of The Endocrine Society.)

The non-collagenous proteins make up only approximately 10% of total bone protein, and can be divided into three major groups:

- proteoglycans
- glycosylated proteins
- γ-carboxylated proteins.

The proteoglycans molecules may be important regulators of bone formation; however, their physiological functions in bone have not been clearly elucidated. The **glycosylated proteins**, such as alkaline phosphatase, osteonectin, osteopontin, fibronectin and bone sialoprotein, probably play a number of different roles, which for many of the proteins have not been well established; however, they may be important in matrix mineralization, bone cell growth and proliferation, and in osteoblast differentiation and maturation. Alkaline phosphatase, which is a zinc-containing metalloenzyme, is an essential enzyme for the normal mineralization of bone. Inherited defects in the molecule result in the condition of hereditary hypophosphatasia, which in its most severe form is lethal in infancy. Zinc deficiency is associated with low circulating levels of alkaline phosphatase.

The **γ-carboxylated proteins** osteocalcin, matrix-Gla-protein, and protein S, are post-translationally modified by the action of vitamin K-dependent γ-carboxylases to form dicarboxylic glutamyl (Gla) residues, which enhance calcium binding. The actual role of these proteins in bone is unclear, but they may inhibit mineral deposition. The measurement of serum levels of osteocalcin is increasingly used as a measure of osteoblastic activity. Clinical vitamin K deficiency reduces the number of carboxylated glutamic acid residues per molecule of osteocalcin.

The **mineral component** of bone is mainly in the form of hydroxyapatite $[Ca_{10}(PO_4)_6(OH)_2]$, which provides stiffness and load-bearing strength to bone. The crystals of hydroxyapatite are approximately 200 Å in length, and form in and around the collagen fibrils, where they grow both by increasing in size and by aggregation. The mechanism by which mineralization occurs is unclear, although it is believed that extracellular matrix vesicles (produced by osteoblasts) initiate mineralization either by removing inhibitors of mineralization, such as pyrophosphate and adenosine triphosphate (ATP), present in the matrix, or by increasing calcium and phosphate concentrations locally to allow crystallization to occur. Although the exact role of alkaline phosphatase produced by osteoblasts in the mineralization process is unclear, it is essential for normal mineralization, as evidenced by the severe mineralization defect seen in children with hypophosphatasia, a disease caused by genetic mutations in the alkaline phosphatase gene.

The hydroxyapatite crystal may take up dietary cations and anions into its lattice. Magnesium or strontium may replace calcium in the crystal lattice, resulting in smaller, less perfect crystals, while fluoride incorporation increases crystal size and decreases solubility. Bisphosphonates, a family of antiresorptive agents, bind to the surface of apatite crystals, preventing resorption. Tetracycline, an antibiotic, also binds avidly to newly formed apatite crystals, resulting in fluorescence of newly deposited bone mineral. This characteristic of tetracycline is used clinically to measure bone mineralization rates and the extent of bone surface undergoing mineralization. If taken during the formation of teeth, tetracyclines result in staining of teeth through their incorporation into the mineralizing enamel.

Bone cells

The important bone cells are **stromal osteoprogenitor cells, osteoblasts, osteocytes, lining cells, and osteoclasts** and their precursors. However, it is becoming increasingly apparent that there is a close interrelationship between the various hemopoietic cells in the bone marrow and bone cells, not only because precursors of bone cells may reside within the marrow but also because of the cross-talk between the various cell types.

Osteoprogenitor cells are found in the periosteum and bone marrow. Various growth factors, cytokines and hormones [including transforming growth factor-β_1 (TGF-β_1), fibroblast growth factor (FGF), a number

of bone morphogenetic proteins and parathyroid hormone (PTH)] are responsible for controlling the proliferation and differentiation of these mesenchymal cells into preosteoblasts, osteoblasts and osteocytes. Both PTH and the active form of vitamin D, 1,25-dihydroxyvitamin D [1,25(OH)$_2$D], are important in controlling the proliferation and differentiation of these bone-forming cells. The control of the development of these cells is complex and beyond the scope of this chapter; however, the reader is referred to a number of reviews for further information.

Osteoblasts are responsible for the secretion of bone matrix and for the production of matrix vesicles, which probably initiate mineralization of the preformed osteoid. During the maturation of the osteoblast, the cell initially secretes collagen and is rich in alkaline phosphatase, but later produces osteocalcin and other matrix proteins, such as osteopontin. As the osteoblast becomes encircled by matrix, it transforms into an osteocyte with cytoplasmic extensions lying in canaliculi connecting with adjacent cells (osteocytes, osteoblasts and lining cells).

Osteoclasts (bone resorbing cells) are derived from hemopoietic stem cells, which have the potential to become macrophages or multinucleated osteoclasts depending on the stimuli received during development. Osteoclasts lie in contact with the mineralized trabecular surface or in Howship's lacunae. These cells are rich in endoplasmic reticulum and Golgi complexes. The cell membrane adjacent to the bone matrix is characterized by a peripheral sealing zone which is rich in integrins, and a central ruffled border which forms a space between the osteoclast and the bone matrix into which lysosomal enzymes (such as tartrate-resistant acid phosphatase and cathepsin K), proteinases (such as collagenase) and hydrogen ions are secreted. The hydrogen ions and enzymes dissolve the mineral and digest the demineralized matrix, the products of which are internalized into the osteoclast, transported across the cell into the extracellular fluid or released through the sealing zone. Hormones that stimulate osteoclast number and activity include parathyroid hormone, 1,25(OH)$_2$D and a number of inflammatory cytokines, while calcitonin reduces osteoclastic activity.

Bone remodeling

Bone is not a dead organ, rather it is continually being resorbed and replaced. This process is known as bone

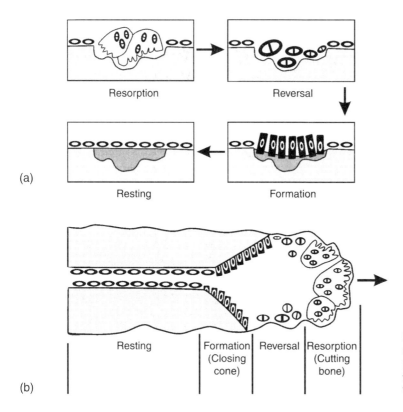

(a)

(b)

Figure 12.3 The bone remodeling cycle. (a) Remodeling at the trabecular bone surface. (b) Remodeling occurring in cortical bone. (Reproduced from Baron, 1999 with permission of Lippincott Williams & Wilkins.)

remodeling (Figure 12.3) and not only helps to maintain bone in optimal condition through repairing microfractures but also is important in serum calcium homeostasis. Bone turnover occurs in discrete packages throughout the skeleton, and the process of resorption followed by replacement is tightly coupled so that in the healthy young adult there is no net loss or gain in bone. As one grows older, and particularly in the postmenopausal period, progressive bone loss occurs as a result of incomplete replacement of the bone that has been resorbed. The control of the rate of bone remodeling, the mechanisms by which the osteoclasts are activated and how the whole process is coupled are areas of intensive investigation, which still have many unanswered questions. The balance between bone formation and resorption is essential in maintaining bone mass (Figure 12.4). Recent studies have provided a better understanding of how the various bone cells are interrelated. For example, osteoblasts control osteoclast precursor development through the production of RANK-ligand, which binds to RANK on osteoclast precursors and stimulates osteoclast proliferation. Osteoprotogerin, a circulating binder of

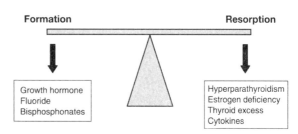

Figure 12.4 Balance between bone formation and resorption, which is essential to maintain bone mass.

RANK-ligand, reduces the amount of RANK-ligand available to bind to osteoclast precursors, thus reducing osteoclast production.

The whole process of remodeling of a particular package of bone takes about 3–4 months, with the resorption process taking about 10 days and the filling in of the cavity taking about 3 months. Systemic hormones, such as PTH, 1,25-$(OH)_2$D and calcitonin, alter bone remodeling mainly through inducing more or fewer remodeling sites in the skeleton. Estrogen deficiency, as occurs at the time of the menopause, causes bone loss mainly through its effect on the osteoblast, preventing complete filling in of the resorption cavity that develops during the remodeling cycle. Excessive bone resorption, either through the formation of excessively deep resorption cavities or through the progressive thinning of trabecular bone with each remodeling cycle, will result in weakening of the trabecular bone structure owing to the loss of connectivity between the various rods and plates that make up the trabecular scaffolding, resulting in progressive risk of minimal trauma fractures. States of very high bone turnover, which may occur in diseases such as Paget's disease or severe primary or secondary hyperparathyroidism, result in the formation of woven rather than lamellar bone. In woven bone the collagen fibers are laid down in a disorganized fashion, resulting in the loss of the normal lamellar structure with a resultant loss in bone strength.

Biochemical assessment of bone remodeling

Since the early 1990s great strides have been made in the development of assays for the measurement of both serum and urine markers of bone formation and resorption, and these have helped in non-invasively assessing bone turnover.

Markers of bone formation

Table 12.1 lists the bone biochemical markers currently available for the assessment of bone turnover.

Total alkaline phosphatase has until recently been the only marker of osteoblastic activity available; however, as serum total alkaline phosphatase also reflects that produced at other sites, in particular the liver,

Table 12.1 Biochemical markers of bone turnover

Formation
- Serum
  - Total alkaline phosphatase (AP)
  - Bone-specific alkaline phosphatase (BSAP)
  - Osteocalcin (OC)
  - Carboxy-terminal propeptide of type I collagen (PICP)
  - Amino-terminal propeptide of type I collagen (PINP)

Resorption
- Serum
  - Cross-linked C-telopeptide of type I collagen (ICTP)
  - Tartrate-resistant acid phosphatase (TRAP)
- Urine
  - Hydroxyproline
  - Free and total pyridinolines (Pyd)
  - Free and total deoxypyridinolines (Dpd)
  - N-telopeptide of collagen cross-links (NTx)
  - C-telopeptide of collagen cross-links (CTx)

elevated total levels do not necessarily reflect an increase in osteoblastic activity. Alkaline phosphatase concentrations are characteristically elevated in all forms of osteomalacia and rickets, in hyperparathyroidism and in Paget's disease. The measurement of **bone-specific alkaline phosphatase** (BSAP) utilizes specific monoclonal antibodies and more accurately reflects an increase in osteoblastic activity. Depressed levels of alkaline phosphatase may occur in zinc deficiency and protein–energy malnutrition, and in inherited disorders of the alkaline phosphatase gene (hereditary hypophosphatasia). **Osteocalcin** is a non-collagenous protein secreted by the mature osteoblast. Thus, serum levels should reflect osteoblastic activity and bone formation. In general, BSAP and osteocalcin values correlate; however, some studies suggest that osteocalcin levels may be normal in patients with rickets despite markedly elevated alkaline phosphatase values. The reasons for this dissociation are unclear.

The **amino- and carboxy-terminal propeptides of type I collagen** (PINP and PICP, respectively) are cleaved and excreted during collagen biosynthesis. Assays against propeptides at both the N- and C-terminals have been developed, but they do not appear to be as useful as either BSAP or osteocalcin in assessing bone formation and osteoblastic activity.

Markers of bone resorption

Unlike the assessment of bone formation, which generally uses serum, the assessment of bone resorption usually requires the measurement of products excreted in urine. The most useful markers are those derived from the breakdown of type I collagen, which occurs during the resorption of bone matrix. The measurement of **hydroxyproline** excretion in urine has until recently been the gold standard; however, hydroxyproline is found not only in collagen derived from bone, but also in collagen from tendons, cartilage and soft tissues. Thus, the amount excreted in urine may reflect the breakdown of other tissues besides bone and that ingested in the diet.

The measurement of hydroxyproline has over the past few years been replaced by the measurement of the **pyridinoline and deoxypyridinoline cross-links of collagen** (Pyd and Dpd, respectively). Dpd is more specific for bone than Pyd, but is less abundant. Currently, the generally used immunoassays measure free Pyd and Dpd, rather than the protein-bound molecules, which may make the interpretation of results difficult if storage or biological variations alter the ratio of free to protein-bound molecules. Similarly, assays have been developed to measure the **N- and C-terminal telopeptides of collagen** in urine.

In serum, an assay is available to measure cross-linked **C-terminal telopeptide of type I collagen**; however, the assay does not appear to be as useful as the measurement of the urinary markers of bone resorption. A reasonably specific marker of osteoclast activity is **tartrate-resistant acid phosphatase** (TRAP), which is secreted into serum. Its measurement is limited by its instability in serum and by the fact that it is not entirely specific for osteoclasts.

Clinical usefulness of biochemical markers of bone turnover

Bone markers are useful in assisting in the diagnosis of metabolic bone disease, such as osteomalacia and rickets, and hyperparathyroidism; however, they have little or no use in the diagnosis of osteoporosis, although they may help in understanding the pathogenesis of osteoporosis and monitoring the response to therapy.

One of the major problems with the use of most of the markers is their great variability from day to day as a result of the need to measure their excretion in urine. Twenty-four-hour urine samples are notoriously difficult to collect accurately, and are thus generally avoided. If one uses a fasting urine specimen, then one needs to relate the excretion of the urine marker to the excretion of creatinine in the same sample. However, creatinine measurements have a built-in variability and vary depending on muscle mass and nutritional status. Compounding the problem is the fact that a number of bone turnover markers have a circadian rhythm; thus,

specimens collected at different times of the day or night may vary markedly. Therefore, samples should be collected at a constant time during the day, and if they are being collected with specimens to assess calcium homeostasis, they should be collected in a fasting state.

Bone turnover markers are probably most useful as a research tool to assess rates of bone turnover in groups of subjects, and in clinical medicine to determine the bone response to an intervention such as drug therapy. They are also most useful when groups of subjects are compared, rather than using them to determine the bone turnover status of an individual.

Assessment of bone mass

One of the techniques used to assess bone health is the measurement of the amount of mineral present in the bone. Before the advent of more advanced techniques, the usual method to assess the amount of mineral in bone was to use radiographs of the lumbar spine or hips and to judge whether the radiographic density appeared to be normal, increased or decreased. The problem with this technique is that one needs to have lost some 30% of bone mineral before it becomes obvious on the routine radiograph and the interpretation is open to considerable subjectivity. The loss of radio-density on radiographs is termed **osteopenia,** which could be due to a loss of bone (matrix and mineral; osteoporosis) or a failure of mineralization of normal amounts of matrix (osteomalacia).

Advances in technology since the early 1980s have resulted in the availability of rapid and accurate methods of assessing bone mass. A number of different techniques have been used to determine bone mass (Table 12.2); however, dual-energy X-ray densitometry

Table 12.2 Techniques used to measure bone mass

Technique	Sites measured	Precision (% CV)	Radiation dose (μSv)
Single-photon absorptiometry (SPA)	Forearm	1–2	<1
Dual-energy X-ray densitometry (DXA)	Spine, hip, forearm, whole body	1–2.5 depending on site	~1–3
Peripheral DXA	Forearm, calcaneus, phalanges	1–1.7	<1
Quantitative computed tomography (QCT)	Spine	2–4	~50
Peripheral QCT	Forearm	~1–2	~1
Quantitative ultrasound (QUS)	Calcaneus, tibia	0.3–5	0

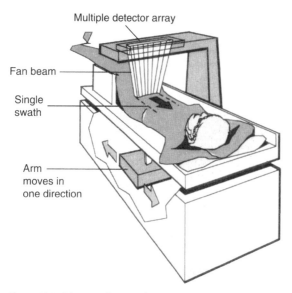

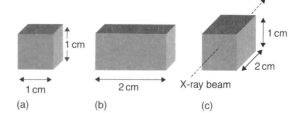

Figure 12.5 Schematic diagram of a dual-energy X-ray densitometer. Note that the collimated X-ray beam moves through the subject from inferior to superior. Using this method, whole-body, lumbar spine, femoral and radial bone mineral content and area may be measured and bone mineral density calculated.

Figure 12.6 The concept of areal bone mineral density (BMD). The three blocks A, B and C represent three blocks of bone of the same volumetric density of x g/cm^3. The projected area of block A is 1 cm^2, block B 2 cm^2 and block C 2 cm^2. Thus, the BMD measured by DXA would be x g/cm^2 for blocks A and B, but $2x$ g/cm^2 for block C, as block C is twice as thick as blocks A and B. Note that BMD measured by DXA is dependent not only on the true bone density (volumetric) but also on the thickness of the bone, which is not directly measured by DXA. The dashed arrow represents the path of the X-ray beam in the three blocks.

> **Box 12.3** Definitions used in densitometry
>
> **Bone mineral content:** The total bone mineral present in a defined area. It is measured in grams.
> **Bone area:** The projected area of bone detected by the attenuation of the X-ray beam. It is measured in cm^2.
> **Bone mineral density:** This is calculated by dividing the measured bone mineral content by the bone area. Thus, it represents an areal bone density and not a volumetric density as the thickness of bone is not determined by DXA. The units are g/cm^2.

(DXA) is the most widely accepted (Figure 12.5). Measurement of bone mass is relevant to assess the degree of osteoporosis/osteopenia, to determine possible fracture risk, and to assess response to therapy or the effect of disease on bone mass.

DXA is generally accepted as the gold standard against which other techniques are measured and has replaced the other techniques in most cases. It measures bone mineral content (BMC) in grams and bone area in cm^2. From these two measurements the so-called bone mineral density (BMD) in g/cm^2 is calculated (Box 12.3). It should be noted that the BMD is an areal bone density and does not measure true volumetric density of bone. Thus, unlike true density, BMD is influenced not only by the true density of bone but also by the volume of bone (Figure 12.6).

An understanding of this is important, as bones with the same volumetric bone density but different volumes will have different BMDs. BMD will increase with increasing bone size without a change in the true bone density. Furthermore, BMD reflects the average areal bone density of the constituents of the particular bone being measured; thus, the value will depend on amount of cortical as well as trabecular bone. Quantitative computed tomography (QCT) has an advantage in that it measures the volumetric density of bone. Furthermore, regions of bone, such as the cortical or trabecular regions, can be selected, thus allowing an assessment of the differential effects of a disease or treatment on the different types of bone. QCT is not more widely used because of the expense of the equipment, its lack of portability and the relatively high radiation dose.

12.3 Bone growth

Bone growth during fetal, childhood and adolescent periods involves not only elongation of long bones by proliferation of the growth plate cartilage, but also growth at the periosteal surfaces of both the long bones and membranous bones. Thus, as bones enlarge they undergo modeling, which involves the resorption of bone in one area and the deposition of bone in another. From the time of birth to closure of the epiphyses and cessation of growth during adolescence, the skeleton increases in length by about three-fold, with quite marked changes in skeletal proportions, with limb length increasing more than trunk length (Figure 12.7).

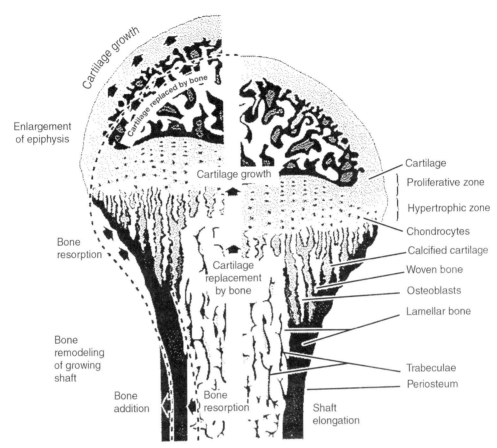

Figure 12.7 Changes associated with longitudinal bone growth of a long bone. Note the modeling that needs to take place in order for the bone to remain the same shape but larger. (Reproduced from St-Arnaud and Glorieux, 1997 with permission of Elsevier Science.)

Skeletal growth rates are not constant throughout childhood. After birth there is a marked deceleration in growth until 3 years of age, when the growth rate plateaus until the onset of puberty. At this time girls have their growth spurt approximately 2 years before boys and fuse their epiphyses earlier than boys.

Hormonal control of skeletal growth

Postnatally, the most important hormones regulating skeletal growth are growth hormone, insulin-like growth factor-1 (IGF-1), thyroid hormone and the sex steroids (Box 12.4).

The control of fetal growth is less clearly understood, but considerable interest in this area has been generated by the important role fetal growth has not only on adult size, but also on the future risk for cardiovascular disease, hypertension and non-insulin-dependent diabetes mellitus. Although genetic factors

Box 12.4 Important hormonal regulators of bone growth

- Growth hormone
- Insulin-like growth factor-1
- Thyroid hormone
- Sex hormones, especially estrogen

play a role in determining fetal growth, the predominant factor is the nutritional, oxygen and hormonal milieu in which the fetus develops. Both IGF-1 and IGF-2 are necessary to achieve normal fetal growth, but the effect of IGF-1 deficiency during fetal life is more severe than that of IGF-2 deficiency.

Growth hormone (GH) probably induces most of its effect on growth through the stimulation of IGF-1 secretion both from the liver and in the growth plate, where it stimulates the proliferation of cartilage cells, resulting in an elongation of long bones. It is possible that the paracrine actions of IGF-1 in the growth plate are more important than the hormonal effects of IGF-1 produced in the liver, as studies using a targeted knockout of the IGF-1 gene in the liver did not show a reduction in the growth-promoting actions of GH. Unlike congenital deficiency of IGF-1, which manifests during fetal development, congenital GH deficiency manifests postnatally with a falling off of growth velocity around 12 months of age. Nutritional deprivation probably causes a reduction in growth velocity through reducing IGF-1 production.

It also appears that IGF-1 may be an important mediator of the effect of sex steroids on bone growth during puberty, as both GH and IGF-1 levels rise during puberty. The rise in GH during puberty is a result of an increase in circulating estrogen concentrations in both boys and girls. In boys it is likely that the increase in estrogens is through the aromatization of testosterone.

Sex steroids play an essential role not only in the growth spurt that occurs during puberty but also in the cessation of growth through the closure of the epiphyses. It appears that at physiological levels circulating estrogen stimulates growth, while at pharmacological levels it suppresses longitudinal growth, possibly through reducing IGF-1 levels. Estrogen is responsible for epiphyseal closure in both boys and girls. Sex steroids have effects not only on the growth plate, but also on the endosteal and periosteal bone surfaces, resulting in an increase in cross-sectional diameter of the long bones. It appears that androgens and estrogen may have different effects on these bone surfaces. Both androgens and estrogen cause an increase in periosteal new bone formation, with resultant widening of the bone, but only estrogen has an effect on the endosteal bone surface, with a consequent increase in cortical bone thickness. Thus, after puberty boys have wider bones than girls (Figure 12.8).

Thyroid hormone is essential for the normal proliferation and maturation of the growth plate. Cretinism or congenital thyroid deficiency is associated with abnormalities of the epiphyses and marked short stature. From a nutritional standpoint, severe iodide deficiency in the mother and infant will manifest with growth failure.

Bone mass accumulation during childhood and adolescence

The skeleton increases its calcium content from birth to the end of adolescence by about 40 times (from 25

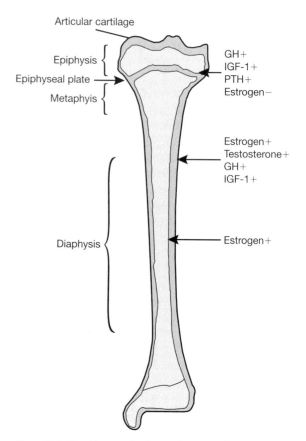

Figure 12.8 Sites of hormonal actions on the growing long bone. Stimulation of bone growth is indicated by +, while inhibition of growth is indicated by − . GH: growth hormone; IGF-1: insulin-line growth factor-1; PTH: Parathyroid hormone.

to 1000 g). A large proportion of this deposition occurs during puberty; however, the proportions gained by boys and girls during this period differ as girls enter puberty earlier than boys. It is estimated that 50% of the total bone mass of the adult female is laid down during puberty, whereas the figure for men is 20%. In Caucasian children, maximal gain in bone mass occurs between 11 and 14 years of age in girls and between 13 and 17 years of age in boys.

The pattern of bone mass accumulation during childhood is similar to that of growth in height, as bone growth accounts for the majority of bone mass accumulation. However, the relationship between BMC and height gain during puberty is not linear, but rather follows a loop pattern (Figure 12.9).

The dissociation between the rates of statural growth and mineral mass accumulation during puberty could

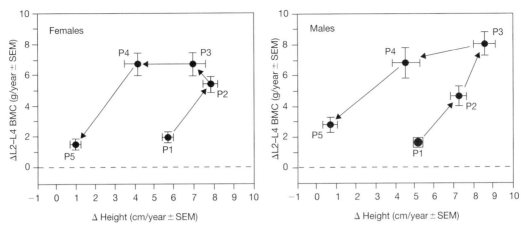

Figure 12.9 Relationship between the changes in bone mineral content (BMC) and height in adolescents grouped according to pubertal stages. Note that in the early stage of puberty (P1) height gain is good but changes in bone mineral density lag behind, while the reverse holds true in the later stages of puberty. (Reproduced from Theintz *et al.*, 1992.)

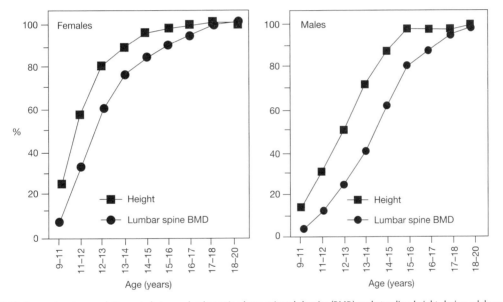

Figure 12.10 Comparison in cumulative gain between lumbar spine bone mineral density (BMD) and standing height during adolescence. The values are expressed as the percentage difference between 18–20-year-old and 9–11-year-old groups. (Reproduced from Fournier *et al.*, 1997 with permission of the American Journal of Clinical Nutrition. © American Society for Clinical Nutrition.)

be viewed as a period of relatively low bone mass (Figure 12.10) and may account for the increase in fracture incidence that occurs round this time. As linear growth slows, bone mass accumulation continues to occur and the deficit is made up.

Peak bone mass

Although longitudinal growth of bone ceases with the fusion of the epiphyses, bone mass continues to accumulate as bone consolidates and periosteal new bone formation continues. The concept of peak bone mass, which is defined as the amount of bone tissue present at the end of skeletal maturation, has assumed considerable significance as there is good evidence that the risk of osteoporotic fractures in later life is inversely related to the amount of bone accumulated during maturation (Box 12.5). Skeletal maturation is considered to occur early in the third decade of life, although the timing of the achievement of peak bone mass may vary slightly between different skeletal sites.

Factors known to influence peak bone mass include heredity, gender, race, nutrition, hormonal status (in particular the sex steroids and IGF-1), exercise and physical weight. By far the most important is the genetic influence, with 50–85% of the variance in peak bone mass at different sites being accounted for by heritability. The role of nutrition and in particular dietary calcium intake during childhood in influencing peak bone mass has been an area of intense investigation and will be discussed later in this chapter. However, a definitive answer on the role of dietary calcium is not yet available. Exercise has been shown to have a modulating influence on peak bone mass, with weight-bearing exercises being the most effective; however, the effect of exercise is relatively small (3–5%). Although small, on a population basis an increase in peak bone mass of this magnitude might have a considerable influence on fracture rates in later life.

There is an increasing gradient of fracture risk with decrease in bone mass, such, for example, that a reduction at the femoral neck of one standard deviation below the young adult mean increases the relative risk of hip fracture by 2.6. Consequently, both peak bone mass and the rate of subsequent bone loss are major determinants of osteoporotic fracture risk in later life. The maximization of peak bone mass by optimizing environmental factors that influence skeletal development during childhood and adolescence is regarded as an important preventive strategy against future fractures.

Conceptually, peak bone mass, as defined by BMC or BMD, contains elements related to the size of the skeleton, to the amount of bony tissue contained within it, to the mineral content of that tissue, and to the degree to which the bony tissue is actively undergoing remodeling. It is, as yet, unclear which of these aspects is most influential in determining future fracture risk.

Gender and ethnic differences in bone mass

Peak bone mass is significantly greater in adult males than females (Figure 12.11). This difference is due to a greater bone size in males than females, rather than due to a difference in true bone density. At birth, boys and girls have similar bone masses and it is only at the onset of puberty that these gender differences develop, owing to the delayed and more prolonged growth spurt in boys.

Ethnic differences in bone mass have been consistently found in studies conducted in the USA, with

---

Box 12.5 Factors influencing peak bone mass

- Genetic
- Race (African–Americans > Caucasians)
- Gender
- Nutritional, e.g. calcium intake
- Physical exercise
- Hormonal status
- Body weight

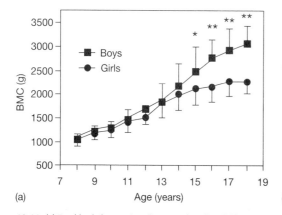

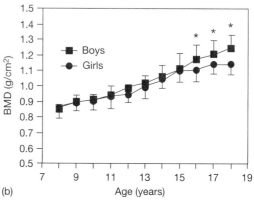

Figure 12.11 (a) Total body bone mineral content (BMC) and (b) areal bone mineral density (BMD) in Caucasian boys and girls from 8 to 18 years. Note the divergence of values between boys and girls developing after the onset of puberty. The effect is more marked for BMC than BMD as true volumetric bone density is similar in boys and girls, the difference in BMD being mainly due to a difference in bone size. (Reproduced from Maynard et al., 1998 with permission of the American Journal of Clinical Nutrition. © American Society for Clinical Nutrition.)

African–Americans having approximately 5–15% greater bone mass at all measured sites than white Americans, after adjusting for body size. These differences are present before the onset of puberty. Thus, it is often assumed that black Africans have similarly elevated bone mass values. Studies in both the Gambia and South Africa have been unable to confirm this. Studies of other ethnic groups have been less detailed, but it appears that Asian women from the Indian subcontinent have similar or lower bone mass than American or European Caucasian women.

Skeletal changes during pregnancy and lactation

Pregnancy and lactation are associated with alterations in calcium and bone metabolism that temporarily affect the mineral content of the skeleton (Box 12.6). These changes are evident from early to mid-gestation and continue through and beyond lactation. In pregnancy, bone resorption and formation rates are increased by 50–200%, and maternal calcium absorption efficiency and urinary calcium excretion are elevated. In lactation, calcium absorption efficiency returns to normal, but there is evidence of renal conservation of calcium in some women. Bone turnover continues to be elevated and differences in the timing of the skeletal response in terms of resorption and formation favor the release of calcium from the skeleton during early lactation, with restitution during and after weaning.

Direct studies of changes in BMC using absorptiometry have been largely restricted to lactating women, because of the small radiation dose involved. Such studies have demonstrated striking reductions in BMC after 3–6 months of lactation, particularly in axial regions of the skeleton, such as the lumbar spine and femoral neck, where decreases average 3–5% (Figure 12.12).

Lactation-associated reductions in BMC are remarkable given that the rate of postmenopausal bone loss is typically 1–3% per year. BMC is recovered later in lactation or after weaning, and at some sites exceeds that measured after parturition. Lactational amenorrhea,

the length of lactation and other aspects of infant-feeding behavior influence the magnitude and temporal pattern of the skeletal response experienced by breast-feeding women. However, the final outcome appears to be similar irrespective of duration of lactation, or indeed whether the woman breast-fed or not. Changes in BMC have been observed during pregnancy, but to date no consistent pattern has emerged. However, substantial increases have been reported in women entering pregnancy while still breast-feeding, suggesting that skeletal changes during pregnancy may depend on the status of the maternal skeleton before conception.

The mechanisms underlying the effects of pregnancy and lactation on calcium and bone metabolism are not fully understood. Originally, it was considered that the observed metabolic changes were due to physiological hyperparathyroidism, driven by the inability of dietary calcium supply to meet the high calcium requirement for fetal growth and breast-milk production. For this reason, women in the past were advised to increase their calcium intake during pregnancy and lactation. It is, however, now generally accepted that this is not the case, first, because PTH concentrations are not elevated during pregnancy and lactation; secondly, because the metabolic changes precede the increased requirement for calcium; and thirdly, because the effects appear to be independent of calcium intake. The fact that the metabolic and skeletal responses to lactation are not related to dietary calcium

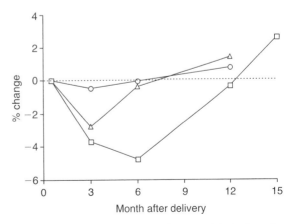

Figure 12.12 Changes in bone mineral content of the lumbar spine during lactation and after weaning. Data are adjusted for scanned bone area. □: Mothers who breast-fed for >9 months, (n =20); △: mothers who breast-fed for 3–6 months, (n =13); ○: mothers who formula-fed (n =11). (Reproduced from Laskey and Prentice, 1999 with permission from the American College of Obstetricians and Gynecologists.)

Box 12.6 Skeletal and mineral changes during pregnancy

- Increased bone turnover
- Increased intestinal calcium absorption
- Increased urinary calcium loss
- Increase in serum 1,25-(OH)$_2$D
- Variable changes in bone mineral content

intake has been confirmed by calcium supplementation studies in populations accustomed to low and medium to high calcium intakes. Direct evidence from supplementation studies in pregnant women is lacking, although studies are in progress. As a consequence of these latest findings, it is no longer considered necessary for a woman to increase her calcium intake during pregnancy and lactation, and this is reflected in recent dietary recommendations, for example by the Department of Health (UK) and the Institute of Medicine Food and Nutrition Board (US/Canada).

Osteoporosis with fractures is a rare complication of pregnancy and lactation. When it does occur, the condition frequently involves the hip or spine, is more common in the first pregnancy and usually resolves spontaneously. The cause is unknown, and most cases are either idiopathic or secondary to warfarin or corticosteroid therapy. There is no evidence that osteoporosis of pregnancy and lactation is a consequence of nutrient deficiencies or that it can be prevented by changes in diet and lifestyle.

12.4 Teeth

Anatomy and development

Humans have two dentitions. The primary dentition, also known as the deciduous dentition, has 20 teeth in four quadrants each with two incisors, one canine and two molars. The permanent dentition contains 32 teeth; each quadrant has two incisors, one canine, two premolars and three molars. The incisors, canines and premolars succeed the overlying primary teeth, but the permanent molar teeth have no predecessors, they develop as the jaws grow beyond the size that accommodates the primary teeth.

Teeth erupt over a wide period, earlier in some individuals than in others. They also erupt in a different sequence in the primary and permanent dentitions, and in the latter between the jaws. In general, mandibular teeth erupt before maxillary teeth. In this chapter mean timings of tooth formation have been rounded off for to make them easier to remember (Table 12.3). There is a considerable range of values depending on the

Table 12.3 Timings of tooth formation and eruption based on Ash's figures

Dentition	Jaw	Order of eruption	Calcification first seen	Crown completed	Eruption	Root completed
Primary	Mandible and maxilla	Central incisor	14 weeks[a]	1½–2½ months	8–10 months	1½ months
		Lateral incisor	16 weeks[a]	2½–3 months	11–13 months	1½–2 months
		First molar	15.5 weeks[a]	5½–6 months	16 months	2¼–2½ months
		Canine	17 weeks[a]	9 months	19–20 months	3¼ months
		Second molar	19 weeks[a]	10–11 months	27–29 months	3 months
Permanent	Mandible		At birth			
		First molar	3–4 months	2½–3 years	6–7 years	9–10 years
		Central incisor	3–4 months	4–5 years	6–7 years	9 years
		Lateral incisor	4–5 months	4–5 years	7–8 years	10 years
		Canine	1¼–2 years	6–7 years	9–10 years	12–14 years
		First premolar	2¼–2½ years	5–6 years	10–12 years	12–13 years
		Second premolar	2½–3 years	6–7 years	11–12 years	13–14 years
		Second molar	8–10 years	7–8 years	11–13 years	14–15 years
		Third molar		12–16 years	17–21 years	18–25 years
	Maxilla		At birth			
		First molar	3–4 months	2½–3 years	6–7 years	9–10 years
		Central incisor	10–12 months	4–5 years	7–8 years	10 years
		Lateral incisor	1½–1¾ years	4–5 years	8–9 years	11 years
		First premolar	2–2¼ years	5–6 years	10–11 years	12–13 years
		Second premolar	4–5 months	6–7 years	10–12 years	12–14 years
		Canine	2½–3 years	6–7 years	11–12 years	13–15 years
		Second molar	7–9 years	7–8 years	12–13 years	14–16 years
		Third molar		12–16 years	17–21 years	18–25 years

[a]In utero.

researcher. As a rule of thumb, the normal range of values in months is about 1 month either side of the mean; year values range about 1 year either side of the mean. Notice in Table 12.3 that calcification of the crowns of primary teeth begins *in utero*.

The anatomy of a typical tooth cross-section is shown in Figure 12.13. A tooth is divided into an anatomical crown and an anatomical root that meet at the neck (cervix). The anatomical crown is that part covered by enamel and the anatomical root is that part covered by cementum. The clinical crown is the portion of the anatomical crown visible in the mouth. The bulk of the tooth consists of calcified enamel and dentin, with a central uncalcified pulp that contains loose connective tissue, nerves and blood vessels.

Composition of enamel, dentin and cementum

Enamel is formed by ectodermal cells (ameloblasts) that disappear once enamel formation is complete. It is highly calcified, approximately 96% inorganic material, 0.8% organic and 3.2% water, arranged as crystals of calcium hydroxyapatite (see Bone matrix). Because the ameloblasts disappear at the completion of enamel formation, if enamel is damaged it cannot re-form. During enamel formation anything that interferes with the ameloblasts or with calcification will produce a poorer quality enamel shown by two visible defects. Hypoplasia is present when the enamel matrix has been poorly formed; it presents as a pit or fissure on the enamel surface. If calcification has been

altered hypocalcification will be seen as opaque, white areas ranging in size from a spot to an entire surface. Highly calcified enamel is transparent, allowing the yellow color of the underlying dentin to be seen; less calcified areas lack this transparency.

The position of enamel hypoplasia or hypocalcification on individual teeth, or on combinations of teeth, in both primary and permanent dentitions, can give a reasonable indication of when development was abnormal. What caused the defect is not so easily decided. Current thought is that excess fluoride is the only nutritional cause that can be diagnosed with reasonable certainty; the majority of other enamel defects are said to be due to transient infections, chronic illness or metabolic conditions such as rickets, but a clear link to the cause is rarely possible. Whatever the cause, there is interference with ameloblast and odontoblast function.

Dentin and cementum are similar in composition to bone, and are less calcified than enamel, being approximately 68% inorganic material, 22% organic and 10% water. Dentin is formed by mesodermal cells (odontoblasts) that retreat towards the pulp as dentin is laid down. They remain after tooth formation is complete and so can form more dentin, called secondary dentin, in response to an irritant such as dental caries or a filling. Secondary dentin and calcifications called pulp stones may also be formed by multipotential cells in the pulp tissue. Dentin itself contains no cells but has fine tubules that contain a portion of the odontoblasts (odontoblast process) left there as the cells retreated towards the pulp while laying down dentin. Secondary dentin may contain trapped cells and does not have tubules. Cementum looks similar to bone and contains entrapped cells (cementoblasts). Cementum attaches the periodontal ligament to the root surface. There is remodeling of the alveolar bone supporting the teeth, as happens elsewhere in the skeleton, but no similar remodeling of tooth tissues takes place.

Development of teeth

The teeth develop from two of the three primary germ layers, ectoderm and mesoderm. Ectoderm gives rise to the enamel of teeth; mesoderm provides the dentin, pulp, cementum and periodontal ligament. By the 37th day of development there is a horseshoe-shaped epithelial thickening in each jaw (the dental lamina). At intervals along this, thickenings develop (the tooth germs). The bottom part of these invaginate to form a

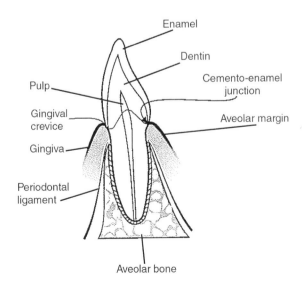

Figure 12.13 Diagram of a longitudinal section of an incisor.

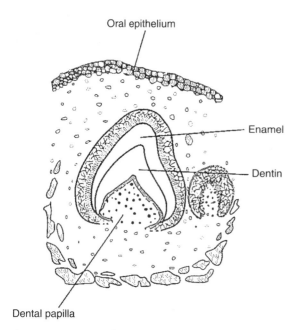

Oral epithelium

Enamel

Dentin

Dental papilla

Figure 12.14 Diagram of the developmental stages of a tooth.

bell-shaped structure around the inner tissue, called the dental papilla. A double layer of cells lining the inner aspect of the bell develops into the outer ameloblasts that lay down enamel from the inside out; and the inner odontoblasts that form dentin as they retreat towards the dental papilla, which is the future pulp area. As these two tissues are deposited the cell layers move apart, the gap being filled with the developing crown. Once the crown is formed the root develops (Figure 12.14).

Eruption

The mechanisms of tooth eruption are complex and still not completely solved. Teeth eventually appear in the mouth through a combination of growth of supporting bone, elongation of the tooth root and growth of the pulp.

Nutrition and teeth

Prenatal nutrition and developing teeth

Surprisingly, prenatal nutrition has very little effect on the developing teeth. Since all of the primary teeth begin to calcify *in utero* they are relatively protected from a lack of calcium; the mother supplies all of the calcium needed whether or not she gains or loses bone during pregnancy.

The movement of tetracyclines and fluoride across the placental barrier has been studied in depth. Cur-

Table 12.4 Recommended dietary fluoride supplement dosage according to drinking water fluoride concentration

Age years	Water fluoride (ppm)		
	<0.3	0.3–0.7	>0.7
Birth–2	0.25	0	0
2–3	0.50	0.25	0
3–13	1.00	0.50	0

The amounts are in mg of fluoride per day (2.2 mg sodium fluoride = 1 mg fluoride ion).

rent opinion is that tetracyclines easily cross the placenta for deposition in the dentin and cementum to produce visible discoloration. In contrast, fluoride does not cross the placenta easily. Fluoride ingestion by the mother must be very high, >3 ppm/day, to produce even mild fluorosis of the primary dentition, and if the mother ingests the usual therapeutic supplemental dose (Table 12.4) this does not raise fluoride levels in the primary teeth developing *in utero*.

Postnatal nutrition and developing teeth

Postnatal nutrition has been shown to affect developing teeth in animal experiments, but effects on humans are less clear. Ingested tetracycline is deposited in developing dentin and cementum to produce a green–gray discoloration that can be seen through the overlying enamel and fluoresces in ultraviolet light.

Adequate calcium in a balanced diet has been stressed to be essential for tooth development after birth, but evidence to support this is lacking. In the 1920s vitamin D deficiency was postulated to produce a 'poorer quality' enamel, but modern research does not support this. Osteoporosis has no effect on the teeth.

Nutrition and dental caries

A direct cause-and-effect relationship between nutritional status and dental caries has not been demonstrated. Both wasting and stunting are associated with retarded exfoliation of the primary teeth and with increased caries rates. What is not clear is whether the increased caries rate is because teeth are present for longer in the mouth and therefore have a longer chance of developing caries, or because the teeth are more susceptible to the disease. Regarding the permanent teeth in the same children, surprisingly, accelerated tooth eruption is seen but still with an increased caries rate. It is believed that a single moderate malnutrition episode

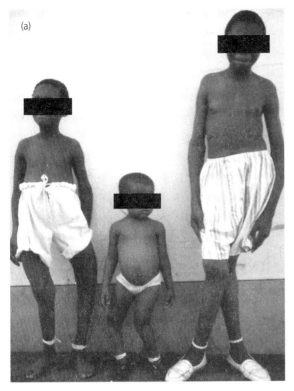
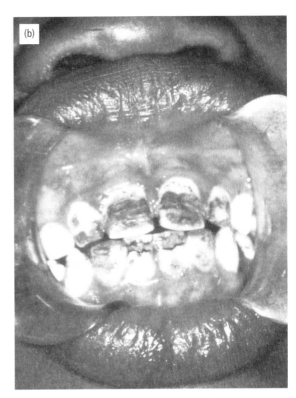

Figure 12.15 (a) Limb deformities in children living in an area associated with endemic fluorosis. (b) Teeth staining due to endemic fluorosis.

under the age of 1 year may alter enamel formation sufficiently to be associated with increased caries later in life, but firm evidence to support this is lacking.

Fluoride and dental fluorosis

Fluoride is regarded by dental associations, dental research organizations and the World Health Organization (WHO) as an essential nutrient that reduces susceptibility to dental caries. The mechanism is complex, but includes formation of calcium fluroapatite through displacement of hydroxyl ions and interference with the metabolism of cariogenic organisms present in dental plaque. Current opinion is that the preventive effect in dental enamel is topical, through adsorption onto enamel crystals in the outer few micrometers of enamel, rather than a systemic deposition into enamel and dentin during tooth development. Some 70% of ingested fluoride is excreted in the urine over 24 h.

Sources of fluoride intake are drinking water and food, as well as fluoridated salt, milk and fluoride-containing dental products such toothpastes, or gels applied topically to teeth. The optimal oral intake of fluoride ion,

that is, the level that gives good protection against dental caries with a low level of dental fluorosis, is approximately 0.5 mg/day. The most cost-effective source is from fluoridated drinking water. For many years the recommended concentration for fluoridated water in temperate climates has been a concentration of 1 ppm of fluoride ion, but because of increased intake from other sources such as fluoridated toothpastes it is now felt that this should be lower to reduce the rate of dental fluorosis. There is not yet general agreement on the level for water fluoridation, other than it will be lower in hot climates in which more water is drunk than the 1 ppm concentration recommended for temperate climates. Regarding fluoride supplementation from tablets, the recommendation of the American Dental Association's Council on Dental Therapeutics is shown in Table 12.4.

Excess fluoride produces dental fluorosis, comprising mottling and staining of teeth as well as surface pitting (Figure 12.15b); the severity of the mottling increases with rising fluoride intake. At a water fluoride ion concentration of 1 ppm about 10% of individuals will show mild mottling (occasional white patches on enamel); the rate is about 20% at a concentration of 2 ppm, thereafter it rises exponentially to 100% at 3 ppm. When very severe mottling is present, enamel is particularly brittle and flakes off the underlying dentin. Caries in such teeth is more frequent than at lower levels of dental fluorosis.

Dental caries

Dental caries is a multifactorial disease. Figure 12.16 summarizes the interaction of teeth, fermentable foods and bacteria that must occur in dental plaque for sufficient time, influenced by an individual's resistance to the disease, for caries to develop.

Bacteria in dental plaque metabolize fermentable carbohydrates into organic acids which demineralize enamel, as well as dentin if in contact with that. The critical pH below which demineralization occurs is pH 5.7. Subsequently, proteolytic enzymes break down the organic component. Remineralization, aided by saliva and fluoride, may happen in the early stages before proteolysis. The more rapidly a food is fermented and the longer a tooth is exposed to a pH below 5.7, the worse is the potential damage. The length of exposure is influenced by a food's inherent retention in the mouth. For example, liquids are cleared from the mouth more rapidly than solids; and foods that stimulate salivary flow though their consistency or chemical properties are cleared more rapidly than bland foods.

The change in pH that is typical is the pattern after a rinse with sucrose. Figure 12.17 shows this Stephan curve after a 10% sucrose rinse in the presence of 24-h-old plaque. After a 1 minute rinse there is a rapid drop in pH within 3 min, followed by a gradual rise back to resting levels over the next 30 min. The return to resting levels is produced by flow of saliva, the buffering action of the salts in saliva and the removal of the food from the mouth. Non-fermentable foods that stimulate saliva flow do not drop the pH below 5.7 and may actually increase it, as in the case of peanuts (Figure 12.17). Since all meals are mixtures of many foods the pH response is complex. Traditional research has reported on eating of single foods and on sequences of food, but not on food mixtures.

The more often the plaque pH is below 5.7, and the longer it remains there, the greater the potential for demineralization and dental caries. Lessening of this risk is the basis for the preventive advice to restrict intake of sticky, fermentable foods to three meals and two snacks per day, together with a reduction in cariogenic organisms in contact with teeth through removal of dental plaque at least once per day.

That sugars, as fermentable carbohydrates, play an etiological role in dental caries is universally accepted, but beyond that statement there is uncertainty on their precise relationship with the disease. In the 1940s results from prospective dietary studies in a Swedish mental institution and an orphanage in Australia, together with national patterns of reduced caries associated with reduced sucrose consumption in

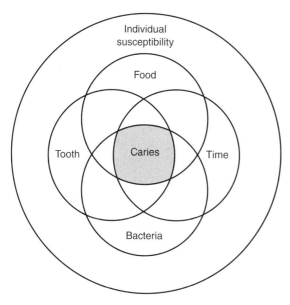

Figure 12.16 Interactions necessary for the development of dental caries.

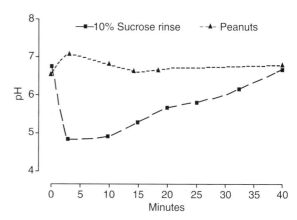

Figure 12.17 Stephan curve after 10% sucrose rinse and 24-h-old dental plaque.

Europe during World War II, suggested a direct causal relationship between sugars, particularly sucrose, and dental caries. This belief has persisted among some scientists to the present day, to the extent that the Committee on Medical Aspects of Food Policy in Great Britain (COMA) recommended that consumption of extrinsic non-milk sugars should not exceed 60 g per person per day. Contrary views are that the Swedish study was far removed from normal eating, and the Australian and World War II results were due to replacement of a highly refined diet with a less refined diet, possibly including protective factors. More recent prospective epidemiological studies have not shown that reductions in fermentable carbohydrates in the general population are accompanied by reductions in dental caries. Indeed, general reductions in dental caries that have occurred over the past 20 years in industrialized countries have happened as fermentable carbohydrate intake has either remained the same or increased. This reduction is held to be the effect of fluoride in toothpastes. National policies to limit sugar intake that some scientists favor are likely to be unattainable, expensive, ineffective and even harmful through an increased intake of fats.

A fair summary of the current opinion on the relationship between fermentable carbohydrates and dental caries is that intake of these in a person at high risk of dental caries plays a more powerful role than in someone at low risk of dental caries. The problem is that risk of dental caries (or resistance to the disease) is a much talked about but ill-understood concept. What is clear from many studies around the world is that about 60% of dental caries occurs in about 20% of people. The reason for this is not known. Targeting of such high-risk persons should be the most cost-effective way of preventing the disease, but as yet identification of high-risk people before dental caries develops remains elusive.

12.5 Nutritional rickets

Nutritional rickets occurs in the pediatric age range, especially in the infant and young child. Although rickets may have a number of different etiologies, nutritional causes are by far the most important globally, and constitute a major public health problem in a number of countries. Despite the ease of its prevention, and the rapidity of its response to treatment, the disease does not receive the attention it should from international agencies and national governments, so children are being left physically handicapped and stunted unnecessarily. In this section the causes, presentation and biochemical and radiological changes associated with nutritional rickets are presented. A brief overview of its treatment and prevention is also provided.

Rickets is a clinical syndrome characterized by a delay in or failure of mineralization of the cartilaginous growth plates in the growing child. These abnormalities result in deformities at the growth plates of rapidly growing bones. Accompanying these changes, there is also a delay in mineralization of newly formed osteoid at the endosteal and periosteal bone surfaces, resulting in an increase in osteoid seam width. These latter abnormalities are features of osteomalacia, which is also characterized by an increase in osteoid surface and volume, an increase in the mineralization lag time and a decrease in tetracycline uptake at the mineralization front. Thus, the disease of rickets is associated with clinical features related to both the growth plate abnormalities of rickets and those of osteomalacia at the various bone surfaces.

Differences between osteoporosis and rickets are listed in Table 12.5.

Causes of rickets

As mentioned above, rickets is primarily a disease characterized by a failure of mineralization of preformed

Table 12.5 Differences between osteoporosis and rickets

	Osteoporosis	Nutritional rickets
Age of presentation	Elderly and postmenopausal women	Infants and young children
Pathology	Loss of bone (mineral: matrix normal)	Failure to mineralize bone matrix (mineral: matrix decreased)
Speed of onset/development	Slow	Rapid
Presentation	Pathological fractures	Limb deformities
Diagnosis	Densitometry assessment or biopsy	Radiographs
Biochemistry	Typically normal	Hypocalemia and elevated alkaline phosphatase

Table 12.6 Classification of the causes of rickets

Calciopenic rickets	Phosphopenic rickets	Inhibition of mineralization
Vitamin D-deficiency	Dietary deficiency, e.g. breast-fed very low-birthweight infant	Aluminum toxicity
Increased vitamin D metabolite catabolism	Inhibition of intestinal phosphate absorption	Fluoride excess
1α-Hydroxylase deficiency	Increased renal loss of phosphate:	Hereditary hypophosphatasia
Renal failure	X-linked hypophosphatemia	1st generation bisphosphonates
Abnormalities of the vitamin D receptor	Fanconi's syndrome	
Dietary calcium deficiency	Distal renal tubular acidosis tumor associated	

The table is not a comprehensive list, but it does highlight the numerous causes of rickets.

matrix. For bone or cartilage matrix to mineralize, the concentrations of both calcium and phosphorus at the mineralization site must be sufficient for the growth and aggregation of the hydroxyapatite crystals, the formation of which are facilitated by the matrix vesicles (from osteoblasts), which actively accumulate calcium and phosphorus ions and remove inhibitors of crystal formation.

Thus, the causes of rickets may be broadly classified into three large groups: those related to an inability to maintain adequate calcium concentrations at the mineralizing bone surface or growth plate (calciopenic rickets), those related to an inability to maintain appropriate phosphorus concentrations (phosphopenic rickets) and those that directly inhibit the process of mineralization (Table 12.6).

From Table 12.6 it is clear that there are numerous causes of rickets, the majority of which are not nutritional in origin and thus will not be considered in this chapter. Nevertheless, nutritional rickets remains the most common form of rickets globally. Until recently, nutritional rickets has been considered to be synonymous with vitamin D-deficiency rickets; however, recent studies suggest that not only is vitamin D deficiency an important cause but so too is a low dietary calcium intake, and the two may act synergistically to exacerbate the risk of developing rickets.

Nutritional rickets: a global perspective

Despite advances in our understanding of calcium homeostasis (see *Introduction to Human Nutrition*, Chapter 9) and vitamin D metabolism (see *Introduction to Human Nutrition*, Chapter 8), nutritional rickets remains a major cause of morbidity and mortality in children in many parts of the world.

Although rickets has been thought of as a disease that originated with the Industrial Revolution in Europe, descriptions of rickets have been attributed to both Homer (900 BC) and Soranus Ephesius (AD 130). Before the Industrial Revolution, rickets was a disease of the children of the aristocracy, as they were frequently kept indoors and excessively clothed if venturing outside. With the rapid growth of cities associated with urban migration, which accompanied the Industrial Revolution, urban slums rapidly developed. The excessive pollution, narrow streets and overcrowding resulted in most young children living in these appalling conditions receiving little or no sunshine. Their mothers likewise were often vitamin D deficient and suffering from osteomalacia, resulting in obstructed labor and neonates being born with no vitamin D stores. In the late nineteenth and early twentieth centuries, several studies described the almost universal prevalence of rickets in young children in Europe. The importance of ultraviolet light in the prevention and treatment of rickets was appreciated in the first quarter of the twentieth century, and with the discovery of vitamin D and its role in the etiology of rickets, the stage was set for the almost complete elimination of vitamin D-deficiency rickets from a number of developed countries through programs of food fortification, vitamin D supplementation and education.

During World War II, the UK introduced vitamin D fortification of a number of foods including milk, cereals and bread. The incidence of rickets fell dramatically, but the program fell into disrepute because of uncontrolled fortification, which was thought to have resulted in an increase in idiopathic hypercalcemia in young infants, although this association has not been conclusively proven. Since then the incidence of nutritional rickets has risen and is particularly a problem among Asian immigrants living in the northern cities of the UK.

In North America, the prevention of rickets through fortification has been more successful. The universal fortification of milk with vitamin D at 400 IU/quart (32 fl oz, approximately 900 ml) since the 1930s has almost eradicated the disease in young children, except in those who are exclusively breast-fed or who are on milk-free diets. However, since the 1980s there have been reports of a resurgence of rickets in at-risk families, in particular in infants who are breast-fed for prolonged periods, in vegan and vegetarian families, and in infants of African–American mothers.

In central Europe and Algeria, rickets has been successfully prevented in infants and young children by the administration of high doses of vitamin D every 3–5 months for the first 2 years of life (*stosstherapie*). Despite the advances that have been made in the prevention of rickets in young children in many developed countries, the disease remains a major problem in a number of developing countries. Not surprisingly, nutritional rickets is more common in those countries at the extremes of latitude, as ultraviolet light exposure is limited for large parts of the year and the cold weather necessitates wearing clothes that cover the majority of the skin surface. Thus, the prevalence of clinical rickets in Tibet has been estimated to be over 60% in children, and similar figures have been obtained from surveys in Mongolia and northern China. Nutritional rickets remains a problem in many countries, despite their lying closer to the equator and being blessed by larger amounts of sunshine than the countries mentioned above. These countries include Sudan, Ethiopia, Nigeria, Algeria, Saudi Arabia, Kuwait and countries in the Middle East. Furthermore, a high prevalence of rickets has been described in young children in areas of Greece and Turkey. Thus, there must be other factors beside high latitude that contribute to predisposing a child to rickets. A number of studies have highlighted poverty, malnutrition, maternal vitamin D deficiency, prolonged breast-feeding and overcrowding as important risk factors.

Cultural and social customs may also aggravate the problem. Several countries have large Muslim communities, which practise 'purdah', thus increasing the risk of vitamin D deficiency in mothers and their young children.

Although the typical age of presentation of vitamin D-deficiency rickets is during the second 6 months of life, reports from a number of developing countries describe clinical signs of rickets in children over the age of 2 years. It is possible that many of these children are suffering from the residual effects of earlier active, but now healed, rickets. However, recent studies from Nigeria, South Africa and Bangladesh have suggested that children outside the infant age group with clinical signs of rickets may be suffering not from vitamin D deficiency, but rather from the effects of low dietary calcium intakes. Calcium intakes of affected children are remarkably similar in the different countries, with intakes estimated to be approximately 200 mg/day. The characteristic features of the diets are the high cereal content and the lack of variety and of dairy product intake. It is unclear how widespread this form of nutritional rickets is; however, low dietary calcium intakes may also exacerbate the severity of vitamin D-deficiency rickets by increasing the catabolism of vitamin D and thus increasing the requirements.

The burden that nutritional rickets places on children globally is unclear, but in those countries in which there is a high prevalence of rickets, a significant proportion of the infant mortality may be directly or indirectly due to the disease. This has clearly been shown in Ethiopia, where it has been estimated that children with rickets have a 13 times higher incidence of pneumonia, which is associated with a 40% mortality. The long-term sequelae of severe rickets are difficult to quantitate, but short stature, residual limb deformities resulting in early osteoarthritis and pelvic deformities in women leading to a high incidence of obstructed labor are some of the problems.

Pathogenesis of vitamin D-deficiency rickets

As mentioned in the section above, the most common cause of nutritional rickets is vitamin D deficiency. To maintain vitamin D sufficiency, people are largely dependent on the conversion in the skin of 7-dehydrocholesterol to vitamin D_3 through the photochemical action of ultraviolet light, as the normal unfortified diet is generally deficient in vitamin D (see *Introduction to Human Nutrition*, Chapter 8). Thus, vitamin D deficiency is most common at the two extremes of life; in young infants who are unable to walk, and in the elderly who are infirm and are unable to go out of doors.

Vitamin D-deficiency rickets is most prevalent in infants and toddlers between the ages of 3 and 18

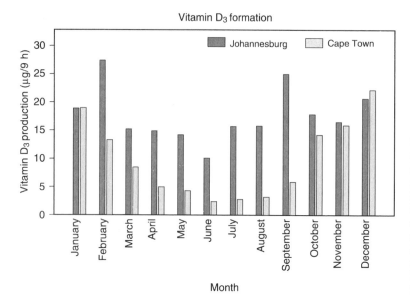

Figure 12.18 Seasonal variation in the production by sunlight of vitamin D₃ from 7-dehydrocholesterol *in vitro* in two cities at different latitudes in the southern hemisphere (Johannesburg, 26° S, and Cape Town, 32° S). Note that production of vitamin D in the two cities during the summer months is similar, but during the autumn and winter months of March to September vitamin D production is minimal in the more southerly city of Cape Town. (Reproduced with permission from Pettifor *et al.*, 1996.)

months, although it may occur at any age if social customs, skin pigmentation and living in countries at extremes of latitude combine to prevent adequate ultraviolet B (UV-B) exposure of the skin. It is uncommon under 3 months of age because the newborn infant is provided with some vitamin D stores as 25-OHD crosses the placenta, umbilical cord values being approximately two-thirds of maternal concentrations. However, the half-life of 25-OHD is only 3–4 weeks, so values fall rapid after birth unless the infant is exposed to ultraviolet light or receives a dietary source of vitamin D. Furthermore, these stores may be inadequate if the mother is vitamin D deficient, resulting in an earlier presentation of rickets or, in the rare case, of the neonate being born with rickets.

Human breast milk typically contains very little of the parent vitamin D or its metabolites. It has been estimated that normal human milk contains the equivalent of approximately 40–60 IU/litre. Assuming that an infant consumes about 650 ml of breast milk daily, the vitamin D intake from that source would only amount to 26–39 IU/day, thus contributing little to the maintenance of the vitamin D status of the exclusively breast-fed infant. Supporting the above conclusions is the finding that serum levels of 25-OHD in exclusively breast-fed infants correlate with their sunshine exposure, highlighting the importance of UV-B exposure, rather than diet, in preventing rickets in breast-fed infants. The amount of sunlight needed to maintain

normal serum concentrations of 25-OHD in the infant appears to be very little, although it will vary according to latitude and season. In Cincinnati, USA, during summer, it has been estimated to vary between 20 min a week for an infant in a nappy only to 2 h a week for an infant fully clothed but without a cap. The reliance on sunlight exposure and the intradermal formation of vitamin D for the maintenance of vitamin D sufficiency in exclusively breast-fed infants has resulted in the presentation of clinical rickets having a strong seasonality in most studies. Rickets is most prevalent in late winter and early spring months (Figure 12.18).

Before the introduction of specially modified cow's milk formulae for the feeding of non-breast-fed infants, breast-feeding was noted to reduce the risk of rickets in young infants. More recent studies, however, consider breast-feeding to be a risk factor. The explanation for this apparent paradox is that breast-milk substitutes are now all required to be vitamin D fortified, thus protecting against vitamin D deficiency. Before the introduction of modified cow's milk formulae, non-breast-fed infants were fed unmodified or diluted cow's milk which, like breast milk, contains very little vitamin D. Further, the calcium:phosphorus ratio of 1:1 and the high phosphate content of cow's milk both adversely affect calcium homeostasis in the relatively vitamin D-deficient infant, resulting in a higher prevalence of clinical rickets.

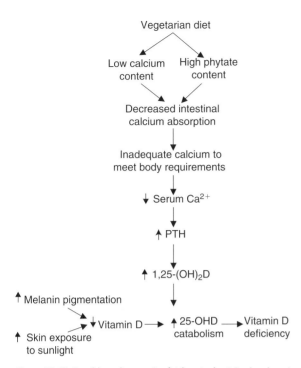

Figure 12.19 Possible pathogenesis of rickets in the Asian immigrant community in northern Europe. The disease is thought to be result of a combination of relative vitamin D insufficiency and inadequate intestinal calcium absorption. PTH: parathyroid hormone.

Although vitamin D deficiency is the ultimate cause of rickets in the Asian community, it is likely that several factors, mentioned earlier, combine to exacerbate the low vitamin D concentrations and the development of rickets. These factors include decreased vitamin D formation in the skin owing to increased skin coverage by clothing and a greater degree of melanin pigmentation than the Caucasian population, a low vitamin D intake, a low dietary calcium content of the mainly vegetarian diet, and poor intestinal absorption of calcium because of the high phytate content of the diet. Low calcium intakes and impaired calcium absorption have been shown to increase vitamin D requirements through an increase in its catabolism as a result of the elevated $1,25\text{-}(OH)_2D$ concentrations (Figure 12.19). Thus, these mechanisms push mild vitamin D insufficiency into frank vitamin D deficiency and rickets unless vitamin D intake or skin exposure to sunlight is increased (Box 12.7). Recommended vitamin D intakes are summarized in Table 12.7 and Box 12.8. Possible strategies to prevent vitamin D deficiency are summarized in Box 12.9.

Box 12.7 Factors predisposing a child to vitamin D deficiency rickets

- Living in a country at high latitude
- Lack of sunlight exposure through overcrowding, social customs, clothing or pollution
- Prolonged breast-feeding without vitamin D supplementation
- Low dietary calcium intake
- Increased melanin pigmentation

Table 12.7 Dietary intakes of vitamin D recommended by British and American expert committees

Age group	UK recommended nutrient intake (μg (IU)/day)	American adequate intake (μg (IU)/day)
0–6 months	8.5 (340)	5.0 (200)
7 months and older toddlers	7 (280)	5.0 (200)
Children and adults	0	5.0 (200)
>65 years (UK) or >70 years (USA)	10 (400)	15 (600)
Pregnancy and lactation	10 (400)	5.0 (200)

Box 12.8 UK recommended vitamin D intakes (1 μg = 40 IU)

0–6 months	8.5 μg/day
7–12 months	7 μg/day
1–3 years	7 μg/day
4–65 years	0 (unless an at-risk group, in which case 10 μg/day)
65+ years	10 μg/day

Box 12.9 Possible strategies to prevent vitamin D deficiency

- Ensure regular skin exposure to sunlight
- Daily vitamin D supplementation
- Intermittent high-dose supplementation (*stosstherapie*)
- Food fortification

Biochemical changes associated with vitamin D deficiency rickets

As discussed in Chapter 8 of *Introduction to Human Nutrition*, in this series, vitamin D plays an important role in maintaining normal calcium homeostasis, mainly through optimizing intestinal calcium absorption. The biochemical hallmark of vitamin D deficiency is a low circulating concentration of 25-OHD, which

Table 12.8 Progression of the biochemical and radiological changes in untreated vitamin D deficiency

	Stage I	Stage II	Stage III
X-ray changes	Nil to slight osteopenia	Mild to moderate changes of rickets	Severe changes of rickets
Serum calcium	Low	Low to normal	Very low
Serum phosphorus	May be normal	Low	Low
Alkaline phosphatase	Normal to mildly elevated	Raised	Very raised
Parathyroid hormone	Normal to mildly elevated	Raised	Very raised

is the major circulating form of the vitamin. In the majority of studies of vitamin D levels in vitamin D-deficiency rickets, 25-OHD levels are reported to be less than 4 ng/ml ($<$10 nmol/l), the normal reference range being $>$12 ng/ml ($>$30 nmol/l). As 1,25-$(OH)_2$D is considered to be the physiologically active metabolite of vitamin D, low levels would be expected to be reported in active vitamin D-deficiency rickets. However, serum 1,25-$(OH)_2$D concentrations are not consistent and low, normal or raised levels have been found in patients. It is suggested that the elevated levels are due to a slight increase in substrate, perhaps through sunlight exposure or dietary intake, causing a transient elevation in 1,25-$(OH)_2$D concentrations. Rapid rises in 1,25-$(OH)_2$D to supraphysiological levels have been documented in vitamin D-deficient subjects after the administration of very small doses of vitamin D or exposure to sunlight.

The biochemical progression of vitamin D deficiency has been divided into three biochemical stages, although there are no sharp boundaries between the stages (Table 12.8). Stage I represents the earliest stage and is characterized by hypocalcemia with normal serum phosphorus, alkaline phosphatase and PTH values. During this phase, the infant may present with features of hypocalcemia; however, clinical or radiological signs of rickets are not seen. Frequently, this stage is not detected clinically. In stage II, secondary hyperparathyroidism has developed and partially corrected the hypocalcemia; thus, serum calcium concentrations may be within the low normal range, but serum phosphorus values are low and alkaline phosphatase concentrations are elevated. In this stage, the typical radiographic features of rickets are found. Stage III is associated with severe clinical and radiological rickets, with hypocalcemia once again occurring and alkaline phosphatase values reaching even higher levels.

Other biochemical features found in vitamin D-deficiency rickets include decreased urinary calcium excretion, decreased renal tubular reabsorption of phosphorus, increased urinary adenosine monophosphate (cAMP) excretion, generalized aminoaciduria and impaired acid excretion, which are all features of hyperparathyroidism. Bone turnover markers are typically increased, with increased excretion of urinary hydroxyproline and pyridinoline cross-links. Characteristically, alkaline phosphatase values are elevated; however, serum osteocalcin has been reported to be within the normal range in untreated rickets.

Histological changes of bone

Histological changes in vitamin D-deficiency rickets occur both at the growth plate and at the endosteal and periosteal bone surfaces. At the growth plate there is a failure of calcification of the longitudinal septa surrounding cartilage cells in the lower hypertrophic zone and the cells fail to undergo apoptosis, while cells in the proliferative zone continue to divide. Blood vessels invading the zone of provisional calcification also cease to proliferate. Thus, the growth plate widens and with the effect of weight bearing and continued proliferation the longitudinal rows of cartilage cells and thus the growth plate become distorted and splayed.

At the endosteal bone surface, newly formed osteoid fails to mineralize; thus, the trabecular surface covered by unmineralized osteoid increases and the osteoid seams widen. Although these features are typical of osteomalacia, they are not pathognomonic unless they are accompanied by the finding of an increase in the mineralization lag time (the time taken for newly laid osteoid to mineralize).

Radiological changes of bone

The radiological changes of rickets are typically seen best at the growth plates of rapidly growing bones; thus, the distal radius and ulna and the femoral and tibial growth plates at the knee are the usual sites examined (Figure 12.20). The characteristic changes

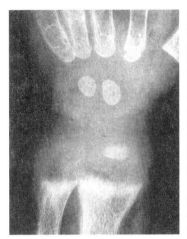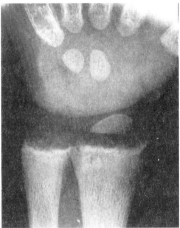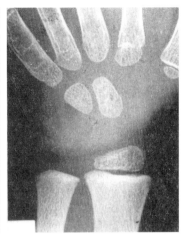

Figure 12.20 Radiographic changes of rickets. Note the progressive improvement in the radiographic picture from left to right in response to vitamin D treatment over a period of 3 months. (Reproduced from Pettifor, 1991 with permission of Lippincott Williams & Wilkins.)

include a loss of the provisional zone of calcification and thus blurring of the demarcation between the metaphysis and the cartilaginous growth plate, widening of the growth plate, and cupping and splaying of the distal metaphysis. The epiphyses typically are poorly mineralized and underdeveloped, resulting in a delay in the bone age compared with chronological age.

The type and position of deformities of the long bones vary depending on the age of the child, the degree of weight bearing and the severity of the rickets. If hypotonia is severe, deformities might not develop until weight bearing occurs with the commencement of treatment. Genu varum (bow legs) tends to occur in young children who develop rickets, as this age group tends to have a normal physiological bowing. In the older child, genu valgum (knock knees) is more common.

Once treatment has commenced, the initiation of radiological healing may be seen within 3 weeks, with the appearance of a broad band of increased density occurring at the position of the provisional zone of calcification at the distal end of the metaphysis (Figure 12.20). Over the following weeks, the epiphyseal plates narrow, the epiphyses mineralize and cortices thicken. Modeling of deformities occurs so that in many situations apparently severe deformities disappear over a period of months.

Clinical presentation

The clinical picture of rickets depends to a certain extent on the age of the child at presentation. Clinical features of hypocalcemia may occur at any age, but are more common in the young infant when they may present with apneic attacks, tetany, convulsions or stridor. Delay in motor milestones and hypotonia are common presentations. Typically, the infant is floppy and sweating and has a protuberant abdomen (Figure 12.21). In severe rickets, hepatosplenomegaly may be present, partially pushed down by the flattened diaphragm, but also enlarged by extramedullary erythropoiesis.

The clinical picture of hypocalcemia and rickets is covered in greater detail in the Clinical Nutrition textbook of this series.

Dietary calcium deficiency

Studies conducted since the 1970s in South Africa and Nigeria have highlighted the importance of low dietary calcium intakes in the pathogenesis of nutritional rickets in vitamin D-replete children outside the infant age group. Prior to these studies, it was believed that low dietary calcium intakes were not responsible for rickets in children, except in a few very unusual situations, when young children with gastrointestinal problems were placed on very restricted diets that were very low in calcium (Figure 12.22).

The hallmark of rickets due to dietary calcium deficiency rather than vitamin D deficiency is the finding of 25-OHD values within the normal range and elevated $1,25\text{-}(OH)_2D$ concentrations in children who are older than those normally at risk of developing vitamin D deficiency (Table 12.9). Further dietary calcium intakes are characteristically low, at about 200 mg/day, devoid of dairy products, and high in phytates and

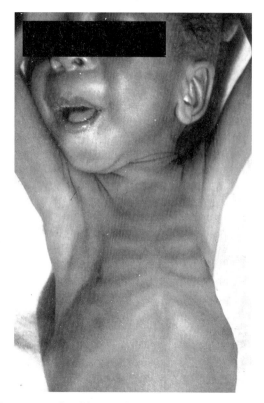

Figure 12.21 Clinical features of an 8-month-old child with vitamin D-deficiency rickets. Note the marked chest deformities and the rather protuberant abdomen. (Reproduced from Pettifor and Daniels, 1997.)

oxalates. In South Africa, the children are usually aged between 6 and 16 years and live in rural parts of the country. Unlike those with vitamin D deficiency, the children with dietary calcium deficiency do not have muscle weakness. In Nigeria, the children are younger than those described from South Africa. They tend to present around 4 years of age, having had symptoms for approximately 2 years. In both countries, medical assistance is generally sought because of progressive lower limb deformities.

Support for the hypothesis that dietary calcium deficiency plays an important role in the pathogenesis of rickets in these children comes from the therapeutic response to calcium supplements (Figure 12.23).

It is not known how widespread the problem of dietary calcium deficiency is. It is likely that children with dietary calcium deficiency have been and continue to be diagnosed as vitamin D deficient and treated with vitamin D and calcium supplements. On this regimen the bone disease will respond, and thus the incidence of dietary calcium deficiency will be severely underestimated. Nevertheless, the apparent scarcity of the clinical disease needs to be confirmed by more detailed studies in developing countries where maize (corn) forms a major part of the cereal staple. Although in both Nigeria and South Africa maize is the staple, recently a report from Bangladesh, where rice

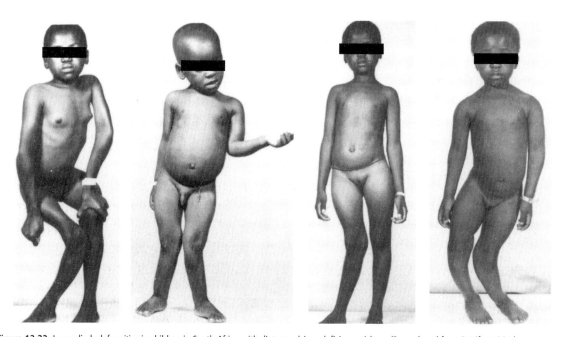

Figure 12.22 Lower limb deformities in children in South Africa with dietary calcium-deficiency rickets. (Reproduced from Pettifor, 1991.)

Table 12.9 Differentiating features between vitamin D deficiency and dietary calcium deficiency rickets

	Vitamin D deficiency	Dietary calcium deficiency
Onset	Usually between 6 and 18 months	Usually after weaning (>2 years)
Hypotonia	Present	Usually not present
Biochemistry:		
– 25-OHD	Usually <10 nmol/l	Usually >25 nmol/l
– 1,25-(OH)$_2$D	Variable (may be low, normal or elevated)	Elevated
Dietary calcium intake	Variable (usual close to RDA)	Low (usually ~200 mg/day)

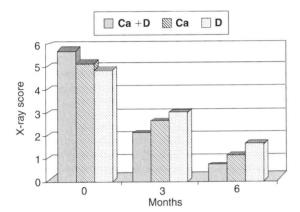

Figure 12.23 Response of randomly assigned Nigerian children with active rickets to treatment with calcium supplements (1000 mg/day), vitamin D (600 000 IU three monthly), or a combination of both over 6 months. The X-ray score reflects the severity of radiographic changes of rickets at the wrist and knee (maximum score = 10). The children who received the calcium supplements with or without vitamin D responded significantly better than those receiving vitamin D alone.

is the cereal staple, has suggested that low dietary calcium intakes may be responsible for an apparent increase in the incidence of rickets in children since the 1980s (Figure 12.24).

Rickets of prematurity

Over the past few decades, rapid advances have been made in the management of very low-birthweight infants, resulting in a marked improvement in survival rates, particularly for infants weighing less than 1000 g at birth. Associated with the increased survival has been an increase in clinical and biochemical evidence of metabolic bone disease in these infants (Box 12.10). The bone disease encompasses a range of abnormalities from radiographic osteopenia to frank rickets and pathological fractures. The major risk factor associated with the development of the disorder is severe immaturity (<1000 g) accompanied by breast-milk or

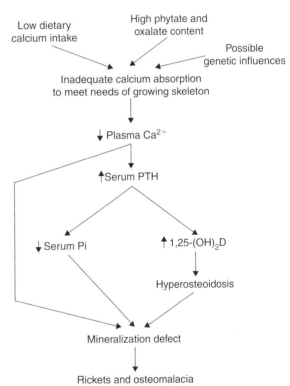

Figure 12.24 Proposed pathogenesis of dietary calcium-deficiency rickets. Note that a combination of factors may play a role in the pathogenesis. PTH: parathyroid hormone; Pi: inorganic phosphate.

soy formula feeding and prolonged illness. Although the pathogenesis is multifactorial, phosphorus depletion due to an inadequate intake plays a major role.

Supplementation of the breast-milk-fed infant with phosphorus rapidly improves the retention of both calcium and phosphorus and corrects the biochemical picture of the phosphorus depletion syndrome. Once an adequate phosphorus intake is assured, the calcium content of breast milk may become a limiting factor, so simultaneous calcium supplementation is often recommended. Care, however, should be exercised as supplemental calcium may precipitate out before being administered to the baby. As vitamin D stores in the newborn infant are limited and many of these very premature low-birthweight infants spend prolonged periods in intensive care units and neonatal nurseries, an adequate vitamin D intake needs to be ensured. It is recommended that vitamin D 800–1000 IU/daily should be provided as a supplement.

12.6 Bone loss with aging

Osteoporosis: a global perspective

The WHO has defined osteoporosis as a condition characterized by low bone mass and microarchitectural deterioration of bone tissue which leads to enhanced bone fragility and a consequent increase in fracture risk. These fractures are most common in the wrist, spinal vertebrae and hip, but they can occur elsewhere in the skeleton. Osteoporosis is further defined by the WHO as a BMC or BMD, measured by absorptiometry, of more than 2.5 standard deviations below the young adult mean. Fractures are the clinically important manifestation of osteoporosis, whereas low bone mass classifies those at risk.

Osteoporosis is a major health problem among older adults. In the UK, over 3 million people are currently affected and approximately 60 000 hip fractures, 50 000 wrist fractures and at least 40 000 vertebral fractures occur each year. One in three British women and one in 12 men over the age of 50 years can expect to experience an osteoporotic fracture during their remaining years. Similarly high fracture rates occur in white populations of northern Europe, the USA and Australasia. However, in other populations, such as those of Africa and China, the incidence is much lower, at least in terms of hip fracture, which is the most reliable statistic available (Figure 12.25). In countries

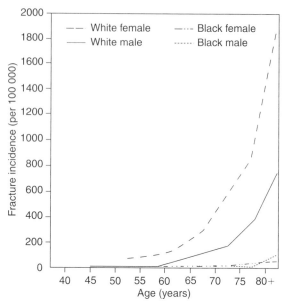

Figure 12.25 Annual incidence of femoral-neck fractures in the Johannesburg population over 40 years of age. The marked ethnic differences in incidence are apparent. (Reproduced from Solomon, 1979 with permission of Elsevier Science.)

where hip fracture rates are high, women are at greater risk than men, while in countries where the incidence of hip fracture is low, men and women are at approximately equal risk. Within countries there are differences between ethnic groups in hip fracture risk. For example, African–Americans and New Zealand Maoris are at lower risk than their Caucasian counterparts, while the incidence of hip fractures in Singapore is highest in the Indian community. However, within all regions and ethnic groups, hip fracture incidence is increasing because of the rise in the number of people surviving to an age when hip fractures are more common. It has been estimated that the global incidence will increase from 1.66 million in 1990 to 6.26 million in 2050 because of the change in demographic profile (Box 12.11).

The pathogenesis of osteoporosis is still a matter of intensive research. Factors that have been implicated include low sex hormone concentrations, especially estrogen withdrawal at the menopause, compromised supply or metabolic handling of calcium and other nutrients, poor vitamin D status and physical inactivity. Low bone mass and propensity to fracture are heritable traits, which makes it likely that there is a strong genetic component in the pathogenesis of the disease. The involvement of a number of candidate genes has been proposed and polymorphisms in these genes are associated with differences in phenotype or gene expression. Examples include the genes encoding for the vitamin D receptor, the estrogen receptor, collagen-1-α_1 and IGF-1. At present, however, there is no convincing evidence of an association between any of these polymorphisms and fracture risk.

There are no accepted explanations for the geographical and ethnic differences in fracture incidence. Effects of differences in diet, sunlight exposure and activity levels have been suggested, as well as genetic influences. The variation in fracture incidence is unlikely to be related to low bone mass per se, since Asian and African people generally have lower BMC than their Western counterparts. This is partly, but not entirely, related to their smaller body and therefore bone size. Global variations in osteoporosis cannot be explained by differences in calcium intake because hip fracture incidence is greatest in countries with the highest calcium intakes, such as those of northern Europe. Differences in skeletal anatomy, metabolism and microarchitecture may be important, such as the shorter hip axis length of Asian and African people relative to their height, and the higher bone turnover and greater trabecular width in the spines of black South Africans.

Postmenopausal osteoporosis

After the attainment of peak bone mass during the second to third decade of life, bone tissue is gradually lost from the skeleton in both men and women. Periosteal bone growth continues, and the tissue that is lost is from endosteal surfaces. In women, this bone loss is accentuated in the 10–15 years that follow estrogen withdrawal at the menopause, when approximately one-third of cortical bone tissue and one-half of cancellous bone tissue is lost.

Bone loss is the net consequence of imbalances between bone resorption and formation resulting from changes in the recruitment, activity and lifespan of

Box 12.12 Features of postmenopausal osteoporosis

- Occurs between 50 and 75 years of age
- Female: male ratio 6:1
- Associated with fractures of the distal forearm and vertebrae
- Associated with estrogen withdrawal
- Associated with excessive osteoclast activity
- Prevented by estrogen replacement

osteoclasts and osteoblasts. Two types of bone loss are often distinguished, postmenopausal (type I) and age-related (type II) osteoporosis, the first being characterised by a relative increase in osteoclast numbers, the latter by a relative decrease in osteoblast numbers. However, the classification of osteoporosis is not clear-cut; both types may coexist or may represent parts of the same continuum. The features of postmenopausal osteoporosis are summarized in Box 12.12.

Postmenopausal, or type I, osteoporosis affects individuals aged 50–75 years and is more common in women than men (ratio 6:1). Accelerated bone loss is associated with reductions in calcium absorption and in circulating concentrations of PTH and 1,25-dihydroxyvitamin D. Fractures occur most commonly at the distal radius (Colles' fracture of the wrist) and in the spinal vertebrae (crush fracture), regions rich in cancellous bone. Estrogen deficiency is regarded as the main pathogenetic factor, and hormone replacement therapy (HRT) is an effective preventive measure. At the cellular level, estrogen withdrawal produces a greater number of active osteoclasts, more bone remodeling sites and deeper excavation of resorption cavities. Trabeculae become perforated and may disappear altogether, which reduces the strength of cancellous bone to withstand compressive forces. A number of antiresorptive agents are available for the treatment of postmenopausal osteoporosis, primarily HRT, bisphosphonates and raloxifene, a selective estrogen receptor modulator.

Age-related osteoporosis

Age-related, or type II, osteoporosis affects women and men over about the age of 70 (ratio 2:1). In general, bone loss is not accelerated and bone turnover may be reduced. Calcium absorption is reduced, 1,25-dihydroxyvitamin D concentrations may be low but PTH levels may be increased. Fractures occur commonly in the proximal femur (hip) and spinal vertebrae (wedge fracture). They are associated with trabecular thinning

---

Box 12.13 Features of age-related oseoprosis

- Occurs generally in people over 70 years of age
- Male: female ratio 2:1
- Involves fractures of the hip and vertebrae
- Associated with impaired osteoblast function
- Associated with decreased intestinal calcium absorption, hyperparathyroidism and poor vitamin D status

Box 12.14 Vitamin D and the elderly

- High prevalence of poor vitamin D status in the elderly
- Poor vitamin D status associated with decreased sunlight exposure, low 7-dehydrocholesterol levels in the skin, poor vitamin D intakes and obesity
- Vitamin D and calcium supplements reduce fracture risk

in cancellous bone and the presence of giant resorption cavities in cortical bone.

Aging is associated with several factors that may result in bone loss and increased bone fragility. These include decreases in physical activity and muscle strength that have direct effects on the skeleton, and also indirect factors via impaired neuromuscular protective mechanisms, which increase the likelihood of falling and of a fall resulting in fracture. Age-related low estrogen and GH concentrations may impair the function and senescence of osteoblasts, resulting in declining bone turnover and osteocyte numbers, which may reduce the ability to repair fatigue microdamage. Secondary hyperparathyroidism caused by declining renal function and compromised vitamin D status may also be important, via direct effects on the skeleton and indirect effects on calcium handling. Calcium and vitamin D supplementation has been shown to reduce the incidence of non-vertebral fractures in elderly men and women. The features of age-related osteoporosis are summarized in Box 12.13.

Low circulating levels of endogenous estrogens are produced in women who are many years postmenopause and these may continue to play an important role in the bone health of older women. Current estrogen use in women aged 65 and older, for example, has been associated with a decreased risk of non-vertebral fractures, especially at the wrist. Similarly in men, some of the skeletal effects of testosterone appear to be mediated through its conversion by aromatase to estrodiol, and this may be one factor involved in male osteoporosis associated with low testosterone concentrations. Recently, it has been proposed that estrogen deficiency is the underlying cause of the late, slow phase of bone loss in postmenopausal women and the continuous phase of bone loss in aging men in addition to the early, accelerated bone loss postmenopause.

Role of vitamin D deficiency

Poor vitamin D status may have a role in the pathogenesis of age-related bone loss and fracture,

although frank osteomalacia is rarely implicated. It is thought that the mechanism for the increase in bone loss and fractures is via the resulting secondary hyperparathyroidism, although the muscle weakness and depression associated with vitamin D deficiency may also be important.

Vitamin D is obtained either from the diet or by endogenous production in the skin by the action of sunlight (see Chapter 8 in *Introduction to Human Nutrition*). The intermediate metabolite 25-hydroxyvitamin D (25-OHD), produced from vitamin D in the liver, is a useful status marker, being responsive to changes in dietary vitamin D and to sunlight exposure. Plasma 25-OHD concentrations decline with age, as a result of decreased endogenous production of the vitamin caused by reduction in the exposure to sunlight, in the tissue content of the precursor, 7-dehydrocholesterol, and in the efficiency of the synthetic process.

Associations have been reported between 25-OHD concentration and BMD in middle-aged and older women. However, vitamin D intervention trials of older people with either bone loss or fracture as outcome have met with mixed success, possibly reflecting differing degrees of vitamin D insufficiency in the various study populations. Trials of calcium and vitamin D together have resulted in a decreased incidence of non-vertebral fractures, but not consistently in the attenuation of bone loss (Box 12.14).

Traditionally, a serum 25-OHD concentration of 25 nmol/l has been used to define the lower end of the normal range, a value higher than that at which clinical osteomalacia is usually seen. Using this cut-off, a significant prevalence of vitamin D insufficiency has been recognized in the elderly populations of UK and elsewhere in Europe, particularly those in residential accommodation. Several recent studies have reported inverse relationships between plasma concentrations of 25-OHD and PTH, suggesting that the rise in PTH that accompanies declining vitamin D status may occur at plasma 25-OHD concentrations higher than the traditional cut-off, especially in older age groups. There are calls to increase the lower cut-off of normality for

25-OHD to match a putative threshold below which the concentration of PTH would be expected to rise. Such a change would substantially increase the numbers of people classified as vitamin D deficient and would, perhaps, prompt greater action to improve vitamin D status. However, on a population basis, there is a wide variation in PTH concentration at any given 25-OHD level and such a threshold has yet to be defined with any certainty. In addition, in the context of age-related bone loss and fragility fractures, it is, as yet, unclear what concentrations of PTH, and hence of 25-OHD, are optimal for long-term bone health.

12.7 Specific nutrients and their effects on bone health

In this section the effects of specific nutrients on bone health will be discussed. It should be borne in mind that isolated nutrient deficiencies are unusual; rather, they reflect an unbalanced diet and therefore may be associated with other less obvious nutrient or energy deficiencies, which could mask or aggravate the apparent effects on bone.

Calcium

Calcium is one of the main bone-forming minerals (99% of the body's approximately 1000 g of calcium is in bone), so an appropriate supply to bone is essential at all stages of life. Only approximately one-third of dietary calcium from a Western-style diet is absorbed, and calcium is lost from the body by urinary excretion and in dermal and gastrointestinal secretions. In estimating calcium requirements, most committees have used either a factorial approach, where calculations of skeletal accretion and turnover rates are combined with typical values for calcium absorption and excretion, or a variety of methods based on experimentally derived balance data. Recommended calcium intakes are shown in Table 12.10. There has been considerable debate about whether current recommended intakes are adequate to maximize peak bone mass and to minimize bone loss and fracture risk in later life, and the controversies continue.

Calcium intake and peak bone mass

Correlations between calcium intake and adult BMC/BMD have been reported from a large number of cross-sectional and retrospective studies, although there are many other studies where no such association

Table 12.10 Dietary intakes of calcium recommended by the British and American expert committees

	UK recommended nutrient intake mg (mmol)/day	American adequate intake mg (mmol)/day
Infants	525 (13.1)	210–270 (5.3–6.8)
Children	350–550 (8.8–13.8)	500–800 (12.5–20.0)
Adolescents		1300 (32.5)
Males	1000 (25.0)	
Females	800 (20.0)	
Adults	700 (17.5)	1000 (25)
Postmenopausal	700 (17.5)	1200 (30)
Pregnancy	700 (17.5)	1000 (25)
Lactation	1250 (31.25)[a]	1000 (25)

[a] May not be necessary.

has been observed. Meta-analyses have concluded that calcium intake is a significant determinant of BMD, but the magnitude of the effect is small, about 1% of the population variance. Interpretation of this association is difficult, however, because few studies have adjusted adequately for the confounding effects of body size.

Supplementation of children with calcium salts results in an increase in bone mineral accompanied by a decrease in bone turnover, possibly indicating fewer remodeling sites at the tissue level, while supplementation with milk appears to increase bone mineral by promoting skeletal growth. Whether either of these interventions ultimately alters peak bone mass and, if so, whether later fracture risk is reduced, has yet to be determined.

Calcium and the postmenopausal period

Calcium supplementation given to women around the time of the menopause has little or no effect on the BMD of cancellous regions of the skeleton, where the greatest loss of bone is occurring at that time, but may cause a modest increase in regions rich in cortical bone.

Calcium intake and bone loss during aging

In older women, calcium supplementation is associated with a higher BMD, by around 1–3%, and with reductions in bone loss in the first 1–2 years after supplementation is started, although it does not prevent some loss from occurring. Longitudinal studies, which follow people prospectively over time, have shown a relationship between customary calcium intake and bone loss in some studies but not others. Case–control studies in Britain, Australia and Canada, populations with medium to high average calcium intakes, have reported no relationship between customary calcium intake and the risk of hip fracture, whereas studies in Hong Kong and southern Europe, where average calcium intakes are lower, have observed an increase in hip fracture risk with declining calcium intake. Cohort studies give similar results. While meta-analyses have suggested an increase in hip fracture incidence with declining calcium intake, this effect appears to be strongest in populations with a comparatively low average calcium intake and suggests that there is a threshold of increasing risk below around 400–500 mg/day.

Long-term studies suggest that the effects of calcium supplementation occur largely in the first 1–2 years. Calcium has antiresorptive properties, and the increase in BMD that accompanies calcium supplementation is thought to reflect a reduction in the activation of new bone remodeling sites, the infilling of current resorption cavities and an increase in the reversible calcium space. Once this process is complete and a new steady state has been achieved, no further increase in BMD occurs and bone loss continues at a similar rate to before. A similar mechanism is thought to underlie the increase in BMD observed during supplementation of children and adolescents with calcium salts. There have been only a few calcium supplementation trials with fracture as an end-point. Results have been modest and inconsistent, but sample sizes have been small. Larger trials of calcium and vitamin D supplementation in elderly people have demonstrated reductions in the incidence of non-vertebral fractures.

In general, the effect of customary calcium intake on the outcome of calcium supplementation has not been investigated. In those studies where it has, no relationship has been noted, except in a study of American women 6 or more years postmenopause, where the effect on BMD and on bone loss was limited to those with a daily calcium intake below 400 mg/day. Taken together with the observational data, this suggests, for women living in Western-style environments, that customary calcium intakes below the UK lower reference nutrient intake (LRNI) of 400 mg/day may not be compatible with long-term bone health. There is, however, no evidence of beneficial skeletal effects of a customary calcium intake above the current UK reference nutrient intake (RNI) for any age group, although calcium supplementation is a recognized adjunct in the treatment of bone loss and the prevention of fracture in vulnerable individuals. Recent committees reviewing the evidence have felt unable to use bone health and fracture outcomes as criteria for calculating RNI values.

Phosphorus

Phosphorus is an essential bone-forming element and, as with calcium, an adequate supply of phosphorus to bone is necessary throughout life. Both calcium and phosphorus are required for the appropriate mineralization of the skeleton, and a depletion of serum phosphate leads to impaired bone mineralization and compromised osteoblast function. However, there is little evidence that, in healthy individuals, the dietary intake of phosphorus limits good bone health, except in the special case of very low-birthweight infants. Although there is a set proportion of calcium and phosphorus in bone (Ca:P = 10:6), the ratio of calcium to phosphorus in the diet can vary over a wide range with no detectable effects on the absorption and retention of either mineral. Reports of correlations between phosphorus intake and BMD are inconsistent and likely to be affected by size-confounding. Concerns have been expressed about the possible adverse effects of the increasingly high intake of phosphorus in Western-style diets, especially in relation to the consumption of carbonated drinks. At present, it seems unlikely that high phosphorus intakes have consequences for long-term bone health.

Magnesium

Magnesium is involved in bone and mineral homeostasis and is important in bone crystal growth and stabilization. In a limited number of studies, magnesium intake has been reported to be positively associated with both BMD and excretion of bone resorption markers in middle-aged women, and short-term increases in BMD have been observed with magnesium supplementation. However, the influence of magnesium nutrition, within the range of normal customary intakes, on long-term bone health is unknown. Magnesium is one of a number of nutrients found in fruit and vegetables which contribute to an alkaline environment and which may promote bone health by a variety of mechanisms (see later in this section), making it difficult to examine the effects of magnesium alone.

Protein intake

High protein intake

On a worldwide basis, high protein intakes have been linked with hip fracture because the consumption of protein, particularly as meat and dairy products, is greatest in countries where hip fractures are common. Protein intake is a determinant of urinary calcium excretion, and animal protein, which is rich in sulfur-containing amino acids, contributes to an acidic environment (see later in this section). There are concerns, but no evidence, that high protein intakes are inadvisable for long-term bone health. For example, when meat is the protein source, the hypercalciuric effect of protein is offset by the hypocalciuric effect of meat phosphorus, and calcium balance is not affected by high-meat diets.

Protein deficiency

Protein deficiency very seldom occurs as an isolated nutrient deficiency; thus, it is difficult to separate out the effects of protein deficiency from those of other nutrient deficiencies that occur in protein energy malnutrition. In children, protein–energy malnutrition is associated with osteopenia and decreased bone growth, which manifests clinically as stunting, a decrease in cortical thickness and a loss of trabecular bone. There is also a delay in bone age due to a delay in the mineralization of the ossification centers, but the epiphyseal plates are narrowed owing to a reduction in cartilage cell proliferation. In the elderly, protein supplements may reduce bone loss, possibly through increasing IGF-1 levels.

In protein–energy malnutrition, the biochemical markers of bone turnover are reduced, as evidenced by a reduction in serum alkaline phosphatase levels and urinary hydroxyproline excretion. A similar reduction in bone turnover is seen at the histological level, with a reduction in osteoblastic and osteoclastic surfaces. Total serum calcium concentrations are often low, in keeping with the reduction in serum albumin values, and serum phosphorus levels may also be markedly reduced. The pathogenesis of the latter changes is ill-understood, although there is evidence of poor renal conservation of phosphate in the child with kwashiorkor.

The long-term consequences of protein deprivation in infancy and childhood on bone health have not been studied, but it appears as though there are few detrimental consequences, as in most countries that have high malnutrition rates, osteoporosis and fractures in adulthood are uncommon.

Vitamin C

Ascorbic acid acts as a cofactor in the hydroxylation of lysine and proline, which are major constituents of

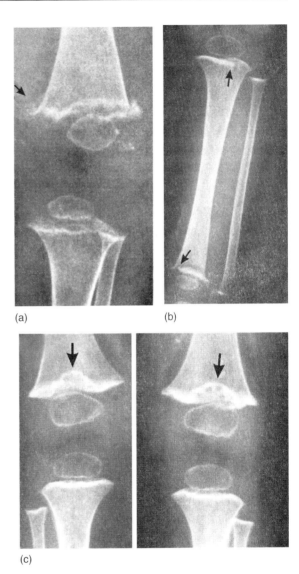

(a)   (b)

(c)

Figure 12.26 Radiographic changes associated with scurvy in children. Advanced scurvy with fractures of thickened, brittle provisional zones of calcification. (a) Multiple infractions in the provisional zone, with peripheral spurring and beginning subperiosteal calcification. (b) Longitudinal fractures of the provisional zones of calcification. (c) Crumpling fractures of the provisional zones of calcification. (Reproduced from Silverman, 1985 with permission from Elsevier Science.)

collagen. Hydroxylation is important in the formation of cross-links between the collagen fibers and the formation of mature collagen. A severe nutritional deficiency of ascorbic acid leads to the clinical picture of scurvy (Figure 12.26); however, the florid syndrome is rarely seen today.

Vitamin K

Vitamin K plays a major role in the γ-carboxylation of glutamic acid residues on a number of proteins (the vitamin K-dependent proteins). The best known of these proteins are the vitamin K-dependent coagulation proteins, but there are also three such proteins in bone; osteocalcin, matrix Gla protein and protein S. The best studied of these is osteocalcin which, unlike the other two bone vitamin K-dependent proteins, is found only in mineralized tissue and synthesized only by osteoblasts and odontoblasts. The characteristic of the γ-carboxylated proteins is their calcium binding activity; thus, osteocalcin is found bound to mineralized matrix. The physiological role of these bone Gla proteins is unclear, but it has been suggested that osteocalcin may inhibit hydroxyapatite formation or control bone resorption.

From a clinical perspective, there are data to suggest that there is an inverse relationship between vitamin K intake and the prevalence of fractures in the elderly. Further, several studies have shown an increase in undercarboxylated osteocalcin (a measure of vitamin K deficiency) in the elderly, and a relationship between the concentration of undercarboxylated osteocalcin and hip fracture rates and BMD. As yet, the data are limited and inconsistent, and no firm conclusions can be drawn.

Similarly, conflicting results have been reported from studies investigating whether or not warfarin, a vitamin K antagonist, is associated with a decrease in bone density and an increased risk of fractures. A recent supplementation study using vitamin K_2 (menatetranone) in elderly osteoporotic patients demonstrated a decrease in clinical fractures and a reduction in the loss of BMD at the lumbar spine over a 2 year period.

Fluoride

The role of fluoride in bone health remains controversial; however, its role in preventing dental caries is not disputed. Over the past 20 years, considerable interest has been generated in the therapeutic role of fluoride in the management of osteoporosis. Although high doses of fluoride increase bone mass and density through stimulating osteoblastic activity and preventing crystal dissolution, there is little evidence at present that it reduces fracture rates.

Some 50% of ingested fluoride is deposited in bone or teeth, where it displaces bicarbonate or hydroxyl ions in hydroxyapatite to form fluoroapatite. Its incorporation in the apatite crystal reduces the ability of the crystal to dissolve, thus in teeth reducing the risk of caries and in bone causing an increase in bone mass. In bone, however, there is little evidence that at physiological concentrations fluoride has any effect on bone mass.

At pharmacological doses, fluoride (approximately 50 mg of sodium fluoride) increases BMD by stimulating bone formation. At higher doses bone formation is abnormal, with features of woven bone appearing. Despite the increase in BMD, particularly at the lumbar vertebrae, there is no conclusive evidence that fracture rates are reduced.

In a number of areas in the world, such as India, South Africa and Tanzania, endemic fluorosis has been reported owing to the chronic ingestion of borehole water with high fluoride concentrations (8–20 mg/l). Typically, the features of endemic fluorosis include joint stiffness, limb deformities and staining of the teeth (Figure 12.15a and b). In children, features of rickets may be seen. Radiologically, there may be osteopenia of the distal ends of the long bones, but the axial skeleton shows osteosclerosis with ligamentous calcification around the joints. The biochemical changes are usually minimal, although hypocalcemia and elevated alkaline phosphatase and parathyroid concentrations have been reported.

Other dietary factors

Many other nutrients and dietary factors may be important for long-term bone health. Among the essential nutrients, plausible hypotheses for involvement with skeletal health, based on biochemical and metabolic evidence, can be made for zinc, copper, manganese, boron, vitamin A, B-vitamins, potassium and sodium. Evidence from physiological and clinical studies is largely lacking. Zinc nutrition is important in infant growth, and associations with BMD have been noted in middle-aged premenopausal women. Copper supplementation ameliorated bone loss in one study of perimenopausal women. A high intake of vitamin A as retinol was associated with hip fracture in Sweden. A higher BMD has been associated with a higher dietary potassium intake, along with other nutrients associated with fruit and vegetable intake. The skeleton acts as a reservoir of alkaline salts for the maintenance of adequate acid–base homeostasis, and foods that promote an alkaline environment, such as fruit and vegetables, may diminish the demand for skeletal salts to balance acid generated from foods such as meat. Sodium is intimately involved in the excretion of calcium through the renal tubules, and a direct relationship is found between urinary sodium and calcium excretion in free-living populations. A high sodium intake may reduce BMD and exacerbate age-related bone loss, but the evidence is not conclusive.

Other components of the diet could also influence bone health. Of these, phytoestrogens are generating interest in that they are naturally occurring plant chemicals with weak estrogenic properties. Phytoestrogens include soy-derived isoflavones, such as genistein and daidzein, and lignans derived from cereals, fruit and vegetables. These compounds are able to bind to both the α- and β-estrogen receptors, and may act as receptor agonists or antagonists depending on the tissue. Studies in animal models suggest that phytoestrogens may prevent bone loss after ovarectomy but, as yet, data from human studies are limited.

Although the evidence of a link between intakes of these dietary components and bone health is not sufficiently secure for firm dietary recommendations, the accumulating picture suggests that current healthy-eating advice to increase potassium intake, to decrease sodium intake and to consume more fresh fruit and vegetables is unlikely to be detrimental to bone health and may be beneficial.

12.8 Lifestyle factors and bone health

Alcohol

Ethanol use increases the risk of fracture through several direct and indirect mechanisms, for example through an increased risk of falls, reduced nutrient intakes with associated malnutrition, increased prevalence of heavy smoking, hypogonadism and a direct inhibition of bone formation. Thus, studies of patients suffering from alcoholism have shown reduced bone density and histological evidence of osteoporosis. Biochemically, the characteristic feature is a reduction in serum osteocalcin; however, reduced serum calcium and vitamin D levels have also been reported.

Whether social drinking (1–2 units/day) is associated with an effect on bone is unclear and inconsistent, with some studies suggesting a positive effect and others suggesting negative effects.

Smoking

Smoking is associated with a small but significant reduction in BMD, particularly in elderly men and women when compared with age-matched controls in the majority of studies. The mechanisms by which smoking reduces bone density are unclear, although a number of possibilities exist including depression of the vitamin D–PTH system, increased alcohol consumption, decreased exercise, reduced free estradiol and decreased body mass.

Physical activity and exercise

Physical activity is an important modulator of bone mass, not only during childhood but also during adulthood and in the elderly. Complete immobilization may result in a loss of some 40% of bone mass. However, exercise added to the normal routine of daily activity may only add a few per cent onto the average bone mass of children and adults. In a meta-analysis of randomized and non-randomized controlled trials conducted over a 30 year period, exercise training programs were found to prevent or reverse bone loss of almost 1% per year in both the lumbar spine and femoral neck in pre- and postmenopausal women. The osteogenic effects of exercise are specific to the anatomical sites at which the mechanical strain occurs. Thus, tennis players have greater bone density in the dominant than in the non-dominant arm. The type of exercise may also make a difference, as swimmers have lower bone density at axial sites than other athletes.

Eating disorders and malabsorption syndromes

Eating disorders (anorexia nervosa and bulimia) are becoming major problems among the adolescent and young adult population of the most developed nations of the world. Beside the obvious adverse effects on nutritional status, these disorders have varying adverse effects on bone. Studies suggest that anorexia nervosa carries with it more severe consequences for bone health than bulimia. Bone loss occurs in the majority of anorexic subjects, with over 50% having bone densities more than 2 SD below age-matched controls. Non-spinal fractures are reported to have a seven-fold increase. It appears that trabecular bone is more severely affected than cortical bone. The pathogenesis of bone loss in anorexia nervosa is multifactorial (Box 12.15); however, estrogen deficiency associated with amenorrhea probably plays a central role. Other contributing factors include malnutrition, IGF-1 deficiency, dehydroepiandrosterone deficiency, increased cortisol levels and possibly associated excessive exercise.

> **Box 12.15** Possible factors responsible for bone loss in anorexia nervosa
>
> - Estrogen deficiency
> - Dehydroepiandrosterone deficiency
> - Undernutrition with associated protein, mineral and vitamin deficiencies
> - Insulin-like growth factor-1 deficiency
> - Increased cortisol levels
> - Excessive exercise

Bulimia appears to affect bone mass less severely than anorexia nervosa. In general, women with bulimia are not as wasted or undernourished as anorectic subjects, nor do they have the same prevalence of amenorrhea. They also appear to be less obsessive about the need for exercise, as in one study only 30% of bulimics exercised regularly, compared with 100% of anorectics. Bulimic subjects who exercise maintain their bone density at weight-bearing sites better than sedentary peers, and have higher bone density than anorectic subjects.

Malabsorption syndromes such as cystic fibrosis (see Clinical Nutrition textbook) and celiac disease are associated with an increased risk of osteoporosis through associated malnutrition, and calcium and vitamin D malabsorption. As life expectancy in subjects with cystic fibrosis increases with the advances that have been made in the control of respiratory complications, minimal trauma fractures are becoming more common.

Inflammatory bowel disease is also associated with an increase in osteoporosis, with approximately 50% of patients estimated to suffer from osteopenia. Factors aggravating the condition include undernutrition, high levels of circulating inflammatory cytokines, lack of exercise and the use of corticosteroids.

Vegetarianism

There is no evidence that a lactovegetarian diet is associated with differences, either detrimental or beneficial, in BMD or fracture risk. There have been few investigations of individuals consuming vegan or macrobiotic diets, but there is some evidence that these may be associated with low BMD. However, interpretation of studies is difficult because of other differences that may be associated with a vegetarian lifestyle which may affect bone health, such as body weight, smoking habits, physical activity patterns and socioeconomic

status. Infants weaned onto macrobiotic diets are at risk of growth retardation and rickets.

Lactose intolerance

Lactose has long been thought to enhance the absorption of calcium, based on animal studies. However, data from human investigations have been inconsistent and recent work suggests that lactose does not have an effect on either calcium absorption or excretion in healthy humans. Lactose intolerance is associated with a low calcium intake, because of avoidance of milk and milk products, and is regarded as a likely risk factor for osteoporosis. Studies with fracture or bone loss as an outcome have produced an inconsistent picture, with some suggesting a modest risk for those with lactose intolerance, but not others.

Body weight, body composition and obesity

Body weight and height are major determinants of BMC and BMD. Small build is a risk factor for vertebral fracture, while tall individuals are more prone to hip fracture (see Section 12.3). Small skeletal size is a recognized risk factor for osteoporosis, although in Scandinavia, taller women are at greater risk of hip fracture. Anatomical variations between adults may reflect the impact of environmental effects at different stages of skeletal development and these may influence later predisposition to fractures. Size in infancy predicts adult BMC, suggesting that the environment *in utero* and early life may be an important modulating factor. Low body weight, especially in connection with anorexia nervosa and the frailty of old age, is associated with an increased risk of fractures, and being overweight with reduced risk. In young people and men, after adjusting for differences in body mass, leanness (a higher lean-to-fat ratio) is associated with higher bone mineral mass, whereas in postmenopausal women, it is fatness (a lower lean-to-fat ratio) that is positively related to bone mineral mass. Various interpretations have been put forward to explain this dichotomy, including the osteogenic effects of muscle in younger people, the shock-absorbing effects of adipose tissue in older people and the possible endogenous production of estrogens by adipose tissue, which may be particularly important in women after the menopause. Recent animal studies have suggested a role for leptin in the control of bone mass. Situations associated with poor leptin signaling are associated with high bone mass.

12.9 Perspectives on the future

Bone research has progressed in leaps and bounds since the 1980s and in the next decade it is likely that a much greater understanding of the genetic and biochemical factors that are important in controlling bone mass and thus the incidence of fragility fractures will develop. These developments will probably offer the pharmaceutical industry an enormous spectrum of therapeutic possibilities for the optimization of bone mass and the treatment of osteoporosis.

From a more nutritional point of view, a lot more needs to be learnt about the factors responsible for bone mass accretion during childhood and adolescence, the development of peak bone mass and bone health in the elderly. Further, the interaction of nutrients, nutritional status, lifestyle, and paracrine and endocrine factors on bone homeostasis need to be explored in greater depth at all stages of the human life cycle. Of increasing interest is the role of micronutrients and non-nutritional compounds in fruit and vegetables, such as vitamin K, phytoestrogens and acid–base balance, on bone homeostasis.

Further reading

Ash MM Jr. Wheeler's Dental Anatomy, Physiology and Occlusion, 7th edn. Philadelphia, PA: WB Saunders, 1993.

Burt BA, Szpunar SM. The Michigan study: the relationship between sugar intake and dental caries over three years. Int Dent J 1994; 44: 230–240.

Baron R. Anatomy and ultrastructure of bone. In: Primer on the Metabolic Bone Disorders and Disorders of Mineral Metabolism, 4th edn (MJ Favus, ed.). Philadelphia, PA: Lippincott Williams and Wilkins, 1999.

Calvo S et al. Molecular basis and clinical application of biological markers of bone turnover. Endocr Rev 1996; 17: 333–368.

Department of Health. Nutritional Aspects of Bone Health: With Particular Reference to Calcium and Vitamin D. Report of the Subgroup on Bone Health, Working Group on the Nutritional Status of the Population of the Committee on Medical Aspects of Food and Nutrition Policy. London: The Stationery Office, 1998.

Dietary sugars and human disease. Report on Health and Social Subjects No. 37. London: Committee on Medical Aspects of Food Policy, 1989.

Favus MJ, ed. Primer on the Metabolic Bone Diseases and Disorders of Mineral Metabolism, 4th edn. Philadelphia, PA: Lippincott Williams and Wilkins, 1999.

Fournier RL et al. Asynchrony between the rates of standing height gain and bone mass accumulation during puberty. Osteoporosis Int 1997; 7: 525–532.

Laskey MA, Prentice A. Obstet Gynecol 1999; 94: 608–615.

Maynard LM et al. Total-body and regional bone mineral content and areal bone mineral density in children aged 8–18 y: the Fels longitudinal study. Am J Clin Nutr 1998; 68: 1111–1117.

Pettifor JM. Calcium, phosphorus and vitamin D. In: Clinical Nutrition of the Young Child (A Ballabriga, O Brusner, J Dobbing et al., eds). New York: Raven Press, 1991.

Pettifor JM. Dietary calcium deficiency. In: Rickets (FH Glorieux, ed.). New York: Raven Press, 1991.

Pettifor JM, Daniels D. Vitamin D deficiency and nutritional rickets in children. In: Vitamin D (D Feldman, FH Glorieux, JW Pike, eds). San Diego, CA: Academic Press, 1997.

Pettifor JM et al. The effect of season and latitude on in vitro vitamin D formation by sunlight in South Africa. S Afr Med J 1996; 86: 1270–1272.

Silverman FH, ed. Caffey's Pediatric X-ray Diagnosis, 8th edn. Chicago, IL: Year Book, 1985.

Solomon L. Bone density in aging Caucasian and African populations. Lancet 1979; ii: 1326–1328.

Sperber GH. Craniofacial Embryology. Dental Practitioner Handbook No. 15, 4th edn. London: Wright, 1989.

St-Arnaud R, Glorieux FH. Vitamin D and bone development. In: Vitamin D (D Feldman, FH Glorieux, JW Pike, eds). San Diego, CA: Academic Press, 1997.

Standing Committee on the Scientific Evaluation of Dietary Reference Intakes, Food and Nutrition Board, Institute of Medicine. Dietary Reference Intakes for Calcium, Phosphorus, Vitamin D and Fluoride. Washington, DC: National Academy Press, 1997.

Symposia of developmental defects of enamel. Adv Dent Res 1989; 3: 87–271.

Theintz G et al. Longitudinal monitoring of bone mass accumulation in healthy adolescents: evidence for a marked reduction after 16 years of age at the level of the lumbar spine and femoral neck in female subjects. J Clin Endocrinol Metab 1992; 75: 1060–1065.

13
The Immune and Inflammatory Systems

P Yaqoob and PC Calder

Key messages

- There is a bidirectional interaction between nutrition, infection and immunity, whereby undernutrition decreases immune defenses against invading pathogens, making an individual more susceptible to infection, but the immune response to an infection can itself impair nutritional status and body composition.
- Practically all forms of immunity are affected by protein–energy malnutrition, but non-specific defenses and cell-mediated immunity are more severely affected than humoral (antibody) responses.
- Micronutrients are required for an efficient immune response and deficiencies in one or more of these nutrients diminish immune function, providing a window of opportunity for infectious agents. However, excessive intakes of some micronutrients may also impair immune function.
- Essential fatty acids have an important role to play in the regulation of immune responses, since they provide precursors for the synthesis of eicosanoids. The balance between n-6 and n-3 polyunsaturated fatty acids may influence the development of immunologically based diseases (particularly inflammatory diseases), although research in this area is not conclusive.
- Deficiencies in essential amino acids are likely to impair immune function, but some non-essential amino acids (e.g. arginine and glutamine) may become conditionally essential in stressful situations.
- Probiotic bacteria have been shown to enhance immune function in laboratory animals and may do so in humans.
- Breast milk has a composition that promotes the development of the neonatal immune response and may protect against infectious diseases.
- There appears to be a range of nutrient intakes over which the immune system functions optimally, but the exact nature of this range is not clear. It is often assumed when defining the relationship between nutrient intake and immune function that all components of the immune system will respond in the same dose-dependent fashion to a given nutrient. This is not correct, at least as far as some nutrients are concerned, and it appears likely that different components of the immune system show an individual dose–response relationship to the availability of a given nutrient.

13.1 Introduction

Associations between famine and epidemics of infectious disease have been noted throughout history: Hippocrates recognized that poorly nourished people are more susceptible to infectious disease as early as 370 BC. In general, undernutrition impairs the immune system, suppressing immune functions that are fundamental to host protection against pathogenic organisms. Undernutrition leading to impairment of immune function can be due to insufficient intake of energy and macronutrients and/or due to deficiencies in specific micronutrients (vitamins and minerals). Often these occur in combination: this is particularly notable for protein–energy malnutrition and deficiencies in micronutrients such as vitamin A, iron, zinc and iodine. Clearly, the impact of undernutrition is greatest in developing countries, but it is also important in developed countries, especially among the elderly, individuals with eating disorders, alcoholics, patients with certain diseases, premature babies and those born small for gestational age. The precise effects of individual nutrients on different aspects of immune function have been notoriously difficult to study. However, it is becoming clear that many nutrients have defined roles in the immune response and that each nutrient has a distinct range of concentrations over which it supports optimal immune function. Lowering the level of the nutrient below this range or increasing it in excess of the range can impair immune function. Thus, the functioning of the immune system is influenced by nutrients consumed as normal components of the diet and appropriate nutrition is required for the host to maintain adequate immune defenses towards bacteria, viruses, fungi and parasites.

Unfortunately, the immune system can become dysfunctional or dysregulated, resulting in inappropriate activation of some components. In some individuals the immune system recognizes a host (self) antigen and then proceeds to direct its destructive activities against host tissues. These diseases are termed chronic inflammatory diseases, and examples are rheumatoid arthritis, psoriasis, systemic lupus erythmatosus, multiple sclerosis, ulcerative colitis and Crohn's disease. In some other individuals the immune system becomes inappropriately sensitized to a normally benign antigen, termed an allergen, and so reacts vigorously when that antigen is encountered. These are the atopic diseases, which include allergies, asthma and atopic eczema. It is now recognized that atherosclerosis has an immunological component and some cancers arise and develop as a result of diminished immunosurveillance. Thus, modulation of immune function by dietary components might be an effective means for altering the course of these diseases. Furthermore, diet may underlie the development of some of these diseases.

This chapter begins with an overview of the key components of the immune system, concentrating on the cells that conduct immune responses, the mechanisms by which they communicate and how the system operates in health and disease. The role of nutrients in the immune system is examined using specific examples, and the cyclic relationship between infection and nutritional status discussed. The main body of the chapter is devoted to an evaluation of the influence of individual macronutrients and micronutrients on immune function.

13.2 The immune system

Innate immunity

The immune system acts to protect the host from infectious agents that exist in the environment (bacteria, viruses, fungi, parasites) and from other noxious insults. The immune system has two functional divisions: the innate (or natural) immune system and the acquired (also termed specific or adaptive) immune system. Innate immunity consists of physical barriers, soluble factors and phagocytic cells, which include granulocytes (neutrophils, basophils, eosinophils), monocytes and macrophages (Table 13.1). Innate immunity has no memory and is therefore not influenced by prior exposure to an organism. Phagocytic cells, the main effectors of innate immunity, express surface receptors specific for bacterial surface antigens. Binding of antigen to the receptors triggers phagocytosis and subsequent destruction of the pathogenic microorganism by complement or by toxic chemicals, such as superoxide radicals and hydrogen peroxide. Natural killer cells also possess surface receptors and destroy

Table 13.1 Components of innate and acquired immunity

	Innate	Acquired
Physicochemical barriers	Skin Mucous membranes Lysozyme Stomach acid Commensal bacteria	Cutaneous and mucosal immune systems Antibodies in mucosal secretions
Circulating molecules	Complement	Antibodies
Cells	Granulocytes Monocytes/macrophages Natural killer cells	Lymphocytes (T and B)
Soluble mediators	Macrophage-derived cytokines	Lymphocyte-derived cytokines

pathogens by the release of cytotoxic proteins. In this way, innate immunity provides a first line of defense against invading pathogens. However, an immune response often requires the coordinated actions of both innate immunity and the more powerful and flexible acquired immunity.

Acquired immunity

Acquired immunity involves the specific recognition of molecules (antigens) on an invading pathogen which distinguish it as being foreign to the host. Lymphocytes, which are subdivided into T- and B-lymphocytes, effect this form of immunity. All lymphocytes (indeed all cells of the immune system) originate in the bone marrow (Figure 13.1). B-lymphocytes undergo further development and maturation in the bone marrow before being released into the circulation, while T-lymphocytes

mature in the thymus. From the bloodstream, lymphocytes can enter peripheral lymphoid organs, which include lymph nodes, the spleen, mucosal lymphoid tissue, tonsils and gut-associated lymphoid tissue. Immune responses occur largely in these lymphoid organs, which are highly organized to promote the interaction of cells and invading pathogens.

The acquired immune system is highly specific, since each lymphocyte carries surface receptors for a single antigen. However, acquired immunity is extremely diverse; the lymphocyte repertoire in humans has been estimated at recognition of approximately 10^{11} antigens. The high degree of specificity, combined with the huge lymphocyte repertoire, means that only a relatively small number of lymphocytes will be able to recognize any given antigen. The acquired immune system has developed the ability for clonal expansion to

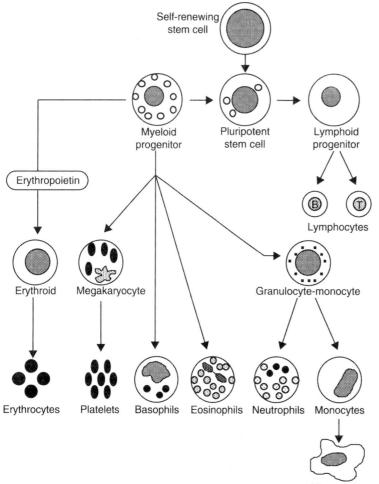

Figure 13.1 Origin of cells of the immune system.

deal with this. Clonal expansion involves the proliferation of a lymphocyte once an interaction with its specific antigen has occurred, so that a single lymphocyte gives rise to a clone of lymphocytes, all of which have the ability to recognize and destroy the antigen causing the initial response. This feature of acquired immunity has often been likened to building up an army to fight a foreign invasion. The acquired immune response becomes effective over several days after the initial activation, but it also persists for some time after the removal of the initiating antigen. This persistence gives rise to immunological memory, which is also a characteristic feature of acquired immunity. It is the basis for the stronger, more effective immune response to re-exposure to an antigen (i.e. reinfection with the same pathogen) and is the basis for vaccination. Eventually, the immune system will re-establish homeostasis using self-regulatory mechanisms which involve communication between cells.

The major features of the acquired immune response are summarized in Box 13.1.

B- and T-lymphocytes

B-lymphocytes are characterized by their ability to produce antibodies, or immunoglobulins, which confer antigen specificity to the acquired immune system (i.e. the antibodies produced by B-lymphocytes are specific for individual antigens). This form of protection against infections is termed humoral immunity and is conducted exclusively by B-lymphocytes. B-lymphocytes carry immunoglobulins, which are capable of binding an antigen, on their cell surfaces. Binding of immunoglobulin with antigen causes proliferation of the B-lymphocyte and subsequent transformation into plasma cells, which secrete large amounts of antibody with the same specificity as the parent cell.

Immunoglobulins (antibodies) are proteins consisting of two identical heavy chains and two identical light chains. Five different types of heavy chain give rise to five major classes of immunoglobulin, IgA, IgD, IgG, IgM and IgE, each of which elicits different components

of the humoral immune response. Antibodies work in several ways to combat invading pathogens. They can 'neutralize' toxins or microorganisms by binding to them and preventing their attachment to host cells, and they can activate complement proteins in plasma, which in turn promote the destruction of bacteria by phagocytes. Since they have binding sites for both an antigen and for receptors on phagocytic cells, antibodies can also promote the interaction of the two components by forming physical 'bridges', a process known as opsonization. The type of phagocytic cell bound by the antibody will be determined by the antibody class; macrophages and neutrophils are specific for IgM and IgG, while eosinophils are specific for IgE. In this way, antibodies are a form of communication between the acquired and the innate immune response; they are elicited through highly specific mechanisms, but are ultimately translated to a form that can be interpreted by the innate immune system, enabling it to destroy the pathogen.

Humoral immunity deals with extracellular pathogens. However, some pathogens, particularly viruses, but also some bacteria, infect individuals by entering cells. These pathogens will escape humoral immunity and are instead dealt with by cell-mediated immunity, which is conferred by T-lymphocytes. T-lymphocytes express antigen-specific T-cell receptors (TCR) on their surface, which have an enormous antigen repertoire. However, unlike B-lymphocytes, they are only able to recognize antigens that are presented to them on a cell surface; this is the distinguishing feature between humoral and cell-mediated immunity. Activation of the TCR results in entry of T-lymphocytes into the cell cycle and, ultimately, proliferation. Activated T-lymphocytes also begin to synthesize and secrete the cytokine interleukin-2 (IL-2), which further promotes proliferation and differentiation by autocrine mechanisms. Thus, the expansion of T-lymphocytes builds up an army of T-lymphocytes in much the same way as that of B-lymphocytes. Effector T-lymphocytes have the ability to migrate to sites of infection, injury or tissue damage. Cytotoxic (CD8) T-lymphocytes eliminate pathogen by secretion of cytotoxic enzymes, which cause lysis of the target cell, or secretion of the antiviral cytokine interferon-γ (IFN-γ), or by inducing apoptosis (suicide) of target cells. Helper (CD4) T-lymphocytes eliminate pathogens by stimulating the phagocytic activity of macrophages and the proliferation of and antibody secretion by B-lymphocytes.

In delayed-type hypersensitivity (DTH), antigen-activated $CD4^+$ T-lymphocytes secrete cytokines, which have several effects, including recruitment of neutrophils and monocytes from the blood to the site of antigen challenge and activation of monocytes to effect elimination of the antigen. This type of cell-mediated immunity forms the primary defense mechanism against intracellular bacteria, such as *Listeria monocytogenes*. The DTH reaction can be induced in humans by contact sensitization with chemicals and environmental antigens or by intradermal injection of microbial antigens, and as such has been widely used as a rapid *in vivo* marker of cell-mediated immunity. Approximately 4 h after initiation, neutrophils infiltrate the site, but this rapidly subsides and by 12 h T-lymphocytes migrate from blood vessels and accumulate in the epidermis. By 48 h macrophages are present in all areas and spongiosis (swelling and thickening of the skin) occurs. The degree of the DTH reaction can be assessed by measuring the thickening of the skin, normally 48 h after exposure to the antigen.

While effective immune responses are highly desirable, some aspects of immunity have undesirable consequences. For example, bactericidal and inflammatory mediators secreted by macrophages are toxic not only to pathogens, but also to host tissues, resulting in unavoidable tissue damage. For this reason, immune responses, and macrophage responses in particular, need to be tightly controlled and the self-regulatory properties of the immune system highly effective.

Communication within the immune system: cytokines

Communication within the acquired immune system and between the innate and acquired systems is brought about by direct cell-to-cell contact involving adhesion molecules and by the production of chemical messengers, which send signals from one cell to another. Chief among these chemical messengers are proteins called cytokines, which can act to regulate the activity of the cell that produced the cytokine or of other cells. Each cytokine can have multiple activities on different cell types. Cytokines act by binding to specific receptors on the cell surface and thereby induce changes in the growth, development or activity of the target cell.

Tumor necrosis factor-α (TNF-α), IL-1 and IL-6 are among the most important cytokines produced by monocytes and macrophages. These cytokines activate neutrophils, monocytes and macrophages to initiate bacterial and tumor cell killing, increase adhesion molecule expression on the surface of neutrophils and endothelial cells, stimulate T- and B-lymphocyte proliferation, and initiate the production of other proinflammatory cytokines (e.g. TNF induces production of IL-1 and IL-6, and IL-1 induces production of IL-6). Thus, TNF, IL-1 and IL-6 are mediators of both natural and acquired immunity and are an important link between them. In addition, these cytokines mediate the systemic effects of inflammation such as fever, weight loss and acute-phase protein synthesis in the liver. Production of appropriate amounts of TNF, IL-1 and IL-6 is clearly important in response to infection, but inappropriate production or overproduction can be dangerous and these cytokines, particularly TNF, are implicated in causing some of the pathological responses that occur in chronic inflammatory conditions (e.g. rheumatoid arthritis and psoriasis).

Helper T-lymphocytes can be subdivided into two broad categories according to the pattern of cytokines they produce (Figure 13.2). It is believed that helper

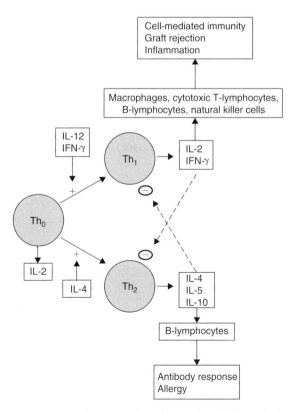

Figure 13.2 Development and cytokine profiles of Th_1 and Th_2 lymphocytes. IL: interleukin; IFN: interferon.

T-cells that have not previously encountered antigen produce mainly IL-2 upon the initial encounter with an antigen. These cells may differentiate into a population, sometimes referred to as Th_0 cells, which differentiate further into either Th_1 or Th_2 cells (Figure 13.2). This differentiation is regulated by cytokines: IL-12 and IFN-γ promote the development of Th_1 cells, while IL-4 promotes the development of Th_2 cells (Figure 13.2). Th_1 and Th_2 cells have relatively restricted profiles of cytokine production: Th_1 cells produce IL-2 and IFN-γ, which activate macrophages, natural killer cells and cytotoxic T-lymphocytes and are the principal effectors of cell-mediated immunity. Interactions with bacteria, viruses and fungi tend to induce Th_1 activity. Since Th_1 cytokines activate monocytes and macrophages, these cytokines may be regarded as proinflammatory. Th_2 cells produce IL-4, which stimulates IgE production, IL-5, an eosinophil-activating factor, and IL-10, which together with IL-4, suppresses cell-mediated immunity (Figure 13.2). Th_2 cells are responsible for defense against helminthic parasites, which is due to IgE-mediated activation of mast cells and basophils. Since Th_2 cytokines suppress Th_1 responses, these cytokines may be regarded as anti-inflammatory. The patterns of cytokine secretion by Th_1 and Th_2 lymphocytes were first demonstrated in mice. It has subsequently been demonstrated that while human helper T-lymphocytes do show differences in cytokine profile, the divisions are not clear and while some cells have a typical Th_1 or Th_2 profile, the majority secrete a mixture of Th_1 and Th_2 cytokines in differing proportions. Thus, the terms 'Th_1 dominant' and 'Th_2 dominant' are commonly used to describe the cytokine profiles of these cells. An interesting feature of Th_1/Th_2 dominance is that once a pattern of cytokine secretion has been established, the dominant arm is able to self-amplify and to antagonize the non-dominant arm. In this way, once a helper T-lymphocyte response has been established, it becomes increasingly polarized towards the dominant phenotype (inflammatory conditions for Th_1 and allergy for Th_2).

Inflammation

Inflammation is the body's immediate response to infection or injury. It is typified by redness, swelling, heat and pain. These occur as a result of increased blood flow, increased permeability across blood capillaries, which permits large molecules (e.g. complement, antibodies, cytokines) to leave the bloodstream and cross the endothelial wall, and increased movement of leukocytes from the bloodstream into the surrounding tissue. Thus, inflammation is an integral part of the innate immune response.

The immune system in health and disease

Clearly, a well-functioning immune system is essential to health and serves to protect the host from the effects of ever-present pathogenic organisms. Cells of the immune system also have a role in identifying and eliminating cancer cells. There are, however, some undesirable features of immune responses.

First, in developing the ability to recognize and eliminate foreign antigens effectively, the immune system is responsible for the rejection of transplanted tissues.

Secondly, the ability to discriminate between 'self' and 'non-self' is an essential requirement of the immune system and is normally achieved by the destruction of self-recognizing T- and B-lymphocytes before their maturation. However, since lymphocytes are unlikely to be exposed to all possible self-antigens in this way, a second mechanism termed clonal anergy exists, which ensures that an encounter with a self-antigen induces tolerance. In some individuals there is a breakdown of the mechanisms that normally preserve tolerance; a number of factors contribute to this, including a range of immunological abnormalities and a genetic predisposition in some individuals. As a result, an inappropriate immune response to host tissues is generated and this leads to autoimmune and inflammatory diseases, which are typified by ongoing chronic inflammation and a dysregulated Th_1 response. Examples of this type of disease include psoriasis, multiple sclerosis and rheumatoid arthritis.

Thirdly, the immune system of some individuals can become sensitized to usually benign antigens from the environment and can respond inappropriately to them. Such antigens can include components of foods or of so-called allergens (e.g. cat or dog fur, house dust mite, some pollens), such that this response can lead to allergies, asthma and related atopic diseases. Although these diseases are often termed chronic inflammatory diseases and are typified by inappropriate recognition of and/or responses to antigens, they have a different immune basis from the diseases described above. Atopic diseases are typically initiated by the production of IgE by B-lymphocytes in response to exposure to an antigen for the first time (this can be present in a variety of forms, e.g. pollen, dust or in foods).

Binding of IgE to specific receptors on the surfaces of mast cells and basophils then occurs (termed sensitization). If the antigen is reintroduced, it will interact with the bound IgE, leading to activation of the cells and the release of both preformed and newly synthesized inflammatory mediators (particularly histamine and the Th_2 cytokines, IL-4, IL-5 and IL-10).

13.3 Why should nutrients affect immune function?

Although the immune system is functioning at all times, specific immunity becomes activated when the host is challenged by pathogens. This activation is associated with a marked increase in the demand of the immune system for substrates and nutrients to provide a ready source of energy, which can be supplied from exogenous sources (i.e. from the diet) and/or from endogenous pools. The cells of the immune system are metabolically active and are able to utilize glucose, amino acids and fatty acids as fuels.

Energy generation involves electron carriers, which are nucleotide derivatives, for example nicotinamide adenine dinucleotide (NAD), flavin adenine dinucleotide (FAD), and a range of coenzymes. The electron carriers and coenzymes are usually derivatives of vitamins: thiamine pyrophosphate is derived from thiamin (vitamin B_1), FAD and flavin mononucleotide from riboflavin (vitamin B_2), NAD from nicotinate (niacin), pyridoxal phosphate from pyridoxine (vitamin B_6), coenzyme A from pantothenate, tetrahydrofolate from folate and cobamide from cobalamin (vitamin B_{12}). In addition, biotin is required by some enzymes for activity. The final component of the pathway for energy generation (the mitochondrial electron transfer chain) includes electron carriers that have iron or copper at their active site.

Activation of the immune response gives rise to the production of proteins (immunoglobulins, cytokines, cytokine receptors, adhesion molecules, acute-phase proteins) and lipid-derived mediators (prostaglandins, leukotrienes). To respond optimally there must be the appropriate enzymic machinery in place (for RNA synthesis and protein synthesis and their regulation) and ample substrate available [nucleotides for RNA synthesis, the correct mix of amino acids for protein synthesis, polyunsaturated fatty acids (PUFA) for eicosanoid synthesis].

An important component of the immune response is oxidative burst, during which superoxide anion radicals are produced from oxygen in a reaction linked to the oxidation of NADPH. The reactive oxygen species produced can be damaging to host tissues and thus antioxidant protective mechanisms are necessary. Among these are the classic antioxidant vitamins, α-tocopherol (vitamin E) and ascorbic acid (vitamin C), glutathione, a tripeptide composed of glutamate, cysteine and glycine, the antioxidant enzymes superoxide dismutase and catalase, and the glutathione recycling enzyme glutathione peroxidase. Superoxide dismutase has two forms, a mitochondrial form and a cytosolic form; the mitochondrial form includes manganese at its active site, whereas the cytosolic form includes copper and zinc. Catalase contains iron at its active site, whereas glutathione peroxidase contains selenium.

Cellular proliferation is a key component of the immune response, providing amplification and memory: before division there must be replication of DNA and then of all cellular components (proteins, membranes, intracellular organelles, etc.). In addition to energy, this clearly needs a supply of nucleotides (for DNA and RNA synthesis), amino acids (for protein synthesis), fatty acids, bases and phosphate (for phospholipid synthesis), and other lipids (e.g. cholesterol) and cellular components. Although nucleotides are synthesized mainly from amino acids, some of the cellular building blocks cannot be synthesized in mammalian cells and must come from the diet (e.g. essential fatty acids, essential amino acids, minerals). Amino acids (e.g. arginine) are precursors for the synthesis of polyamines, which have roles in the regulation of DNA replication and cell division. Various micronutrients (e.g. iron, folic, zinc, magnesium) are also involved in nucleotide and nucleic acid synthesis.

Thus, the roles for nutrients in immune function are many and varied and it is easy to appreciate that an adequate and balanced supply of these is essential if an appropriate immune response is to be mounted.

13.4 Assessment of the effect of nutrition on immune function

There is a wide range of methodologies by which to assess the impact of nutrients on immune function. Assessments can be made of cell functions *ex vivo* (i.e. of the cells isolated from animals or humans subjected

Table 13.2 Assessment of the effect of nutrition on immune function

In vivo measures
  Size of lymphoid organs
  Cellularity of lymphoid organs
  Numbers of cells circulating in bloodstream
  Cell-surface expression of molecules involved in immune response
    (e.g. antigen presentation)
  Circulating concentrations of Ig specific for antigens after an
    antigen challenge
  Concentration of secretory IgA in saliva, tears and intestinal
    washings
  Delayed-type hypersensitivity response to intradermal application
    of antigen
  Response to challenge with live pathogens (mainly animal studies;
    outcome usually survival)
  Incidence and severity of infectious diseases (widely used in
    human studies)
Ex vivo measures
  Phagocytosis by neutrophils and macrophages
  Oxidative burst by neutrophils and macrophages
  Natural killer cell activity against specific target cells (usually
    tumor cells)
  Cytotoxic T-lymphocyte activity
  Lymphocyte proliferation (following stimulation with an antigen
    or mitogen)
  Production of cytokines by lymphocytes and macrophages
  Production of immunoglobulins by lymphocytes
  Cell-surface expression of molecules involved in cellular activation

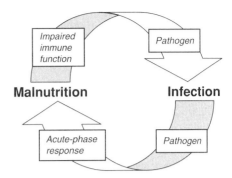

Figure 13.3 Cyclic relationship between malnutrition and infection. Undernutrition impairs immune defenses, lowering resistance to invading pathogens. In turn, infection alters nutrient status and contributes to the undernourished state.

to dietary manipulation and studied in short- or long-term culture) or of indicators of immune function *in vivo* (e.g. by measuring the concentrations of proteins relevant to immune function in the bloodstream or the response to an immunological challenge). Table 13.2 lists some examples of methods used for the assessment of immune function.

13.5 Impact of infection on nutrient status

Undernutrition decreases immune defenses against invading pathogens and makes an individual more susceptible to infections. However, the immune response to an infection can itself impair nutritional status and body composition. Thus, there is a bidirectional interaction between nutrition, infection and immunity (Figure 13.3).

Infection impairs nutritional status and body composition in the following ways.

Infection is characterized by anorexia

Reduction in food intake (anorexia) can range from as little as 5% to almost complete loss of appetite. This can lead to nutrient deficiencies even if the host is not deficient before the infection and may make apparent existing borderline deficiencies.

Infection is characterized by nutrient malabsorption and loss

The range of infections associated with nutrient malabsorption is wide and includes bacteria, viruses, protozoa and intestinal helminths. Infections that cause diarrhea or vomiting will result in nutrient loss. Apart from malabsorption, nutrients may also be lost through the feces as a result of damage to the intestinal wall caused by some infectious agents.

Infection is characterized by increased resting energy expenditure

Infection increases the basal metabolic rate during fever: each 1°C increase in body temperature is associated with a 13% increase in metabolic rate, which significantly increases energy requirements. This places a significant demand on nutrient supply, particularly when coupled with anorexia, diarrhea and other nutrient losses (e.g. in urine and sweat).

Infection is characterized by altered metabolism and redistribution of nutrients

The acute-phase response is the name given to the metabolic response to infections and it includes the onset of fever and anorexia, the production of specific acute-phase reactants, and the activation and proliferation of immune cells. This catabolic response occurs with all infections, even when they are subclinical, and serves to bring about a redistribution of nutrients away from

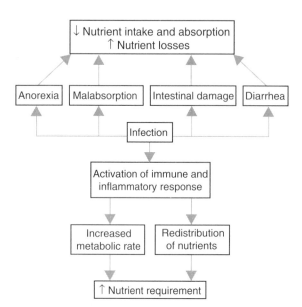

Figure 13.4 Impact of infection on nutritional status.

skeletal muscle and adipose tissue and towards the host immune system. This redistribution is mediated by the production of proinflammatory cytokines by leukocytes and associated endocrine changes. Amino acids, mobilized from skeletal muscle, are used by the liver for the synthesis of acute-phase proteins (e.g. C-reactive protein) and by leukocytes for the synthesis of immunoglobulin and cytokines. The average loss of protein over a range of infections has been estimated to be 0.6–1.2 g/kg body weight per day.

It is clear that the inflammatory cytokines mediate many of the effects that lead to compromised nutritional status following an infection, including anorexia, increased energy expenditure and redistribution of nutrients, while malabsorption and maldigestion are brought about by the pathogen itself. The result is that an increased nutrient requirement coincides with reduced nutrient intake, reduced nutrient absorption and nutrient losses (Figure 13.4).

13.6 Malnutrition and immune function

Protein–energy malnutrition

Protein–energy malnutrition, although often considered a problem solely of developing countries, has been described in even the most affluent of countries. Moderate malnutrition in the developed world is

encountered among the elderly, anorexics and bulimics, premature babies, hospitalized patients and patients with various disease conditions [e.g. cystic fibrosis, acquired immunodeficiency syndrome (AIDS) and some cancers]. It is important to recognize that protein–energy malnutrition often coexists with micronutrient deficiencies, and poor outcome of intervention can result from a lack of awareness of multiple deficiencies.

Practically all forms of immunity may be affected by protein–energy malnutrition but non-specific defenses and cell-mediated immunity are more severely affected than humoral (antibody) responses. Protein–energy malnutrition causes atrophy of the lymphoid organs (thymus, spleen, lymph nodes, tonsils) in laboratory animals and humans. There is a decline in the number of circulating lymphocytes, which is proportional to the extent of malnutrition, and the proliferative responses of T-lymphocytes to mitogens and antigens is decreased by malnutrition, as is their synthesis of IL-2 and IFN-γ and the activity of natural killer cells. Production of cytokines by monocytes (TNF-α, IL-6 and IL-1β) is also decreased by malnutrition, although their phagocytic capacity appears to be unaffected. The *in vivo* skin response to challenge with specific antigens is reduced by malnutrition. However, numbers of circulating B-lymphocytes and immunoglobulin levels do not seem to be affected or may even be increased by malnutrition; it has been suggested that underlying infections may influence these observations.

Low birthweight

The fetus accumulates several nutrients, including zinc, copper, iron and vitamin A, during the last trimester of pregnancy, particularly during the last 6–8 weeks. Premature babies are therefore born with lower nutrient reserves than term infants. There is transfer of IgG from mother to fetus beyond 32 weeks of gestation, which means that babies delivered prematurely have low serum IgG concentrations. This is thought to contribute to the high frequency of respiratory infections and sepsis in low birthweight babies, which may be exacerbated by the poor nutritional status.

Anorexia nervosa and bulimia nervosa

Anorexia nervosa is characterized by a marked fear of fatness, a disturbed perception of body size and image, and an obsessive desire to lose increasing amounts of weight. In anorexia nervosa the appetite will often remain normal until late in the course of the illness; binge eating and purging may be a characteristic. Patients with bulimia nervosa also obsessively pursue thinness, but in this disease there is often rapid consumption of a large quantity of food usually followed by purging; periods of fasting and excessive exercise may also be used.

Although impairment of immune function does exist in anorectic patients, it appears to be less severe than that seen in protein–energy malnutrition. This may be because, in contrast to subjects with protein–energy malnutrition, anorectics usually consume sufficient levels of protein and fat (though not carbohydrate or energy) and have only moderate vitamin and mineral deficiencies. The degree and nature of immune impairment seen in patients with anorexia nervosa and bulimia nervosa differ widely between patients and this may reflect the extent of the nutritional deprivation, the stage of the disease and the precise nature of the hormonal abnormalities induced.

13.7 The influence of individual micronutrients on immune function

Much of what is known about the impact of single nutrients on immune function comes from studies of deficiency states in animals and humans, and from controlled animal studies in which the nutrients are included in the diet at known levels. There is now overwhelming evidence from these studies that particular nutrients are required for an efficient immune response and that deficiencies in one or more of these nutrients diminish immune function and provide a window of opportunity for infectious agents. It is logical that multiple nutrient deficiencies might have a more significant impact on immune function, and therefore resistance to infection, than a single nutrient deficiency. What is also apparent is that excess amounts of some nutrients also impair immune function and decrease resistance to pathogens. Thus, for some nutrients there may be a relatively narrow range of intake that is associated with optimal immune function.

Vitamin A

The vitamin A (or retinoid) family includes retinol, retinal, retinoic acid and esters of retinoic acid. Vitamin A deficiency is accompanied by an increased incidence and severity of infectious diseases and some cancers, and this has been linked to an impaired immune response.

Almost all immune responses studied have been shown to be impaired by vitamin A deficiency.

Vitamin A is essential for maintaining epidermal and mucosal integrity; vitamin A-deficient mice have histopathological changes in the gut mucosa consistent with a breakdown in gut barrier integrity and impaired mucous secretion, both of which would facilitate entry of pathogens through this route. There is also a decline in mucosal immunity in vitamin A-deficient animals. Vitamin A also regulates keratinocyte differentiation and vitamin A deficiency induces changes in skin keratinization, which may explain the observed increased incidence of skin infection.

The impact of vitamin A deficiency on infectious disease has been studied widely in the developing world. Vitamin A deficiency is associated with increased morbidity and mortality in children, and appears to predispose to respiratory infections, diarrhea and severe measles. Although vitamin A deficiency increases the risk of infectious disease, the interaction is bidirectional such that infections can lead to vitamin A deficiency: diarrhea, respiratory infections, measles, chickenpox and human immunodeficiency virus (HIV) infection are all associated with the development of vitamin A deficiency.

Replenishment of vitamin A in deficient individuals leads to restoration of lymphoid organ development, circulating immune cell populations, immune cell functions and the DTH response. There are suggestions that high levels of vitamin A in the diet might enhance immune responsiveness above 'normal'. However, very high doses of vitamin A can sometimes decrease immune function, leading to the conclusion that the response of the immune system to vitamin A is bell-shaped, and that there is a narrow range of doses which produce optimal immune function, while lower intakes or excessive intakes result in suboptimal immune function.

If vitamin A deficiency impairs immune function and decreases host resistance to infection, then it is logical to assume that providing vitamin A should diminish the incidence and severity of infectious disease. While this is the case for mortality related to measles and diarrheal disease, vitamin A supplementation appears to offer little protection against respiratory tract infections.

Carotenoids

The carotenoids are a group of over 600 naturally occurring pigmented compounds that are widespread in plants, although fewer than 30 carotenoids occur commonly in human foodstuffs. Early studies reported that feeding β-carotene to rats increased their resistance to infections, that providing carotenoids to children improved severe ear infections, and that dietary carotenoids appeared to protect against lung and skin cancers. However, detailed studies investigating the effects of carotenoids on parameters of immune function (e.g. lymphocyte proliferation, natural killer cell activity, cytotoxic T-cell activity, expression of cell-surface molecules on monocytes, DTH) have generally not been consistent, with some studies showing benefit and others showing no effect. Further confusion in the area arose when three major intervention trials showed no benefit or an increase in lung cancer in smokers receiving β-carotene supplementation. This area requires further research.

Folic acid and B-vitamins

Folic acid deficiency in laboratory animals causes thymus and spleen atrophy, and decreases circulating T-cell numbers, the activity of cytotoxic T-lymphocytes and spleen lymphocyte proliferation, but does not alter phagocytosis or the bactericidal capacity of neutrophils. In contrast, vitamin B_{12} deficiency decreases phagocytosis and the bactericidal capacity of neutrophils.

Vitamin B_6 deficiency in laboratory animals causes thymus and spleen atrophy, and decreases lymphocyte proliferation and the DTH response. In a study in healthy elderly humans a vitamin B_6-deficient diet (3 μg/kg body weight per day or about 0.17 and 0.1 mg/day for men and women, respectively) for 21 days resulted in a decreased percentage and total number of circulating lymphocytes, decreased T- and B-cell proliferation in response to mitogens and decreased IL-2 production. Repletion at 15 or 22.5 μg/kg body weight per day for 21 days did not return the immune functions to starting values; however repletion at 33.75 μg/kg body weight per day (about 1.9 and 1.1 mg/day for men and women, respectively) returned immune parameters to starting values. Providing a larger dose of 41 mg vitamin B_6/day for 4 days caused a further increase in lymphocyte proliferation and IL-2 production. This comprehensive study indicates that vitamin B_6 deficiency impairs human immune function, that the impairment is reversible by repletion, and that lymphocyte functions are enhanced at levels of vitamin B_6 above those typical of habitual consumption.

Vitamin C

Vitamin C is a water-soluble antioxidant found in high concentrations in circulating leukocytes and appears to be utilized during infections. As with vitamin B_6, the effects of vitamin C on immune function are very much dependent on dosage, and confusion has arisen as a result of attempts to compare studies where different doses have been used. However, one study investigated the effect of vitamin C at different levels in the diet on immune function in a group of young, healthy, non-smokers. The subjects first increased their vitamin C intake by 250 mg/day for 4 days, when baseline measurements were made, and then reduced their vitamin C intake to 5 mg/day for 32 days: the vitamin C-deficient diet decreased mononuclear cell vitamin C content by 50% and decreased the DTH response to seven recall antigens, but did not alter lymphocyte proliferation. Adding back vitamin C at 10, 20, 60 or 250 mg/day (each for 28 days) did not induce recovery of the DTH response, even though the mononuclear cell vitamin C content returned to baseline. These data suggest that optimal immune function is not achieved at the vitamin C intakes recommended in most countries.

Numerous studies of vitamin C and the common cold have been carried out; there is general agreement that vitamin C reduces the severity of symptoms following infection, but not the incidence of infection itself. The protective role of vitamin C may be related to enhanced clearance of the virus by increased IFN production.

Vitamin D

The active form of vitamin D is 1,25-dihydroxy vitamin D_3 and is referred to here as vitamin D. Vitamin D receptors have been identified in most immune cells, suggesting that it has immunoregulatory properties. Experiments involving the addition of vitamin D to isolated cells in culture have indicated that it suppresses some components of acquired immunity and enhances some components of natural immunity. The potential immunosuppressive effects of vitamin D have been tested in animal models of autoimmunity and transplantation. These studies showed that dietary vitamin D prolongs the survival of skin grafts in mice and heart transplants in rats, but causes toxicity. Vitamin D deficiency resulted in increased susceptibility of mice to the autoimmune disease experimental allergic encephalomyelitis (a model of multiple sclerosis) and administration of vitamin D, before and after the induction of this disease in mice and rats prevented its development.

Unfortunately, studies of vitamin D and human immune function are few in number and inconsistent; this area requires clarity and further research.

Vitamin E

Vitamin E is the major lipid-soluble antioxidant in the body and is required for protection of membrane lipids from peroxidation. Free radicals and lipid peroxidation are immunosuppressive; thus, it is considered that vitamin E should act to optimize and even enhance the immune response. Except in premature infants and the elderly, clinical vitamin E deficiency is rare in humans, although many individuals have vitamin E intakes below the recommended daily intake in many countries. Cigarette smoking imposes free radical damage and smokers have increased levels of indicators of free radical damage to lipids, low levels of lung and serum vitamin E, increased numbers of neutrophils and macrophages in the lung, increased reactive oxygen species production by phagocytes and depressed immune responses. Thus, cigarette smokers have a higher vitamin E requirement than non-smokers.

A positive association exists between plasma vitamin E levels and DTH responses, and a negative association has been demonstrated between plasma vitamin E levels and the incidence of infections in healthy adults over 60 years of age. There appears to be particular benefit of vitamin E supplementation for the elderly; a comprehensive study demonstrated increased DTH responses in elderly subjects supplemented with 60, 200 and 800 mg vitamin E/day, with maximal effect at a dose of 200 mg/day. This dose also increased the antibody responses to hepatitis B, tetanus toxoid and pneumococcus vaccinations. This 'optimal' dose of 200 mg vitamin E/day is well in excess of a typical recommended dose; thus, it appears that adding vitamin E to the diet at levels beyond those normally recommended enhances some immune functions above normal, and it has even been argued that the recommended intake for vitamin E is not adequate for optimal immune function. However, as with many other micronutrients, doses that are hugely in excess of normal requirements may suppress the immune response; indeed, the 800 mg vitamin E/day supplement decreased some of the antibody responses to below those of the placebo group.

Zinc

Zinc deficiency in animals is associated with a wide range of immune impairments. Zinc deficiency has a marked impact on bone marrow, decreasing the number of nucleated cells and the number and proportion of cells that are lymphoid precursors. In patients with zinc deficiency related to sickle-cell disease, natural killer cell activity is decreased, but can be returned to normal by zinc supplementation. In acrodermatitis enteropathica, which is characterized by reduced intestinal zinc absorption, thymic atrophy, impaired lymphocyte development and reduced lymphocyte responsiveness and DTH are observed. Moderate or mild zinc deficiency or experimental zinc deficiency (induced by consumption of <3.5 mg zinc/day) in humans results in decreased thymulin activity, natural killer cell activity, lymphocyte proliferation, IL-2 production and DTH response; all can be corrected by zinc repletion.

Low plasma zinc levels can be used to predict the subsequent development of lower respiratory tract infections and diarrhea in malnourished populations. Indeed, diarrhea is considered a symptom of zinc deficiency and several studies show that zinc supplementation decreases the incidence of childhood diarrhea. However, as with vitamin A supplementation, most studies fail to show a benefit of zinc supplementation in respiratory disease in malnourished populations. In contrast, low-birthweight infants supplemented with 5 mg zinc/day for 6 months have been shown to suffer a lower incidence of gastrointestinal and respiratory infections, which have been related to increased cell-mediated immunity. The reasons for the discrepancy in both cases (i.e. vitamin A and zinc) are not entirely clear, but may be due to other nutrient deficiencies being present in supplementation studies carried out in malnourished populations, which would undoubtedly influence the outcome.

Although increasing zinc intake enhances immune function, excessive intakes impair immune responses. For example, giving 300 mg zinc/day for 6 weeks to young adult humans decreased lymphocyte and phagocyte function. High zinc intakes can result in copper depletion, and copper deficiency impairs immune function (see below).

Copper

Although overt copper deficiency is believed to be rare in humans, modest deficiency is likely to be present among some populations. Zinc and iron impair copper uptake, so that taking high doses of these might induce mild copper deficiency. Copper deficiency has been described in premature infants and in patients receiving total parenteral nutrition. The classic example of copper deficiency is Menkes' syndrome, a rare congenital disease which results in the complete absence of ceruloplasmin, the copper-carrying protein in the blood. Children with Menkes syndrome have increased bacterial infections, diarrhea and pneumonia. Human studies involving subjects on a low copper diet result in decreased lymphocyte proliferation and IL-2 production, while copper administration reverses many of the effects of copper deficiency, including spleen lymphocyte responsiveness and IL-2 production; however, as with many other micronutrients, excess copper can be immunosuppressive.

Iron

Iron deficiency has multiple effects on immune function in laboratory animals and humans. Iron-deficient individuals have normal phagocytic function, but there is impaired ability to kill bacteria by neutrophils, probably as a result of an alteration in respiratory burst. Iron deficiency is associated with gastrointestinal and respiratory infections.

Despite the suppressive effects of iron deficiency on immune responses, iron supplementation can be associated with an increased risk of infection. For example, if iron-deficient individuals who have compromised resistance to infection are given large doses of iron parenterally or orally, an exacerbation of infection and death can occur. This has, unfortunately, been learnt at great cost in studies where:

- iron administration to low birthweight babies increased the incidence of septicemia
- the incidence of infections among Somali nomads was increased by iron supplementation
- Chilean children who received iron-fortified milk (12 mg iron/liter) had a 20% higher incidence of diarrhea than those who received a control milk containing 1 mg iron/liter
- Bangladeshi children who received supplemental iron (15 mg/day for 15 months) in addition to vitamins A, D and C had 26% more days with diarrhea than children who received the vitamins alone.

The detrimental effects of iron administration may occur because microorganisms require iron and

providing it may favor the growth and replication of the pathogen. Indeed, it has been argued that the decline in circulating iron concentrations that accompanies infection is an attempt by the host to 'starve' the infectious agent of iron. There are several mechanisms for witholding iron from a pathogen in this way. Lactoferrin has a higher binding affinity for iron than do bacterial siderospores, making bound iron unavailable to the pathogen. Furthermore, once lactoferrin reaches 40% saturation with iron, it is sequestered by macrophages. It is notable that breast milk contains lactoferrin, which may protect against the use of free iron by pathogens transferred to an infant.

The situation regarding iron status and malaria is particularly complicated, since red blood cells host this parasite; thus, host stores of iron and the invading pathogen coincide. This might explain the observations that malaria is more common in iron-replete than iron-deficient individuals, and that the levels of malaria infection and the severity of the disease are increased by iron supplementation. Indeed, it could be argued that lowering iron status might improve malaria outcome: this is borne out by the observation that iron chelation therapy enhances the clearance of parasites and accelerates the effect of antimalarials.

Selenium

Selenium is found in high concentrations in the liver, spleen and lymph nodes. Selenium deficiency in laboratory animals decreases a range of immune functions and increases susceptibility to bacterial, viral, fungal and parasitic challenges. Selenium deficiency does not affect the ability of neutrophils or macrophages to engage in phagocytosis, but it does diminish the ability of the cells to kill microorganisms once they have been ingested. Selenium supplementation studies in animals demonstrate that selenium increases antibody titers in response to immunization and antigen challenges, lymphocyte proliferation, IFN-γ production, natural killer cell activity, DTH response and rejection of skin allografts, and decreases susceptibility to infections. In humans, selenium deficiency results in decreased circulating IgG and IgM concentrations.

Micronutrient combinations and resistance to infection

Given that individual micronutrients have impressive effects on immune function, it is important to consider the effects of supplementation with micronutrient combinations, which is much more likely to occur in a real situation. In a study investigating this question, elderly humans given a multinutrient mix containing the US recommended daily allowances of vitamins A, B_6, B_{12} and D, thiamin, riboflavin, niacin, folate, iron, zinc, copper, selenium, iodine, calcium and magnesium, and higher than the US recommended daily allowances of vitamin C (80 mg/day), vitamin E (44 mg/day) and β-carotene (16 mg/day) for 12 months had a higher antibody response to influenza vaccine and less infection-related illness than the placebo group.

Micronutrients and human immonodeficiency virus infection

Many individuals with HIV infection consume less than the recommended daily allowance for a range of micronutrients. Nutrient intake by patients with HIV infection may be decreased as a result of loss of appetite, aversion to food and throat infections, while vomiting, diarrhea and malabsorption may also contribute to deficiencies. The prevalence of micronutrient deficiencies (based largely on concentrations in the plasma or serum) varies widely depending on the population and the stage of the disease, but it appears that deficiencies in vitamins A, B_6, B_{12}, C, D and E, β-carotene, selenium and zinc are common.

Micronutrient deficiencies may increase oxidative stress and compromise host immunity, so contributing to HIV disease progression. However, the effect of supplementation to HIV-infected patients with either single or multiple micronutrients is not clear, perhaps because of the complex nature of the disease.

Micronutrients and asthma and allergy

Respiratory diseases such as asthma impose oxidant stress on the individual as a result of inappropriate production of reactive oxygen species (e.g. superoxide and hydroxyl radicals, hydrogen peroxide, hypochlorous acid). These reactive species damage host tissues, upregulate the production of inflammatory cytokines and adhesion molecules, thereby amplifying the inflammation, induce bronchoconstriction, elevate mucus secretion and cause microvascular leakage. Oxidant stress can deplete cells and tissues of antioxidants, if they are not replenished sufficiently through the diet. Furthermore, a low dietary intake of antioxidants may exacerbate the problem by allowing reactive species generation to proceed unchecked. Among the important

---

Box 13.2 Key points: micronutrients

- Micronutrient deficiencies are common in the developing world, but also occur in the developed world, especially among the elderly, premature infants and patients with certain diseases
- Micronutrient deficiencies impair immune function: all aspects of immunity can be affected
- Micronutrient deficiencies make the host more susceptible to infections
- Providing micronutrients to deficient individuals can restore immune function and resistance to infections in some situations
- Increasing the intake of some micronutrients (vitamin A, vitamin E, β-carotene, zinc) above the levels normally recommended may enhance immune function
- Excess amounts of some micronutrients (vitamin A, zinc, iron) impair immune function
- Some diseases are characterized by oxidant stress and this will be compounded by micronutrient deficiencies
- Insufficient intake of micronutrients may contribute to the progression of diseases that have a strong oxidative stress component

---

antioxidants to consider are vitamins C and E (vitamin C is the major antioxidant present in the airway surface of the lung), glutathione, the glutathione recycling enzyme glutathione peroxidase, and the enzymes that remove superoxide and hydrogen peroxide (superoxide dismutase and catalase, respectively); glutathione peroxidase, superoxide dismutase and catalase contain selenium, copper and zinc, and iron, respectively. Low dietary intakes of selenium, vitamin C and vitamin E have been shown to increase the risk of asthma.

The use of vitamin C in asthma and allergy has been investigated in a number of studies, half of which support its use, while the other half demonstrate no benefit. The effects of selenium are similarly unclear, and while vitamin E has been shown to improve symptoms in animal models of asthma, human studies to verify this are lacking.

The roles that micronutrients play in immunity are summarized in Box 13.2.

13.8 Dietary fat and immune function

Fatty acids in the diet

Fatty acids consist of hydrocarbon chains, which may be saturated (no double bonds), monounsaturated (one double bond) or polyunsaturated (more than one double bond). Fatty acids have systematic names, but most also have common names and are described by a shorthand nomenclature. This nomenclature indicates the number of carbon atoms in the chain, the number of double bonds in the chain and the position of the first double bond from the methyl-terminus of the chain. The position of the first double bond in the hydrocarbon chain is indicated by the n-7, n-9, n-6 or n-3 portion of the shorthand notation for a fatty acid. Thus, in an n-6 fatty acid the first double bond is located on carbon number 6 counted from the methyl-terminus and in an n-3 fatty acid the first double bond is located on carbon number 3 counted from the methyl-terminus. Note that the n notation is sometimes referred to as ω or omega.

Saturated fatty acids and most monounsaturated fatty acids can be synthesized in mammalian tissues from non-fat precursors, such as glucose or amino acids. However, mammals cannot insert double bonds before carbon number 9 in oleic acid. Thus, mammals cannot convert oleic acid (18:1n-9) into linoleic acid (18:2n-6). Likewise, mammals cannot convert linoleic acid into α-linolenic acid (18:3n-3). It is because linoleic acid and α-linolenic acid cannot be synthesized by mammals that they are termed essential fatty acids. Furthermore, mammalian cells cannot interconvert n-6 and n-3 fatty acids. However, desaturases and elongases, which are present in mammalian cells, are able to extend and insert further double bonds into linoleic and α-linolenic acids which have been consumed in the diet, generating families of n-6 and n-3 fatty acids (Figure 13.5). Derivatives of the essential fatty acids formed in this way are described as conditionally essential. The major product of n-6 fatty acid metabolism is arachidonic acid (20:4n-6), while the major end-products of n-3 fatty acid metabolism are eicosapentaenoic acid (EPA; 20:5n-3) and docosahexaenoic acid (DHA; 22:6n-3); these fatty acids are incorporated into cell membranes to a significant extent.

Plant tissues and plant oils tend to be rich sources of linoleic and α-linolenic acids. For example, linoleic acid comprises over 50%, and often up to 80%, of the fatty acids found in corn, sunflower, safflower and soybean oils. Rapeseed and soybean oils are good sources of α-linolenic acid, since this fatty acid contributes between 5 and 15% of total fatty acids. The intake of longer chain PUFA is not known precisely, but EPA and DHA are found in relatively high proportions in the tissues of oily fish (e.g. herring, mackerel, tuna, sardines) and in the commercial products 'fish oils', which are a preparation of the body oils of oily fish or liver oils of lean fish. Note that in the absence of significant

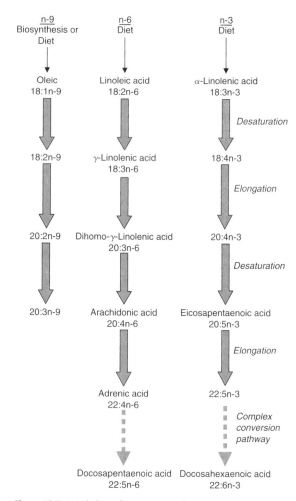

Figure 13.5 Metabolism of n-6 and n-3 polyunsaturated fatty acids.

consumption of oily fish, α-linolenic acid is the major dietary n-3 fatty acid.

Essential fatty acid deficiency and immune function

Animal studies have shown that deficiencies in both linoleic and α-linolenic acids result in decreased thymus and spleen weight, lymphocyte proliferation, neutrophil chemotaxis, macrophage-mediated cytotoxicity and DTH response compared with animals fed diets containing adequate amounts of these fatty acids. Thus, the immunological effects of essential fatty acid deficiency appear to be similar to the effects of single micronutrient deficiencies, although there are no human studies to confirm this (essential fatty acid deficiency is very rare in humans). However, essential fatty acid deficiency would be expected to have a similar effect, because cells of the immune system require PUFA for membrane synthesis and as precursors for the synthesis of eicosanoids (see below).

Amount of dietary fat and immune function

High-fat diets have been reported to result in diminished immune cell functions (both natural and cell-mediated immunity) compared with low-fat diets, but the precise effect depends on the exact level of fat used in the high-fat diet and its source. Furthermore, reductions in total dietary fat intake to below 30% of total energy enhance many immune responses, including lymphocyte proliferation, natural killer cell activity and cytokine production.

Eicosanoids: a link between fatty acids and the immune system

The conversion of 20-carbon atom PUFA to a group of mediators termed eicosanoids provides the key link between fatty acids and immune function. The membranes of most cells contain large amounts of arachidonic acid, which is the principal precursor for eicosanoid synthesis. Arachidonic acid in cell membranes can be mobilized by various phospholipase enzymes, most notably phospholipase A_2, and the free arachidonic acid can subsequently act as a substrate for cyclooxygenase (COX), forming prostaglandins (PG) and related compounds, or for one of the lipoxygenase (LOX) enzymes, forming leukotrienes (LT) and related compounds (Figure 13.6). There are many different compounds belonging to each class of eicosanoid and

they are each formed in a cell-specific manner. For example, monocytes and macrophages produce large amounts of PGE_2 and PGF_2, neutrophils produce moderate amounts of PGE_2 and mast cells produce PGD_2. The LOX enzymes have different tissue distributions, with 5-LOX being found mainly in mast cells, monocytes, macrophages and granulocytes, and 12- and 15-LOX being found mainly in epithelial cells.

Prostaglandins are involved in modulating the intensity and duration of inflammatory and immune responses. PGE_2 has a number of proinflammatory effects, including the induction of fever and erythema, increasing vascular permeability and vasodilatation and enhancing pain and oedema caused by other agents such as histamine. However, PGE_2 also suppresses lymphocyte proliferation and natural killer cell activity, and inhibits the production of TNF-α, IL-1, IL-6, IL-2 and IFN-γ; thus, in these respects PGE_2 is immunosuppressive and anti-inflammatory. LTB_4 increases vascular permeability, enhances local blood flow, is a potent chemotactic agent for leukocytes, induces the release of lysosomal enzymes, enhances the generation of reactive oxygen species, inhibits lymphocyte proliferation, promotes natural killer cell activity and can enhance the production of inflammatory cytokines. Thus, arachidonic acid gives rise to a range of mediators that may have opposing effects to one another, so the overall physiological effect will be governed by the nature of the cells producing the eicosanoids, the concentrations of the mediators, the timing of their production and the sensitivities of target cells to their effects.

Consumption of fish oil results in a decrease in the amount of arachidonic acid in the membranes of most cells in the body, including those involved in inflammation and immunity. This means that there is less substrate available for synthesis of eicosanoids from arachidonic acid. Furthermore, EPA competitively inhibits the oxygenation of arachidonic acid by COX. Thus, fish oil feeding results in a decreased capacity of immune cells to synthesize eicosanoids from arachidonic acid. In addition, EPA is itself able to act as a substrate for both COX and 5-LOX (Figure 13.7), giving rise to derivatives that have a different structure from those produced from arachidonic acid (i.e. 3-series PG and thromboxanes and 5-series LT). Thus, the EPA-induced suppression of the production of arachidonic-acid derived eicosanoids is mirrored by an elevation of the production of EPA-derived eicosanoids. The eicosanoids produced from EPA are often less

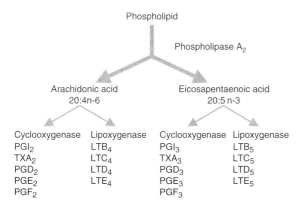

Figure 13.6 Synthesis of eicosanoids from polyunsaturated fatty acids. PG: prostaglandin; TX: thromboxane; LT: leukotriene.

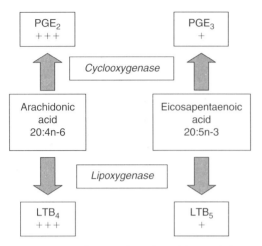

Figure 13.7 Potency of eicosanoids synthesized from arachidonic acid versus eicosapentaenoic acid. PG: prostaglandin; LT: leukotriene.

biologically potent than the analogs synthesized from arachidonic acid, although the full range of biological activities of these compounds has not been investigated. LTB_5 is only about 10% as potent as a chemotactic agent and in promoting lysosomal enzyme release as LTB_4. LTB_5 can partially inhibit LTB_4-mediated superoxide formation and chemotaxis. The reduction in the generation of arachidonic acid-derived mediators that accompanies fish oil consumption has led to the idea that fish oil is anti-inflammatory and may affect immune function in general.

Linoleic acid, α-linolenic acid and immune function

Saturated fatty acids have little impact on immune function, whereas linoleic acid has the potential to suppresses lymphocyte and natural killer cell activities. These effects may be exerted via the production of PGE_2 from arachidonic acid, which is derived from linoleic acid. Although PGE_2 is well known for its proinflammatory properties, it has several immunosuppressive activities. It is apparent, however, that both a deficiency and an excess of linoleic acid can lead to suppressed immune function, depending on the absolute level of fat in the diet (essential fatty acid deficiency leads to impaired immune function, but high-fat diets also suppress immunity).

The precise effect of α-linolenic acid on lymphocyte functions depends on the level of linoleic acid and the total PUFA content of the diet. Adding linseed oil (providing about 15 g α-linolenic acid/day) to a low-fat diet

(total fat provided 29% energy) has been shown to result in a significant decrease in human blood lymphocyte proliferation and in the DTH response after 6 weeks. Thus, as for linoleic acid, it appears that both a deficiency and an excess of α-linolenic acid can lead to suppressed immune function.

Fish oil and immune function

Since EPA leads to decreased PGE_2 production (see above), it is often stated that fish oil consumption should reverse the effects of PGE_2. However, the situation is likely to be more complex than this because PGE_2 is not the sole mediator produced from arachidonic acid and the range of mediators produced have varying, sometimes opposite, actions (see above). Furthermore, EPA will give rise to mediators, which also have varying actions. Thus, the overall effect of fish oil feeding cannot be predicted solely on the basis of an abrogation of PGE_2-mediated effects. The recognition of this complexity appears to be borne out by experimental observations. A large number of animal studies on the effects of fish oil on inflammation and immunity indicate that fish oil decreases a wide range of immune cell responses when fed at high levels. It has become clear that the observed effects of fish oil are different to those that are predicted solely on the basis of a decrease in PGE_2 production or indeed on production of eicosanoids *per se*. Thus, there are likely to be other mechanisms of action of fish oil that do not involve eicosanoids and have not yet been fully defined. It is also worth noting that most animal studies investigating the effects of fish oil have used amounts far in excess of those that could be consumed by humans.

Supplementation of the diet of healthy human volunteers with fish oil-derived n-3 PUFA has been shown, in general, to support the idea that fish oil (at the levels used experimentally) exerts a range of immunological effects, although not all studies agree. The most consistent effects of fish oil include diminished recognition of, and response to, host antigen, decreased movement of leukocytes towards sites of inflammatory activity, decreased binding of leukocytes to endothelial cells and their movement from the bloodstream to the subendothelial space, and decreased cellular activation and the release of chemoattractants, cytokines, eicosanoids and reactive species. Fish oil is clearly anti-inflammatory at levels provided in human studies; however, these levels would require the consumption of at least six standard 1 g fish oil capsules per day (this would provide approximately 2 g EPA plus DHA). There is a considerable lack of human studies that seek to determine the dose dependence of fish oil on immune function.

Fish oil and infection

If fish oil were immunosuppressive it would be expected to diminish host defense. Some animal studies support this suggestion, while others do not. Since the response to microbial infections is predominantly a Th_1-mediated response (or at least requires Th_1-type cytokines such as IFN-γ), the reduced survival of laboratory animals fed large amounts of fish oil to bacterial challenges suggests that fish oil suppresses the Th1 response *in vivo*. However, fish oil also decreases the metabolic responses to bacterial infection, including fever, anorexia and weight loss, and can, in some situations, increase survival following a challenge by limiting inflammatory damage (mainly the action of proinflammatory cytokines) to the host. The outcome of fish oil supplementation in infections is therefore complex and will depend on the balance between effects on the immunological response to the pathogen and effects on the metabolic response to infection in the host.

Dietary fat and Th_1 skewed immunological diseases

Chronic inflammatory diseases are characterized by a dysregulated Th_1-type response and often by an inappropriate production of arachidonic acid-derived eicosanoids, especially PGE_2 and LTB_4. The effects of fish oil outlined above suggest that it might have a role in prevention and therapy of chronic inflammatory diseases. There has been a number of clinical trials assessing the benefits of dietary supplementation with fish oils in several chronic inflammatory diseases in humans. In some of these studies, in particular clinical trials of rheumatoid arthritis, anti-inflammatory effects of fish oil were observed (e.g. lowered LTB_4, IL-1 and C-reactive protein production), which were associated with clinical improvements and a lower requirement of anti-inflammatory drugs. However, other chronic inflammatory conditions, such as multiple sclerosis and systemic lupus erythematosus, are unaffected or only marginally affected by fish oil treatment, suggesting that the therapeutic effect of fish oil in inflammatory conditions is not universal.

Dietary fat and Th_2 skewed immunological diseases

Eicosanoids synthesized from arachidonic acid play a role in atopic diseases: PGD_2, LTC_4, D_4 and E_4 are produced by the cells that mediate pulmonary inflammation in asthma, such as mast cells, and are believed to be the major mediators of asthmatic bronchoconstriction. The role of arachidonic acid as a precursor for eicosanoid synthesis has highlighted its significance in the etiology of asthma. However, arachidonic acid appears to have a dual role in asthma, since PGE_2 regulates the activities of macrophages and lymphocytes; its actions in this context inhibit the production of the Th_1-type cytokines IL-2 and IFN-γ without affecting the production of the Th_2-type cytokines IL-4 and IL-5, and stimulate B-cells to produce IgE. These observations are important since they suggest that PGE_2 is involved the development of the allergic disease.

Linoleic acid consumption has increased dramatically in developed countries since the mid-1960s and this period of increased intake coincides with the period over which the incidence of childhood allergy has increased. There has therefore been speculation that increased vegetable oil (and hence linoleic acid) consumption results in increased cellular arachidonic acid levels, which increases the capacity for PGE_2 production, which in turn alters the balance of Th_1 and Th_2 cytokines to encourage the development of asthma and other allergic diseases.

The notion that elevated arachidonic acid levels are associated with allergic disease is opposed by the frequently reported abnormalities in fatty acid composition of blood, cells and milk from atopic mothers and/or their offspring. Lowered proportions of arachidonic acid have been observed in plasma, epidermal and erythrocyte phospholipids, and adipose tissue of patients with atopic dermatitis, in cord blood T-cells and mononuclear cells of newborn infants at risk of atopy, and in the breast milk and colostrum of mothers with a history of atopic dermatitis. These observations have been taken to suggest that a deficiency in δ^6-desaturase plays a role in these diseases. Such a deficiency would result in an imbalance between different members of the n-6 PUFA family and between the n-6 and the n-3 PUFA families. Rather than atopic disease being driven by an excess of arachidonic acid, an alternative suggestion is that PGE_2 plays a role in thymic T-cell development and in controlling T-cell activity, and that this regulation is diminished in atopics, owing to a decreased availability of arachidonic acid. This area has not yet been resolved and requires further work.

The roles that dietary fats play in immunity are summarized in Box 13.3.

13.9 Dietary amino acids and related compounds and immune function

Sulfur amino acids and related compounds

Sulfur amino acids are essential in humans. Deficiency in methionine and cysteine results in atrophy of the thymus, spleen and lymph nodes and prevents recovery from protein–energy malnutrition. When combined with a deficiency of isoleucine and valine, also essential amino acids, sulfur amino acid deficiency results in severe depletion of gut lymphoid tissue, very similar to the effect of protein deprivation.

Glutathione is a tripeptide that consists of glycine, cysteine and glutamate (from glutamine), and is recognized to have antioxidant properties. Glutathione concentrations in the liver, lung, small intestine and

immune cells fall in response to inflammatory stimuli (probably as a result of oxidative stress), and this fall can be prevented in some organs by the provision of cysteine in the diet. Although the limiting precursor for glutathione biosynthesis is usually cysteine, the ability of sulfur amino acids to replete glutathione stores is related to the protein level of the diet. Glutathione can enhance the activity of human cytotoxic T-cells, while depletion of intracellular glutathione diminishes lymphocyte proliferation and the generation of cytotoxic T-lymphocytes.

Taurine is a sulfonated β-amino acid derived from methionine and cysteine metabolism, but is not a component of proteins. Taurine transfer to the fetus occurs throughout gestation, but especially over the last 4 weeks, and neonates have a reduced capacity to synthesize taurine. Thus, taurine levels are low in premature and low-birthweight babies. In humans, plasma taurine concentrations are decreased by trauma and sepsis. Taurine is present in high concentrations in most tissues and particularly in cells of the immune system; in lymphocytes it contributes 50% of the free amino acid pool. The role of taurine within lymphocytes is not clear. In neutrophils taurine appears to play a role in maintaining phagocytic capacity and microbicidal action through interaction with myeloperoxidase, an enzyme involved in respiratory burst. Taurinechloramine is formed by complexing of taurine with hypochlorous acid (HOCl) produced by myeloperoxidase. Hypochlorous acid, although toxic to bacteria, causes damage to host tissues and it has been proposed that the formation of taurinechloramine is a mechanism to protect the host from this damage. Although taurine appears not to affect mediator production by macrophages, taurinechloramine decreases PGE_2, TNF-α and IL-6 production by macrophages.

Arginine

Arginine is a non-essential amino acid in humans and is involved in protein, urea and nucleotide synthesis, and adenosine triphosphate (ATP) generation. It also serves as the precursor of nitric oxide, a potent immunoregulatory mediator that is cytotoxic to tumor cells and to some microorganisms. In laboratory animals arginine decreases the thymus involution associated with trauma, promotes thymus repopulation and cellularity, increases lymphocyte proliferation, natural killer cell activity and macrophage cytotoxicity, improves DTH, increases resistance to bacterial infections, increases survival to sepsis and burns, and promotes wound healing. There are indications that arginine may have similar effects in humans, although these have not been tested thoroughly. There is particular interest in the inclusion of arginine in enteral formulae given to patients hospitalized for surgery, trauma and burns, since it appears to reduce the severity of infectious complications and the length of hospital stay. However, in many of the clinical studies carried out in these patients, the enteral formulae used have contained a variety of nutrients with immunomodulatory actions, so it has been difficult to ascribe beneficial effects to any one nutrient alone.

Glutamine

Glutamine is the most abundant amino acid in the blood and in the free amino acid pool in the body; skeletal muscle is considered to be the most important glutamine producer in the body. Once released from skeletal muscle, glutamine acts as an interorgan nitrogen transporter. Important users of glutamine include the kidney, liver, small intestine and cells of the immune system. Plasma glutamine levels are lowered (by up to 50%) by sepsis, injury and burns, and following surgery. Furthermore, the skeletal muscle glutamine concentration is lowered by more than 50% in at least some of these situations. These observations indicate that a significant depletion of the skeletal muscle glutamine pool is characteristic of trauma. The lowered plasma glutamine concentrations that occur are likely to be the result of demand for glutamine (by the liver, kidney, gut and immune system) exceeding the supply, and it has been suggested that the lowered plasma glutamine contributes, at least in part, to the impaired immune function that accompanies such situations. It has been argued that restoring plasma glutamine concentrations in these situations should restore immune function. As with arginine, there are animal studies to support this. Clinical studies, mainly using intravenous infusions of solutions containing glutamine, have also reported beneficial effects for patients undergoing bone marrow transplantation and colorectal surgery, patients in intensive care and low-birthweight babies, all of whom are at risk from infection and sepsis. In some of these studies, improved outcome was associated with improved immune function. In addition to a direct immunological effect, glutamine, even provided parenterally, improves gut barrier function in patients at risk of infection. This would have the benefit of decreasing

---

Box 13.4 Key points: amino acids and immunity

- Deficiencies in essential amino acids are likely to impair immune function
- A key role of sulfur amino acids is in maintaining levels of the antioxidant glutathione and so in preventing oxidative stress
- Some classically non-essential amino acids (arginine, glutamine) may become essential in stress situations

---

the translocation of bacteria from the gut and eliminating a key source of infection.

The roles that dietary amino acids play in immunity are summarized in Box 13.4.

13.10 Probiotics and immune function

Indigenous bacteria are believed to contribute to the immunological protection of the host by creating a barrier against colonization by pathogenic bacteria. This barrier can be disrupted by disease and by the use of antibiotics, so allowing easier access to the host gut by pathogens. It is now believed that this barrier can be maintained by providing supplements containing live 'desirable' bacteria; such supplements are termed probiotics. Probiotic organisms are found in fermented foods including traditionally cultured dairy products and some fermented milks. The organisms included in commercial probiotics include lactic acid bacteria (*Lactobacillus acidophilus*, *Lactobacillus casei*, *Enterococcus faecium*) and *Bifidobacteria*. These organisms only colonize the gut temporarily, making regular consumption necessary. In addition to creating a barrier effect, some of the metabolic products of probiotic bacteria (e.g. lactic acid and a class of antibiotic proteins termed bacteriocins produced by some bacteria) may inhibit the growth of pathogenic organisms. Probiotic bacteria may also compete with pathogenic bacteria for nutrients and may enhance the gut immune response to pathogenic bacteria. Despite the extensive animal studies, which suggest enhancement of immune function by probiotics, the effects of probiotic bacteria on human immune function are still controversial. Some benefits in the incidence and severity of diarrhea have been reported, but measurements of immune function have been very limited.

The roles that probiotics play in immunity are summarized in Box 13.5.

13.11 Breast-feeding and immune function

The composition of breast milk

Breast milk is the best example of a foodstuff with immune-enhancing properties. Milk contains a wide range of immunologically active components, including cells (macrophages, T- and B-lymphocytes, neutrophils), immunoglobulins (IgG, IgM, IgD, sIgA), lysozyme (which has direct antibacterial action), lactoferrin (which binds iron, so preventing its uptake by bacteria), cytokines (IL-1, IL-6, IL-10, IFN-γ, TNF-α, transforming growth factor-β), growth factors (epidermal growth factor, insulin-like growth factor), hormones (thyroxin), fat-soluble vitamins (vitamins A, D, E), amino acids (taurine, glutamine), fatty acids, amino sugars and nucleotides. Breast milk also contains factors that prevent the adhesion of some microorganisms to the gastrointestinal tract and so prevents bacterial colonization. Human breast milk contains factors that promote the growth of useful bacteria (e.g. *Bifidobacteria*) in the gut; this factor is absent from the milk of all other species. The content of many factors varies among milks of different species, and is different between human breast milk and many infant formulae. Human milk is rich in immunoglobulins the antimicrobial proteins lactoferrin and lysozyme, vitamins A, D and E, PUFA, free amino acids and nucleotides; in contrast, cow's milk either lacks or contains much lower amounts of many of these factors.

Breast-feeding, immune function and infection

Breast-feeding is thought to play a key role in the prevention of infectious disease, particularly diarrhea and gastrointestinal and lower respiratory infections, in both developing and developed countries. In addition to preventing infectious disease, breast-feeding enhances the antibody responses to vaccination. Several studies have examined the effect of breast-feeding versus formula-feeding on risk of death due to infectious diseases in developing countries. A meta-analysis of these studies, published in the Lancet in 2000 (see Further reading), suggested that infants who are not breast-fed have a six-fold greater risk of dying from infectious diseases in the first 2 months of life than those who are breast-fed. However, it appears that this protection decreases steadily with age, as infants begin complementary feeding, so that by 6–11 months, the protection afforded by breast-feeding is no longer apparent. Breast-feeding may provide better protection against diarrhea (up to 6 months of age) than against deaths due to respiratory infections. There are also geographical influences on the protection afforded by breast-feeding; in some continents, protection can be observed throughout the first year of life, whereas in others it is much more short-lived.

The roles that breast-feeding plays in immunity are summarized in Box 13.6.

13.12 Perspectives on the future

Deficiencies of total energy or of one or more essential nutrients, including vitamins A, B_6, B_{12}, C and E, folic acid, zinc, iron, copper, selenium, essential amino acids and essential fatty acids, impair immune function and increase susceptibility to infectious pathogens. This occurs because each of these nutrients is involved in the molecular and cellular responses to challenge of the immune system. Providing these nutrients to deficient individuals restores immune function and improves resistance to infection. For several nutrients the dietary intakes that result in greatest enhancement of immune function are greater than recommended intakes. However, excessive intake of some nutrients also impairs immune responses. Thus, four potential general

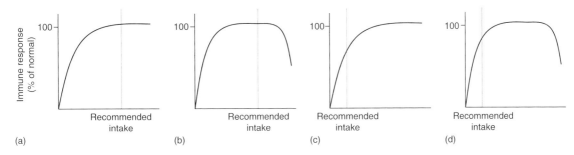

Figure 13.8 Four possible relationships between nutrient intake and immune function. All patterns assume that a deficiency of the nutrient impairs the immune response. In pattern (a) the immune response is maximal, in terms of relationship to the intake of the nutrient under study, at the recommended level of intake and intakes somewhat above the recommended intake do not impair immune function. In pattern (b) the immune response is maximal, in terms of relationship to the intake of the nutrient under study, at the recommended level of intake and intakes somewhat above the recommended intake impair immune function. In pattern (c) the immune response is submaximal, in terms of relationship to the intake of the nutrient under study, at the recommended level of intake and intakes somewhat above the recommended intake do not impair immune function. In pattern (d) the immune response is submaximal, in terms of relationship to the intake of the nutrient under study, at the recommended level of intake and intakes somewhat above the recommended intake impair immune function.

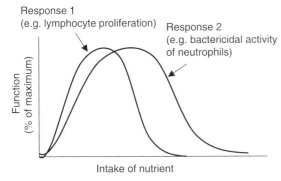

Figure 13.9 Dose–response relationships of different immune functions to the same nutrient may not be identical.

relationships between the intake of a nutrient and immune function appear to exist (Figure 13.8). It is often assumed when defining the relationship between nutrient intake and immune function that all components of the immune system will respond in the same dose-dependent fashion to a given nutrient. This is not correct, at least as far as some nutrients are concerned, and it appears likely that different components of the immune system show an individual dose–response relationship to the availability of a given nutrient (Figure 13.9).

Although outside the scope of this chapter, it is important to consider the role of hormones in regulating immune function during malnutrition. An inadequate supply of nutrients to the body may cause physiological stress, leading to an elevation in the circulating concentrations of glucocorticoids and catecholamines. Both classes of hormones have an inhibitory effect on immune function and may therefore be important factors when considering the relationship between nutrient supply and immunological outcome.

It is now appreciated that the supply of nutrients that are not considered to be essential according to traditional criteria may also influence immune function; this is particularly notable for the amino acids glutamine and arginine, and may indicate that a re-evaluation of the definitions of essentiality, nutrient requirements and nutrient status is required for some dietary components.

Finally, an early point of contact between nutrients and the immune system occurs within the intestinal tract. Relatively little is known about the relationship between nutrient status and the function of the gut-associated immune system. This is of particular relevance when considering adverse reactions to foods: the role of immunoregulatory nutrients in responses to food components and in sensitization to food-borne allergens is largely unknown. An understanding of the interaction between nutrients, the types of bacteria that inhabit the gut, and gut-associated and systemic immune responses is only now beginning to emerge.

The term 'optimal immune function' is often used in the literature without careful thought about its definition. An optimal immune response to any given nutrient measured by one marker will not necessarily be optimal according to a second marker of immune function (Figure 13.9). Furthermore, the effect of a given nutrient on immune response may be altered by levels of other nutrients. For these reasons, the natural desire to 'optimize' the immune response may not be realistic. At best, it is reasonable to expect that correction of marginal deficiencies will improve immunity, but further enhancement using micronutrient supplements cannot be guaranteed and in excessive doses is likely to be detrimental. At the other extreme, there is interest in the potential therapeutic effect of nutrients in diseases involving dysregulation of the immune system (e.g. n-3 fatty acids in rheumatoid arthritis). In some, but by no means all cases, there is supportive evidence for this approach. Between these extremes there are many unanswered questions, but it is clear that the study of the modulation of immune function by nutrients has important implications in both developing and developed countries.

Further reading

Alexander JW. Immunonutrition: the role of ω-3 fatty acids. Nutrition 1998; 14: 627–633.

Bendich A. Antioxidant vitamins and human immune responses. Vitam Horm 1996; 52: 35–62.

British Nutrition Foundation. Report of the Task Force on Unsaturated Fatty Acids. London: British Nutrition Foundation, 1992.

Chandra RK. 1990 McCollum Award Lecture. Nutrition and immunity: lessons from the past and new insights into the future. Am J Clin Nutr 1991; 53: 1087–1101.

Scrimshaw NS, SanGiovanni JP. Synergism of nutrition, infection and immunity: an overview. Am J Clin Nutr 1997; 66: 464S–477S.

WHO Collaborative Study Team on the Role of Breastfeeding on the Prevention of Infant Mortality. Lancet 2000; 355: 451–455.

14
Phytochemicals

A Cassidy and FS Dalais

Key messages

- Phytochemicals, also known as phytonutrients, are plant-based compounds with a number of physiological functions in mammalian systems.
- They are classified as: the phenolic phytochemicals (the flavonoids), other phenolic phytochemicals (tannins, stilbenes and lignans), carotenoids, phytosterols, and sulfur-containing compounds (sulfides and glucosinolates).
- Phytochemicals can have beneficial effects in a range of diseases, including cardiovascular disease and cancer, as well as immune function.
- There is still incomplete knowledge about their metabolism, bioavailability, mode of action, dose response and in some cases the actual compounds responsible for the health benefit.

14.1 Introduction

Fruits and vegetables are rich sources of micronutrients and dietary fiber, but they also contain a wide variety of secondary metabolites which provide the plant with color, flavor, antimicrobial and insecticidal and other such properties. Many of these potentially protective plant compounds, termed phytochemicals, are now receiving increased attention. Phytochemicals, also known as phytonutrients, are plant-based compounds with a number of physiological functions in mammalian systems. Many of them are ubiquitous throughout the plant kingdom and hence are present in our daily diet. Among the most important classes are the carotenoids, flavonoids, and more complex phenolics, phytosterols and the glucosinolates, which are classified based on their chemical and structural characteristics. This chapter will focus on the different classes of phytochemicals and their relationship to human diseases.

14.2 Historical perspective

The belief that plants and plant foods held properties other than nutritional ones stems back to early civilizations. Egyptian culture, for example, used a number of teas and herbs for healing of disease. A report on diet and cancer from the Food and Nutrition Board of the US National Academy of Science in the early 1980s, together with other studies in the mid-1980s, highlighted the fact that there were compounds in our diet that protected us against cancer. In the early 1990s came a number of epidemiological studies which further emphasized the relationship between vegetable and fruit consumption and cancer. Since then, a large number of studies have strongly illustrated the possibility that phytochemicals in vegetables and fruits may play a role in reducing the risk of cancer, as well as a number of other chronic health conditions such as cardiovascular disease.

Nutrition research is only beginning to understand how many of these naturally occurring compounds work. Like many nutrients, phytochemicals can have adverse effects as well as beneficial effects on human health, depending on the biochemical nature of the compound (whether it is retained in the body or absorbed and excreted rapidly in urine). When phytochemicals were first discovered, they were mainly considered to be toxic or as antinutrients. It is true that some phytochemicals prevent the absorption of certain nutrients, but the focus has now changed to examining the beneficial properties of these compounds.

To date, about 30 000 phytochemicals have been identified, of which 5000–10 000 are present in the food that we consume. Even though it is hard to quantify the dietary intake of phytochemicals, it has been estimated that the average diet contains a daily dose of about 1.5 g.

Phytochemicals are classified based on their chemical structure and/or functional attributes. The list below is by no means exhaustive, but relates to phytochemicals that have been more commonly studied in cell, animal and human models, and consumed as part of our daily diet.

14.3　The phenolic phytochemicals

Flavonoids

Flavonoids form part of the largest category of phytochemicals, the phenolic phytochemicals. The term 'phenolic' encompasses a variety of plant compounds containing an aromatic ring with one or more hydroxyl groups. Many phenolics occur in nature with a sugar group attached to them, hence making them water soluble.

The phenolics are plant secondary metabolites, derived from the acetate and shikimate pathways. As will be discussed below, phenolics are partly responsible for the color, taste and smell of many foods, be they desirable or undesirable. They are influenced by factors such as growing conditions, cultivar, ripeness, processing (i.e. fermentation and cooking) and storage.

Flavonoids have a 15-carbon structure made up of two phenolic rings connected by a three-carbon unit. Flavonoids are grouped into anthocyanins and anthoxanthins. Anthocyanins include molecules of red, blue and purple pigments, while anthoxanthins include colorless or white to yellow molecules such as flavonols and flavones. The six anthoxanthins are discussed first: flavonols, flavones, flavanols, as one group; flavanones and chalcones as a second group; and isoflavones as a third group.

Flavonols, flavone and flavanols

Flavonols, together with flavones and flavanols, make up the three major subclasses of flavonoids and are the most widely distributed of flavonoids. Common flavonols include quercetin, kaempferol and myricetin, and they occur in highest levels in onions, apples, tea and kale (Figure 14.1 and Table 14.1). Two important flavones include luteolin and apigenins, found in

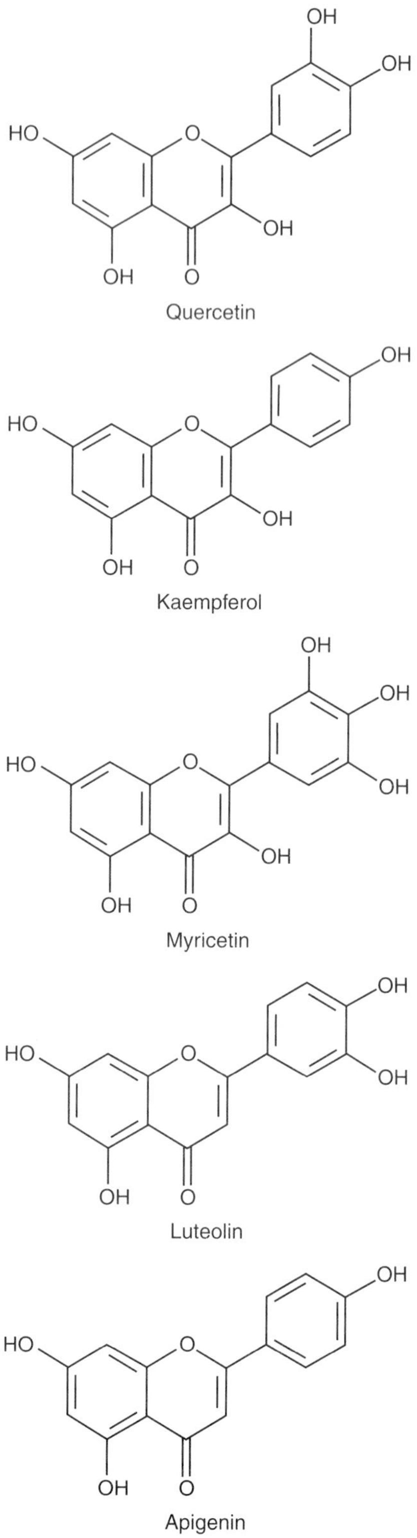

Quercetin

Kaempferol

Myricetin

Luteolin

Apigenin

Figure 14.1 Chemical structure of flavonols and flavones.

Table 14.1 Main groups of flavonoids, the individual compounds and food sources (Reproduced from Nijveldt et al. (2001) with permission of the American Journal of Clinical Nutrition. © American Society for Clinical Nutrition.)

Group	Compound	Food sources
Flavones	Apigenin	Apple skins
	Chrysin	Berries
	Kaempferol	Broccoli
	Luteolin	Celery
	Myricetin	Fruit peels
	Rutin	Cranberries
	Sibelin	Grapes
	Quercetin	Lettuce
		Olives
		Onions
		Parsley
Flavanones	Fisetin	Citrus fruit
	Hesperetin	Citrus peel
	Narigin	
	Naringenin	
	Taxifolin	
Catechins	Catechin	Red wine
	Epicatechin	Tea
	Epigallocatechin gallate	
Anthocyanins	Cyanidin	Berries
	Delphinidin	Cherries
	Malvidin	Grapes
	Pelargonidin	Raspberries
	Peonidin	Red grapes
	Petunidin	Red wine
		Strawberries
		Tea
		Fruit peels with dark pigments
Isoflavones	Genistein	Soy
	Daidzein	

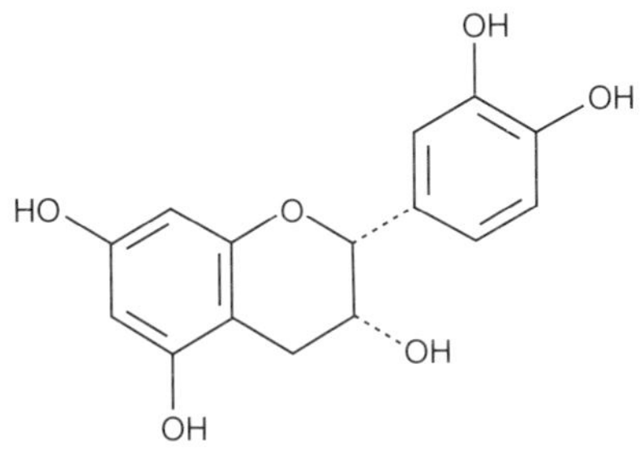

Figure 14.2 Chemical structure of the flavanol epicatechin.

Table 14.2 Concentration of flavonones and flavones in various foods

Compound	Food or beverage	Concentration
Quercetin	Onions	300 mg/kg
	Kale	100 mg/kg
	Apples	20–70 mg/kg
	Black tea	10–25 mg/l
	Red wine	5–15 mg/l
	Fruit juices	<5 mg/l
Kaempferol	Kale	211–470 mg/kg
Luteolin	Celery (stalks and leaves)	5–20 mg/kg
Apigenin	Celery (stalks and leaves)	15–60 mg/kg

that they lack an oxygen molecule at the 4-position of the C ring. The principal flavanols include catechin, epicatechin and gallocatechin (Figure 14.2). These compounds are often found as esters with gallic acid and are known as epicatechin gallate and epigallocatechin gallate. Flavanols are also known as flavan-3-ols or catechins. They are found in many plant foods, notably tea, red wine and apples (Table 14.1).

Improvements in analytical instrumentation and methodologies have made the analysis and identification of these compounds more reliable, precise and sensitive. Many of the flavonoids occur in plants bound to sugars as glycosides, with a minority also occurring in the free unbound or aglycone form. For this reason, extraction techniques have been developed to cleave the sugar group from the flavonoid before analysis by high performance liquid chromatography (HPLC) or liquid chromatography–mass spectrometry (LCMS). Various studies have analyzed the flavonoid content of a number of vegetables, fruits and drinks, such as tea, wine and fruit juices. As mentioned previously, it is hard to estimate the daily intake of these compounds given their complexity, their presence in so many foods and the fact that they are influenced by a number of external factors such as the environment in which they are grown and the various cultivars. The formation of flavonols and flavones is dependent on light and they tend to be more concentrated in leaves and other parts of the plant exposed to sunlight. High concentrations of flavonols are found in the skin of fruits. Quercetin levels are generally below 10 mg/kg in most vegetables, but are found in high concentrations in a number of vegetables, fruits and drinks, as are other flavonoids (Table 14.2).

Flavanols occur in a number of plant foods, but tea is probably the most substantial source in most countries. Tea, both black and green, contains small amounts of catechin, epicatechin and gallocatechin,

celery (Figure 14.1 and Table 14.1). The structural difference between these two classes of flavonoids is that flavones lack a hydroxyl group on the 3-position of the C ring. Flavanols differ from the above flavonoids in

Table 14.3 Concentration of flavanols in black and green tea

Compound	Beverage	Concentration (mg/kg)
Epicatechin gallate	Black tea	8–110
Epigallocatechin	Black tea	5–90
	Green tea	20–290
Epigallocatechin gallate	Black tea	20–230
	Green tea	60–400

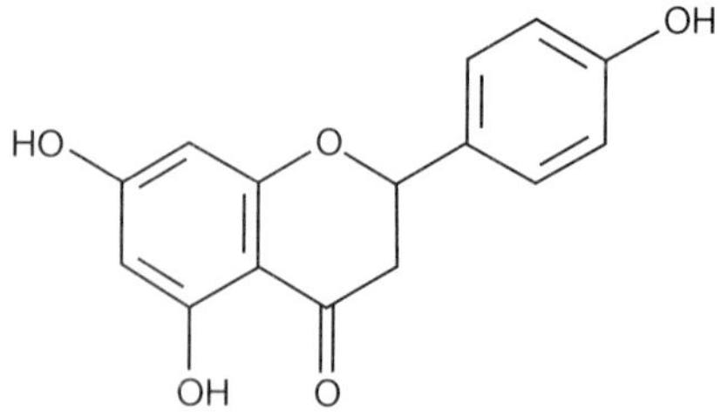

Figure 14.3 Chemical structure of the flavanone naringenin.

and large amounts of epicatechin gallate, epigallocatechin and epigallocatechin gallate (Figure 14.2 and Table 14.3). In addition, red wine has been reported to contain high levels of catechin and epicatechin. Given the range of concentrations, it is hard to estimate the daily consumption of these compounds. The intake of flavonols, flavones, flavanols, and flavanones has been estimated to be 23 mg to 28 mg/day.

Several studies have examined the metabolism and health effects of flavonols, flavones and flavanols. It was long thought that because these compounds were bound to sugars, only the aglycones, or unbound fractions, could be absorbed. Animal studies have shown that bacteria in the colon can hydrolyze the sugar group, but they also degrade the now free aglycones, hence making absorption minimal. In ileostomy patients, quercetin glycoside absorption from onions was better than the free form, 52% compared with 24%. In normal subjects, different rates of absorption were observed, possibly owing to the bioavailability being different depending on the food. Studies on flavanols (catechin) using radiolabeling have demonstrated that 50% of the administered radioactivity is excreted in urine, suggesting that flavanols are readily absorbed. Absorbed compounds seem to be extensively metabolised through the liver while unabsorbed compounds are degraded in the colon.

Flavanones and chalcones

Flavanones and chalcones are described as minor flavonoids because of their limited occurrence, even though they are sometimes present in significant concentrations in foods. These two flavonoid groups are closely related because flavanones can be converted to chalcones in alkaline media and the opposite can occur in acidic environments.

Flavanones are commonly found in citrus fruits. Examples include hesperetin (lemon, lime and mandarin) and naringenin (grapefruit) (Figure 14.3).

Neohesperidin and naringin are responsible for the bitter taste of oranges and grapefruits. In terms of levels, these compounds are found in higher concentrations in the skin of the fruits than in the flesh or juice. Given the easy conversion of chalcones to flavanones, chalcones are limited in nature. Naringenin chalcone, for example, is present in tomato skin, juice, paste and tomato sauce.

Similar to the flavonoids described previously, flavanones and chalcones occur mostly as glycosides. Like other flavonoids, the glycosides tend not to be absorbed until the aglycones are formed from the action of the gut microflora. Studies measuring the urinary excretion of naringenin have demonstrated that individuals consuming grapefruit juice containing 200 mg of naringin excreted 30 mg of naringenin glucuronide daily. These flavanone aglycones have also been shown to be degraded by human and animal intestinal microflora to simpler phenols and phenolic acids, as discussed later.

Given that lipid peroxidation and oxygen free radicals are thought to be involved in conditions such as atherosclerosis, cancer and inflammation, the primary health focus for flavonoids is their antioxidant properties. Among other studies, the Zutphen Study highlighted the link between flavonoids and cardiovascular disease. *In vitro* studies have shown that flavonoids are scavengers of lipid peroxy radicals, superoxide anions and singlet oxygen. They also inhibit cyclooxygenase, which is turn reduces platelet aggregation and thrombosis. Quercetin is an inhibitor of low-density lipoprotein (LDL) oxidation.

In the hypercholesterolemic hamster, the combination of a flavonone-rich citrus extract and ascorbic acid decreased lipids and other lipid-related factors related to atherosclerosis. In colon cancer-induced rats, the flavonone hesperidin has been shown to decrease the

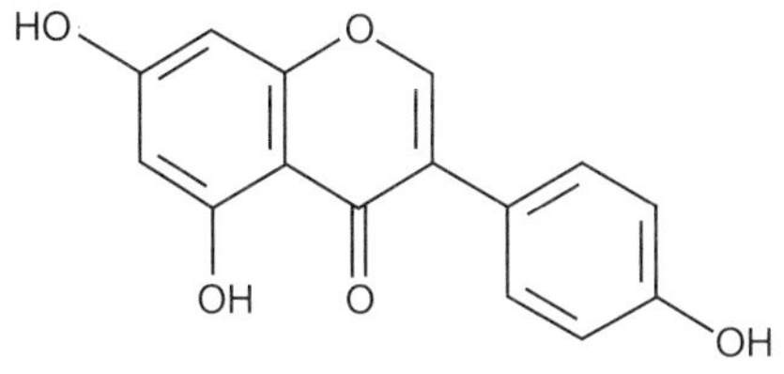

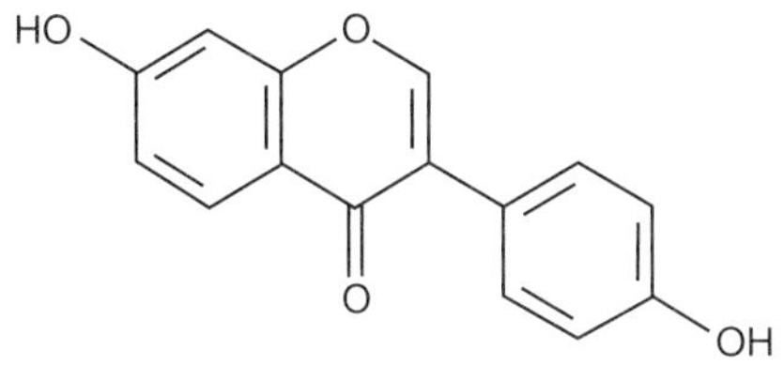

Figure 14.4 Chemical structure of the isoflavones genistein and daidzein.

incidence of tumors and inhibit the development of aberrant crypt foci.

Isoflavones

Isoflavones are flavonoids, but are also called phytoestrogens because of their estrogenic activity. Structurally, they exhibit a similarity to mammalian estrogens and bind to estrogen receptors α and β. Apart from basic structural similarities, the key to their estrogenic effect is the presence and the distance between the hydroxyl groups on the A and B rings. They are classified as estrogen agonists, but also as estrogen antagonists since they compete with estrogen for receptors. They have also been demonstrated to have mechanisms that are independent of the estrogen receptor.

Isoflavones are found in legumes, with soy being the principal dietary source. Like most flavonoids, they are present in plants mainly as glycosides, with concentrations ranging from 0.1 to 3.0 mg/g. Consumption levels of isoflavones are hard to estimate, but recent data suggest that populations that consume high levels of soy, such as the Japanese, ingest between 20 and 50 mg/day. As glycosides (malonyl, acetyl or β-glycosides), the isoflavones are inactive. Common estrogenically active isoflavones include genistein, daidzein and glycitein (these are all aglycones) (Figure 14.4).

The metabolism and absorption of isoflavones require hydrolyzation by intestinal glycosidases, which in turn release the aglycones. These are absorbed or further metabolized to other estrogenic or non-estrogenic compounds. The plasma half-life of these compounds is about 7–8 h, with levels ranging from 50 to 800 ng/ml in adults consuming soy foods. Isoflavones are mainly excreted in urine conjugated to glucuronic acid or sulfate. Fermented food products such as tempe (commonly consumed in Indonesia) contain high levels of the aglycones.

In humans, various factor affect the biological effect of isoflavones, such as the medium of administration, chemical form, metabolism, bioavailability, level of exposure, and the hormonal and dietary state of the individual. Isoflavones have potential health beneficial effects in cardiovascular disease, cancer, osteoporosis and the menopause. These have been illustrated in many *in vitro* and animal studies, but to date results in human studies are inconsistent, possibly for the reasons listed above. Whether the isoflavones are the active components responsible for these effects remains to be elucidated, but to a certain extent it seems that they have actions of their own and also act together with other components in soy. From the cardiovascular perspective, a meta-analysis highlighted the link between soy consumption and its lipid-lowering effects. Like other flavonoids, isoflavones are also antioxidants, adding to their potential cardiovascular beneficial effects.

Given their estrogenic activity, it has been hypothesized that isoflavones may act similarly to hormone replacement therapy (HRT). Studies have examined the role of high soy-based diets and isoflavones in isolation on hot flushes and other menopausal symptoms. The consensus is that foods high in isoflavones have physiological effects in menopausal women, but the health effects cannot be attributed to isoflavones alone. There does not seem to be any effect of isoflavones given in isolation. Despite the limited number of studies, the evidence also seems to support a benefit for bone preservation in menopausal women, but no firm conclusions can be drawn. Human date on the effects of isoflavones on cancer are scarce, and because of their estrogenic activity there is some concern over their effects in estrogen-dependent cancers such as breast cancer. To date, breast cancer case–control studies have illustrated a potential protective effect for isoflavones, while other studies have shown a potential increased risk. More work is needed in this area.

Anthocyanins

Anthocyanins are one of the most important groups of water-soluble pigments in plants. Like other flavonoids, they occur principally as glycosides and are responsible for red, blue, purple and shades in between; the color is dependent on other pigments and pH. It has been difficult to quantify anthocyanins by their molar absorptivity, depending on pigments and pH, as well as the balance between colorless and colored forms. Processing, cooking and physical damage to the food also transform them, making quantification even harder.

Anthocyanins have been identified in over 27 families of food plants. In the USA, consumption has been estimated at 215 mg during summer and 180 mg during winter. However, the regular consumption of red wine would result in much higher levels of consumption from the grapes. Human data on the absorption and metabolism of anthocyanins are scarce. The 'French paradox' suggested that components of red wine were responsible for protection against cardiovascular disease, highlighting the fact that anthocyanins may be responsible for this effect. However, there are no data on their intact absorption. The animal data also suggest limited absorption of anthocyanins. Given the analytical limitations and lack of research in this area, not much can be said about the health benefits of these compounds.

Other phenolic phytochemicals

Tannins

Tannins differ from the phenolics in that they are compounds of high molecular weight. They are highly hydroxylated and can form insoluble complexes with carbohydrates and proteins. The term tannin is derived from its tanning properties; it forms stable tannin–protein complexes in animal hides, as in leather. Over the past 30 years, much of the literature on tannins has been on their antinutritive effects, but the evidence below illustrates that they also have potential health benefits.

Tannins can be divided into two major groups, hydrolyzable and condensed tannins. Hydrolyzable tannins are readily hydrolyzed with acid, alkali, enzymes and hot water. The principal hydrolyzable tannins are gallic acid (Figure 14.5) and its condensation product hexahydroxydiphenic acid. They can be further subdivided into gallotannins and ellagitannins, which are derived from gallic acid and hexahydroxydiphenic acid, respectively. Condensed tannins, also known as proanthocyanidins, are high molecular weight compounds which are far more common in the diet than the hydrolyzable tannins. One of the key features of

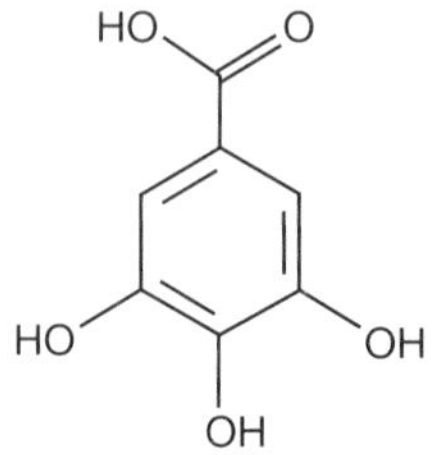

Gallic acid

Figure 14.5 Chemical structure of the hydrolyzable tannin gallic acid.

condensed tannins is that they yield anthocyanidins when heated in acidic media, hence the name proanthocyanidins.

Tannins are found in a wide range of cereals, fruits and nuts. Structurally, they possess over 10 phenolic groups and 5–7 aromatic rings per 1000 units of relative molecular mass. Their complex polymer structure makes them hard to analyze, making it difficult to estimate the amounts consumed, their digestibility and their physiological effects. It has been shown, however, that tannins are extensively recovered in the feces of rats fed diets high in apple pulp. This indigestibility may work in favor of tannins for their health effects. Many of the compounds listed in previous sections show antioxidant activity and are soluble phenolic compounds. However, recent studies have shown that proanthocyanidins and high molecular weight hydrolyzable tannins could be 15–30 times more potent than simple phenolics in antioxidative activity.

The effects of tannins on lipid metabolism has not been studied extensively. Proanthocyanidins have been shown to increase fecal fat excretion, while grape tannins and tannic acid increase high-density lipoprotein (HDL) cholesterol and decrease low-density lipoprotein (LDL) cholesterol concentrations in the rat model. Hydrolyzable tannins also have anticarcinogenic effects *in vitro* and in animal models.

Stilbenes

Stilbenes are present in a wide range of plant and are synthesized from cinnamic acid derivatives. Their production in plants is positively associated with resistance to mold and they are produced in response to microbial infection or stress. The major active component is *trans*-resveratrol and most studies to date have concentrated on the physiological effects of this stilbene (Figure 14.6).

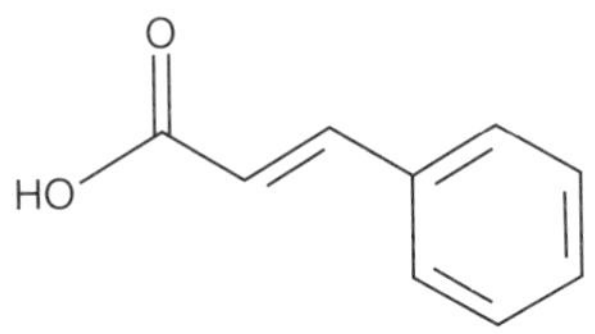

Figure 14.6 Chemical structure of stilbenes.

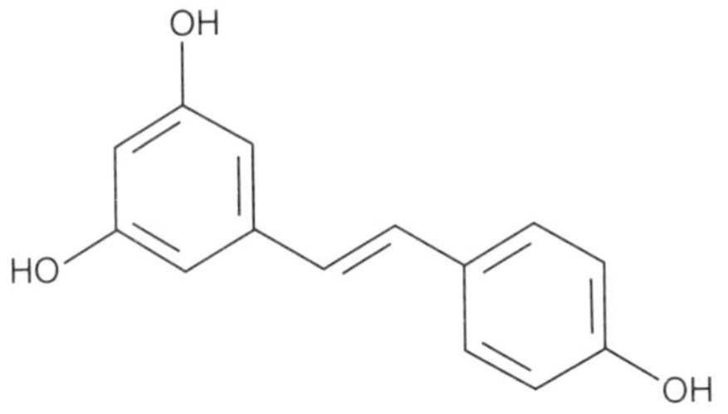

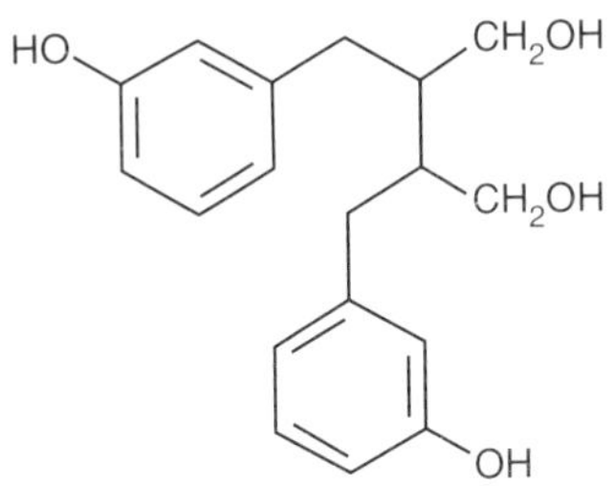

Figure 14.7 Chemical structure of mammalian lignans.

In folk medicine, including Chinese medicine, humans have used medicinal plants containing resveratrol for many years. Based on the quantitative data currently available, the major dietary sources of stilbenes are grapes, grape juices, wine, peanuts and peanut butter. They are predominantly located in the skin and in general are absent or only present in low amounts in fruit flesh. In wines the levels of resveratrol depend on the grape variety, climatic conditions of the harvest and the ecological procedures used; however, studies suggest that the levels in red and white grape skins are comparable. The extent of maceration of skins and seeds during fermentation is the key determinant of the stilbene concentration in the wine, but the yeast strains and fining agents used and the time spent in oak barrels also alter levels. Red wines contain the highest levels of *trans*-resveratrol, with approximately 8 mg/l, but levels vary depending on the grape variety. Levels in rose wines range between 1.38 and 2.93 mg/l, while levels in white wines are generally low since during the wine-making process minimal contact is made with the grape skins, which are the main source of resveratrol.

Lignans

Lignans are phenolic compounds that are present in many plant species. Although they are present in high concentrations in linseed (flaxseed) they are also present in measurable amounts in many of the cereals, pulses, fruits and vegetables commonly consumed in the Western world. Although the levels of lignans are generally low on an individual food basis, their ubiquity in the plant kingdom suggests that they may well be an important source of phytoestrogens, particularly to consumers of high plant-based diets (e.g. vegans and vegetarians). The structure of lignans in plants is different to the structure of the mammalian lignans which are formed as a result of microbial metabolism in the gut. The lignan precursors (secoisolariciresinol, matairesinol) are present in plants as glycoside conjugates, but following ingestion microbial enzymes convert these precursors to enterodiol and enterolactone (Figure 14.7). Confirmation of a bacterial source for the production of the mammalian lignans (enterodiol and enterolactone) was shown many years ago when humans administered selective antibiotic therapy over a 6–8 day period immediately showed a decrease in enterodiol and enterolactone excretion and after 2–3 days urinary excretion of the metabolites was undetectable. In common with estrogens and isoflavones, the lignans undergo efficient enterohepatic circulation; they are absorbed from the intestinal tract, then transported via the portal vein system to the liver, where they undergo conjugation with glucuronic acid. This more water-soluble conjugate is then excreted via the kidneys and by the biliary route, where it is present primarily as the non-glucuronide conjugate in urine and bile.

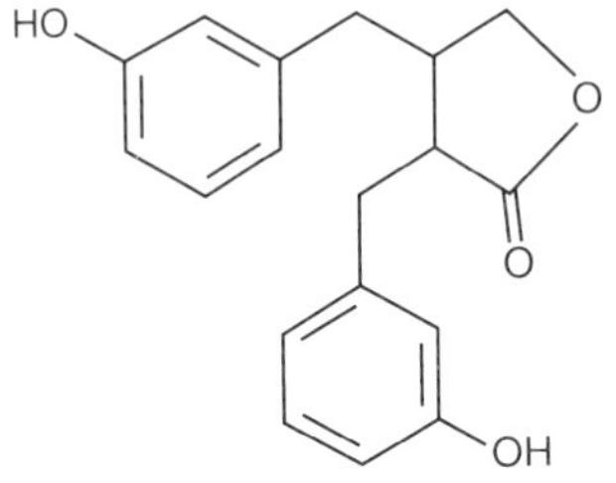

Epidemiological studies have shown positive correlations between the intake of fiber-rich foods and urinary lignan excretion. This is not surprising given the richest dietary sources of lignan precursors (pulses, legumes, fruit and vegetables). To date, several animal studies have addressed the potential anticancer effects of these compounds, but interest in the biological effects of lignans in relation to human health has received little attention compared with the isoflavone class.

14.4 Carotenoids

Carotenoids are the most abundant pigments responsible for bright colors such as red, orange and yellow in many of the fruits and vegetables that we eat. They also provide coloration in certain species of insects, birds and crustaceans, such as the orange of lobster shells. Carotenoids protect cells against photosensitization and act as light-absorbing pigments during photosynthesis, and β-carotene has been shown to be a precursor to vitamin A. Approximately 600 carotenoids have been identified in nature, of which about 50 contain provitamin A activity. Carotenoids such as the carotenes are hydrocarbons which contain oxygenated xanthophylls consisting of eight isoprenoid units. They have a high number of double bonds in their polyisoprenoid structure, thus making isomerization possible to produce mono- or poly-*cis* isomers, even though most carotenoids occur in the *trans* configuration. Humans cannot synthesize carotenoids and are thus dependent on dietary sources. Carotenoids are usually fat soluble and once ingested are released from complex proteins, incorporated into micelles and transported to the intestinal mucosa. Provitamin A carotenoids are then cleaved to produce vitamin A, while unconverted carotenoids are absorbed directly into the blood. Carotenoids are transported in the circulation by LDL. The major circulating carotenoids include β-carotene, α-carotene, lycopene, β-cryptoxanthin, lutein and zeaxanthin (Figure 14.8).

The early epidemiological studies suggesting the link between fruit and vegetable consumption and the reduction in the risk of certain cancers highlighted the carotenoids, notably β-carotene, as potential candidates for this protective effect. Since then, intervention studies with β-carotene have shown that it does not have a protective effect against cancer (lung cancer); however, carotenoids may serve as an indicator of a healthy lifestyle. There are other areas of interest where carotenoids may be involved.

The area of carotenoid research seems to be more developed in terms of randomized, placebo-controlled trials than research into other phytochemicals. While the epidemiological association between β-carotene and lung cancer has been strong and consistent, the evidence regarding other carotenoids and other diseases such as cardiovascular disease, prostate cancer, breast cancer and age-related macular degeneration is less clear.

With regard to cardiovascular disease and breast cancer, the majority of recent studies show no statistically significant relationship with β-carotene. The early evidence on the potential protective effects of lycopene and prostate cancer has not been supported by subsequent studies. Similarly, the early indication of a protective effect of lutein and zeaxanthin on age-related macular degeneration has failed to be replicated in subsequent studies.

Several pathways have been proposed for the potential effects of carotenoids. One that is common to many phytochemicals is the antioxidative pathway. To date the evidence is conflicting, with no clear antioxidant activity for carotenoids.

Much of the evidence for the health-beneficial effects of carotenoids stems from epidemiological studies. As previously stated, they may serve as markers of a healthy lifestyle, and are indicative of fruit and vegetable consumption. Carotenoids seem to have health effects, but may have no effect in isolation (e.g. β-carotene and lung cancer), and they may need to be in a food matrix and/or consumed with other foods to provide health benefits.

14.5 Phytosterols

Over 250 plants have been reported to contain measurable levels of phytosterols. The nutritional interest in these compounds relates to the fact that they have a similar structure to cholesterol, with differences in the side-chain, and therefore have the potential to act as 'natural' dietary cholesterol-lowering agents. Sitosterol is the major sterol in plant materials, but stigmasterol, campesterol, brassica and avena sterols also occur in many plant materials (Figure 14.9). Similarly cholesterol in mammalian cells, they play an important role in the structure and function of cell membranes and are incorporated into membranes; they regulate the fluidity of membranes and may play a role

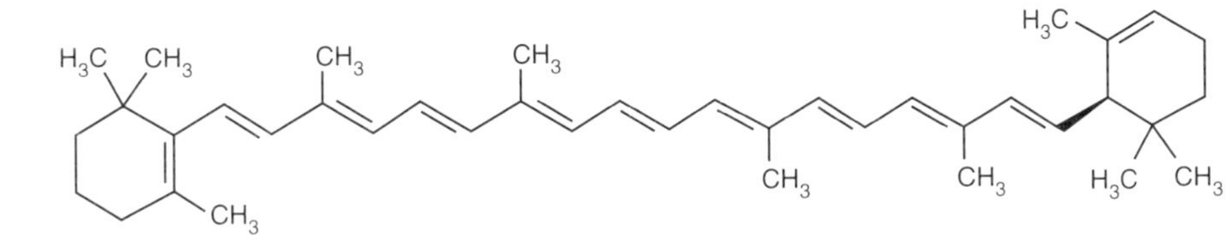

Figure 14.8 Chemical structure of carotenoids.

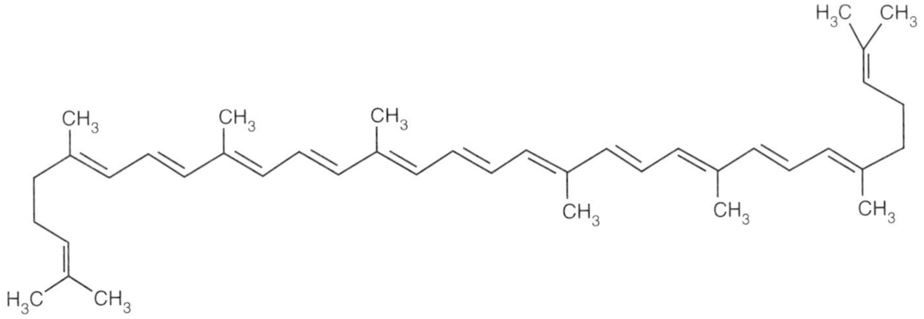

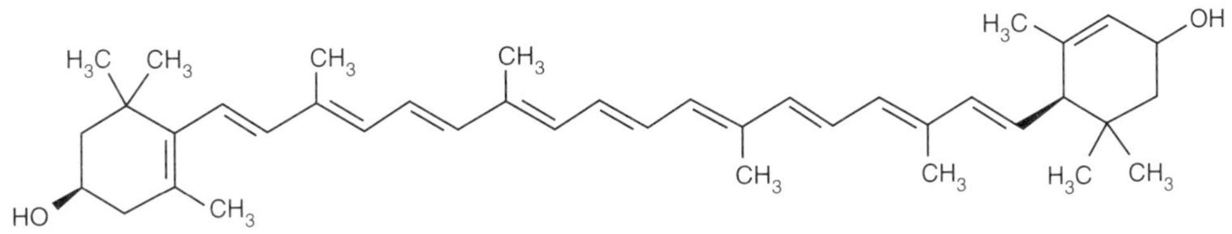

in the adaptation of membranes to temperature. Within the plant they also play a key role in cell differentiation and proliferation, and their accumulation in seeds and oils suggests that they are important in the growth of new cells and shoots.

The richest natural sources of these compounds are vegetable oils (and products derived from oils) but cereal grains (cereal-based products) and nuts also contain measurable amounts. Recent studies suggest that total estimated intake ranges from 146 to 405 mg/day, but intake in vegetarians is up to three times higher. This difference has been reflected in serum levels, 350 μg/dl in vegetarians versus 270 μg/dl in non-vegetarians, and studies suggesting that biliary clearance is higher in vegetarians.

In the 1950s large amounts of plant sterols (up to 50 g/day) were fed to patients with hypercholesterolemia to lower their serum cholesterol levels. However, interest in their clinical use declined because they were poorly soluble and concerns were expressed over the potential causation of phytosterolemia from increased intake. The development of fat-soluble plant stanol esters in the early 1990s unmasked the potential for relatively small (1.5 g/day) and safe doses to have hypocholesterolemic effects in human studies. The popularity of stanol esters for cholesterol lowering renewed the interest in using plant sterols for that purpose, and clinical data showed that the addition of phytosterols to the diet lowered cholesterol even in normocholesterolemic subjects. Studies suggest that the dose of plant sterols is important, with 2 g/day offering the ideal dose for cholesterol lowering, higher doses do not appear to enhance efficacy. However, higher doses seem to interfere with the absorption of other phytochemicals such as carotenoids and other lipid-soluble compounds.

One of the major metabolic effects of consuming dietary plant sterols relates to the inhibition of absorption and subsequent compensatory stimulation of the synthesis of cholesterol. The ultimate effect is a lowering of cholesterol as a result of the enhanced elimination of cholesterol in stools.

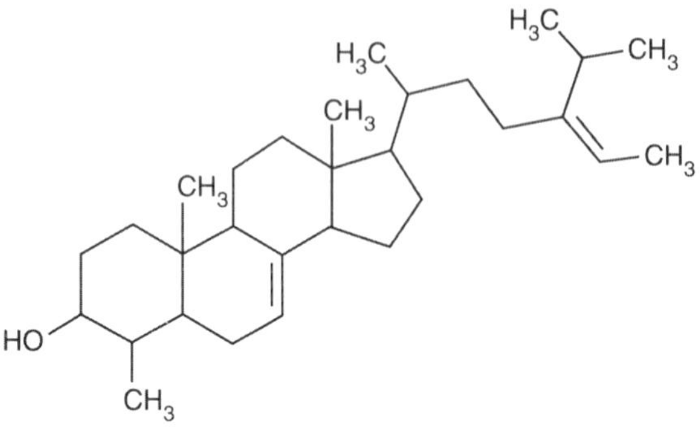

Sitosterol

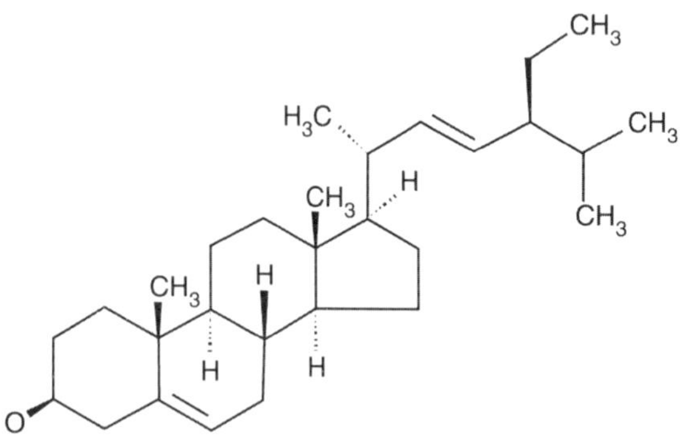

Stigmasterol

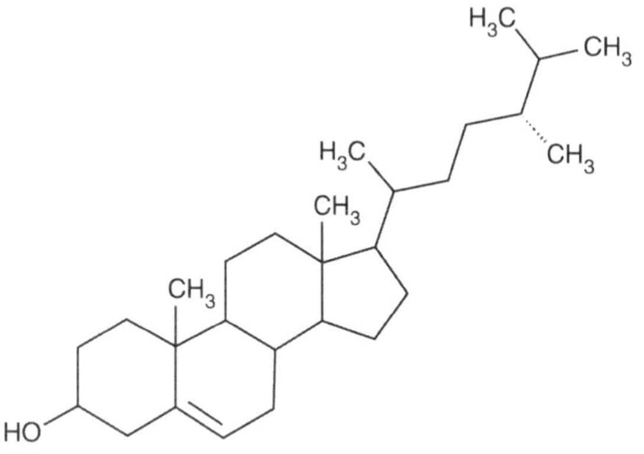

Campesterol

Figure 14.9 Chemical structure of phytosterols.

14.6 Sulfur-containing compounds

Sulfides

Sulfur-containing compounds (the allium family) may have a number of health beneficial properties. Sulfides are found in large quantities in garlic and other bulbous plants. The main component, which is believed

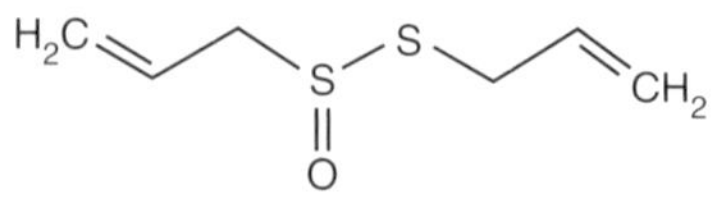

Allicin

Figure 14.10 Chemical structure of allicin.

to be the active component, is allicin, formed by the combination of its precursor, alliin, with the enzyme allinase (Figure 14.10).

These compounds are volatile and are responsible for the well-known garlic odor. Garlic cloves can contain up to 4 g of alliin/kg of fresh weight, but no exact dosage is known for its health benefits. A large amount of work has been carried out on the metabolism of allicin in animal models and in humans, and to date there is still debate as to mode of action of these compounds. This, however, has not prevented scientists from carrying out human clinical trials, as well as *in vitro* and animal studies, on the effects of garlic and allicin on various health end-points. Human studies have shown that garlic consumption may have beneficial effects on cholesterol, blood pressure, platelet aggregation and coagulation time. Garlic may also have antibiotic properties. More work is still needed, as plants such as garlic also contain a number of other bioactive compounds.

Glucosinolates

Glucosinolates are a large group of sulfur-containing compounds present in brassica vegetables. When the plant tissue is damaged by food preparation or chewing, the glucosinolates are hydrolyzed by endogenous enzymes (myrosinase) to release a range of breakdown products including isothiocyanates, thiocyanates and indoles. Isothiocyanates, also referred to as 'mustard oils', are hot and bitter compounds with an acrid smell.

Humans are sensitive to the strong flavours associated with glucosinolate breakdown products and these compounds are therefore important determinants of flavor in many important brassicas. Allyl isothiocyanate is largely responsible for the characteristic hot flavors of mustard and horseradish, and the glucosinolates sinigrin and progoitrin are responsible for the bitterness of brussel sprouts and other brassica vegetables. Glucosinolate breakdown products exert a variety of toxic and antinutritional effects in several animal species; the adverse effects on thyroid metabolism are a noted example. They are goitrogenic in animals, but these effects can be mitigated to some extent by increasing levels of iodine in the diet. However, this goitrogenicity has limited the exploitation of brassica feedstuffs for domestic livestock. These compounds may induce goitrogenic effects in humans, but there is little epidemiological evidence to suggest that this is an important cause of human disease. In a study where 150 g of Brussels sprouts was added to volunteer diets, there was no effect on thyroid hormone levels, presumably because cooking had inactivated myrosinase and thus reduced the biological availability of the goitrogenic breakdown products to subclinical levels.

Evidence is emerging that brassica vegetables may have important anticarcinogenic effects associated with the biological activity of glucosinolate breakdown products. The World Cancer Research Fund review of the role of diet in cancer prevention concluded that diets rich in cruciferous vegetables probably protect humans specifically against cancers of the colon, rectum and thyroid and, when consumed as part of a diet rich in other types of vegetables, against cancer at other sites. This epidemiological evidence is consistent with a host of experimental studies, which from the 1960s onwards have indicated that glucosinolate breakdown products exert anticarcinogenic effects in experimental animal models. The mechanism to explain these effects relates to the ability of glucosinolate breakdown products (e.g. the isothiocyanates and sulfuraphane) to modulate the activities of phase I (e.g. cytochrome P450) and phase II (e.g. glutathione S-transferase, UDP- glucuronyl transferase) biotransformation enzymes, which together catalyze a variety of hydrolytic, oxidation and reduction reactions (phase I), the products of which are then available for conjugation reactions (phase II).

14.7 Phytochemical toxicity

The concept that phytochemicals are potentially beneficial to human health is rapidly gaining both scientific and public credence. Although in the future sufficient convincing evidence may well be available to prove potential health benefits from the consumption of some of the phytochemicals addressed in this chapter, for several other phytochemicals there is clear evidence of toxicity to animals and occasionally to humans. For the majority of the currently identified phytochemicals there are limited data on safe levels or optimal levels of intake for health benefits, and it is crit-

ical that these margins are more clearly defined in future research.

14.8 Perspectives on the future

As illustrated throughout this chapter, the area of phytochemicals and nutrition is one that is relatively embryonic. Phytochemicals are involved in a number of diseases, ranging from cardiovascular disease to cancer, as well as immune function. There is still much to be learnt about their metabolism, bioavailability, mode of action, dose response and, in some cases, the actual compounds responsible for the health effect. The research has focussed on foods as well as individual components of food to help us to further our knowledge in the above fields. Given the limited information to date, there are no recommended dietary intakes for phytochemicals, but consumers should consume a wide variety of foods that incorporate the various phytochemicals to maximize disease prevention. Further research is required to define optimal doses for potential health effects, and to define 'safe' levels of intakes for many of these phytochemicals. Many of these compounds should be viewed as pharmaceutical compounds, because although they occur naturally they still require the same levels of proof of efficacy and safety in use as synthetic pharmaceutical agents. With the current drive towards supplementation and the use of genetically modified technology to enhance levels of 'desirable' compounds in foods, it is paramount that further research is conducted to add to our knowledge on the importance of enhancing our diet with specific phytochemicals for potential health benefits.

Further reading

Bravo L. Polyphenols: chemistry, dietary sources, metabolism, and nutritional significance. Nutr Rev 1998; 56: 317–333.

Howard BV, Kritchevsky D. Phytochemicals and cardiovascular disease. A statement for healthcare professionals from the American Heart Association. Circulation 1997; 95: 2591–2593.

King A, Young G. Characteristics and occurrence of phenolic phytochemicals. J Am Dietetic Assoc 1999; 99: 213–218.

Nijveldt RJ, van Nood E, van Noorn DEC et al. Am J Clin Nutr 2001; 74: 418–426.

Olson JA, Krinsky NI. Introduction: the colorful, fascinating world of the carotenoids: important physiologic modulators. FASEB J 1995; 9: 1547–1550.

Steinmetz KA, Potter JD. Vegetables, fruit, and cancer prevention: a review. J Am Dietetic Assoc 1996; 96: 1027–1039.

15
The Control of Food Intake

A Drewnowski and F Bellisle

Key messages

- Food intake is governed by physiological signals and by factors in the environment.
- Physiological signals affecting food intake involve a feedback mechanism that responds to energy requirements to maintain energy homeostasis.
- Neurotransmitters, hormones and brain peptides play a crucial role in appetite and satiety.
- Important motivational factors include hunger, satiety, satiation and palatability. Food palatability has been measured in terms of pleasantness, intention to eat or the amount of food consumed. Satiation has been measured in terms of fullness, reduced hunger, reduced palatability or reduced amount of food consumed.
- Important elements of eating behavior include meal size, meal frequency and the interval between eating occasions.
- The energy density of the diet may be a key factor in the control of food intake.
- In affluent societies where food is overabundant, a greater understanding of the control of food intake in the treatment of obesity and overweight is required.

15.1 Introduction

Human energy intake and body weight are thought to be determined by one or more homeostatic mechanisms. According to this theory, body weight can only fluctuate within narrow limits around a physiological set-point. The worldwide epidemic of obesity poses a challenge to this conventional view. The prevalence of obesity has risen sharply since the 1980s, both in the USA and worldwide. By current estimates [The Third National Health and Nutrition Examination Survey in the USA (NHANES III)], one in two American adults is overweight, with a body mass index (BMI) >25, and one in three is obese (BMI >30). Given that human physiology has not changed and the genetic pool remains the same, the explanation must lie in reduced physical activity and altered eating habits.

Ready access to plentiful, palatable and affordable foods is one potential explanation for rising obesity rates. This environmental view implies that the sheer availability of food may override any regulatory mechanism we possess. Energy intakes and food choices may be controlled by the energy density of the diet or its palatability, or by some other aspect of the global food supply. In particular, the consumption of refined grains, added sugars and fat has been linked to rising rates of obesity, diabetes and coronary heart disease.

The questions are how energy intake is determined, by what mechanisms, and to what extent? A related question is whether separate control mechanisms exist for the consumption of macronutrients, carbohydrate, protein and fat. While physiological mechanisms may serve to protect us from energy deficits, some researchers now suggest that internal defenses against excess food consumption are deficient or may be absent altogether. Exploring behaviors relevant to the control of food intake is the principal theme of this chapter.

15.2 Theories of control

Early theories of control were based on the premise that a feedback mechanism accounted for the fact that eating behaviors covered energy needs in an apparently regulated fashion.

© 2003 A Drewnowski and F Bellisle. For more information on this topic visit www.nutritiontexts.com

- The glucostatic theory of energy intake, developed by Mayer (1953), posited that food consumption was triggered by a decrease in the availability of glucose to tissues. The rate of glucose utilization was more important than its actual level in the blood.
- The lipostatic theory proposed by Kennedy (1953) suggested that body fat was the key substance that regulated eating behavior. This theory remained speculative until the discovery of leptin, a hormone secreted by the adipose tissue, which provides signals to the brain.
- An aminostatic theory suggested that amino acid metabolites were the crucial agents determining satiety. This is reflected in current work on the satiating value of protein-rich foods.
- The hepatostatic theory, enunciated by Russek (1971), focussed on the metabolic activity of the liver during fasting as opposed to absorptive phases.
- The thermostatic theory proposed by Brobeck (1948) suggested that the heat generated during digestion led to a rise in temperature that inhibited eating behavior.

While there was evidence to support all of the above theories, some mechanisms were clearly more applicable to short-term eating behaviors, while others were more likely to be involved in the long-term control of body weight. In addition, the theories implied that the consumption of fat, carbohydrate and protein might be regulated separately, in addition to the regulation of energy. The theories shared the common premise that energy intake was controlled by a feedback mechanism that responded primarily to energy needs.

For any individual, variations in daily energy needs are primarily a function of changes in physical activity, given that the amount of energy expended on basal metabolism and thermogenesis stays relatively constant. Food consumption is the behavioral mechanism meant to ensure energy balance between intake and expenditure. In theory at least, daily energy intakes of sedentary people should only vary within very narrow limits. In practice, a person's food intake can vary greatly from one day to the next and there is little evidence for a tight control mechanism. On the contrary, weekly records of all foods consumed by healthy adults confirm that daily food intakes are highly variable. In addition, studies that provide subjects with extra dietary energy in the form of set meals or preloads only rarely observe a downward adjustment in energy intake at a subsequent

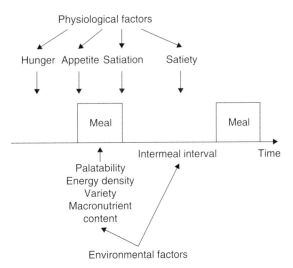

Figure 15.1 Physiological and environmental factors involved in the control of food intake.

meal. Moreover, the nutrient composition of foods and beverages consumed does not lead to adjustments in the intake of other constituents of the diet. Whereas the control of food intake should reflect homeostatic mechanisms, these have been difficult to demonstrate under experimental conditions or in field studies.

15.3 The neuroscience of food intake

Human eating behavior responds to both physiology and the environment (Figure 15.1). The question is, how do metabolic factors interact with the food environment to shape habitual eating behaviors? Whereas early studies focussed on the hypothalamus as the critical brain system (see Chapter 8), recent progress in neuroscience has led to a better understanding of neurotransmitters, hormones and brain peptides involved in appetite and satiety. These studies mostly focussed on laboratory animals, with only a few studies conducted in humans. Many different neurotransmitters, some acting at the level of the brain, contribute to the control of food intake, and the list grows daily.

- Serotonin is thought to have a specific role in carbohydrate appetite and in the promotion of satiety. Pharmacological agents, serotonin reuptake blockers, have been used to suppress carbohydrate cravings and to help weight management among the obese.
- Dopamine mediates food reward and is thought to be involved in food cravings.

- Endogenous opiate peptides or endorphins are thought to mediate the pleasure response to sugar and fat. Endorphin blockade by naloxone, an opiate antagonist, reduced taste preferences and the consumption of preferred sweet and high-fat foods.
- Neuropeptide Y (NPY), synthesized by neurons of the arcuate nucleus projecting to the paraventricular nucleus of the hypothalamus, is a potent stimulant of food intake, and may be particularly effective in promoting consumption.

Other neuropeptides are present both in the brain and in peripheral tissues. For example, cholecystokinin (CCK) is mostly found in the endothelial cells of the intestine. Its release following a meal is associated with satiety. It has been suggested that CCK acts by delaying gastric emptying, thereby increasing gastric distension, which reinforces the feelings of satiation. Other important hormones and neuropeptides include the following.

- Insulin is a hypoglycemic factor and is essential for the cellular utilization of glucose in most tissues (excluding the brain). Insulin is secreted by the pancreas a few minutes after the beginning of a meal. The action of insulin is thought to potentiate the satiating effects of CCK. Peripheral insulin is transported across the blood–brain barrier by an active transport system. Central insulin may affect food intake by modulating the effect of intestinal peptides on meal size. After weight loss, peripheral and central insulin levels decrease, thus making the brain less sensitive to the satiating effects of CCK: such a mechanism could contribute to stabilizing body-fat stores over time. The central action of insulin becomes less potent under conditions of a high-fat diet. Locally, insulin antagonizes NPY. Fasting increases NPY biosynthesis in the hypothalamus, provided that insulin levels are low.
- Leptin is a hormone secreted mainly by adipocytes. Prior to leptin's discovery in 1995, some researchers had suggested that the level of insulin present in the brain reflected the amount of the adipose mass and influenced food intake accordingly. Lystin was initially thought to be a feedback signal from adipose tissue that would suppress eating. However, the effects of leptin on food intake are still unclear. Contrary to expectations, the levels of circulating leptin are elevated in obese people, suggesting that the problem is not leptin deficiency but leptin resistance. In general,

administration of exogenous leptin to overweight people has failed to reduce either energy intakes or body weight. There is also a risk that injections of exogenous leptin may worsen leptin resistance. Novel strategies for weight reduction aim to improve leptin sensitivity.

- Glucagon, a hormone secreted at mealtime by the pancreas, is a well-known satiety factor. It probably exerts its action via glucosensitive cells located in the liver.
- Bombesin acts in a similar fashion to CCK and may stimulate endogenous CCK release. Injections of exogenous bombesin inhibit food intake in humans.
- Somatostatin, another gastrointestinal hormone, also inhibits food intake in animals.
- Calcitonin strongly suppresses food intake when administered peripherally or centrally.
- Ghrelin, a peptide related to the growth hormone, increases with food deprivation and may be the physiological signal triggering a meal.

Although these factors have a major impact on the eating behavior of animals under laboratory conditions, their influence on human eating habits in a natural setting is unclear.

15.4 Motivational states

Humans consume food several times per day. Ideally, people should begin to eat when they are hungry and stop when they are satiated. Whereas the term hunger denotes an internal state of energy depletion and a general motivation to eat, the term appetite is more correctly defined as a desire to consume a given food. Satiety is commonly defined as a state of energy repletion following a meal. While initiation of eating has been linked with a transient drop in plasma glucose and increased free fatty acid levels, increased satiety has been linked with rising CCK and plasma insulin concentrations. However, the correspondence between the underlying physiology and hunger and satiety states is not always clear. Moreover, people often eat when they are not hungry. Food choices and amounts consumed are strongly influenced by environmental factors, such as the taste of foods. The term 'taste' denotes not just the four basic tastes, sweet, sour, salty and bitter, but also food aroma and its texture. A pleasure or hedonic component is also involved. A food's appeal combines its palatability, defined as an integral property of the food itself, and the individual's predisposition to consume, as measured by some index of appetite.

The principal function of taste is to orient the person towards a suitable source of dietary energy and away from potential toxins or poisons. In general, the more preferred or palatable foods are those that deliver maximum energy per unit weight or volume. Many of these foods are sweet or rich in fat, or both. The sensory pleasure response to sweet taste is present at birth, and young children tend to select those foods that are both familiar and sweet. Studies also show that the acceptance of novel flavors by children is greatest when those flavors are paired with a rich source of energy, most often starch or fat. In contrast, infants and children will avoid any food with a bitter taste, including many vegetables.

Palatability and satiation have opposite effects on food intake during a meal. Whereas palatability increases appetite and therefore food consumption, satiation decreases motivation to eat, leading to a faster termination of eating. Some researchers make a further distinction between satiation, which leads to meal termination and reduced meal size, and post-meal satiety, which delays the onset of the next meal. The concept of sensory-specific satiety or flavor fatigue explains why foods that are similar in taste or appearance to those recently consumed are rated less pleasant than newly presented foods. For example, the perceived pleasantness of sweet taste is reduced following the ingestion of sweet glucose solutions, a phenomenon described in the literature as negative aliesthesia. Sensory-specific satiety may help to explain why variety seeking is a characteristic feature of human eating habits.

The concepts of hunger, palatability, and satiation are closely intertwined. In some studies, these variables have served as proxy measures of each other. Food palatability has been measured in terms of rated pleasantness, intention to eat or the amount of food consumed. Satiation has been measured in terms of fullness, reduced hunger, reduced palatability or reduced amount of food consumed. In other words, given the reciprocal nature of palatability and satiation measures, the most palatable foods would be the least satiating and vice versa. The creation of highly palatable and satiating foods – one of the goals of the food industry – may be a contradiction in terms.

15.5 The preload paradigm

A number of studies have used the preload paradigm to study adjustments in energy intake following an experimental meal of variable composition. The two principal manipulations were to increase preload volume but keep energy constant, and to keep volume constant and manipulate preload energy. This was achieved by adding water or by manipulating nutrient content, often by using aspartame, Olestra or dietary fiber. Preload meals would then be followed by one or more test meals, using a within-subject design. On some occasions, respondents' intakes were also measured later during the day.

In general, people who best compensated for missing preload calories were children and young adults with high energy needs. Those respondents increased energy intakes during the next test meal, most often lunch. In contrast, studies of normal-weight adult men and women showed that providing excess dietary energy as preload led to little or no downward adjustment during a subsequent test meal. Overweight and restrained women also failed to compensate for energy provided in the form of breakfast preloads. Excess energy consumed at breakfast time led to higher overall energy intakes for that day. Some researchers believe, furthermore, that extra energy provided in the form of liquids, as opposed to solid foods, is not compensated for at all. A recent study showed no differences in later food consumption following the ingestion of mineral water, flavored mineral water, or mineral water sweetened with either aspartame or sucrose.

Given that people generally consume three or four meals per day, daily energy intake is largely determined by meal size. Meal size is critically influenced by the palatability and energy density of foods, as well as by the variety of the foods available. However, meal size can also depend on such non-regulatory factors as chronic dietary restraint, number of people present, time of day, time of week and time of year, as well as food-related attitudes and beliefs. The number of meals consumed each day can also be influenced by environmental variables.

15.6 The role of energy density

One key factor in the control of food intake is the energy density of the diet. Energy density of foods, measured in terms of available energy per unit weight (kJ/g), is largely determined by the food's water content. While foods such as chocolate or potato chips generally provide 5 kcal/g or more, raw vegetables and fruit, salad greens, soups and beverages tend to provide no more than 0.1–0.5 kcal/g. Energy-dense foods are dry and often contain fat, sugar or starch. In contrast, low energy-density foods are more likely to contain water, protein or fiber. The concepts of energy density, palatability and satiation are also closely linked. Foods are palatable because their energy density is high. As a rule, energy-dense foods such as chocolate are palatable but not satiating, whereas foods with lower energy density, such as spinach, are more satiating but less palatable.

Under *ad libitum* conditions in the laboratory, people tend to consume a constant weight or volume of food as opposed to a constant amount of energy. Daily energy intakes would then depend on food choices and on the energy density of the diet. Since bulky, low-energy-density foods provide fewer calories per unit weight, they should, in theory, lead to reduced energy intakes and therefore weight loss. Lowering the energy density of the total diet is thought to be a viable approach to weight reduction.

Past and present guidelines for weight control have long suggested replacing energy-dense foods with less energy-dense whole grains, vegetables and fruit. However, high-energy-density foods are more palatable and more appealing, especially to the younger consumer. It is only with age that energy needs decline and so does the mean energy density of the diet. Analyses of the NHANES II data set showed that the mean energy density of the diet dropped from a high of 1.2 kcal/g in childhood and adolescence to a low of 0.75 kcal/g among adult women in the 45–54-year age group. This reduction in energy density was achieved by an increase in the consumption of vegetables and fruit. In this way, the behavioral adaptation to reduced energy needs involved a shift in food choices and eating habits.

15.7 Psychosocial factors

In affluent societies, where the availability of food is not an issue, the primary influences on food choice are taste (palatability), cost and convenience. Taste factors predispose the consumer towards good-tasting foods, often those that contain fat, sugar and salt. Concerns over food costs predispose the consumer towards foods that provide maximum dietary energy at lowest cost. Such foods often contain added sugar and fat. Concerns with convenience and labor-saving predispose the consumer towards packaged foods, many of which also contain fat, sugar and salt. Concerns with nutrition and health and the seeking of dietary variety play a subsidiary role. Psychosocial and environmental factors may have more of an impact on food choices

and eating habits than do physiological mechanisms. Current dietary trends reflect how the food industry has adapted to these consumer needs.

15.8 Implications for aging and body-weight management

As people age, they generally become both heavier and fatter. At the same time energy intake declines, as does energy expenditure. Older adults consume less energy and tend to consume fewer energy-dense foods. Consumption of vegetables and fruits increases with age, whereas the consumption of added sugars declines. The decline in energy needs is largely accounted for by a sharp drop in physical activity rates. An age-associated decline in bitter taste responsiveness has been linked to increased acceptance of some bitter-tasting vegetables and fruit. A decline in sensory-specific satiety is said to be the cause of reduced variety seeking and, at times, a more monotonous diet.

Among healthy older adults, the increase in body weight can stay within narrow limits. Studies showing that body weights of French adults increased by 10 kg between the ages of 20 and 60 years suggest that mechanisms controlling body weight can operate with an impressive degree of precision. Since 1 kg of body weight corresponds to 7000 kcal of food energy, the mean imbalance between energy intake and expenditure comes to 1750 kcal per year, or less than 5 kcal/day. Other studies showed that starvation and weight loss were followed by an eventual recovery of body weight up to, or even above, pre-diet levels. These observations have led to the hypothesis that a 'ponderostat' mechanism was responsible for keeping body weight at its physiological set-point.

However, the concept of a set-point was more valuable in principle than in practice. While the body weights of some people are stable, others show a great degree of fluctuation. Weight cycling or yo-yo dieting is a common phenomenon, and while some people manage to maintain a more or less fixed level of body fat, others do not. The current consensus is that while a physiological set-point may defend the body from excessive weight loss, physiological mechanisms protecting the body from excessive weight gain are less effective and less precise.

A better understanding of the control of human food intake is needed for the more effective treatment of obesity and overweight. Current approaches to weight management are based on the premise that food intake is controlled with some degree of precision. Most of them involve some kind of a feedback mechanism.

- Serotonin reuptake blockers (SSRIs) are intended to restore serotonin imbalance, halt carbohydrate cravings, and lead to a reduction in both food intake and body weight.
- Leptin administration is supposed to mimic the body's signals regarding excess fat storage, leading to a reduction in food intake and weight loss.
- Proposed manipulations of satiety using energy density of the diet are also based on the premise that food intake responds to metabolic or physiological events.

However, none of these interventions has managed to reduce growing obesity rates. The failure of existing strategies opens up the interesting possibility that body weight is loosely controlled rather than tightly regulated. If innate or learned regulatory mechanisms are imprecise or absent altogether, then obesity may reflect the overwhelming influence of environmental factors. As such, obesity is a medical issue and a public health problem. The observed association between obesity and the socioeconomic gradient requires novel intervention strategies to impact food policy and affect the modern food supply.

15.9 Perspectives on the future

While decades of studies on food intake behavior have shown that control mechanisms do exist, it is not clear to what extent they affect human dietary behaviors in affluent societies. From the evolutionary perspective, it is not altogether surprising that physiological mechanisms that were critical to survival under conditions of energy shortage are now inadequate to cope with energy excess. Future research should focus on the environmental factors that predispose certain individuals, but not others, to become obese, with special emphasis on socioeconomic factors, education and income. New studies show that diet structure and diet quality are directly related to diet cost and that the observed health disparities may be linked to an unequal access to a healthy diet. Elucidating the interaction between physiological factors and the economics of food choice is the next challenge for obesity and nutrition research.

Further reading

Bellisle F, Perez C. Low-energy substitutes for sugars and fats in the human diet: impact on nutritional regulation. Neurosci Biobehav Rev 1994; 18: 197–205.

Blundell JE, Lawton CL, Cotton JR et al. Control of human appetite: implications for the intake of dietary fat. Annu Rev Nutr 1996; 16: 285–319.

Campfield LA. Socratic debate: cognitive is more important than physiological regulation of appetite: con argument. In: Progress in Obesity Research, Vol. 7 (A Angel, H Anderson, C Bouchard et al., eds), pp. 359–365. London: John Libbey, 1996.

Drewnowski A. Taste preferences and food intake. Annu Rev Nutr 1997; 17: 237–253.

Green SM, Blundell JE. Subjective and objective indices of the satiating effect of foods. Can people predict how filling a food will be? Eur J Clin Nutr 1996; 50: 798–806.

16
Overnutrition

L Bandini and A Flynn

Key messages

Obesity
- The prevalence of obesity is increasing throughout the world in both affluent and poorer countries, and has become a worldwide health problem because of its association with increased morbidity from many chronic diseases.
- Obesity can be identified by the measurement of skinfold thicknesses and by calculating body mass index, although both of these methods have their limitations.
- Although there are genetic components to obesity, the increased prevalence observed over the past 30 years cannot be attributed solely to a change in the genes.
- An increase in the incidence of obesity can be attributed to environmental factors which lead to increased energy intake and/or to decreases in physical activity that have resulted in a positive energy balance.
- As industrialization and technology increase, further decreases in physical activity are expected.

- If these decreases in energy expenditure are not reversed or compensated for by a decrease in energy intake, the epidemic of obesity, with its associated health consequences, is likely to continue.

Vitamin and mineral overconsumption
- For a number of vitamins and minerals adverse health effects can result when the capacity for homeostasis is exceeded by continuing high dietary intakes.
- The tolerable upper intake level (UL) is a dietary reference standard that may be used to evaluate the risk of excessive intakes of vitamins and minerals in groups and as a guide to individuals for the maximum level of the usual intake of micronutrients.
- The UL for nutrients may be derived based on the principles of risk assessment, and UL have been established recently for several vitamins and minerals by authorities in a number of countries.

Section I: Obesity

16.1 Introduction

Obesity is defined as an excess of body fat. Overweight refers to an excess of body weight. The amount of body fat changes with age and development, and differs between males and females. Therefore, criteria for defining obesity and overweight need to be based on both age and gender.

16.2 Identification

Body fat can be measured precisely by laboratory methods such as dual-energy X-ray absorptiometry (DEXA), total body water and hydrodensitometry (see Chapter 2 on body composition in *Introduction to Human Nutrition*). These methods give an estimate of total body fat, or adipose tissue, in the body. Because people of different sizes will have different amounts of body fat, a diagnosis of obesity cannot be made on the basis of absolute amounts of fat. For example, a person who has 20 kg of body fat and weighs 60 kg has a percentage body fat of 33%. A second person who has 25 kg of fat but weighs 80 kg will be 31.3% fat. The first person has less total fat but a higher percentage body fat than the second person. Although obesity is defined as an excess of body fat, techniques for directly assessing body fatness are not available for clinical use. Furthermore, there are no defined criteria for diagnosing obesity from measures of body fatness. Thus, identifying obese persons in clinical practice is not based on percentage body fat but rather on measures that correlate with body fat. The most common methods used in clinical assessment are skinfold thickness and body mass index (BMI).

16.3 Skinfold thickness

The identification of clinical measures of overweight and obesity that accurately reflect body fat has been an area of much research and discussion. Measures of triceps skinfold (TSF) thickness represent a measure of subcutaneous fatness (fat underneath the skin). Studies have shown that measures of TSF thickness correlate well with body fatness in both children and adults, and are used to identify people who are overweight or obese. However, two assumptions are made when TSF thickness measures are used to assess body fatness. The first is that the triceps skinfold is representative of subcutaneous fatness. The second is that subcutaneous fatness is correlated with total body fat. These assumptions are not always valid. In disease states, or in individuals with significant amounts of visceral fat (fat around the internal organs), changes in body fat distribution may alter the relationship of TSF thickness with total body fat. A significant limitation of using TSF thickness to measure body fatness is that extensive training is required to perform the measurement correctly. Furthermore, it is harder to measure TSF accurately in obese people. Therefore, as a person becomes fatter, the reliability of these measures decreases. These limitations make the method less useful for identifying obesity in a clinical setting.

Other investigators have measured skinfold thickness at several subcutaneous sites, including the subscapular, suprailiac, abdominal, bicep and tricep areas, and have developed equations to calculate body fatness from the sum of several skinfolds. Although the use of equations where skinfold thickness is measured in several sites is probably more representative of subcutaneous fat than TSF thickness alone, skinfold measures cannot identify individuals with significant amounts of visceral fat.

Equations combining skinfold thickness, circumferences such as waist, and body weight and height have also been developed to estimate body fatness.

16.4 Body mass index

Adults

Over the past decade a considerable amount of research has been done to evaluate the usefulness of BMI as a measure to identify overweight and obesity.

$$BMI = weight\ in\ kg/height\ in\ meters\ squared$$

A man who is 172 cm tall and weighs 89 kg will have a BMI of 30.1: BMI = $(85\,kg/1.72\,m^2)$
Another man who is also 172 cm tall and weighs 73 kg will have a BMI of 24.7: BMI = $(73\,kg/1.72\,m^2)$.

Studies have shown that BMI, although not a direct measure of fatness, is significantly correlated with body fat measured by laboratory methods, including hydrodensitometry, isotope dilution and total body potassium (see *Introduction to Human Nutrition*). One of the major advantages of using BMI as a measure of overweight or obesity is that it can be derived from measures of height and weight. It is much easier to obtain reliable measures of weight and height than skinfold thickness. However, BMI cannot distinguish whether the excess weight is due to fat or due to muscle mass. Thus, the use of BMI to identify overweight individuals may result in misclassification for individuals with increased muscle mass, such as heavyweight boxers or wrestlers.

The World Health Organization (WHO) has classifications for overweight and obesity in adults based on BMI (1997) (Table 16.1). The same cut-off points are also recommended by the US National Institutes of Health (NIH). In the NIH clinical guidelines for the identification, evaluation and treatment of overweight and obesity in adults, evidence is presented showing an increase in morbidity and mortality at or above the cut-off points used for identifying overweight (BMI ≥ 25) and obesity (BMI ≥ 30). This document provides justification for choosing the cut-off points indicated in Table 16.1.

Children and adolescents

Many countries use BMI to identify overweight and obesity in children and adolescents. Cut-off points for obesity vary among countries. While numerous countries use their own reference population to define obesity, others may use reference populations from other countries. In the USA, a task force on obesity recommended the use of age and gender BMI percentiles to identify overweight children and adolescents. A BMI greater than the 85th and 95th percentile for age and gender are identified as overweight and obese, respectively (Barlow and Dietz, 1998). Recently, an international task force (Cole *et al.*, 2000) proposed international reference standards to identify obesity in children. These standards are based on data from six countries, including Brazil, Great Britain, Hong Kong, the Netherlands, Singapore and the USA.

Measures of weight for height have often been used to identify obesity in children and adolescents. Charts prepared by the US National Center for Health Statistics have been used to identify children who are overweight, that is, above the 95th percentile of weight for height (Hamill, 1979). There is considerable controversy over the use of US growth reference charts for identifying overweight and underweight children in other countries.

The growth charts historically available for children do not provide weight-for-height reference values during adolescence. Weight-for-height percentiles are often extrapolated from weight-for-age and height-for-age data. Recently, the Centers for Disease Control in the USA published revised growth charts (http://www.cdc.gov/growth_charts). These revised growth charts now include new reference charts for BMI based on age and gender and are recommended for the identification of overweight children in the USA. They provide percentile curves for BMI and include the 3rd and 97th percentiles for age and gender.

16.5 Energy balance

Obesity is the result of a long-term energy imbalance where energy intake exceeds energy expenditure (Table 16.2). This leads to a positive energy imbalance and an increase in body fat stores.

- Obesity ultimately results from a positive energy imbalance.
- Positive energy imbalance results from:
  - an increase in energy intake with no change in energy expenditure
  - a decrease in energy expenditure with no change in energy intake
  - an increase in energy intake and a decrease in energy expenditure.

Efforts to understand the etiology of obesity have focussed on differences in energy intake and energy expenditure among obese and non-obese individuals. Either an increase in energy intake or a decrease in energy expenditure are potential factors that could contribute to an energy imbalance.

Energy intake

A considerable amount of research has gone into examining whether people who are obese consume more energy than non-obese people. The majority of studies of energy intake in obese and non-obese children and adults do not show differences in energy intake between obese and non-obese people. These studies have been questioned because there is uncertainty about whether the reported energy intakes of subjects in these studies are accurate. Until the development of the doubly labeled water (DLW) method

Table 16.1 Classification of overweight and obese in adults according to body mass index (BMI)

Classification	BMI (kg/m^2)
Underweight	<18.5
Normal range	18.5–24.9
Overweight	≥25
Preobese	25–29.9
Obese class I	30.0–34.9
Obese class II	35.0–35.9
Obese class III	≥40.0

Used with permission from WHO (1997).

Table 16.2 Energy balance

Energy balance	Energy intake = Energy expenditure	Maintenance of fat stores
Positive energy imbalance	Energy intake > Energy expenditure	Increase in fat stores
Negative energy imbalance	Energy intake < Energy expenditure	Decrease in fat stores

for the measurement of energy expenditure, it was not possible to assess unobtrusively the validity of dietary reporting. Now, using the DLW technique, measures of daily energy expenditure can be made simultaneously with measures of energy intake. If an individual is in energy balance, energy expenditure should equal energy intake. However, recent studies using DLW to measure energy expenditure indicate substantial underreporting of energy intake in both obese and non-obese people. These studies suggest that comparisons of energy intake among obese and non-obese individuals are often inaccurate and cannot be used to determine whether obese individuals eat more than non-obese individuals.

Energy expenditure

Resting metabolic rate (RMR) accounts for a major proportion of daily energy expenditure. Its contribution to energy expenditure varies among individuals, but in sedentary adults accounts for between 60 and 70% of daily energy expenditure. The remaining 30–40% of daily energy expenditure that is not due to RMR is the energy spent on activity and the thermic effect of food (TEF). In children, this will also include the energy cost for growth. Energy expenditure is discussed in detail in *Introduction to Human Nutrition*.

Components of energy expenditure

Components of energy expenditure are:

- resting metabolic rate
- thermic effect of food
- physical activity
- growth.

Since the 1980s, many studies have been conducted to compare resting energy expenditure, the TEF and daily energy expenditure among obese and non-obese people. Studies have not shown significant differences in resting energy expenditure between obese and non-obese adults or children. Studies on the TEF are equivocal, with some suggesting that energy expenditure may be decreased in the obese and others showing no differences between obese and non-obese people. Although the TEF contributes only a small percentage to daily energy expenditure (6–10%), small differences over a long period could potentially lead to a significant energy imbalance. Studies of daily energy expenditure which include RMR, TEF and physical activity among obese and non-obese people have not found differences

in total energy expenditure between the two groups. It is possible that some individuals may increase their daily energy expenditure significantly by constant fidgeting. This non-exercise activity-related thermogenesis (NEAT) may contribute to variable energy needs among individuals. It remains unclear, however, whether individuals with high NEAT are less likely to become overweight. Although these studies have not found differences in the obese state, differences may exist among individuals before they become obese (preobese state). When an individual gains weight, resting metabolic rate (RMR) and daily energy expenditure increase. Part of this increase is due to an increase in fat-free mass. Thus, a defect in energy expenditure in the preobese state may be normalized with weight gain.

Diet-induced thermogenesis

In the 1980s considerable research focussed on the role of diet-induced thermogenesis (DIT) in maintaining energy balance. DIT refers to an increase in energy expenditure in response to overeating. If energy expenditure were increased in response to an excess intake of energy, the excess energy would be dissipated as heat, and obesity could be prevented. It has been hypothesized that lean individuals could compensate for excess energy intake by burning the excess energy as heat, whereas obese individuals would be metabolically more efficient and store the excess energy as fat. Results of overfeeding studies in which energy expenditure was measured have found little evidence for DIT in obese or non-obese individuals.

Stock (1999) suggested that the role of DIT in regulating energy balance is secondary to its role in eliminating non-essential energy for individuals consuming low nutrient-dense diets and that in our society only recently has food become so accessible that the role of DIT in maintaining energy balance has become significant. Stock calculated the theoretical cost of weight gain in many of these overfeeding studies that reported little evidence of DIT and argued that 84% of subjects in these studies exhibit some increase in DIT.

Substrate oxidation

The three macronutrients, carbohydrate, protein and fat, are oxidized to carbon dioxide and water and can provide energy for metabolic needs. Because the human body has a limited storage capacity for excess carbohydrate, a lack of storage capacity for excess protein and a large capacity to store excess fat, with excess energy intake, intakes of carbohydrate and protein will be oxidized preferentially to fat. Thus, fat oxidation will be decreased and the excess fat will be stored. As shown in the energy balance equation (Table 16.2), when energy intake is greater than energy expenditure body fat stores will increase. Thus, excess energy intake from any of the macronutrients will result in a positive gain of body fat stores.

The non-protein respiratory quotient (RQ) indicates the contribution of carbohydrate and fat being oxidized in the body. The RQ of carbohydrate is 1.0 and the RQ of fat 0.71. An individual with a higher RQ is burning more carbohydrate than fat, compared with a person with a lower RQ. When a person is in energy balance, the amount of carbohydrate and fat oxidized should be the same as that obtained from the diet. It has been suggested, however, that factors other than the proportion of macronutrients in the diet, such as age and gender, may affect RQ as well as thermogenesis and food intake. Some studies have suggested that fat oxidation may be reduced in obese individuals. It remains unclear whether substrate oxidation influences energy intake, and its role in the development of obesity is the subject of present research.

Overall, studies of energy expenditure do not support the hypothesis that there is a defect in metabolism in the already obese state. However, several genetic and environmental factors may increase an individual's risk of developing obesity.

16.6 Etiology

Genetic factors

Heritability of body fatness

Evidence suggests that there is a genetic component to obesity. Studies examining fatness similarities among twins and other biological siblings have shown that similarities are strongest for monozygotic twins (MZ), then dizygotic (DZ) twins, and then other siblings. Heritability of fatness has been examined by assessing MZ and DZ twins living in similar or different environments and in adopted children separated from their biological parents. BMI was used to assess body fatness. Studies of twins and adoptees both found that heredity was a major determinant of BMI. This observation supports a strong genetic component to fatness. However, because families share the same environment, it is difficult to determine how much of the similarity

in fatness is due to genetic factors and how much is due to environmental factors.

Genetic basis to energy balance

A genetic basis to energy balance would be expected to show its effect on energy intake, energy expenditure, or both. In the 1950s it was suggested that the body fat stores are regulated and that signals in the body provide feedback to the area of the brain controlling food intake and energy expenditure. These signals would be released in proportion to the body's adipose tissue stores. Therefore, if body fat stores increased, a compensatory mechanism would be initiated that would result in a decrease in energy intake. The discovery of leptin in 1994 provides a possible mechanism to support early theories of models for body-weight regulation.

Studies in mice have shown that a defect in the gene for leptin is associated with obesity, increased food intake and a reduction in metabolic rate. The role of leptin in body-weight regulation in humans is not fully understood. Leptin is thought to be involved in weight regulation through a series of complex interactions with other neurohormones involved in appetite regulation.

One potential role for leptin in weight regulation is through the action of uncoupling proteins (UCP), which are involved in DIT. UCPs provide heat without generating adenosire triphosphate (ATP) by uncoupling oxidation and phosyphorylation. Thus, when food is oxidized, the energy is dissipated as heat rather than converted to ATP. In animals, DIT occurs in brown adipose tissue (BAT). Because adult humans do not have significant amounts of BAT, it was assumed that UCPs were not important for humans. Recently, however, UCPs have been found in adult human tissues. Considerable research is presently underway to identify the role that UCPs may play in human body-weight regulation.

Plasma levels of leptin are positively associated with fat mass. In general, the more adipose tissue an individual has, the higher their leptin level will be. This suggests that human obesity is not associated with a decrease in leptin. It is hypothesized that obesity may be associated with a resistance to leptin. Thus, individuals with leptin resistance may have normal or high leptin levels, but may not be responsive to these levels of leptin.

The role of leptin in energy expenditure is another area of intense research. Clinical studies are examining the relationship of leptin levels to energy expenditure in both children and adults. More research is needed to clarify the role that leptin plays in body weight regulation.

Heritability of energy expenditure

Because some of the variability in RMR, TEF and daily energy expenditure is genetic. It has been suggested that individuals who have low energy expenditure may have an inherited risk for the development of obesity. The major determinant of RMR is fat-free mass. Age and gender also contribute to variability in RMR.

Studies have examined whether children of obese parents have a decreased RMR compared with children of non-obese parents. The results of these studies are conflicting. More research is needed to determine whether children of obese parents have a lower RMR and whether a low RMR increases their risk for becoming obese.

Racial differences in the prevalence of obesity have led to speculation that there may be ethnic differences in energy expenditure. Because of the high prevalence of obesity reported in African–American children and adults, many studies have been conducted to compare the energy expenditure of African–Americans and Caucasians. These studies have examined RMR, total energy expenditure and substrate oxidation. Although most studies comparing RMR in African–Americans and Caucasians report a reduced RMR in African–Americans, some do not. Even if these differences are established they cannot be interpreted to suggest that a low metabolic rate causes obesity. Longitudinal studies are needed to determine whether these reductions in RMR lead to an increase in weight gain over time and thus contribute to the higher prevalence of obesity seen in African–Americans compared with Caucasians. There are limited data on RMR in other ethnic groups.

Studies comparing substrate oxidation rates between African–Americans and Caucasians are few and contradictory. More studies are needed to determine whether African–Americans oxidize fat at lower rates and whether this lower rate of oxidation contributes to increased body weight.

Only a few studies have compared the energy spent on physical activity and daily energy expenditure among African–American and Caucasian individuals. These studies are equivocal. As with RMR, a reduction in the energy spent on physical activity or total energy expenditure cannot be interpreted as the cause of obesity.

Again, longitudinal studies are needed to determine whether reductions in energy expenditure, either RMR, the energy spent on physical activity or total daily energy expenditure, in the preobese state, are associated with increases in body weight. The results of the few longitudinal studies to date are equivocal. Many longitudinal studies are currently being conducted to test the hypothesis that a low RMR or total daily energy expenditure is a risk factor for the development of obesity.

Environmental factors

Although genetic factors may increase the susceptibility of an individual to obesity, obesity is ultimately due to a positive energy balance, which occurs when energy intake exceeds energy expenditure for a prolonged period. Thus, the interaction between genetics, that is, an increased susceptibility to obesity, and an environment that promotes increased energy intake and/or decreased energy expenditure, can lead to obesity.

Environmental factors that may contribute to obesity are those factors that can influence either energy intake or energy expenditure. In this section, environmental factors that may increase food intake and decrease energy expenditure will be discussed.

Energy intake

Dietary factors that may increase energy intake include:

- fat
- energy density
- glycemic index
- variety
- fiber.

It has been hypothesized that diets high in fat may lead to obesity. Diets high in fat have been targeted as the culprit for excess energy intake owing to the high energy density and palatability of fat. However, there is considerable controversy regarding the relationship between high-fat diets and obesity.

Studies in metabolic units that have monitored the food intakes of subjects support the hypothesis that energy intakes will be higher on a high-fat diet. Studies such as these are conducted in laboratory settings for short periods. These studies do not allow generalization to subjects living at home in an unrestricted environment. Thus, there may be additional factors that affect energy intake in free-living subjects that are not readily apparent in the laboratory such as accessibility to food, social factors, and opportunities for physical activity. Furthermore, changes occurring over a few days or weeks in the laboratory may not be maintained over longer periods.

For example, a study was conducted for 20 weeks on an outpatient basis where the food was prepared in a metabolic kitchen. Results showed that higher energy intakes were needed to maintain weight on a lower fat diet in both non-obese and obese women. These data suggest that the macronutrient composition of the diet may be important in weight regulation.

The association of overweight (BMI $\geq$ 25) with the percentage of energy from fat in the diet has been examined in 20 different countries. A positive association was found between energy intake from fat and the proportion of the population that is overweight. One of the limitations of these ecological data, however, is that there is no information available at the individual level. Therefore, it is not clear whether it is the people who are eating the high-fat diets who are obese.

Overall, epidemiological studies examining the relationship between high-fat diets and weight gain are conflicting. In the USA, between 1976–1980 and 1988–1991, the percentage of energy from fat in the diet has decreased but the prevalence of obesity has increased. The Second National Health and Nutrition Examination Survey, conducted in 1976–1980 (NHANES II), found that the average intake of energy from fat in Americans 2 years of age and older was 36%. The NHANES III (phase 1) study conducted from 1988 to 1991 found that the average intake of calories from fat was 34%. The two surveys also assessed the prevalence of overweight in children and adults. In the NHANES II survey the prevalence of overweight in adults was 25.4%. In the NHANES III (phase 1) survey, the prevalence was higher, 33.2%. Similar patterns were seen in children. Thus, in the USA, the prevalence of obesity is rising despite a concurrent decrease in the percentage of energy from fat. Again, these data do not tell us anything about the diets of those individuals who are obese.

The question of whether high-fat diets lead to increased energy intake is further complicated by the fact that fat has a higher energy density than carbohydrate. As a result, the energy content of food high in fat is greater than the energy content for the same weight of a food high in carbohydrate. Some researchers have suggested that energy-dense diets promote weight gain and that it is the energy density of food, not the fat content, that is associated with weight gain.

Other factors hypothesized to be associated with excessive energy intake are diets with a high glycemic index, diets with low fiber content and the large variety of food choices available to consumers. Considerable research is currently being conducted to determine whether any of these dietary factors may be associated with obesity.

In addition, other environmental factors such as increased accessibility to food, lower cost of fast foods, and increased availability of food outside the home may lead to increased energy intake. For example, in the USA many high-energy food items are more accessible and less costly than fresh fruit and vegetables. In the USA, vending machines are located in recreational facilities, schools and office buildings. Although there may be a wide variety of foods in the vending machines, the choices are limited with respect to nutrients. Furthermore, most vending machines are usually filled with high-energy, low-nutrient-dense foods or carbonated soft drinks and juices in 12–20 oz (560 ml) portions, providing 1.5–2.5 servings.

The way in which food is packaged and sold often makes it more economical to buy the larger size of an item, although the larger portion may be excessive. For example, soft drinks are often purchased in 20 oz (560 ml) bottles. Although the nutrition label reads 2–2.5 servings, the consumer may not be aware of this. Such marketing strategies and advertising on television and billboards encourage the consumption of high-energy, low-nutrient-dense foods.

The availability of meals and food outside the home may also contribute to excess energy intake. Portion sizes in restaurants are often large. Fast-food restaurants generally provide high-fat meals with increased energy. All of these environmental factors can promote a positive energy balance.

Inactivity

The energy spent on physical activity is a major determinant of daily energy expenditure. Decreases in physical activity will consequently decrease energy expenditure. If the energy spent on physical activity is decreased without a concomitant decrease in energy intake, a positive energy imbalance will result. An example of the secular trends in diet and activity in relation to obesity in Britain is shown in Figure 16.1. Although there has been a decline in total energy intake, there has also been an increase in sedentary behavior such as television viewing. In addition, there has been an increase in the number of cars per household, which suggests that activity may have decreased further.

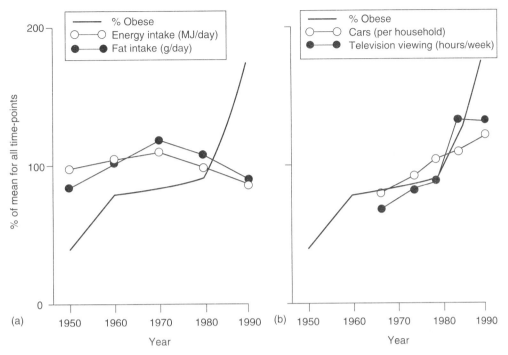

Figure 16.1 Secular trends in (a) diet and (b) activity in relation to obesity in Britain. Reproduced from Prentice AM, Jebb SA. Obesity in Britain, gluttony or sloth? BMJ 1995; 311: 437–439 with permission of BMJ Publishing Group.

Television viewing is a major sedentary behavior in our current lifestyle. As the amount of time spent watching television increases, the amount of time spent in physical activity will decrease. Some studies suggest that television viewing contributes to inactivity and increases the risk of obesity. Furthermore, television commercials for food may increase snacking during viewing time.

In developed countries, other environmental factors have resulted in decreased activity among individuals. In addition to television viewing, computers, video games and online shopping have resulted in less physical activity at home and in the workplace. Cars have reduced the amount of walking time, even for short distances. Food preparation has been made easier by labor-saving devices. These advances in technology have contributed to a more sedentary lifestyle and thus a decrease in daily energy expenditure.

Safety issues may contribute to the decline in physical activity in children and adults. Many children live in areas where it is unsafe to walk to school or play outside, contributing to a decrease in physical activity and an increase in sedentary behavior. In many communities, adults may not have a safe place to walk or exercise after work.

In an environment where energy intake is increased and energy expenditure is reduced, and genetic factors exist that may increase an individual's susceptibility to obesity, the interaction between genetics and environment may lead to a positive energy balance.

A good example of this can be seen in the Pima Indians living in Arizona. There is a significantly higher BMI in Pima Indians living in Arizona than a related group of Pima Indians living in Mexico. The diet of the Arizona Pima Indians is typical of a Western diet, being higher in fat and lower in complex carbohydrates than the traditional diet of the Mexican Pimas. In addition, the Mexican Pimas engage in strenuous physical activity to meet their daily needs, while the Arizona Pimas are less physically active. This combination of a high-fat diet and decreased physical activity in this genetically susceptible population has contributed to a high prevalence of obesity.

16.7 Pathological syndromes

Although obesity is rarely the result of a metabolic disorder, there are pathological syndromes in which it is the result of a metabolic disorder. These cases account for only a small percentage of obese individuals and

include Prader–Willi syndrome, Laurence–Moon–
Bardet Biedl syndrome, hypothyroidism, Alsrom–
Hallgren syndrome, Carpenter syndrome, Cohen
syndrome, Cushing's syndrome, growth hormone
deficiency and polycystic ovary syndrome.

16.8 Consequences of obesity

Physiological effects of excess fat

Obesity increases the risk for many chronic diseases,
including:

- cardiovascular disease (e.g. stroke and hypertension)
- type II diabetes mellitus
- gallbladder disease
- some types of cancers
- respiratory illnesses
- reproductive problems.

Individuals who are obese are at increased risk for
many types of chronic diseases. Obesity is a risk factor for cardiovascular disease, including coronary heart
disease, hypertension and stroke, and type II diabetes
mellitus. Individuals with these chronic diseases are at
higher risk for mortality than individuals who do not
have these chronic diseases.

The risk for other diseases is increased as well. Obese
individuals are at risk for the development of gallbladder disease, some types of cancer (i.e. breast, ovarian,
cervical cancer in postmenopausal women, colorectal),
respiratory illnesses (i.e. sleep apnea, Pickwickian
syndrome), and reproductive problems. They may
develop osteoarthritis and low back pain, which may
limit mobility and reduce independence in activities of
daily living, thus impacting on the quality of life.

Obese children and adolescents show elevations in
cardiovascular disease risk factors such as increases in
cholesterol levels, blood glucose and blood pressure.
These risk factors tend to cluster in individuals and
track from childhood to adulthood. There are reports
that the incidence of type II diabetes, once thought to
be an adult disease, is increasing in children and adolescents. This is concerning given the increasing
prevalence of childhood obesity in many countries
throughout the world.

Not all obese people will develop these diseases.
The risk that an obese individual will develop any of
these health consequences associated with obesity may
be influenced by other factors, including genetics,
smoking, fat distribution and level of fitness.

Fat distribution

As early as the 1950s, an association between upper
body fat obesity and metabolic complications such as
diabetes and arteriosclerosis was recognized, with diabetes and arteriosclerosis being more common in individuals with upper body obesity than those with lower
body obesity. In the 1980s, numerous studies were conducted that showed a significant relationship between
upper body obesity, assessed by the ratio of waist to
hip circumference, and metabolic abnormalities such
as glucose intolerance, insulin resistance and abnormal
lipid levels. Now known as the metabolic syndrome,
the insulin resistance syndrome or syndrome X, this
syndrome is a cluster of metabolic abnormalities
including hyperinsulinemia, impaired glucose tolerance, hypertension, hypertriglyceridemia, decreases in
high-density lipoprotein (HDL) levels, increases in
apolipoprotein B, and increases in small, dense lipoprotein levels, and is associated with upper body obesity.

Individuals with upper body obesity have increased
amounts of subcutaneous abdominal adipose tissue as
well as increased amounts of visceral adipose tissue.
The subcutaneous adipose tissue that is associated with
upper body obesity is directly underneath the skin
around the abdominal area. Visceral adipose tissue or
intra-abdominal tissue surrounds the internal organs.
Excess visceral adiposity is thought to be responsible
for the metabolic abnormalities associated with upper
body fatness, but the relationship between visceral
adiposity and metabolic abnormalities is not fully
understood. Because visceral adipose tissue drains via
the portal venous system, the liver receives all of the
metabolic products from visceral fat, including free
fatty acids. As fat stores increase there will be more free
fatty acids. It has been speculated that the direct exposure of the liver to high levels of free fatty acids may
be related to hepatic insulin resistance (Matsuzawa *et
al.*, 1995).

Visceral adipose tissue can only be measured using
computed tomographic (CT) scans and magnetic resonance imaging (MRI).

Waist circumference appears to be a good marker for
upper body obesity. Because fat distribution, like BMI,
appears to be an independent risk factor for the morbidity of obesity, it is recommended that waist circumference be measured in addition to BMI to identify
people at risk for obesity. Waist circumferences greater
than 102 cm in men and 88 cm in women are associated
with an increased risk of metabolic complications. More
research is needed to determine the relationship

between increased visceral adipose tissue and metabolic abnormalities, including lifestyle factors that may be beneficial in preventing the metabolic syndrome.

Psychological effects

The psychosocial effects of obesity on both children and adults can be substantial. Obese people are often viewed as lazy overeaters who lack the willpower to diet and exercise. This misunderstanding of the causes of obesity leads to negative attitudes towards obese individuals. Obese children and adolescents often experience discrimination and teasing from other children. Obese adults have reported being discriminated against in the workplace and in college acceptance.

16.9 Perspectives on the future

Future research will help to identify the questions of what factors increase an individual's susceptibility to obesity. Longitudinal studies will help to determine whether a low energy expenditure is a risk factor for the development of obesity. Research should focus on genetic and physiological factors that influence food intake and energy expenditure. Understanding the causal factors associated with obesity are critical for prevention and treatment.

In addition to the societal attitudes towards obese persons, there are data to suggest that individuals who are overweight may have a lower self-esteem and are more likely to be depressed. More research is needed to understand the psychological effects of obesity

The mechanisms associated with increased upper body obesity and metabolic abnormalities are not clearly understood. Further research in this area is needed to determine the mechanisms linking abdominal fatness and the metabolic abnormalities observed.

There are few population-based data on the risk of obesity in many ethnic groups, including Hispanic and Asian people. More work needs to be done to identify the risk factors for obesity in different cultures.

Section II: Vitamin and mineral overconsumption

16.10 Introduction

The increased availability of fortified foods and the increased use of dietary supplements in many countries has led to increased interest in the adverse health effects that may arise from overconsumption of vitamins and minerals. It is well recognized that such adverse effects can occur with high intakes of some vitamins and minerals. While it is generally considered that the risk of such effects is low, the incidence of such occurrences in different populations is generally not known with any certainty. In some countries, for example in the European Union and North America, the need to protect consumer health through regulating the addition of vitamins and minerals to foods and nutritional supplements has led to the establishment of scientifically based upper limits of intake for these micronutrients.

16.11 Adverse effects of vitamins and minerals: concepts

Failure of homeostasis

Vitamins and essential minerals are subject to homeostatic control, through which body content is regulated. This reduces the risk of depletion of body pools that could lead to deficiency when intakes are low. It also reduces the risk of excessive accumulation in tissues that could lead to adverse effects when intakes are high. A measure of protection against potential adverse effects of high intakes is provided by adaptation of homeostatic control mechanisms; for example, limiting absorption efficiency, adaptation of metabolic processes, or enhancing excretion in feces, urine, skin or lungs (Box 16.1).

However, for a number of micronutrients the capacity for homeostasis may be exceeded by continuing high dietary intakes. This can lead to abnormal accumulation in tissues, or overloading of normal metabolic or transport pathways.

Threshold dose

For nutrients no risk of adverse health effects is expected unless a threshold dose (or intake) is exceeded. Thresholds for any given adverse effect vary among members of the population. In general, for nutrients there are insufficient data to establish the distribution of thresholds in the population for individual adverse effects.

Variation in sensitivity of individuals

Sensitivity to adverse effects of micronutrients is influenced by physiological changes and common conditions associated with growth and maturation that occur during an individual's lifespan. Even within relatively homogenous lifestage groups, there is a range of sensitivities to adverse effects (e.g. sensitivity is influenced by body weight and lean body mass). Some subpopulations have extreme and distinct vulnerabilities owing to genetic predisposition or certain metabolic disorders or disease states (Box 16.2).

Effect of bioavailability

Bioavailability of a nutrient relates to its absorption and utilization, and may be defined as its accessibility to normal metabolic and physiological processes.

Bioavailability influences the usefulness of a nutrient for physiological functions at physiological levels of intake, and the nature and severity of adverse effects at excessive intakes. There is considerable variation in nutrient bioavailability in humans; for instance, the chemical form of a nutrient may have a large influence on bioavailability. Other modulating factors include the nutritional status of the individual, nutrient intake level, interaction with other dietary components and the food matrix (e.g. consumption with or without food). For example, high zinc intakes increase the synthesis in intestinal mucosal cells of metallothionein, a protein that avidly binds copper and reduces its absorption.

Tolerable upper intake level

While dietary reference standards have been established over many years for evaluation of the nutritional adequacy of dietary intakes, it is only in recent years that the need for dietary reference standards for evaluating and managing the risk of excessive intakes of vitamins and minerals has been recognized. Such reference standards have been established for a number of vitamins and minerals and are referred to as tolerable upper intake levels (sometimes also called upper safe levels).

The tolerable upper intake level (UL) is the maximum level of total chronic daily intake of a nutrient (from all sources, including foods, water, nutrient supplements and medicines) judged to be unlikely to pose a risk of adverse health effects to almost all individuals in the general population. 'Tolerable' connotes a level of intake that can be tolerated physiologically by humans. ULs may be derived for various lifestage groups in the population (e.g. adults, pregnant and lactating women, infants and children). The UL is not a recommended level of intake but is an estimate of the highest (usual) level of intake that carries no appreciable risk of adverse health effects.

The UL is meant to apply to all groups of the general population, including sensitive individuals, throughout the lifestage. However, it is not meant to apply to individuals receiving the nutrient under medical supervision or to individuals with predisposing conditions that render them especially sensitive to one or more adverse effects of the nutrient, such as those with genetic predisposition or certain disease states.

The term adverse health effect may be defined as any significant alteration in structure or function or any impairment of a physiologically important function that could lead to an adverse health effect in humans.

16.12 Derivation of the tolerable upper intake level

Risk assessment

ULs can be derived for nutrients using the principles of risk assessment that have been developed for biological and chemical agents. Risk assessment is a systematic means of evaluating the probability of occurrence of adverse health effects in humans from an excess exposure to an environmental agent (in this case nutrients in food and water, nutrient supplements and medicines). The hallmark of risk assessment is the requirement to be explicit in all of the evaluations and judgments that must be made to document conclusions.

In general, the same principles of risk assessment apply to nutrients as to other food chemicals, but it is recognized that vitamins and minerals possess some characteristics which distinguish them from other food chemicals (Box 16.3).

The steps involved in the application of risk assessment principles to the derivation of ULs for vitamins and minerals are summarized in Figure 16.2 and explained in more detail below.

Hazard identification

This involves the collection, organization and evaluation of all information pertaining to the adverse health effects of a given nutrient, and summarizes the evidence concerning the capacity of the nutrient to cause one or more types of adverse health effect in humans.

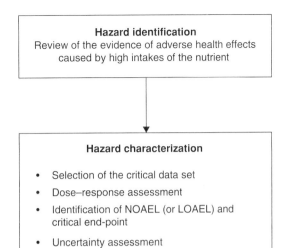

Figure 16.2 Steps in the development of the tolerable upper intake level (UL). NOAEL: no observed adverse effect level; LOAEL: lowest observed adverse effect level.

Human studies provide the most relevant data for hazard identification and, when they are of sufficient quality and extent, are given the greatest weight. Other experimental studies (in experimental animals and *in vitro* studies) may also be used. Key issues that are addressed in the data evaluation include the extent to which there is evidence of adverse health effects on humans and whether the relationship established by the published human data is causal, mechanisms of adverse effects, quality and completeness of the database, and identification of distinct and highly sensitive subpopulations.

Hazard characterization

As intake of a nutrient increases, a threshold is reached above which increasing intake increases the risk of adverse health effects. This is illustrated diagrammatically in Figure 16.3.

Hazard characterization involves the qualitative and quantitative evaluation of the nature of the adverse health effects associated with a nutrient. This includes a dose–response assessment, which involve determining the relationship between nutrient intake (dose) and adverse health effect (in terms of frequency and severity). Based on these evaluations, a UL is derived, taking into account the scientific uncertainties in the data. ULs may be derived for various lifestage groups within the population.

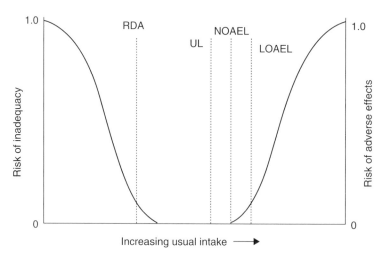

Figure 16.3 Theoretical description of health effects of a nutrient as a function of level of intake. As intakes increase above the tolerable upper intake level (UL) the risk of adverse effects incerases. RDA: recommended daily allowance; NOAEL: no observed adverse effect level; LOAEL: lowest observed adverse effect level.

Dose–response assessment

The dose–response assessment involves a number of key components.

Selection of the critical data set

The data evaluation process results in the selection of the most appropriate or critical data set(s) for deriving the UL. The critical data set defines the dose–response relationship between intake and the extent of the adverse health effect known to be the most relevant to humans. Data on bioavailability need to be considered and adjustments in expressions of dose–response are made to determine whether any apparent differences in dose–response between different forms of a nutrient can be explained. The critical data set should document the form of the nutrient investigated, the route of exposure, magnitude and duration of intake, and the intake that does not produce adverse health effects, as well as the intake that produces adverse health effects.

Identification of the no observed adverse effect level or lowest observed adverse effect level and critical end-point

The no observed adverse effect level (NOAEL) is the highest intake of a nutrient at which no adverse effects have been observed. The NOAEL can be identified from evaluation of the critical data set. If there are no adequate data demonstrating a NOAEL, then a lowest observed adverse effect level (LOAEL, the lowest intake

at which an adverse effect has been demonstrated) may be used. Where different adverse health effects (or end-points) occur for a nutrient, the NOAELs (or LOAELs) for these end-points will differ. The critical end-point is the adverse health effect exhibiting the lowest NOAEL (i.e. the most sensitive indicator of a nutrient's adverse effects). The derivation of a UL based on the most sensitive end-point will ensure protection against all other adverse health effects.

Uncertainty assessment

There are usually several scientific uncertainties associated with extrapolation from the observed data to the general population and several judgments must be made in deriving uncertainty factors to account for the individual uncertainties. The individual uncertainty factors may be combined into a single composite uncertainty factor for each nutrient, and applying this (composite) uncertainty factor (UF) to a NOAEL (or LOAEL) will result in a value for the derived UL that is less than the experimentally derived NOAEL, unless the uncertainty factor is 1.0. The larger the uncertainty, the larger the UFs and the lower the UL.

UFs are used to account for imprecision of the data, lack of data and adequacy of the data on variability between individuals. There are several potential sources of uncertainty, including:

- interindividual variation and sensitivity with respect to the adverse effect

- extrapolation from experimental animal data to humans
- if a NOAEL is not available, a UF may be applied to account for the uncertainty in deriving a UL from the LOAEL
- using a subchronic NOAEL to predict chronic NOAEL.

The UFs are lower with higher quality data and when the adverse effects are extremely mild and reversible. For example, for magnesium a UF of 1.0 may be used since the adverse effect (osmotic diarrhea) is relatively mild and reversible, there is a sufficiently large amount of data available relating magnesium intake level to this adverse effect in humans to cover adequately the range of interindividual variation in sensitivity, and a clear NOAEL can be established. In contrast, for vitamin B_6 a UF of 4 may be used since the adverse effect (neurotoxicity) is potentially severe, there are only limited data, mainly from inadequate studies of insufficient duration, relating vitamin B_6 intake level to this adverse effect in humans, and no clear NOAEL can be established.

In the application of uncertainty factors there should be cognizance of nutritional needs, e.g. the derived UL should not be lower than the recommended intake.

Derivation of tolerable upper intake levels

The UL is derived by dividing the NOAEL (or LOAEL) by the (composite) UF. ULs are derived for different lifestage groups using relevant data. In the absence of data for a particular lifestage group, extrapolations are made from the UL for other groups on the basis of known differences in body size, physiology, metabolism, absorption and excretion of a nutrient. For example, when data are not available for children and adolescents, extrapolations are usually made on the basis of body weight using the reference weights for adults and children in the population.

To the extent possible, ULs are derived for separate lifestage groups (e.g. infants, children, adults, the elderly, and women during pregnancy or lactation). Although within relatively homogeneous lifestage groups there is a range of sensitivities to adverse health effects due, for example, to differences in body weight and lean body mass, it is generally not possible to make a distinction between males and females in establishing ULs for adults or children.

Table 16.3 Examples of tolerable upper intake levels (ULs) for vitamins and minerals

Nutrient	UL (adults)	Adverse effect
Retinol	3000 μg	Teratogenicity, hepatotoxicity
Vitamin D	50 μg	Hypercalcemia
Vitamin E	1000 mg	Hemorrhagic effects
Vitamin B_6	25 mg	Sensory neuropathy
Folic acid	1000 μg	Progression of neuropathy or masking of anemia in B_{12} deficiency
Vitamin C	2000 mg	Osmotic diarrhea, gastrointestinal disturbances
Calcium	2500 mg	Milk alkali syndrome
Magnesium	250 mg (supplemental)	Osmotic diarrhea
Phosphorus	4000 mg	Hyperphosphatemia
Iron	45 mg (supplemental)	Gastrointestinal effects
Zinc	40 mg	Reduced copper status
Copper	10 mg	Hepatotoxicity
Manganese	11 mg	Neurotoxicity
Selenium	300 μg	Clinical selenosis: brittle nails, hair loss
Iodine	1100 μg	Thyrotoxicosis

ULs taken from US Food and Nutrition Board and EU Scientific Committee on Food.

The derivation of ULs for the normal healthy population, divided into various lifestage groups, accounts for normally expected variability in sensitivity, but it excludes subpopulations with extreme and distinct vulnerabilities due to genetic predisposition or other considerations. (Including these would result in ULs that are significantly lower than are needed to protect most people against the adverse effects of high intakes.) Subpopulations needing special protection are better served through the use of public health screening, health-care providers, product labeling or other individualized strategies. The extent to which a subpopulation becomes significant enough to be assumed to be representative of a general population is an area of judgment and risk management.

It should be noted that derivation of a UL does not take into account possible adverse effects of acute bolus dosages. In general, adverse effects from acute or short-term intake require much greater intake levels than those arising from long-term or chronic exposure.

ULs have been derived for a number of vitamins and minerals (Table 16.3) and examples of the derivation of UL for selenium and vitamin D are given in Boxes 16.4 and 16.5. Adverse effects associated with

Box 16.4 Derivation of UL for selenium

- Chronic selenosis has been described in regions of high soil selenium in China. Symptoms include hair and nail brittleness and loss, skin rash, mottled teeth, garlic-breath odor and neurological disturbances including peripheral anesthesia, with numbness, convulsions, paralysis and motor disturbances in more severe cases.
- The high prevalence of selenosis in Enshi, South China, provided an opportunity for the study of the dose–response relationship of selenium intake to selenosis in 350 adults during the 1980s. Toxic effects occurred with increasing frequency as selenium intake increased above 850 μg/day. Lowering selenium intake in affected individuals led to the disappearance of symptoms. The LOAEL for clinical symptoms of selenosis is about 900–1000 μg Se/day and a NOAEL of 850 μg/day can be established.
- A UF of 3 may be used to cover uncertainties in the data (the NOAEL used was derived from a study on a large number of subjects and is expected to include sensitive individuals; although the toxic effect is not severe, it may not be readily reversible). This leads to a UL of 300 μg/day for adults.
- This UL may also be applied to pregnant and lactating women as there is no evidence to indicate that there is increased sensitivity of the fetus or breast-fed infant to high levels of maternal selenium intake.
- Owing to insufficient data on adverse effects of selenium in children, extrapolation from the UL for adults to children on a body-weight basis may be performed to derive a UL for children.

Box 16.5 Derivation of UL for vitamin D

- Vitamin D toxicity has been described in individuals consuming excessive amounts of vitamin D-containing supplements. The effects observed include damage to kidney and other soft tissues such as blood vessels, heart and lungs, owing to calcification. This results from hypercalcemia caused by a vitamin D-induced increase in calcium absorption in the gastrointestinal tract and calcium resorption from bone. Elevated serum 25-hydroxyvitamin D (an indicator of vitamin D status) levels may be used to confirm that the hypercalcemia is vitamin D induced.
- Data from controlled studies of the response of serum 25-hydroxyvitamin D to increasing intakes of vitamin D intake in human subjects may be used to establish the dose–response. A NOAEL of 100 μg/day can be established as the highest intake that does not result in elevation of serum 25-hydroxyvitamin D above the upper end of the reference range.
- A UF of 2 may be used to cover uncertainties in the data (i.e. to cover the range of interindividual sensitivity in the population). This leads to a UL of 50 μg/day for adults. This UL may also be applied to pregnant and lactating women as there is evidence to suggest that there is no increased sensitivity of the fetus or breast-fed infant to this level of maternal vitamin D intake.
- Although there are insufficient data for adverse effects of vitamin D in children, a UL of 50 μg/day may be used for children of 10 years and older and, for children aged 1–9 years, extrapolation from the UL for adults on a body-weight basis may be performed to derive a UL.

Box 16.6 Vitamin C high intakes: myths and facts

- Vitamin C is often taken in large amounts (500 mg/day or more) for presumed health benefits. Evidence to date does not support a role for high doses of vitamin C in prevention of the common cold, although there is a moderate benefit in terms of duration and severity of episodes in some groups. Although there is epidemiological evidence to suggest a protective effect of vitamin C against cardiovascular disease, some cancers (e.g. stomach, lung) and cataract, such benefits have not been established unequivocally.
- It has been suggested that antioxidants such as vitamin C may act as pro-oxidants at high intake levels. This is partly based on *in vitro* observations that ascorbic acid may interact with free iron or copper to promote lipid peroxidation or oxidative damage to DNA. However, this hypothesis has not been substantiated *in vivo*, where both iron and copper are normally tightly bound to transport and storage proteins and are unavailable to participate in such redox reactions.
- Reports of increased urinary oxalate excretion and kidney stone formation with high intakes of vitamin C have not been confirmed. Such effects are considered unlikely given the limited intestinal absorption of vitamin C at doses greater than 200 mg/day.
- A UL of 2000 mg/day may be derived based on osmotic diarrhea and related gastrointestinal disturbances that arise from the osmotic effect of unabsorbed vitamin C passing through the intestine when the capacity of the saturable absorption system has been exceeded.

high intakes of vitamin C, β-carotene and vitamin A are outlined in Boxes 16.6–16.8. While ULs are usually based on total intake of a nutrient, in some cases adverse health effects have been associated with intake from a particular source, such as supplements, rather than total intake, and in such cases the UL is based on intake from these sources only. For many nutrients there are no systematic studies of the adverse health effects of high intakes and UL is derived from limited data. Experience has shown that it is not always possible to establish a UL for a micronutrient using the science-based risk-assessment approach. Such a situation can arise for different reasons:

- evidence of the absence of any adverse health effects at high intakes
- lack of evidence of any adverse effect; this does not necessarily mean that there is no potential for adverse effects resulting from high intake
- evidence of adverse effects but insufficient data on which to base a dose–response assessment.

Box 16.7 β-Carotene supplementation and smoking

- Prospective epidemiological studies have shown that higher consumption of carotenoid-containing fruits and vegetables and higher plasma levels of carotenoids, including β-carotene, are associated with a lower risk of a number of cancers and cardiovascular disease.
- Several long-term intervention studies with supplemental β-carotene have not shown a reduction in chronic disease risk. Indeed, two of the studies carried out in the 1990s reported an increase in lung cancer associated with supplemental β-carotene (20–30 mg/day for 4–8 years) in current smokers. However, another study reported that supplementation with 25 mg/day β-carotene for up to 12 years (including smokers and non-smokers) showed no excess of lung cancer.
- No other adverse effects have been described for β-carotene. For example, no toxic effects have been reported from the therapeutic use of β-carotene at high doses (about 180 mg/day) over many years for the treatment of erythropoietic protoporphyria, a photosensitivity disorder. Carotenodermia, a yellowish discoloration of the skin, is a harmless and well-documented effect of excess intake of β-carotene and other carotenoids.
- At present the data on the potential for β-carotene to produce increased lung cancer are conflicting and not sufficient for a dose–response assessment and derivation of a UL. However, caution is advised in the use of β-carotene supplements.
- This does not conflict with dietary advice for fruit and vegetable consumption (e.g. five or more servings per day) since this provides much lower intakes of β-carotene (3–6 mg/day), which is also of lower bioavailability, than the supplemental intake levels associated with possible adverse effects (20 mg/day or more).

Box 16.8 Vitamin A toxicity

- High intakes [in excess of 3000 μg retinol equivalents (RE)/day] of preformed vitamin A (retinol and related compounds) appear to be teratogenic in humans, resulting in craniofacial malformations and abnormalities of the central nervous system (except for neural tube defects), thymus and heart. Evidence for this includes epidemiological studies on vitamin A intake level and pregnancy outcome, established teratogenicity in humans of therapeutic use of retinoic acid (a vitamin A metabolite), as well as established teratogenicity of vitamin A in a number of animal species.
- Hepatotoxicity is one of the most severe outcomes of chronic intake of high dosages of vitamin A (generally in excess of about 15 000 μg RE/day in supplements or in rich food sources such as liver and liver oils), arising from overload of the storage capacity of the liver for the vitamin.
- Some epidemiological studies have indicated that intakes of vitamin A in excess of 1500 μg RE/day may reduce bone mineral density and increase the risk of osteoporosis and hip fractures in some population groups, particularly in pre- and postmenopausal women. However, other studies have not found such an effect and this conflicting evidence is not adequate to establish a causal relationship or a UL.
- A UL of 3000 μg RE/day may be derived for women of reproductive age based on epidemiological data on the occurrence of birth defects in infants of exposed mothers. For other adults a UL of 3000 μg RE/day may be derived based on case reports of hepatotoxicity arising from prolonged overconsumption of vitamin A.

16.13 Use of tolerable upper intake levels as dietary reference standards

The UL is a dietary reference standard that can be used for both the evaluation and management of risk of excessive intake of vitamins or minerals in individuals or populations. The UL is not in itself an indication of risk. However, the UL can be applied to data derived from intake assessment (e.g. the distribution of usual total daily nutrient intakes among members of the general population) to identify those individuals or population groups at risk and the circumstances in which risk is likely to occur. In general, risk is considered to be the probability of an adverse effect (and its severity) and will depend on the fraction of the population exceeding the UL and the magnitude and duration of such excesses.

Individuals

It is not possible to identify a single risk-free intake level for a nutrient that can be applied with certainty to all members of a population. However, if an individual's usual nutrient intake remains below the UL there is no appreciable risk of adverse effects from excessive intake. At usual intakes above the UL the risk of adverse effects increases with increasing level of intake. However, the intake at which a given individual will develop adverse health effects as a result of taking large amounts of a nutrient is not known with certainty. The UL can be used as a guide for the maximum level of usual intake of individuals, although it is not a recommended intake. Occasional excursions above the UL are possible without an appreciable risk of adverse health effects.

Groups

The proportion of the population with usual intakes below the UL is likely to be at no appreciable risk of adverse health effects due to overconsumption, while the proportion above the UL may be at some risk, the magnitude of which depends on the magnitude and duration of the excess. The UL is derived to apply to the most sensitive members of the general population. Thus, many members of the population may regularly consume nutrients at or even somewhat above the UL without experiencing adverse effects. However, because it is not known which individuals are most sensitive, it is necessary to interpret the UL as applying to all individuals.

In the management of risk of excessive intake of vitamins or minerals in individuals or populations the UL can be used in several ways. For example, it may be used for setting maximum levels of addition of vitamins and minerals to foods or nutritional supplements such that the risk of excessive intake in the population is minimized. It is also a useful basis for providing information and advice to individuals or groups on maximum intake levels of nutrients, such as in the labeling of nutritional supplements.

16.14 Perspectives on the future

The application of science-based risk-assessment methods to the establishment of upper intake levels for vitamins and minerals represents a significant advance in providing dietary reference standards for evaluating and managing the risk of overconsumption of these nutrients. These reference standards will be increasingly used in nutritional surveillance as studies on nutrient intakes in populations pay greater attention to the possibility of overconsumption of micronutrients resulting from the wider use of nutritional supplements and consumption of fortified foods in some countries.

This field is still limited by a lack of good data on dose–response relationships for adverse health effects of micronutrients in humans. To improve the understanding of such effects research is needed to provide better knowledge of the physiological effects of micronutrients at the molecular, cellular and whole-body levels, and of the kinetics of their absorption, metabolism and excretion at different dietary levels of intake.

Further reading

Obesity

Barlow SE, Dietz WH. Obesity evaluation and treatment: expert committee recommendations. The Maternal and Child Health Bureau, Health Resources and Services Administration, and the Department of Health and Human Services. Pediatrics 1998; 102: E29.

Boss O, SS, Paoloni-Giacobino A *et al*. Uncoupling protein-3: a new member of the mitochondrial carrier family with tissue-specific expression. FEBS Lett 1997; 498: 39–42.

Bray G, PB, Popkin BM. Dietary fat intake does affect obesity! Am J Clin Nutr 1998; 68: 1157–1173.

Cole TJ, BM, Flegal KM, Dietz WH. Establishing a standard definition for child overweight and obesity worldwide: international survey. BMJ 2000; 320: 240.

Fleury C, NM, Neverova M, Collins S *et al*. Uncoupling protein-2: a novel gene linked to obesity and hyperinsulinemia. Nat Genet 1997; 15: 269–272.

Hamill PV, 'Drizd TA, Johnson CL, Reed RB, Roche AF, Moore WM. Physical growth: National Center for Health Statistics percentiles. Am J Clin Nutr 1979; 32(3): 607–629.

Levien JA, Eberhardt NL, Jensen MD. Role of non-exercise activity thermogenesis in resistance to fat gain in humans. Science 1999; 283: 212–214.

Matsuzawa Y, Shimomura I, Nakamura T, Keno Y, Kotani K, Tokunaga K. Pathophysiology and pathogenesis of visceral fat obesity. Obesity Research 1995; 3(Suppl. 2) 187S–194S.

Prentice AM, Jebb SA. Obesity in Britain, gluttony or sloth? BMJ 1995; 311: 437–439.

Stock MJ. Gluttony and thermogenesis revisited. Int J Obes Relat Metab Disord 1999; 23(11): 1105–1117.

Vitamin and mineral overconsumption

European Commission Scientific Committee on Food. Tolerable Upper Intake Levels for Vitamins and Minerals, 2000/01. http://www.europa.eu.int/comm/food/fs/sc/scf/index_en.html

FAO/WHO (Food and Agricultural Organization of the UN/World Health Organisation, Expert Consultation) 1995. Application of Risk Analysis to Food Standards Issues. Recommendations to the Codex Alimentarius Commission (ALINORM 95/9, Appendix 5).

Food and Nutrition Board, Institute of Medicine, National Academy of Sciences. Dietary Reference Intakes. Washington, DC: National Academy Press, 1997–2001. http://www.nap.edu/

Food and Nutrition Board, Institute of Medicine, National Academy of Sciences. Dietary Reference Intakes: Applications in Dietary Assessment: A Report of the Subcommittees on Interpretation and Uses of Dietary Reference Intakes and Upper Reference Levels of Nutrients, and the Standing Committee on the Scientific Evaluation of Dietary Reference Intakes, Food and Nutrition Board. Washington, DC: National Academy Press, 2001. http://www.nap.edu/catalog/9956.html

World Health Organization. Trace Elements in Human Nutrition and Health. Geneva: WHO (Prepared in Collaboration with the FAO of the UN and the IAEA), 1996.

17
Undernutrition

Mario Vaz

Key messages

- Undernutrition within the context of chronic energy deficiency (CED) may be defined as a steady state at which a person is in energy balance, although at a 'cost'.
- Classification of CED is based on the extent of the reduction of body mass index and physical activity level. Socioeconomic status can also contribute to CED, and should be taken into account when appropriate.
- To maintain homeostasis, the body adapts in CED to lower energy intake to ensure survival. Individuals with CED have lower body weights, fat-free mass and fat stores. These changes in body composition conserve energy expenditure in CED.

- Several components of daily energy expenditure are altered in CED: resting metabolic rate, physical activity and thermogenesis.
- The nervous and endocrine systems are key regulatory mechanisms that favor energy conservation in CED.
- In humans the physiological or functional consequences of CED include reduced muscle strength and endurance, reduced immunity and altered autonomic nervous function. Each of these has important implications for lifestyle and health status.

17.1 Introduction

Close to 800 million people in the world are believed to be undernourished. There are, however, large regional differences in the prevalence of undernutrition. This chapter will focus predominantly on adult undernutrition. Malnutrition in children is dealt with in the *Clinical Nutrition* textbook in this series.

17.2 Definition and classification of undernutrition

Undernutrition encompasses a wide range of macronutrient and micronutrient deficiencies. Micronutrient deficiencies, for instance, include those of water-soluble vitamins (thiamìn, riboflavin and niacin), fat-soluble vitamins (e.g. vitamin A and vitamin D) and minerals (e.g. iodine and iron). Deficiencies of these micronutrients, if severe, lead to classic clinical presentations. Niacin deficiency, for instance, leads to pellagra, characterized by 'Cassal's necklace', a typical skin lesion around the neck.

Iodine deficiency is associated with a 'goiter', a swelling of the thyroid gland. Iron deficiency, which is widespread throughout the world and particularly in developing countries, is associated with anemia. Detailed discussions of micronutrient deficiencies are dealt with in the relevant chapters dedicated to these nutrients in *Introduction to Human Nutrition*. This chapter deals primarily with energy deficiency.

In 1988, James, Ferro-Luzzi and Waterlow drew a distinction between acute energy deficiency (AED) and chronic energy deficiency (CED). AED was defined as 'a state of negative energy balance, i.e. a progressive loss of body energy'. This occurs in a variety of clinical conditions associated with acute weight loss, including anorexia nervosa, cancer and malabsorption disorders. In contrast, CED was defined as a 'steady state at which a person is in energy balance although at a "cost"'. Issues pertaining to AED are dealt with in Chapter 5 in Section 5.7, on the metabolic consequences of starvation.

One way to identify individuals who are energy deficient is to assess their actual energy intakes in relation

Table 17.1 Classification of chronic energy deficiency (CED) according to body mass index (BMI) and physical activity level (PAL)

	Normal		Chronic energy deficiency			
			Grade I		Grade II	Grade III
BMI	⩾18.5	17.0–18.4	17.0–18.4	16.0–17.0	16.0–17.0	<16.0
PAL[a]	–	⩾1.4	<1.4	⩾1.4	<1.4	–

Modified from James *et al.* (1988) and data reproduced with permission.
[a] In this system, PAL is calculated as the measured energy intake or expenditure divided by basal metabolic rate.

to what is 'adequate'. The problem is clearly to delineate what is adequate. An adequate energy intake might reasonably be seen as the amount of energy that is required to sustain life's processes under reasonable conditions of activity. On this basis, if we were to define adequate as the amount of energy required to sustain an individual with a sedentary physical activity pattern, we could then identify an individual whose intake falls below this level.

Individuals of different body sizes have different basal metabolic rates (BMR), and BMRs can now be estimated using prediction equations. During the course of a day a sedentary individual expends a total energy that is about 1.4 times the BMR. This multiplicative factor of BMR is called a physical activity level (PAL). The actual PAL of an individual can be computed as the daily energy intake divided by the BMR. Thus, individuals who have a PAL of <1.4 are clearly obtaining insufficient energy to support a sedentary lifestyle. Incidentally, studies have shown that a PAL of less than 1.4 is only seen in individuals who spend less than 4–5 h a day on their feet. In energy balance, energy intake is equal to the energy expended, and thus PAL can also be computed as the daily energy expenditure divided by the BMR. The identification of individuals with CED would be enhanced if we could combine the measurement of PAL with an additional, independent factor that reflects energy deficiency.

With energy deficiency there is a reduction in body weight and in energy stores [fat and fat-free mass (FFM)]. A simple index of body energy stores is the body mass index (BMI): weight (kg)/height^2 (m). Thus, theoretically, BMI could be used to identify individuals who are energy deficient. The problem is to define the BMI cut-off. Based on the range of BMIs in healthy populations and on studies identifying the functional consequences of a low BMI, the lower limit of a desirable BMI has been fixed at 18.5 kg/m^2.

Table 17.1 provides a classification of CED based on the two principles outlined in the earlier paragraphs. It categorizes CED, based on a combination of a low PAL (signifying an inadequate energy intake) and a low BMI (signifying inadequate energy stores).

Individuals with marginally lower energy stores (BMI 17.0–18.4) but adequate energy intakes (PAL ⩾1.4) are deemed normal. If, however, individuals have both marginally lower energy stores (BMI 17.0–18.4) and lower than adequate energy intakes (PAL < 1.4), they are categorized as grade I CED.

In several situations, the estimations of energy intake or energy expenditure become impractical. Under these circumstances, in developing countries, the combination of BMI with an index of socioeconomic status has been used to identify CED. The assumption is that individuals of a low socioeconomic status are more likely to be at risk of energy deprivation. The problems of this system of identifying CED are that local socioeconomic scales have to be devised, and these must be subjected to periodic revision to take into account changing economic and social conditions.

In situations where a large population needs to be surveyed, BMI alone may be used as a simple, but objective anthropometric indicator of nutritional status of the adult population. When applied to large numbers of people (populations), BMI is sensitive to socioeconomic status and to seasonal fluctuations in food consumption levels, and has been recommended as the method of choice to assess the numbers of people who are undernourished worldwide.

To summarize, in different situations, CED may be identified on the basis of:

- a combination of BMI and PAL
- a combination of BMI and socioeconomic status
- BMI alone.

17.3 Adaptation and chronic energy deficiency

When there is a sudden change in the internal environment of cells and tissues, the body calls on regulatory processes to maintain the constancy of the internal environment. This maintenance of internal constancy is called homeostasis. When the change in the internal or external environment is for a longer period, the body may need to evoke greater changes, in both structure and function, in order to survive. Adaptation is, thus, the process by which an organism maintains physiological activity and survives when there is a sustained alteration in the environment with respect to one or more parameters. These adaptive processes remain in place so long as the alteration in the environment persists. While this simplistic overview of adaptation may suggest that adaptation is without any detrimental consequences, this chapter will demonstrate that adaptation does indeed have a 'cost'.

- Adaptation is the response of the body to a sustained perturbation in the environment, with the aim of ensuring function and survival.
- Adaptation persists for as long as the perturbation is maintained.
- Every adaptation has a cost.

In CED, the sustained environmental perturbation is a lower energy intake. It is conceivable that the body adapts to this situation, to ensure the survival of the individual. A suitable adaptation would be somehow to limit energy expenditure so that the individual remains in energy balance, albeit at a lower energy intake. Interest in the patterns of energy expenditure in CED subjects has, in part, been due to anecdotal evidence that many of these individuals are involved in heavy physical activity (laborers, coolies, agricultural workers, etc.), despite their limited energy intakes. This apparent discrepancy suggests that CED subjects evoke energy-saving mechanisms to function adequately and to survive. The potential mechanisms that aid in the conservation of energy in CED are discussed below.

17.4 Changes in body composition in chronic energy deficiency

Before proceeding further, it is worthwhile to have a picture of what individuals with CED look like in terms

Table 17.2 Anthropometric characteristics of a subject with chronic energy deficiency (CED) compared with a well-nourished subject

	CED	Well-nourished
Weight (kg)	42	69
Height (cm)	160	175
Body mass index (kg/m²)	**16.5**	**22.5**
Fat (%)	10	20
Fat mass (kg)	4	14
Fat-free mass (kg)	38	55

of their body composition. This is illustrated in Table 17.2, which compares a typical male CED individual with his well-nourished counterpart.

Table 17.2 indicates that individuals with CED have lower body weights, fat free mass (FFM) and fat stores. In addition, individuals with CED subjects may be shorter, and this is taken as evidence of long-standing energy depriva-tion, dating back to the years of linear growth. These changes in body composition help to conserve energy in CED. For instance, the lower body weight results in a lower energy cost of physical activity, particularly with weight-bearing activities. The reduction in metabolically active FFM ensures a lower BMR, in absolute terms. A reduction in these two major components of daily energy expenditure results in considerable energy saving for the individual who is chronically energy deficient. Later, we shall see that the benefits of the changes in body composition in the individual with CED which favor energy conservation are offset by some derangements in normal physiology. In contrast to the energy-saving benefit of a lower body weight and a lower FFM, the reduction in fat stores, and the attendant loss in heat insulation, would be expected, if anything, to enhance energy expenditure during cold exposure. This is discussed in greater detail later in this chapter.

17.5 Energy metabolism in chronic energy deficiency

Many researchers have attempted to determine whether CED subjects have energy-saving mechanisms that are independent of the loss in body weight and FFM. This inference could be made if the metabolic rate per unit of metabolically active tissue were lower than in well-nourished subjects. The most easily measurable form of metabolically active tissue is the FFM. Studies conducted so far have targeted most components of daily energy expenditure and these are discussed in greater detail below.

Basal metabolic rate/resting metabolic rate

Classic studies on acute energy deprivation by Benedict, Keys *et al.*, and Grande indicated that semi-starvation was associated with a reduction in resting metabolic rate (RMR). This reduction was explained both by a reduction in body weight and by a reduction in the metabolic activity of the tissues (metabolic efficiency). These findings have been replicated in more recent studies on obese subjects with restricted diets. The varying duration of energy restriction, however, makes comparisons between these studies difficult, particularly since there is some evidence that the reduction in RMR may occur in two phases. An initial phase of 2 or 3 weeks is associated with enhanced metabolic efficiency, while the further reduction in RMR with continued energy restriction beyond this period is largely accounted for by a loss of active tissue mass.

Chronically energy-deficient subjects also have reduced BMRs in absolute terms. 'Metabolic efficiency' in early studies, right up to the 1980s, was essentially determined by dividing BMR by the active tissue mass (usually FFM). Some, but not all studies, showed a decrease in BMR/kg FFM. In recent years, there have been detailed discussions on whether this computation of metabolic efficiency is appropriate. While the relationship between BMR and FFM is linear, there is a positive intercept, which means that smaller individuals have a higher BMR/kg FFM. This higher BMR/kg FFM may, in part, be related to the fact that the proportion of muscle mass lost from FFM is substantially more than the proportion of viscera. Resting skeletal muscle mass is metabolically less active than viscera. Thus, the relatively higher viscera to muscle mass ratio in CED would be associated with a higher BMR/kg FFM.

A more appropriate statistical method to adjust BMR for FFM is the analysis of covariance (ANCOVA). In this method, it is assumed that since there is a linear relationship between FFM and BMR, changes in x (FFM) will affect the mean value of y (BMR). However, since x (FFM) is different between well-nourished and CED subjects, it follows that differences in y (BMR) between the two groups will be explained at least in part by the differences in x (FFM). The ANCOVA attempts a comparison of the BMRs of the two groups at the same FFM.

More recent studies in CED that have used this statistical method have indicated that BMR is reduced in CED when adjusted for FFM using an ANCOVA.

Thus, CED subjects have a lower BMR, largely due to a lower body weight and a reduced active tissue mass. There is some evidence of increased metabolic efficiency in CED in terms of a reduced BMR when adjusted for FFM.

Physical activity

One of the ways in which an individual with CED could conserve energy is by being less physically active. This is, in fact, what has been observed in laboratory experiments involving semistarvation for a long duration. It is more difficult to establish whether individuals with CED reduce their physical activity under free-living conditions. Earlier studies used the laborious method of time-and-motion analysis. In this method, trained observers accompany subjects and note their activities in a diary for the entire duration of a day or several days. The development of the doubly labeled water technique (see Chapter 2 of Introduction to Human Nutrition) has allowed for the estimation of free-living energy expenditure and, consequently, also of PALs. There are some data to suggest that individuals of low BMI can sustain high levels of physical activity at least over the periods of measurement. There is a possibility, however, particularly in largely agrarian societies, that CED subjects may show large seasonal variations in physical activity.

Another way in which CED subjects may conserve energy is by an enhanced 'efficiency'. There are many ways in which efficiency is defined in exercise physiology. One of the more common terms is 'mechanical efficiency'. Mechanical efficiency is expressed as a percentage, and is the ratio of external work performed, to the energy expended. The mechanical efficiency of performing activities such as climbing stairs and cycling is in the region of about 20–25%. The rest of the energy expended is dissipated as heat. Several laboratory studies in CED subjects have assessed mechanical efficiency during stepping, treadmill walking and cycling. When viewed together, there is no compelling evidence, yet, to support the notion that CED subjects have a greater mechanical efficiency.

It is also conceivable that CED subjects may minimize the energy cost of physical activity by performing tasks in such a manner that reduces unnecessary movements, or results in a better balance of loads ('ergonomic efficiency'). In Africa, for instance, women of the Luo and

Kikuyu tribes can carry substantial loads with great economy. The possibility of an enhanced ergonomic efficiency in CED subjects needs to be investigated further.

Following strenuous, sustained, physical exercise, energy expenditure may be elevated for up to 24 h. This enhanced energy expenditure is sometimes called the excess postexercise oxygen consumption (EPOC). There is some evidence that EPOC is reduced in CED subjects, both in the immediate period following exercise and in the delayed period of about 12 h after exercise.

To summarize, CED subjects may potentially conserve energy in relation to physical activity by the following means:

- decreased physical activity
- increased mechanical efficiency
- enhanced ergonomic efficiency
- reduced EPOC.

A more detailed account of physical activity in provided in Chapter 18.

Thermogenesis

The thermic effect of food (TEF) comprises approximately 10% of daily energy expenditure and is defined as the rise in energy expenditure following the consumption of food. There are many factors that determine TEF, including the size and composition of the meal, the palatability of the food and the antecedent dietary intake. Because there is a very limited amount of data on TEF in CED, it is difficult to comment on whether TEF is reduced in this state. There is some evidence that the TEF/kg FFM in CED subjects following a mixed meal is higher than in their well-nourished counterparts. Intercountry comparisons have demonstrated that Gambian men (not necessarily of low BMI) in the 'hungry' season have a lower TEF than Europeans.

On exposure to cold, individuals rely on both heat-conserving and heat-generating mechanisms to maintain body temperature. The heat-conserving mechanisms include the insulation provided by subcutaneous fat and vasoconstriction of peripheral blood vessels, particularly in skin and skeletal muscle. Vasoconstriction limits the amount of warm blood that is brought to the surface of the body. Thus, less heat is lost from the body. Heat-generating mechanisms include non-shivering thermogenesis (NST) and shivering. NST is largely mediated by the sympathetic nervous system,

which enhances a whole host of metabolic processes including glycogenolysis in liver and muscle, gluconeogenesis and lipolysis. NST has been studied under laboratory conditions by infusing either epinephrine (adrenaline) or norepinephrine (noradrenaline) intravenously into volunteers. These studies suggest that thermogenesis to exogenously administered catecholamines may be lower in CED subjects. On exposure to mild cold, CED subjects are able to thermoregulate adequately. Greater vasoconstriction of the peripheral blood vessels and an earlier onset of NST compensate for the lack of fat insulation. With more intense cold, however, undernourished subjects show reduced thermogenesis and are unable to thermoregulate adequately. Any energy conservation is therefore offset by their increased susceptibility to hypothermia in response to cold exposure. There is speculation that the high number of deaths during cold waves in developing countries may be related to this factor.

Protein metabolism in relation to energy expenditure

There have been few studies in CED that have explored the relationship of protein metabolism and energy expenditure. The impetus for these investigations is the knowledge that protein synthesis contributes substantially to the BMR. Thus, a reduction in protein synthetic rates could conceivably reduce BMR and result in energy conservation. The studies demonstrate that while BMR and protein synthesis are both lower than in well-nourished subjects in absolute terms, there are no differences when protein turnover (synthesis and breakdown) is expressed per kilogram of FFM.

Energy expenditure during pregnancy

Pregnancy and lactation place increased energy demands on the mother. This is a situation where CED subjects are particularly vulnerable. Studies carried out on Gambian women have indicated that BMR is depressed during the first 18 weeks of gestation and that the total metabolic costs over 36 weeks of pregnancy are far lower than in well-nourished women in Western populations. These results imply some energy-saving mechanisms. In this particular study, however, the vast majority of women had BMIs in excess of 18.5. In contrast to the findings in the Gambia, studies on well-nourished pregnant Indian women, as well as Chinese and Malay women in Asia, failed to identify any conservation of energy during pregnancy. One of the consequences of a low BMI in pregnant women is the birth of babies of low birth weight. This is of importance because a low birth weight is associated with increased infant mortality. In addition, low birthweight babies may be more susceptible to chronic disease if they survive into adulthood. The metabolism of pregnancy and lactation is dealt with in greater detail in Chapter 6.

17.6 Regulatory processes in chronic energy deficiency

The two large regulatory systems in the body are the nervous system and the endocrine (hormonal) system, and both can modulate metabolic rate.

One of the components of the nervous system that has been studied fairly extensively in relation to metabolic activity is the sympathetic nervous system (SNS). Classic studies by Young and Landsberg demonstrated a reduction in SNS activity in animal models with underfeeding, and an enhanced SNS activity with overfeeding. Pharmacological studies demonstrated that virtually all components of daily energy expenditure, including BMR, were reduced when SNS activity was blocked. Thus, a hypothesis has emerged that attempts to explain a putative reduction in metabolic activity in CED on the basis of diminished SNS activity. Short-term underfeeding experiments in humans support the hypothesis of a reduced SNS activity with reduced energy intakes. In CED too, there is evidence of reduced SNS activity. There have, however, been no studies that have measured metabolic rates in CED in the presence of SNS blockade.

Among the hormones, one that particularly stands out in terms of metabolic regulation is thyroid hormone (thyroxine). Indeed, there was a time before thyroxine levels could be measured in blood, when hypothyroidism was diagnosed on the basis of a reduced BMR. Thyroid hormone exists in two forms, T_4 and T_3. Of these, T_3 is biologically more active and is derived from T_4. Several studies have demonstrated that T_3 is reduced with starvation and acute underfeeding experiments, and that this is, in part, due to a reduced conversion of T_4 to T_3. Alteration in thyroid hormone status has been incompletely characterized in CED.

Several other hormones, such as glucagon, glucocorticoids, growth hormone, insulin-like growth factors and progesterone, could potentially modulate metabolic rate. The role of these hormones in CED has not been studied adequately.

17.7 Functional consequences of energy deficiency

This section explores some of the consequences of energy deficiency in terms of the cost of adaptation. Table 17.3 summarizes this in terms of functional changes and real-life consequences.

Muscle function

Several laboratory studies have demonstrated that CED is associated with a reduction in muscle strength as well as muscle endurance. The reduction in muscle strength is to a large extent associated with a reduction in muscle mass. Some studies have, however, indicated that the loss in strength persists even after correcting for muscle mass. In other words, muscle strength per unit muscle area or mass is less than in well-nourished subjects. This suggests that there are functional changes in skeletal muscle with CED.

Skeletal muscle is made up of two large categories of muscle fiber types. Type I fibers are increased in marathon runners and are important for endurance. Type II muscle fibers are increased in weightlifters and are a determinant of muscle strength. In undernutrition, there is a decline in type II fibers and this may account for the decline in muscle strength. There are also reports of a conversion of type II fibers to type I fibers. This has a benefit in energetic terms, because the type I fibers use less adenosine triphosphate (ATP) during muscle contraction than type II fibers. In addition to the changes in muscle fiber type, undernutrition is associated with a reduction in sources of energy within skeletal muscle, such as glycogen, ATP and phosphocreatinine. A reduction in these energy sources could impair muscle function.

Table 17.3 Real-life consequences of physiological functional changes that occur in chronic energy deficiency (CED)

Functional changes in CED	Real-life consequences
Reduced muscle strength and endurance	Decreased work performance and earning capacity
Reduced immunity	More infections, increased sickness, loss of working days
Altered autonomic nervous function	Possibly altered drug dosage requirements. Consequences with aging/improved nutritional status not known

In real life, the consequence of diminished skeletal muscle function in CED is reduced work performance and physical work capacity. Thus, for instance, sugar-cane cutters in Colombia who are taller and heavier and have higher FFMs are more productive. The height deficit in CED may be an additional disadvantage since taller individuals have greater limb lengths, which may provide greater leverage during manual tasks.

Immune function

There is considerable evidence to indicate that acute energy deficiency is associated with diminished immune function. Immune function is of two types. Cellular immunity, which is mediated by the T-lymphocyte, is involved predominantly in defense against viruses, fungi and protozoa. Antibodies produced by the B-lympho-cytes mediate humoral immunity. Several studies suggest that cellular immunity is more affected than humoral immunity in children with protein– energy malnutrition. The consequence of a reduced immunity is an increased susceptibility to infection. Individuals with a low BMI thus tend to be sick for a greater number of days in the year. Healing may also be delayed following surgery, and the period of hospitalization may be prolonged. In addition, mortality increases sharply in those individuals who are of low BMI, especially below a BMI of $16 \, \text{kg/m}^2$.

Autonomic nervous function

Earlier in this chapter, we discussed how changes in sympathetic nervous function could help in the conservation of energy in CED. In CED there is evidence that sympathetic nervous activity is reduced. There is also some evidence that parasympathetic nervous activity (the other arm of the autonomic nervous system) is increased.

Nerves act by releasing chemical messengers called neurotransmitters. These neurotransmitters in turn act on certain proteins on cell membranes called receptors, which then produce a cellular response. When the level of a neurotransmitter is high, the number of receptors reduces so as to maintain a constant cellular response. Conversely, when the neurotransmitter level is low, the number of receptors increases. Many drugs used in clinical practice act on the receptors of the autonomic nervous system. Because autonomic nervous activity (both sympathetic and parasympathetic) is altered in CED, the receptor number is also altered. If drugs are administered that act on these receptors, the response of the drug is likely to be higher or lower than normal,

depending on whether the receptor number is increased or decreased. Thus, the required dose of drugs acting on the autonomic nervous system may be altered in CED. In summary, therefore, the conservation of energy in the CED subject is largely due to a reduction in body size and in metabolically active tissue. Metabolic efficiency in CED contributes to energy saving in a rather small way. The adaptation of the CED subject to lowered energy intakes is not, however, without its costs, as highlighted in the preceding section.

17.8 Perspectives on the future

This chapter has highlighted some issues in CED for which we have an incomplete understanding. This section raises some of the issues with which health-care professionals will have to deal in the future. Much of what follows is speculative, and the reader is encouraged to pick up the leads and delve further into the issues that have been raised.

Chronic energy deficiency and aging

Young CED subjects have a diminished SNS activity. As people age, their blood vessels become stiffer. This stiffness in the blood vessels results in a reduced distensibility to increases in arterial pressure (a reduced arterial compliance). Since the body's sensors for blood pressure are essentially mechanoreceptors located in the blood-vessel wall, the ability of the body to sense changes in pressure within these vessels becomes impaired (reduced baroreflex sensitivity). Whenever there is a fall in blood pressure, as for instance when a person stands up suddenly, the SNS is activated to constrict blood vessels and restore the blood pressure to normal. Because elderly people have reduced baroreflex sensitivity, their resting sympathetic nervous activity is increased as a compensatory mechanism. Elderly individuals who have impaired SNS activity may suffer from postural and postprandial hypotension. In these situations, elderly subjects are sometimes unable to maintain blood pressure when standing up or after a meal. They complain of dizziness or light-headedness and may even have falls. It is not known what happens to CED subjects when they age. Will they continue to show a relatively reduced SNS activity in an attempt to conserve energy? If so, will they be more prone to postural and post-prandial hypotension?

Improved nutrition in chronic energy deficiency

Is increasing food intake the answer to CED? Many developing countries are now undergoing a nutritional transition, related to increased economic growth and a departure from traditional diets. The result is that people are becoming heavier and fatter. Obesity is a risk factor for many diseases, including coronary artery disease and diabetes. Earlier in the chapter a typical CED subject with a BMI of 16.5 was described. If this same individual were to gain weight to achieve a BMI of 25, his body weight at this BMI would be 64 kg, a gain of almost 22 kg. A substantial portion of this is likely to be fat. Individuals with a BMI near $25 \, kg/m^2$ are conventionally considered to be at the upper end of the normal BMI range. How should this CED individual be evaluated? Should he be considered at higher risk of developing heart disease and diabetes because of his weight and fat gain, despite his normal BMI?

Small babies now, larger problems later?

As mentioned earlier, low birthweight babies are seen more often in mothers with a low BMI. These babies also have a higher mortality. What happens to babies of low birth weight who survive into adulthood? Barker showed that low birthweight babies in the UK had a higher prevalence of high blood pressure, diabetes and coronary heart disease when they grew up to be adults. The mechanism by which this happens is not fully understood. The increased prevalence of diabetes has been linked to poor fetal growth, resulting in a reduced number of pancreatic β-cells, which produce insulin. Will developing countries where low birth weights are fairly common have to face the increased burden of diabetes, hypertension, and so on, as lifespans increase? How can we dissect out the contributions of poor fetal growth from environmental factors that are operative after birth? Will continued CED into adulthood be protective against these diseases? The intriguing possibility of fetal undernutrition affecting health in adulthood remains to be elucidated, particularly within the context of CED.

Further reading

Della Bianca P, Jequier E, Schutz Y. Lack of metabolic and behavioural adaptation in rural Gambian men with low body mass index. Am J Clin Nutr 1994; 60: 37–42.

James WPT, Ferro-Luzzi A, Waterlow JC. Eur J Clin Nutr 1988; 42: 969–981.

Norgan NG, Ferro-Luzzi A. Human adaptation to energy undernutrition. In Handbook of Physiology. Section 4. Environmental Physiology Vol. II (MJ Fregly, CM Blatteis, eds), pp. 1391–1409. New York: Oxford University Press for The American Physiological Society, 1996.

Soares MJ, Piers LS, Shetty PS, Jackson AA, Waterlow JC. Whole body protein turnover in chronically undernourished individuals. Clin Sci 1994; 86: 441–446.

Soares MJS, Shetty PS. Basal metabolic rates and metabolic economy in chronic undernutrition. Eur J Clin Nutr 1991; 45: 363–373.

Waterlow JC. Metabolic adaptation to low intakes of energy and protein. Annu Rev Nutr 1986; 6: 495–526.

18
Exercise Performance

AE Jeukendrup and LM Burke

Key messages

- The most important component of energy expenditure for athletes who are in training is exercise. Energy expenditure can amount up to 36 MJ/day for endurance athletes.
- Carbohydrate plays a crucial role in the diet of most athletes as it restores muscle and liver glycogen. Carbohydrate loading has been shown to increase muscle glycogen stores and endurance capacity.
- Carbohydrate feeding in the hour before the start of exercise can enhance performance. Some individuals, however, may be prone to develop hypoglycemia.
- Carbohydrate ingested during exercise (longer than 45 min) improves exercise performance by maintaining blood glucose concentration and high rates of carbohydrate oxidation, spares liver glycogen and may in some conditions spare muscle glycogen. Carbohydrates may also have central effects, although this has not been established.
- Muscle glycogen stores can be restored effectively by eating a high-carbohydrate meal or snack providing at least 1 g/kg carbohydrate within 15–30 min of finishing the exercise session. This is important when the schedule calls for rapid recovery between prolonged training sessions (<8 h recovery).
- A diet containing 7–10 g carbohydrate/kg body weight usually results in maintenance of muscle glycogen stores on a 24 h basis in trained athletes.
- Although the hypothesis that chronic high-fat diets may increase the capacity to oxidize fat and improve exercise performance during competition is attractive, there is currently no evidence to support this.
- Both endurance and strength athletes may have increased protein requirements. The recommendation for protein intakes for strength athletes is therefore generally 1.6–1.7 g/kg body weight per day and for endurance athletes 1.2–1.8 g/kg body mass per day. However, these increased requirements are normally easily met by the high energy intake by these athletes.
- Low body fat and low body weight are important in many sports, especially at the elite level. If loss of body fat is required, a realistic rate loss of about 0.5 kg/week should be chosen and both short-term and long-term goals should be set.
- Low iron status in athletes is overdiagnosed from single measures of low hemoglobin and ferritin levels. A major problem is the failure to recognize that the increase in blood volume that accompanies training will cause a dilution of all the blood contents. This hemodilution, often termed 'sports anemia', does not impair exercise performance.
- Dehydration can have dramatic effects on performance. Endurance performance is reduced but dehydration also affects sports with short duration, high-intensity exercise and skill sports. Severe dehydration can result in heat injury, characterized by excessive sweating, headache, nausea, dizziness, and reduced consciousness and mental function. When the core temperature rises to over 40°C, heat stroke may develop, characterized by hot, dry skin, confusion and loss of consciousness.
- Hyperhydration can reduce the thermal and cardiovascular strain of exercise. Hyperhydration can be induced by having subjects drink large volumes of water or water–electrolyte solutions for 1–3 h before exercise. However, much of the fluid overload is rapidly excreted and so expansions of the body water and blood volume are only transient.
- Fluid intake may be useful during exercise longer than 30–60 min, but there is no advantage during strenuous exercise of less than 30 min in duration.
- Plasma volume is more rapidly and completely restored in the postexercise period if sodium chloride (77 mmol/l or 450 mg/l) is added to the water consumed. This sodium concentration is similar to the upper limit of the sodium concentration found in sweat, but is considerably higher than the sodium concentration of many commercially available sports drinks, which usually contain 10–25 mmol/l (60–150 mg/l).
- Ingestion of 150% or more of weight loss is required to achieve normal hydration within 6 h following exercise.
- The nutrition supplement market has grown incredibly

in the last few years. However, there is little or no evidence to support the use of the vast majority of these supplements in sport.
- Oral creatine supplementation of 20 g/day for 5–6 days increases the muscle total creatine content in men by about 20% (30–40% of the increase is phosphocreatine). A subsequent daily dose of 2 g is enough for

maintenance of this increased concentration. Creatine loading increases the amount of work performed during single and repeated bouts of short-lasting, high-intensity exercise. Besides weight gain, creatine does not seem to have major side-effects. However, the long-term effects of creatine ingestion are unknown and therefore caution must be exercised.

18.1 Introduction

The relation between nutrition and physical performance has fascinated people for a long time. In Ancient Greece athletes had special nutrition regimes to prepare for the Olympic Games. It has become clear that different types of exercise and different sports will have different energy and nutrient requirements and therefore food intake must be adjusted accordingly. Certain nutritional strategies can enhance performance, improve recovery and result in more profound training adaptations. More recently, special drinks and energy bars have been developed and these have been marketed as sports foods. There is also a considerable amount of quackery in sports nutrition and a large number of nutrition supplements is on the market with claims to improve performance and recovery. This chapter will first review the nutritional demands of exercise in relation to the physiological demands. Strategies to improve exercise performance are then discussed. Finally practical applications will be discussed and detailed advice will be provided where possible.

18.2 Energy expenditure during physical activity

In resting conditions cells need energy to function: ionic pumps in membranes need energy to transport ions across cell membranes and the muscle fibers of the heart need energy to contract. During exercise the energy expenditure may increase several-fold, mainly because skeletal muscle requires energy to contract. In some cases the energy provision can become critical and continuation of the exercise is dependent on the availability of energy reserves. Most of these reserves must be obtained through nutrition. In endurance athletes, for example, energy depletion (carbohydrate depletion) is one of the most common causes of fatigue. Carbohydrate intake is essential to prevent early fatigue as a result of carbohydrate depletion.

Definition and assessment methods

There are several ways to measure (or estimate) human energy expenditure:

- direct calorimetry
- indirect calorimetry:
  - closed circuit spirometry
  - open circuit spirometry (douglas bag technique, breath-by-breath technique, portable spirometry)
- doubly labeled water
- labeled bicarbonate
- heart-rate monitoring
- accelerometry
- observations, records of physical activity, activity diaries, recall.

The methods range from direct but complex measurements of heat production (direct calorimetry) to relatively simple indirect metabolic measurements (indirect calorimetry), and from very expensive tracer methods (doubly labeled water) to relatively cheap and convenient rough estimations of energy expenditure (heart-rate monitoring and accelerometry). For a detailed analysis of these methods the reader is referred to Chapter 2 of the *Introduction to Human Nutrition* textbook in this series.

The most important component of energy expenditure for athletes who are in training is exercise. Basal metabolic rate (BMR) and diet-induced thermogenesis (DIT) become relatively unimportant when athletes train for 2 h/day or more. Energy expenditure during physical activity ranges from 20 kJ/min for very light activities to 100 kJ/min for very high-intensity exercise.

Energy expenditure and substrate use

Energy can be defined as the potential for performing work or producing force. Force production by skeletal muscles requires adenosine triphosphate (ATP). This compound contains energy in its phosphate bonds and upon hydrolysis of ATP this energy is released and is used to power all forms of biological work. In muscle, energy from the hydrolysis of ATP by myosin ATPase is used for muscle contraction. The hydrolysis of ATP yields approximately 31 kJ of free energy per mole of ATP degraded to ADP and inorganic phosphate (Pi):

$$ATP + H_2O \rightarrow ADP + H^+ + Pi$$
$$-31 \text{ kJ per mole of ATP}$$

The stores of ATP are very small and would only be sufficient for about 2 s of maximal exercise. The body therefore has various ways to resynthesize ATP. The different mechanisms involved in the resynthesis of ATP for muscle force generation include:

- phosphocreatine breakdown
- glycolysis, which involves metabolism of glucose-6-phosphate, derived from muscle glycogen or blood-borne glucose
- the products of carbohydrate, fat, protein and alcohol metabolism can enter the tricarboxylic acid (TCA) cycle in the mitochondria and be oxidized to carbon dioxide and water (aerobic metabolism). This process is known as oxidative phosphorylation and yields energy for the synthesis of ATP.

The rate of energy delivery from phosphocreatine is very fast, somewhat slower from glycolysis and much slower from aerobic metabolism. Within the muscle fiber, the concentration of phosphocreatine is about three or four times greater than the concentration of ATP. When phosphocreatine is broken down to creatine and inorganic phosphate by the action of the enzyme creatine kinase, a large amount of free energy is released. The phosphocreatine can be regarded as a back-up energy store: when the ATP content begins to fall during exercise, the phosphocreatine is broken down, releasing energy for restoration of ATP. During very intense exercise (8–10 s maximal exercise) the phosphocreatine (PCr) store can be almost completely depleted.

$$PCr + ADP + H^+ \leftrightarrow ATP + Cr$$
$$-43 \text{ kJ per mole of PCr}$$

Under normal conditions, muscle clearly does not fatigue after only a few seconds of effort, so a source of energy other than ATP and phosphocreatine must be available. This is derived from glycolysis, which is the name given to the pathway involving the breakdown of glucose (or glycogen), the end-product of this series of chemical reactions being pyruvate. This process does not require oxygen, but does result in energy in the form of ATP. In order for the reactions to proceed, however, the pyruvate must be removed; in low-intensity exercise when adequate oxygen is available to the muscle, pyruvate is converted to carbon dioxide and water by oxidative metabolism in the mitochondria. In some situations the pyruvate is removed by conversion to lactate, a reaction that does not involve oxygen. The net effect of glycolysis can thus be seen to be the conversion of one molecule of glucose to two molecules of pyruvate, with the net formation of two molecules of ATP and the conversion of two molecules of NAD^+ to NADH. If glycogen rather than glucose is the starting point, three molecules of ATP are produced, as there is no initial investment of ATP when the first phosphorylation step occurs. An 800 m runner, for example, obtains about 60% of the total energy requirement from anaerobic metabolism, and may convert about 100 g of carbohydrate (mostly glycogen, and equivalent to about 550 mmoles of glucose) to lactate in less than 2 min. The amount of ATP released in this way (three ATP molecules per glucose molecule degraded, about 1667 mmol of ATP in total) far exceeds that available from phosphocreatine hydrolysis. This high rate of anaerobic metabolism not only allows a faster steady-state speed than would be possible if aerobic metabolism alone had to be relied upon, but also allows a faster pace in the early stages before the cardiovascular system has adjusted to the demands and the delivery and utilization of oxygen have increased in response to the exercise stimulus.

During exercise lasting for several minutes up to several hours carbohydrate and fat are the most important fuels. These two energy sources are stored in the human body and can be mobilized from these stores when the demand increases. Both carbohydrate and fat are broken down to acetyl-coenzyme A (acetyl-CoA), which will then enter a series of reactions referred to as the tricarboxylic acid (TCA) cycle or Krebs cycle. In essence, the most important function of the TCA cycle is to generate hydrogen atoms for their subsequent passage to the electron transport chain by means of NADH and $FADH_2$. The aerobic process of electron transport–oxidative phosphorylation regenerates ATP from ADP, thus conserving some of the chemical potential energy contained within the original substrates in the form of high-energy phosphates. As long

Table 18.1 Availability of substrates in the human body (Estimated energy stores of fat and carbohydrate in an 80 kg man with 15% body fat)

Substrate		Weight (kg)	Energy (kcal)
Carbohydrates	Plasma glucose	0.02	78
	Liver glycogen	0.1	388
	Muscle glycogen	0.4	1550
	Total (approximately)	0.52	2000
Fat	Plasma fatty acid	0.0004	4
	Plasma triacylglycerols	0.004	39
	Adipose tissue	12.0	100 000
	Intramuscular triacylglycerols	0.3	2616
	Total (approximately)	12.3	106 500

Adapted from Jeukendrup *et al.* (1998).
Values given are estimates for a 'normal' man and not those of an athlete, who might be leaner and have more stored glycogen. The amount of protein in the body is not mentioned, but this would be about 10 kg (40 000 kcal); mainly located in the muscles.

as there is an adequate supply of oxygen and substrate is available, NAD^+ and FAD are continuously regenerated and TCA metabolism proceeds. This system cannot function without the use of oxygen.

Carbohydrate is stored in the liver and muscle (Table 18.1). The liver contains approximately 80 g of carbohydrate in the form of glycogen and skeletal muscle contains approximately 300–800 g (depending on muscle mass and diet). These stores are relatively small compared with the very large fat stores (mainly in subcutaneous adipose tissues). Even a lean athlete will have 4–7 kg of fat. Every gram of glycogen stored in liver or muscle is stored with 2.7 g of water. In addition, fat contains more than twice as much energy per gram as carbohydrate (36 kJ versus 16 kJ). Therefore, fat provides far more fuel per unit of weight than carbohydrate. In fact if we could only use the available carbohydrate as a substrate, we would probably only run between 20 and 30 km, whereas with fat as the only fuel, we could theoretically run between 1000 and 2000 km.

At rest and during low-intensity exercise, fat is often the substrate of choice. As the exercise intensity increases carbohydrate, and in particular muscle glycogen will become more and more important. Figure 18.1 displays the most important sources of fuel utilized during exercise. During low-intensity exercise, plasma fatty acids provide approximately one-third of the total energy. Glucose derived from the liver accounts for approximately 10% at low intensities but becomes more and more important at higher exercise intensities. Muscle glycogen is relatively unimportant

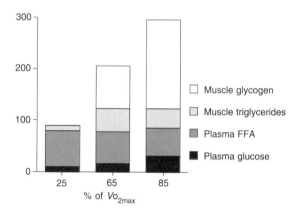

Figure 18.1 Substrate utilization at different exercise intensities. (Data adapted from Romijn *et al.*, 1993.)

at low intensities [40% maximal aerobic power ($V_{O_2\,max}$)] but is by far the most important fuel during high-intensity exercise (70–90% $V_{O_2\,max}$). Fat oxidation is usually the predominant fuel at low exercise intensities, whereas during high exercise intensities carbohydrate is the major fuel.

In absolute terms, fat oxidation increases as the exercise intensity increases from low to moderate intensities, even though the percentage contribution of fat may actually decrease (Figure 18.2). For the transition from light to moderate-intensity exercise, the increased fat oxidation is a direct result of the increased energy expenditure. At higher intensities of exercise (>75% $V_{O_2\,max}$) fat oxidation will be inhibited and both the relative and absolute rates of fat oxidation will decrease

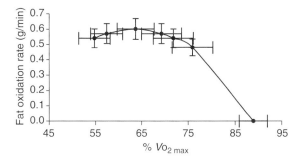

Figure 18.2 Fat oxidation as a function of exercise intensity in trained men. (Adapted from Achten and Jeukendrup, 2002.)

to negligible values. Above approximately 65% $V_{O_2 max}$, fat oxidation decreases despite high rates of lipolysis. The blood flow to the adipose tissue may be decreased (owing to sympathetic vasoconstriction) and this may result in a decreased removal of fatty acids from adipose tissue. During high-intensity exercise, lactate accumulation may also increase the re-esterification and inhibit the oxidation of fatty acids.

Carbohydrate and fat are always oxidized as a mixture, and whether carbohydrate or fat is the predominant fuel depends on a variety of factors.

- *Exercise intensity*: at higher exercise intensities more carbohydrate and less fat will be utilized. Carbohydrate can be utilized aerobically at rates up to about 4 g/min. The breakdown during very high-intensity exercise can amount to 7 g/min.
- *Duration of exercise*: fat oxidation increases and carbohydrate oxidation decreases as the exercise duration increases. Typical fat oxidation rates are between 0.2 and 0.5 g/min, but values of over 1.0–1.5 g/min have been reported after 6 h of running. The contribution of fat to energy expenditure can even increase to as much as 90%. This increased fat oxidation is likely to be caused by a reduction in muscle glycogen stores towards the later stages of prolonged exercise.
- *Level of aerobic fitness*: After endurance training the capacity to oxidize fatty acids increases and fat oxidation at the same absolute and relative exercise intensity is higher.
- *Diet*: substrate utilization usually reflects the diet. A high-carbohydrate diet will promote carbohydrate oxidation, whereas a low-carbohydrate diet will reduce body carbohydrate stores and result in lower rates of carbohydrate oxidation.

- *Carbohydrate intake before or during exercise*: after an overnight fast most of the energy requirement is covered by the oxidation of fatty acids derived from adipose tissue. Lipolysis in adipose tissue is mostly dependent on the concentrations of hormones (epinephrine to stimulate lipolysis and insulin to inhibit lipolysis). At rest a large percentage (about 70%) of the fatty acids liberated after lipolysis will be re-esterified within the adipocyte and approximately 30% of the fatty acids will be released into the systemic circulation. Resting plasma fatty acids concentrations are typically between 0.2 and 0.4 mmol/l. As soon as exercise is initiated, the rate of lipolysis and the rate of fatty acid release from adipose tissue are increased. During moderate-intensity exercise lipolysis increases approximately three-fold, mainly because of an increased β-adrenergic stimulation. In addition, during moderate-intensity exercise the blood flow to adipose tissue is doubled and the rate of re-esterification is halved. Blood flow in skeletal muscle is increased dramatically and therefore the delivery of fatty acids to the muscle is increased.

18.3 Carbohydrate and performance

Carbohydrate fuel plays a major role in the performance of many types of exercise and sport. The depletion of body carbohydrate stores is a cause of fatigue or performance impairment during exercise, particularly during prolonged (>90 min) sessions of submaximal or intermittent high-intensity activity. This fatigue may be seen both in the muscle (peripheral fatigue) and in the brain and nervous system (central fatigue). Unfortunately, total body carbohydrate stores are limited, and are often substantially less than the fuel requirements of the training and competition sessions undertaken by athletes. Therefore, sports nutrition guidelines promote a variety of options for increasing carbohydrate availability for an exercise session. These strategies include consuming carbohydrate before, during and in the recovery period between prolonged exercise bouts.

Many studies show that exercise is improved by strategies that enhance or maintain carbohydrate status during exercise. Exercise scientists find it convenient to measure performance by having the athlete exercise in a laboratory, often on a bike or running treadmill, at a steady workrate. They measure the time for which the athlete can exercise until they fatigue, or the point at which they fail to keep up with this workrate. Technically, this measurement should be called exercise capacity or endurance. Although these studies are relatively easy to conduct and can show the beneficial effects of a dietary intervention, they do not necessarily mimic the real demands of a sporting event. After all, in most races, the athlete tries to cover a set distance as fast as possible rather than exercise until they are exhausted. Studies that try to simulate a real event, especially in the field rather than in the laboratory, are harder to conduct. The most complicated types of performance belong to unpredictable team games or sports involving complex decision-making and motor skills. It is hard to find a way to measure adequately all the components of performance, and it is complicated to organize a protocol in which the same event is conducted twice, before and after an intervention, or with a treatment and a placebo. Despite the difficulties in conducting studies, strategies that enhance carbohydrate availability have been shown to enhance cycling and running endurance, cycling and running performance, and the performance of complex games such as in tennis, soccer and ice hockey. There is also some evidence that the benefits from combining two strategies that enhance carbohydrate availability; for example, a combination of eating a high-carbohydrate meal before the event and consuming carbohydrate during the event, are additive. Studies of single-carbohydrate strategies or combinations of strategies need to be conducted over a greater range of sports and exercise events so that scientists can give more detailed advice to athletes.

Recent studies have provided preliminary evidence that there are other benefits from high-carbohydrate eating strategies apart from increasing fuel stores for exercise. For example, a growing number of investigations has reported performance benefits when carbohydrate is consumed before and during high-intensity exercise of around 1 h. In these situations, the athlete's body carbohydrate stores should already be sufficient to fuel the event, so it is not clear why additional carbohydrate would provide an advantage. It is possible that carbohydrate intake improves the function of the brain and central nervous system, making the athlete feel better during the exercise task. Further research is needed to confirm and explain the effects.

Finally, carbohydrate intake during and after exercise appears to assist the immune response to exercise.

Cellular immune parameters are often reduced or compromised after a prolonged workout. However, some studies have shown that carbohydrate intake can decrease or prevent this outcome. Whether this actually leads to an improvement in the immune status and health of athletes (e.g. fever sick days) remains to be seen and would require a sophisticated long-term study.

Fueling up before exercise

Carbohydrate stores in the muscle and liver should be well-filled prior to exercise, particularly in the competition setting where the athlete wants to perform at their best. The key factors in glycogen storage are dietary carbohydrate intake and, in the case of muscle stores, tapered exercise or rest. In the absence of muscle damage, muscle glycogen stores can be returned to normal resting levels (to 350–500 mmol/kg dry weight muscle) with 24–36 h of rest and an adequate carbohydrate intake (7–10/kg body weight per day). Normalized stores appear adequate for the fuel needs of events of less than 60–90 min in duration (e.g. a soccer game, half-marathon or basketball game). Supercompensated glycogen levels do not enhance performance in these events.

Carbohydrate loading is a special practice that aims to maximize or supercompensate muscle glycogen stores up to twice the normal resting level (e.g. ∼ 500–900 mmol/kg dry weight). The first protocol was devised in the late 1960s by Scandinavian sports scientists who found, using muscle biopsy techniques, that the size of pre-exercise muscle glycogen stores affected endurance during submaximal exercise. Their series of studies found that several days of a low-carbohydrate diet depleted muscle glycogen stores and reduced cycling endurance compared with a mixed diet. However, following up with a high-carbohydrate intake over several days caused a supercompensation of muscle glycogen stores and prolonged the cycling time to exhaustion. These pioneering studies produced the 'classical' 7 day model of carbohydrate loading. This model consists of a 3–4 day depletion phase of hard training and low carbohydrate intake, finishing with a 3–4 day loading phase of high carbohydrate eating and exercise taper (i.e. decreased amounts of training). Early field studies of prolonged running events showed that carbohydrate loading enhanced sports performance, not by allowing the athlete to run faster, but by prolonging the time for which race pace could be maintained.

Further studies undertaken on trained subjects have produced a modified carbohydrate loading strategy. The muscle of well-trained athletes has been found to be able to supercompensate its glycogen stores without a prior depletion or glycogen-stripping phase. For well-trained athletes at least, carbohydrate loading may be seen as an extension of fueling up, involving rest/taper and high carbohydrate intake over 3–4 days. The modified carbohydrate loading protocol offers a more practical strategy for competition preparation, by avoiding the fatigue and complexity of the extreme diet and training protocols associated with the previous depletion phase. Typically, carbohydrate loading will postpone fatigue and extend the duration of steady state exercise by around 20%, and improve performance over a set distance or workload by 2–3%.

Pre-event meal

Food and fluids consumed in the 4 h before an event may help to achieve the following sports nutrition goals:

- to continue to fill muscle glycogen stores if they have not fully restored or loaded since the last exercise session
- to restore liver glycogen levels, especially for events undertaken in the morning where liver stores are depleted from an overnight fast
- to ensure that the athlete is well-hydrated
- to prevent hunger, yet avoid gastrointestinal discomfort and upset during exercise
- to include foods and practices that are important to the athlete's psychology or superstitions.

Consuming carbohydrate-rich foods and drinks in the pre-event meal is especially important in situations where body carbohydrate stores have not been fully recovered and/or where the event is of sufficient duration and intensity to deplete these stores. The intake of a substantial amount of carbohydrate (~200–300 g) in the 2–4 h before exercise has been shown to enhance various measures of exercise performance compared with performance undertaken after an overnight fast.

However, some experts have suggested that carbohydrate intake before exercise may have negative consequences for performance, especially in the hour before exercise. Carbohydrate intake causes a rise in plasma insulin concentrations, which in turn suppresses the availability and oxidation of fat as an exercise fuel. The final result is an increased reliance on carbohydrate

oxidation at the onset of exercise, leading to faster depletion of muscle glycogen stores and a decline in plasma glucose concentration. There has been considerable publicity surrounding one study from the 1970s, which found that subjects performed worse after consuming carbohydrate in the hour before exercise than when they cycled without consuming anything. This has led to warnings that carbohydrate should not be consumed in the hour before exercise. However, a far greater number of studies have shown that any metabolic disturbances following pre-exercise carbohydrate feedings are short-lived or unimportant. These studies show that carbohydrate intake in the hour before exercise is associated with a neutral effect or a beneficial performance outcome.

Nevertheless, there is a small subgroup of athletes who experience a true fatigue, associated with a decline in blood glucose levels, if they start to exercise within the hour after consuming a carbohydrate snack. This problem can be avoided or diminished by a number of dietary strategies.

- Consume a substantial amount of carbohydrate (>75 g) rather than a small amount, so that the additional carbohydrate more than compensates for the increased rate of carbohydrate oxidation during the exercise.
- Choose a carbohydrate-rich food or drink that produces a low glycemic index (GI) response (that is, a low blood glucose and insulin response) rather than a carbohydrate source that has a high GI (producing a large and rapid blood glucose and insulin response).
- Consume carbohydrate throughout the exercise session.

Some sports scientists have suggested that all athletes will benefit from the choice of low GI rather than high GI carbohydrate foods in the pre-event meal. This theory is based on the idea that low GI foods will provide a more sustained release of carbohydrate energy throughout the exercise session, and create less of a metabolic disturbance during exercise because of a reduced insulin response. However, the balance of studies has failed to find performance benefits following the intake of a low GI pre-exercise meal compared with an equal amount of high GI carbohydrate, even when metabolic differences between low GI and high GI meals were noted. Furthermore, it has been shown that when carbohydrate is ingested during exercise according to sports nutrition guidelines, any metabolic or performance effects arising from the choice of a low GI or high GI pre-event meal are overridden.

Therefore, each athlete must judge the benefits and the practical issues associated with pre-exercise meals in their particular sport or situation. The type, timing and quantity of pre-event meals should be chosen according to the athlete's individual circumstances and experiences. Foods with a low-fat, low-fiber and low to moderate protein content are the preferred choice for the pre-event menu since they are less likely to cause gastrointestinal upsets. Liquid meal supplements or carbohydrate containing drinks and bars are a simple snack for athletes who suffer from pre-event nerves or have an uncertain competition timetable. Examples of carbohydrate-rich foods and drinks that are often used in pre-event meals are listed in the Box 18.1.

Carbohydrate intake during exercise

Numerous studies show that the intake of carbohydrate during prolonged sessions of moderate-intensity or intermittent high-intensity exercise can improve endurance (i.e. prolong time to exhaustion) and performance. As reviewed above, there is also some evidence that carbohydrate intake may benefit shorter duration high-intensity sports, or the immune response to prolonged exercise. Even when there is no significant benefit from consuming carbohydrate during exercise, performance is not adversely affected. Although there is some evidence that increasing carbohydrate availability causes glycogen sparing in slow-twitch muscle fibers during running, the major mechanisms to explain the benefits of carbohydrate feeding during prolonged exercise are the maintenance

of plasma glucose concentration (sustaining brain function) and the provision of an additional carbohydrate supply to allow the muscle to continue high rates of carbohydrate oxidation.

Investigations into different types of carbohydrate show that there are no important differences in the oxidation of moderate to high GI carbohydrate sources consumed during prolonged, moderate-intensity exercise. Carbohydrate consumed during exercise is oxidized in small amounts during the first hour of exercise ($\sim 20\,g$) and thereafter reaches a peak rate of around 1 g/min. Even ingestion of very large amounts of carbohydrate will not result in higher oxidation rates. In general, a carbohydrate intake of 60 g/h is recommended, with carbohydrate feedings starting well in advance of fatigue/depletion of body carbohydrate stores. Ingestion of more than 60 g/h will not have an additive effect and may even cause gastrointestinal distress. In the world of sport, athletes consume carbohydrate during exercise using a variety of foods and drinks, and a variety of feeding schedules. Sports drinks [commercial solutions providing 4–8% carbohydrate (4–8 g carbohydrate/100 ml), electrolytes and palatable flavors] are particularly valuable since these allow the athlete to replace their fluid and carbohydrate needs simultaneously. Such drinks will be discussed in greater detail in the section below. Each sport or exercise activity offers particular opportunities for fluid and carbohydrate to be consumed throughout the session, whether it be from aid stations, supplies carried by the athlete, or at formal stoppages in play such as time-outs or half-time breaks. The athlete should be creative in making use of these opportunities.

Postexercise refueling

Restoration of muscle glycogen concentrations is an important component of postexercise recovery and is challenging for athletes who train or compete more than once each day. The main dietary issue in glycogen synthesis is the amount of carbohydrate consumed. The optimal carbohydrate intake for glycogen storage is 7–10 g/kg body weight per day. However, there is some evidence that moderate and high GI carbohydrate-rich foods and drinks may be more favorable for glycogen storage than some low GI food choices. Glycogen storage may occur at a slightly faster rate during the first couple of hours after exercise; however, the main reason for encouraging an athlete to consume carbohydrate-rich meals or snacks soon after exercise is that effective refueling does not start until a substantial amount of carbohydrate ($\sim 1\,g/kg$ body weight) is consumed. When there is limited time between workouts or events (e.g. hours or less) it makes sense to turn every minute into effective recovery time by consuming carbohydrate as soon as possible after the first session. However, when recovery time is longer, immediate carbohydrate intake after exercise is unnecessary and the athlete can afford to follow their preferred and practical eating schedule as long as goals for total carbohydrate intake are met over the day.

Certain amino acids have a potent effect on the secretion of insulin, which is a stimulator of glycogen resynthesis. For this reason the effects of adding amino acids and proteins to a carbohydrate solution have been investigated. One study compared glycogen resynthesis rates after ingestion of carbohydrate, protein or carbohydrate plus protein. As expected, very little glycogen was stored when protein alone was ingested, and glycogen storage was increased when carbohydrate was ingested. But most interestingly, glycogen storage was further increased when carbohydrate was ingested together with protein. However, other studies have shown that if the amount of ingested carbohydrate is high, addition of protein or amino acids has no further effect. Nevertheless, recovery goals also include attention to the immune system, muscle building and injury repair. Therefore, it may be useful to eat nutrient-rich forms of carbohydrate foods and drinks during the recovery period to provide a range of valuable nutrients.

Everyday eating for recovery

Although strategies to promote carbohydrate availability have been shown to enhance performance and recovery after a single bout of exercise, it has been difficult to demonstrate that a long-term period of high carbohydrate eating will promote better training adaptations and long-term performance than a moderate carbohydrate diet. Theoretically, inadequate carbohydrate intake during repeated days of exercise will lead to gradual depletion of muscle glycogen stores and impairment of exercise endurance. This theory, based on observations of reduced muscle glycogen levels following successive days of running, is summarized in Figure 18.3. Several studies have been undertaken to compare refueling and performance on high-carbohydrate diets and moderate-carbohydrate diets for periods of 7 days to 4 weeks. Although these studies

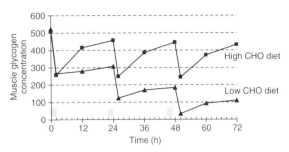

Figure 18.3 Muscle glycogen concentration after 3 days of hard training with a high-carbohydrate (CHO) or a mixed diet. (Adapted from Costill *et al.*, 1971.)

show that high-carbohydrate diets are better at promoting muscle glycogen restoration, superior performance has not been clearly demonstrated. Some scientists have suggested that this means that high-carbohydrate diets are not really needed by endurance athletes. Others feel that the lack of clear evidence is a reflection of problems with the design of the studies; for example, not being conducted over sufficient time to see a separation in performance, or not having a measurement of performance that is sensitive enough to detect small but real differences. Further carefully conducted studies are needed to find the answers. In the meantime, in view of the evidence that supports the benefits of carbohydrate availability on acute exercise performance, it is sensible for the current sports nutrition guidelines to promote a high-carbohydrate diet during periods of prolonged strenuous training or competition.

Dietary guidelines for the general population make recommendations for carbohydrate intake as a percentage of dietary energy intake (e.g. to increase carbohydrate to >55% of total energy intake). Some sports nutrition experts have followed this terminology. However, athletes undertaking strenuous exercise have carbohydrate requirements based principally on muscle fuel needs, which are quantifiable according to the size of the athlete and the duration of their exercise program. Therefore, it makes sense, and is more practical, to be consist in describing carbohydrate goals in terms of grams per kilogram of the athlete's body weight. This allows the athlete to work out their carbohydrate requirement for a given situation (e.g. 7 g/kg for a 70 kg athlete =490 g). Meals and menus can then be constructed using information on food labels or in food composition tables to achieve this carbohydrate target. General eating patterns that help to achieve a high carbohydrate intake are summarized in Box 18.2.

18.4 Fat metabolism and performance

At rest and during exercise skeletal muscle is the main site of oxidation of fatty acids. In resting conditions, and especially after fasting, fatty acids are the predominant fuel used by skeletal muscle. During low-intensity exercise, metabolism is elevated several-fold compared with resting conditions and fat oxidation is increased. When the exercise intensity increases, fat oxidation increases further, until exercise intensities of about 65% $V_{O_2\,max}$, after which a decline in the rate of fat oxidation is observed. In contrast to carbohydrate metabolism, which increases as a function of the aerobic workrate, fat oxidation is reduced at high exercise intensities (Figure 18.2).

Fat oxidation and diet

Diet has marked effects on fat oxidation. In general, a high-carbohydrate, low-fat diet will reduce fat oxidation, whereas a high-fat, low-carbohydrate diet will increase fat oxidation. It might be argued that in most of these studies the effects were seen because of the effects of the last meal, which is known to have a marked effect on substrate utilization. However, several days of a high-fat, low-carbohydrate diet will affect substrate utilization even when followed by a day of high-carbohydrate meals. The results indicate that there are chronic effects of diet that cannot directly be explained by substrate availability. In one study, when subjects consumed a high-fat diet or a high-carbohydrate diet for 5 days, followed by 1 day on a high-carbohydrate diet, the 1 day with high carbohydrate intake replenished glycogen stores in both conditions and muscle glycogen concentrations were identical. Yet there were large differences in substrate utilization between the two diets. Respiratory exchange ratio (RER) changed from 0.90 to 0.82 after 5 days on a high-fat diet. After consuming a high-carbohydrate diet for 1 day RER was still lower than baseline values (0.87). Since these changes were not caused by differences in substrate availability (muscle glycogen), they are likely to be related to metabolic adaptations in the muscle.

In conclusion, chronic diets can have marked effects on metabolism. These effects seem only partly

Box 18.2 Guidelines for achieving a high carbohydrate intake

- Be prepared to be different: Westernized eating plans are not suffiiciently high in carbohydrates for many athletes.
- Base meals and snacks around the following nutritious carbohydrate foods, so that these take up at least half of the room on the plate: whole-grain breads and breakfast cereals; rice, pasta, noodles and other grain foods; fruits; starchy vegetables (e.g. potatoes, corn); legumes (lentils, beans, soy-based products) and sweetened dairy products (e.g. fruit-flavored yogurt, fruit smoothies).
- Be wary that many foods commonly believed by athletes to be carbohydrate rich are actually high-fat foods (e.g. cakes, take-away foods, chocolates and pastries). Be aware of low-fat eating strategies.
- Use sugar and sugar-rich foods as a palatable and compact source of carbohydrate, especially to add to a nutritious carbohydrate-rich meal, or to supply carbohydrates during and after exercise.
- When carbohydrate and energy needs are high, increase the *number* of meals and snacks, rather than the *size* of meals. Be organized to have snacks on hand in a busy day.
- Choose lower fiber choices of carbohydrate-rich foods to provide a compact fuel source when energy needs are high, or to provide a better tolerated pre-event meal.
- Note that carbohydrate-rich drinks (e.g. fruit juices, soft drinks, fruit/milk smoothies) are also a compact source for special situations or high-carbohydrate diets. This category includes many of the supplements made specially for athletes (e.g. sports drinks, liquid meal supplements, carbohydrate gels, sports bars).
- Fuel up for competition with 24–36 h of exercise taper and high carbohydrate intake (7–10 g/kg per day). Extend this preparation to 72 h, to 'carbohydrate load' in preparation for endurance events (>90 min duration). Specialist dietary advice from a sports dietitian may be needed to achieve high-carbohydrate intake goals.
- Consume carbohydrates during training and competition sessions of greater than 90 min duration, and experiment to see whether this helps during high-intensity sessions of ~60 min. Sports drinks will look after fluid and carbohydrate needs simultaneously, being specially designed to deliver these nutrients rapidly. Design a feeding protocol that provides 60 g carbohydrate per hour to optimize carbohydrate delivery.
- Begin effective recovery of muscle glycogen stores by eating a high-carbohydrate meal or snack providing at least 1 g/kg carbohydrate within 15–30 min of finishing the exercise session. This is important when the schedule calls for rapid recovery between prolonged training sessions (<8 h recovery). Nutritious carbohydrate-rich foods and drinks can provide protein and other nutrients that may also be useful in recovery.

related to the effects of diets on substrate availability. Adaptations at the muscular level, which result in changes in substrate utilization in response to a diet, may occur in as little as 5 days.

Fat intake during exercise

Long-chain triglycerides

Nutritional fats include triglycerides (containing mostly C16 and C18 fatty acids), phospholipids and cholesterol, of which only triglycerides can contribute to any extent to energy provision during exercise. In contrast to carbohydrates, nutritional fats reach the circulation only slowly since they are potent inhibitors of gastric emptying. Furthermore, the digestion in the gut and absorption of fat are also rather slow processes compared with the digestion and absorption of carbohydrates. Bile salts, produced by the liver, and lipase secreted by the pancreas are needed for the breakdown of the long-chain triglycerides (LCT) into glycerol and three long-chain fatty acids. The fatty acids are then transported in chylomicrons via the lymphatic system, which ultimately drains into the systemic circulation. Long-chain dietary fatty acids typically enter the blood 3–4 h after ingestion.

The fact that these long-chain fatty acids enter the circulation in chylomicrons is also important, and it is generally believed that the rate of breakdown of chylomicron-bound triglycerides by muscle is relatively slow. It has been suggested that the primary role of these triglycerides in chylomicrons is the replenishment of intramuscular fat stores after exercise. The usual advice, therefore, is to reduce the intake of fat during exercise to a minimum. Many 'sports bars' or 'energy bars', however, contain significant amounts of fat and it is therefore advisable to check the food label before choosing an energy bar.

In summary, LCT ingestion during exercise is not desirable because it slows gastric emptying, and because the triglycerides only slowly appear in the systemic circulation in chylomicrons, which are believed to be a less important fuel source during exercise.

Medium-chain triglycerides

Medium-chain fatty acids have different properties to long-chain fatty acids, and it has been suggested that medium-chain fatty acids could be a useful energy source during exercise. Medium-chain fatty acids contain 8–10 carbons, whereas long-chain fatty acids contain 12 or more carbons. Medium-chain triglycerides (MCT) are more polar and therefore more soluble in water, and they are more rapidly digested and absorbed in the intestine than LCT. Furthermore, medium-chain fatty acids follow the portal venous system and enter the liver directly, while long-chain fatty acids are passed into the systemic circulation slowly via the lymphatic system. MCT is normally present in our diet in very small quantities, with few natural sources. MCT is usually synthesized from coconut oil.

Unlike LCT, MCT are rapidly emptied from the stomach, rapidly absorbed and metabolized, and may be a valuable exogenous energy source during exercise, in addition to carbohydrates It has been suggested that MCT ingestion may improve exercise performance by elevating plasma fatty acid levels and sparing muscle glycogen. However, the ingestion of 30 g of MCT has no effect on plasma fatty acid concentration, glycogen sparing or exercise performance. Ingestion of larger amounts of MCT is likely to cause gastrointestinal distress and therefore cannot be recommended.

Therefore, MCT do not appear to have the positive effects on performance that are often claimed.

Fasting

Fasting has been proposed as a way to increase fat utilization, spare muscle glycogen and improve exercise performance. In rats, short-term fasting increases plasma epinephrine and norepinephrine concentrations, stimulates lipolysis and increases the concentration of circulating plasma fatty acids. This, in turn, increases fat oxidation and 'spares' muscle glycogen, leading to a similar, or even increased running time to exhaustion in rats. In humans, fasting also results in an increased concentration of circulating catecholamines, increased lipolysis, increased concentration of plasma fatty acids and a decreased glucose turnover. Muscle glycogen concentrations, however, are unaffected by fasting for 24 h when no strenuous exercise is performed. Although it has been reported that fasting had no effect on endurance capacity at low exercise intensities (45% $V_{O_2 max}$), performance may be significantly impaired at intensities higher than 50% V_{O_2} max. The observed decrease in performance was not reversible by carbohydrate ingestion during exercise. Liver glycogen stores will be substantially depleted after a 24 h fast and therefore euglycemia may not be as well maintained during exercise, compromising brain function.

In summary, fasting increases the availability of lipid substrates, resulting in increased oxidation of fatty acids at rest and during exercise. However, since the liver glycogen stores are not maintained, exercise performance is impaired.

High-fat diets

In 1939, Christensen and Hansen demonstrated that a high-fat diet for 3–5 days resulted in impaired exercise capacity. This is likely to be related to the decreased muscle glycogen concentrations that can be expected after a high-fat, low-carbohydrate diet. Fat oxidation increases with such a diet, but this may merely be the result of the lack of availability of carbohydrate as an energy source.

Early studies reported that adaptation to a high-fat diet for 4–6 weeks resulted in increased fat oxidation and a maintenance of endurance capacity. However, these studies are difficult to interpret because of the small subject numbers and the variation in the results. Nevertheless, it is remarkable that performance was not reduced in all subjects, even though muscle glycogen levels measured before exercise were decreased by almost 50%. In at least some cases it appears that the increased capacity for fat oxidation can compensate for the low availability of muscle glycogen. However, other studies have shown that a fat-adaptation period beyond 4 weeks causes a decrease in exercise performance, which cannot be reversed by a week on a high-carbohydrate diet. These results indicate that the reduction in performance might be caused by an impairment of the adaptations achieved by the training program.

More recent research has shown that worthwhile adaptations to a high-fat diet occur in as little as 5–6 days, providing a more practical period for undertaking major dietary changes, and perhaps an opportunity to gain benefits without causing long-term inhibition of the training process. Another twist is the concept of 'dietary periodization', where the period of adaptation to a high-fat diet is followed by acute carbohydrate feeding. This strategy might induce enzymic adaptations in the muscle while also allowing optimization of pre-exercise glycogen stores. In a series of studies performed to test this possibility, trained cyclists received a high-fat diet for a relatively short period (5–6 days) followed by a day of carbohydrate loading on the following day. At the end of the period, metabolism and performance were monitored over a series of exercise tasks. The results showed that there were no benefits to the performance of endurance cycling tasks (2–3 h) but a trend towards perfor-mance improvement for ultraendurance events (5 h). Further research is needed.

In conclusion, although the hypothesis that chronic high-fat diets may increase the capacity to oxidize fat and improve exercise performance during competition is attractive, there is currently no evidence to support this. From a health perspective, eating large amounts of fat has been associated with the development of obesity and cardiovascular disease. Exposure to high-fat diets has also been associated with insulin resistance. Whether this is also true for athletes who are physically active and have a greater capacity to oxidize fat, has yet to be determined. Because there is limited information about the negative effects of high-fat diets for athletes and the effects of these diets on performance are unclear, caution should be exercised when recommending high-fat diets to athletes.

18.5 Effect of exercise on protein requirements

There is still considerable debate about how much dietary protein is required for optimal athletic performance. This interest in protein (meat) probably dates back to Ancient Greece. There are reports that athletes in Ancient Greece, in preparation for the Olympic Games, consumed large amounts of meat. This believe stems partly from the large proportion of the total protein in a human body (about 40%). Muscle also accounts for 30–50% of all protein turnover in the body. Both the structural proteins that make up the myofibrillar proteins and the proteins that act as enzymes within a muscle cell change as an adaptation to exercise training. Indeed, muscle mass, muscle protein composition and muscle protein content will change in response to training. Therefore, it is not surprising that meat has been popular as a protein source for athletes, especially strength athletes.

Non-essential amino acids can be synthesized from essential and non-essential amino acids. This is important in situations with inadequate dietary protein intake. In muscle, the majority of amino acids are incorporated into tissue proteins, with a small pool of free amino acids. This pool undergoes turnover, receiving free amino acids from the breakdown of protein and contributing amino acids for protein synthesis. Protein breakdown in skeletal muscle serves two main purposes:

- to provide essential amino acids when individual amino acids are converted to acetyl-CoA or TCA cycle intermediates.

- to provide individual amino acids that can be used elsewhere in the body for the synthesis of neuro-transmitters, hormones, glucose and proteins.

Clearly, if protein degradation rates are greater than the rates of synthesis, there will be a reduction in protein content; conversely, muscle protein content can only increase if the rate of synthesis exceeds that of degradation.

Increased protein requirements

Exercise, especially endurance exercise, results in increased oxidation of the branched chain amino acids (BCAA), which are essential amino acids and cannot be synthesized in the body. Therefore, increased oxidation would imply that the dietary protein requirements are increased. Some studies in which the nitrogen balance technique was used showed that the dietary protein requirements for athletes involved in prolonged endurance training were higher than those for sedentary individuals. However, these results have been questioned.

It has been estimated that protein may contribute up to about 15% to energy expenditure in resting conditions. During exercise this relative contribution is likely to decrease because energy expenditure is increased and most of this energy is provided by carbohydrate and fat. During very prolonged exercise when carbohydrate availability becomes limited the contribution of protein to energy expenditure may amount up to about 10% of total energy expenditure. Thus, although protein oxidation is increased during endurance exercise, the relative contribution of protein to energy expenditure remains small. Protein requirements may be increased somewhat, but this increased need may be met easily by a moderate protein intake. The research groups that advocate an increased protein intake for endurance athletes usually recommend a daily intake of 1.2–1.8 g/kg body weight. This is about twice the level of protein intake that is recommended for sedentary populations.

There are reports of increased protein breakdown after resistance exercise. The suggested increased dietary protein requirements with resistance training are related to increased muscle bulk (hypertrophy) rather than increased oxidation of amino acids. Muscle protein breakdown is increased after resistance training, but to a smaller degree than muscle protein synthesis. The elevations in protein degradation and synthesis are transient. Protein breakdown and

synthesis after exercise are elevated at 3 and 24 h after exercise, but return to baseline levels after 48 h. These results seem to apply to resistance exercise and high-intensity dynamic exercise.

There is controversy as to whether strength athletes really need to eat large amounts of protein. The nitrogen balance studies that have been conducted on such athletes have been criticized because they generally have been of short duration and a steady-state situation may not be established. The recommendation for protein intakes for strength athletes is therefore generally 1.6–1.7 g/kg body weight per day. Again this seems to be met easily with a normal diet and no extra attention to protein intake is needed. Protein supplements are often used, but are not necessary to meet the recommended protein intake.

Amino acid versus protein intake

In the past the amino acid needs of the body were primarily met by ingestion of whole proteins in the diet. However, over the past few years the supplementation of individual amino acids has become increasingly popular. This is the result of technological advances that have made it possible to manufacture food-grade ultrapure amino acids, but also reflects the general interest in the pharmacological and metabolic interactions of free-form amino acids in various areas of clinical nutrition. Here, individual amino acids are used to reduce nitrogen losses and improve organ function in traumatized and critically ill patients. The results of these studies have been applied to populations of athletes and healthy individuals, where intake of separate amino acids is claimed to improve exercise performance, stimulate hormone release and improve immune function, among a variety of other positive effects.

However, amino acid metabolism is very complex. One amino acid can be converted into another and amino acids may influence nerve impulse transmission as well as hormone secretion. The composition of specific amino acid mixtures or even high-protein diets may lead to nutritional imbalances, because overload with one amino acid may reduce the absorption of other amino acids.

18.6 Physique and sports performance

Physical characteristics, such as height, body weight, muscle mass and body fat levels, can all play a role in the performance of sport. An athlete's physique is determined by inherited characteristics, as well as the conditioning effects of their training program and diet. Often, 'ideal' physiques for individual sports are set, based on a rigid set of characteristics of successful athletes. However, this process fails to take into account that there is considerable variability in the physical characteristics of sportspeople, even between elite athletes in the same sport. Therefore, it is dangerous to establish rigid prescriptions for individuals, particularly with regard to body composition. Instead, it is preferable to nominate a range of acceptable values for body fat and body weight within each sport, and then monitor the health and performance of individual athletes within this range. These values may change over the athlete's career.

Some athletes easily achieve the body composition suited to their sport. However, others may need to manipulate characteristics such as muscle mass or body fat levels through changes in diet and training. It is important for an athlete to identify a suitable and realistic body-fat goal, and to achieve this desired change in a suitable period using sensible methods. Descriptions of the various methods of body composition assessment are found elsewhere in this text. For athletes, the criteria for choosing a certain technique should include the validity, reliability and sensitivity of the method. Some methods are best suited to laboratory studies, while methods that are accessible and inexpensive can be used in the field by athletes and coaches. In practice, useful information about body composition can be collected from anthropometric data such as skinfold (subcutaneous) fat measurements, and various body girths and circumferences. Coaches or sports scientists who make these assessments on athletes should be well trained so that they have a small degree of error in repeating measurements. Regular monitoring of the body composition of an athlete can determine their individual 'ideal' physique at different times of the training and competition calendar. It can also monitor their success in achieving these ideals.

18.7 Weight maintenance and other body-weight issues

Losing weight

Many sports dietitians note that losing body weight or, more precisely, losing body fat, is the most common reason for an athlete to seek nutrition counseling. A small body size is useful to reduce the energy cost of activity, to improve temperature regulation in hot conditions, and to allow mobility to undertake twists and turns in a confined space. This physique is characteristic of athletes such as gymnasts, divers and marathon runners. A low level of body fat enhances the power to weight ratio over a range of body sizes, and is a desirable characteristic of many sports that require weight-bearing movement, particularly against gravity (e.g. distance running, mountain biking and uphill cycling, jumps and hurdles). However, low body-fat levels are also important for esthetic sports such as diving, gymnastics and figure skating, where judging involves appearance as well as skill.

There are many common situations in which an athlete's body-fat level increases above their healthy or ideal range. A common example is the athlete who comes back from an injury or a break from training several kilograms of body fat in excess of their usual playing weight. Where it is warranted, loss of body fat by an athlete should be achieved by a gradual program of sustained and moderate energy deficit, achieved by a decrease in dietary energy intake and, perhaps, an increase in energy expenditure through aerobic exercise or activity (see Box 18.3). However, many athletes in weight or fat-conscious sports strive to achieve very low body-fat levels, or to reduce body-fat levels below what seems their natural or healthy level. Although weight-loss efforts often produce a short-term improvement in performance, this must be balanced against the disadvantages related to having very low body-fat stores or following unsafe weight-loss methods. Excessive training, chronic low energy and nutrient intake, and psychological distress are often involved in fat-loss strategies and may cause long-term damage to health, happiness or performance.

Athletes should be encouraged to set realistic goals for body weight and body fat. These are specific to each individual and must be judged by trial and error over a period of time. 'Ideal' weight and body-fat targets should be set in terms of ranges, and should consider measures of long-term health and performance, rather than short-term benefits alone. In addition, the athlete should be able to achieve their targets while eating a diet that is adequate in energy and nutrients, and free of unreasonable food-related stress. Some racial groups or individuals naturally carry very low levels of body fat, or can achieve these without paying a substantial

Exercise performance 363

Box 18.3 Strategies for eating to lose body fat

- Identify individual 'ideal' body fat and body weight targets that are consistent with good health and performance, and are achievable.
- If loss of body fat is required, plan for a realistic rate loss of about 0.5 kg/week, and set both short-term and long-term goals.
- Examine current exercise and activity plans. If training is primarily skill or technique based, or a sedentary lifestyle between training sessions is observed, the athlete may benefit from scheduling in some aerobic exercise activities. This should always be done in conjunction with the coach.
- Take an objective look at what the athlete is really eating by arranging to keep a food diary for a period (e.g. a week). Many athletes who feel that they 'hardly eat anything' will be amazed at their hidden eating activities.
- Reduce typical energy intake by an amount that is appropriate to produce loss of body fat (e.g. 2–4 MJ or 500–1000 kcal/day) but still ensures adequate food and nutrient intake. An athlete should not reduce their energy intake below 5–6 MJ or 1200– 1500 kcal/day unless supervised by a sports dietitian. Meals should not be skipped; rather, food should be spread over the day, particularly to allow for efficient refueling after training sessions.
- Target occasions of overeating for special attention. Useful techniques include making meals filling by choosing high-fiber and low glycemic index forms of foods, fighting the need to finish everything on the plate, and spreading food intake over the day so that there is no need to approach meals feeling extreme hunger.
- Focus on opportunities to reduce intake of fats and oils. Such strategies include choosing low-fat versions of nutritious protein foods; minimizing added fats and oils in cooking and food preparation, and enjoying high-fat snack and sweet foods as occasional treats rather than everyday foods.
- Be moderate with alcohol intake (and perhaps sugar), since these may represent 'empty' kilojoules. Since alcohol intake is associated with relaxation, it is often associated with unwise eating.
- Focus on nutrient-rich foods so that nutrient needs can be met from a lower energy intake. A broad-range, low-dose vitamin/mineral supplement should be considered if daily energy intake is to be restricted below 6 MJ or 1500 kcal for prolonged periods.
- Be aware of inappropriate eating behavior. This includes eating when bored or upset, or eating too quickly. Stress or boredom should be handled using alternative activities.
- Be wary of supplements that promise weight loss. There are no special pills, potions or products that produce safe and effective weight loss. If something sounds too good to be true, it probably is.
- Note that a sports dietitian can assist athletes who are having difficulties with weight-loss goals, or would like a supervised program. Expert advice is needed for those who are struggling with an eating disorder or disordered eating behavior.

penalty. Furthermore, some athletes vary their body-fat levels over a season, so that very low levels are achieved only for a specific and short time. In general, however, athletes should not undertake strategies to minimize body-fat levels unless they can be sure there are no side-effects or disadvantages. Most importantly, the low body-fat levels of elite athletes should not be considered natural or necessary for recreational and subelite performers.

It is suggested that there is a higher risk of eating disorders, or disordered eating behaviors and body perceptions, among athletes in weight-division sports, or sports in which success is associated with lower body-fat levels than might be expected in the general community. Females seem at greater risk than males, reflecting the general dissatisfaction of females in the community with their body shape, as well as the biological predisposition for female athletes to have higher body-fat levels than male athletes, despite undertaking the same training program. Even where clinical eating disorders do not exist, many athletes appear to be restrained eaters, reporting energy intakes that are considerably less than their expected energy requirements. An adequate intake of energy is a prerequisite for many of the goals of sports nutrition.

Recently, the female athlete triad, the coexistence of disordered eating, disturbed menstrual function and suboptimal bone density, has received considerable publicity. This will be discussed in greater detail in the section below. Expert advice from sports medicine professionals, including dietitians, psychologists and physicians, is important in the early detection and management of problems related to body composition and nutrition.

Making weight

Some sports involve weight divisions in competition, with the goal of matching opponents of equal size and strength. Examples include combative sports (boxing, judo, wrestling), light-weight rowing and weight-lifting. Unfortunately, the culture and common practice in these sports is to try to compete in a weight division that is considerably lighter than normal training body weight. Athletes then 'make weight' over the days before the competition by dehydrating (via saunas, exercising in 'sweat clothes' and diuretics), and restricting food and fluid intake. The short-term penalties of these behaviors include the effect of dehydration and inadequate fuel status on performance. Long-term penalties include psychological stress, chronic inadequate nutrition and effects on hormone status. In 1997 three deaths were recorded among college wrestlers in the USA as a result of severe weight-making practices.

Athletes in these sports should be guided to make better choice of the appropriate competition weight division, and to achieve necessary weight loss by safe and long-term strategies to reduce body-fat levels.

Gaining muscle mass

Gain of muscle mass is desired by many athletes whose performance is linked to size, strength or power. Increases in muscle mass and strength occur during adolescence, particularly in males. In addition, many athletes pursue specific muscle hypertrophy gains through a program of progressive muscle overload. The main nutritional requirement for gain of muscle mass while undertaking a strength-training program is additional energy intake. This is required for the manufacture of new muscle tissue and other tissues needed to support it, as well as to provide fuel for the training program that supplied the stimulus for this muscle growth. Many athletes do not achieve an adequate energy intake to support these goals. Box 18.4 provides some practical strategies to address this challenge.

18.8 Vitamins and minerals

The daily requirement for at least some vitamins and minerals is increased beyond population levels in people undertaking a strenuous exercise program. The potential reasons for this increased requirement are increased loss through sweat, urine and perhaps feces, and through increased production of free radicals. Unfortunately, at present the additional micronutrient requirements of athletes cannot be quantified. The key factors ensuring an adequate intake of vitamins and minerals are a moderate to high energy intake and a varied diet based on nutritious foods. Dietary surveys show that most athletes report dietary practices that easily supply vitamin and minerals in excess of recommended daily allowances (RDAs) and are likely to meet any increases in micronutrient demand caused by training. However, not all athletes eat varied diets of adequate energy intake, and may need help to improve both the quality and quantity of their food selections.

Studies of the micronutrient status of athletes have not revealed any significant differences between indices in athletes and sedentary controls. The results suggest that athletic training, *per se*, does not lead to micronutrient deficiency. These data should, however,

---

Box 18.4 Strategies for eating to increase muscle mass

- Ensure that the athlete is following a well-devised weight training program that will stimulate muscle development and growth.
- Set goals for weight and strength gain that are practical and achievable. Continued increases of 2–4 kg/month are generally considered a good return.
- Be organized: apply the same dedication to the eating program as is applied to training, in order to increase their intake of nutrient-dense foods and supply a daily energy surplus of approximately 2–4 MJ (500–1000 kcal). This additional food should supply carbohydrate to fuel the training sessions, and adequate protein and micronutrients for the development and support of new tissue.
- Increase the number of times that they eat rather than the size of meals. This will enable greater intake of food with less risk of 'overfilling' and gastrointestinal discomfort. A supply of nutritious, high-carbohydrate snacks should be available between meals, particularly after training sessions.
- Avoid excessive intake of fiber, and include the use of 'white' cereals with less bulk (e.g. white rice, white bread). It is often impractical to consume a diet that is solely based on whole-grain and high-fiber foods.
- Make use of high-energy fluids such as milkshakes, fruit smoothies or commercial liquid meal supplements. These drinks provide a compact and low-bulk source of energy and nutrients, and can be consumed with meals or as snacks, including before or after a training session.
- Be aware that many athletes do not eat as much – or more importantly, as often – as they think. It is useful to examine the actual intake of athletes who fail to gain weight yet report 'constant eating'. Commitments such as training, sleep, medical/physiotherapy appointments, work or school often get in the way of eating opportunities. A food record will identify the hours and occasions of minimal food intake. This information should be used to reorganize the day, or to find creative ways to make nutritious foods and drinks part of the activity.

---

be interpreted very carefully since most indices are not sensitive enough to detect marginal deficiencies. Overall, generalized vitamin and mineral supplementation for all athletes is not justified. Furthermore, studies do not support an increase in performance with such supplementation, except in the case where a pre-existing deficiency was corrected.

The best management for the athlete with a high risk of suboptimal intake of micronutrients is to provide nutrition education to improve their food intake. However, a low-dose, broad-range multivitamin/mineral supplement may be useful where the athlete is unwilling or unable to make dietary changes, or when the athlete is traveling to places with an uncertain food supply and eating schedule.

Antioxidant vitamins

Exercise has been linked with an increased production of free oxygen radical species capable of causing cellular damage. A sudden increase in training stress (such as an increase in volume or intensity) or a stressful environment (training in hot conditions or at altitude) is believed to increase the production of these free oxygen radicals, leading to an increase in markers of cellular damage. Supplementation with antioxidant vitamins such as vitamin C or vitamin E is suggested to increase antioxidant status and provide protection against this damage.

The literature on the effects of antioxidant supplementation on antioxidant status, cellular damage and performance is complex and confusing. Some, but not all, studies show that acute supplementation during periods of increased stress may provide bridging protection until the athlete is able to adapt his or her own antioxidant status to meet this stress. It is possible that subtle benefits occur at a cellular level, which are too small to translate into detectable performance benefits. Whether ongoing supplementation is necessary for optimal training adaptations and competition performance of athletes is also unknown. Again, any benefits may be too small to detect.

Iron

Minerals are the micronutrients at most risk of inadequate intake in the diets of athletes. Inadequate iron status can reduce exercise performance via suboptimal levels of hemoglobin, and perhaps iron-related muscle enzymes. Reductions in the hemoglobin levels of distance runners first alerted sports scientists to the issue of iron status of athletes. However, more recent research has raised the problem of distinguishing true iron deficiency from alterations in iron status measures that are caused by exercise itself. Low iron status in athletes is overdiagnosed from single measures of low hemoglobin and ferritin levels. A major problem is the failure to recognize that the increase in blood volume that accompanies training will cause a dilution of all the blood contents. This hemodilution, often termed sports anemia, does not impair exercise performance.

Nevertheless, some athletes are at true risk of becoming iron deficient. The causes are essentially the same as for members of the general community: a lower than desirable intake of bioavailable iron and/or increased iron requirements or losses. Iron requirements may be increased in some athletes owing to growth needs, or to increased losses of blood and red blood cell destruction. However, the most common risk factor among athletes is a low-energy and/or low-iron diet, with females, restricted eaters, vegetarians and athletes eating high-carbohydrate, low-meat diets being likely targets.

Iron is found in a range of plant and animal food sources in two forms. Heme iron is found only in animal foods containing flesh or blood, whereas organic iron which is found both in animal foods and plant foods. Whereas heme iron is relatively well absorbed from single foods and mixed meals (15–35% bioavailability), the absorption of non-heme iron from single plant sources is low and variable (2–8%). The bioavailability of non-heme iron, and to a lesser extent heme ion, is affected by other foods consumed in the same meal. Factors that enhance iron absorption include vitamin C, peptides from fish, meat/and chicken, alcohol and food acids, while factors that inhibit absorption include phytates, polyphenols, calcium and peptides from plant sources such as soy protein. The absorption of both heme and non-heme iron is increased as an adaptive response in people who are iron deficient or have increased iron requirements. While the iron bioavailability studies from which these observations have been made have not been undertaken on special groups such as athletes, it is generally assumed that the results can be applied across populations of healthy people.

The assessment of total dietary iron intake of athletes is not necessarily a good predictor of their iron status; the mixing and matching of foods at meals plays an important role by determining the bioavailability of dietary iron intake. For example, in two groups of female runners who reported similar intakes of total dietary iron, the group that reported regular intake of meat was estimated to have a greater intake of absorbable iron and showed higher iron status than a matched group of runners who ate meat only occasionally.

Low iron status, indicated by serum ferritin levels lower than 20 ng/ml, should be considered for further assessment and treatment. Present evidence does not support that low iron status without anemia reduces exercise performance. However, many athletes with such low iron stores, or a sudden drop in iron status, frequently complain of fatigue and an inability to recover after heavy training. Many of these respond to strategies that improve iron status or prevent a further decrease in iron stores.

Evaluation and management of iron status should be undertaken on an individual basis by a sports medicine expert. Prevention and treatment of iron deficiency may include iron supplementation, with a recommended therapeutic dose of 100 mg/day of elemental iron for 2–3 months. However, the management plan should include dietary counseling to increase the intake of bioavailable iron, and appropriate strategies to reduce any unwarranted iron loss. Many athletes self-prescribe iron supplements; indeed, mass supplementation of athletes with iron has been fashionable at various times. However, these practices do not provide the athlete with the opportunity for adequate assessment of iron losses and expert dietary counseling from a sports dietitian. Dietary guidelines for increasing iron intake should be integrated with the athlete's other nutritional goals, such as a need for high carbohydrate intake or reduced energy intake (Box 18.5).

Calcium

Weight-bearing exercise is considered to be one of the best protectors of bone health. Therefore, it is puzzling to find reports of low body density in some female athletes, notably distance runners. However, a serious outcome of menstrual disturbances in female athletes is the high risk of either direct loss of bone density or failure to optimize the gaining of peak bone mass during early adulthood. Individually or in combination, these problems involved in the female athlete triad (disordered eating, menstrual dysfunction and reduced bone status) can directly impair athletic performance. Significantly, they will reduce the athlete's career span by increasing their risk of illness and injury, including stress fractures. Long-term problems may include an increased risk of osteoporosis in later life.

Optimal nutrition is important to correct factors that underpin the menstrual dysfunction, as well as those that contribute to suboptimal bone density. Adequate energy intake and the reversal of disordered eating or inadequate nutrient intake are important. A team approach involving a sports physician, sports dietitian, psychologist and/or psychiatrist, a coach and the family may be needed to treat the athlete with disordered eating or eating disorders.

Adequate calcium intake is important for bone health, and requirements may be increased to 1200–1500 mg/day in athletes with impaired menstrual function. Again, strategies to meet calcium needs must

---

Box 18.5 Strategies to meet iron and calcium needs

- Include heme iron-rich foods (red meats, shellfish, liver) regularly in meals, at least three to five times per week. These can be added to high-carbohydrate meal (e.g. meat sauce on a pasta dish; liver pâté in a sandwich).
- Enhance the absorption of non-heme iron (found in whole-grains, cereal foods, eggs, leafy green vegetables, etc.) by including a vitamin C food or meat/fish/chicken at the same meal. For example, a glass of orange juice may be consumed with breakfast cereal, or a small amount of lean meat can be added to beans to make a chilli con carne.
- Be aware that some foods (excess bran, strongly brewed tea) interfere with iron absorption from non-heme iron foods. Athletes who are at risk of iron deficiency should avoid these items, or separate them from meals.
- Take iron supplements only on the advice of a sports dietitian or doctor. They may be useful in the supervised treatment and prevention of iron deficiency, but are not a substitute for dietary improvements.
- Eat at least three servings of dairy foods a day, where one serving is equal to 200 ml of milk or a 200 g carton of yogurt. Low-fat and reduced-fat types are available. Dairy products can be added to a high-carbohydrate meal (e.g. milk on breakfast cereal, cheese in a sandwich).
- Use fortified soy products (soy milk, yogurts) when the athlete is unable to eat dairy products.
- Allow extra calcium for athletes who are growing, having a baby or breast-feeding. Dairy intake should be increased to four or five serving a day. Female athletes who are not having regular menstrual cycles also require extra calcium and should seek expert advice from a sports physician.
- Note that fish eaten with its bones (e.g. tinned salmon, sardines) is also a useful calcium source, and can also accompany a high-carbohydrate meal (e.g. salmon casserole with rice).
- Athletes who are vegetarian, or unable to eat dairy or soy products and red meat in these amounts, should seek the advice of a sports dietitian. With assistance they may find creative ways or the use of other foods to meet iron and calcium needs, or to use mineral supplements correctly.

---

be integrated into the total nutrition goals of the athlete. Where adequate calcium intake cannot be met through dietary means, usually through the use of low-fat dairy foods or calcium-enriched soy alternatives, a calcium supplement may be considered (see Box 18.5).

18.9 Fluid and electrolyte loss and replacement in exercise

Water has many important functions in the human body. Approximately 55–60% of the body is comprised of water. The total water content of the human body is between 30 and 50 liters. Every day we excrete water (sweat, urine, evaporative losses), while water intake may vary from 1 liter to about 12 liters per day. Water turnover can be very high in some conditions, but the total body water content is remarkably constant and rarely exceeds variations of 1 liter. However, during exercise and especially during exercise in hot conditions, sweat rates (and thus water losses) may increase dramatically and dehydration may occur (i.e. the body is in negative fluid balance). Dehydration can have an enormous impact on physical and mental function, and increases the risk of heat illness. Even mild dehydration can result in reduced exercise capacity.

Fluid losses

Exercise (muscle contraction) causes an increase in heat production in the body. Muscle contraction during most activities is only about 15–20% efficient. This means that of all the energy produced only about 15–20% is used for the actual movement and the remainder is lost as heat. For every liter of oxygen consumed during exercise approximately 16 kJ of heat is produced and only 4 kJ is actually used to perform mechanical work. If this heat was not dissipated the body would soon overheat.

When a well-trained individual is exercising at 80–90% $V_{O_2 max}$, the body's heat production may be more than 1000 W (i.e. 3.6 MJ/h). This could potentially cause the body core temperature to increase by 1°C every 5–8 min if no heat could be dissipated. As a result, body core temperature could approach dangerous levels in less than 20 min.

There are several mechanisms to dissipate this heat and to maintain body core temperature in a relatively narrow range: 36–38°C in resting conditions and 38–40°C during exercise and hot conditions. The most important cooling mechanism of the body is sweating, although radiation and convection can also contribute. Sweat must evaporate from the body surface to exert a cooling effect. Evaporation of 1 liter of water from the skin will remove 2.4 MJ of heat from the body. Although sweating is a very effective way to dissipate heat, it may cause dehydration if sweat losses are not replenished. This may cause further problems for the athlete: progressive dehydration impairs the ability to sweat and, therefore, to regulate body temperature. Body temperature rises more rapidly in the dehydrated state and this is commonly accompanied by a higher heart rate during exercise.

Fluid losses are mainly dependent on three factors:

- the ambient environmental conditions (temperature, humidity)
- the exercise intensity
- the duration of exercise and the duration of the heat exposure.

The environmental heat stress is determined by the ambient temperature, relative humidity, wind velocity and solar radiation. The relative humidity is the most important of these factors, since a high humidity will severely compromise the evaporative loss of sweat. Often sweat will drip off the skin in such conditions, rather than evaporate. This means that heat loss via this route will be less effective.

It is important to note that problems of hyperthermia and heat injury are not restricted to prolonged exercise in a hot environment: heat production is directly proportional to exercise intensity, so that very strenuous exercise, even in a cool environment, can cause a substantial rise in body temperature.

To maintain water balance, fluid intake must compensate for the fluid loss that occurs during exercise. Fluid intake is usually dependent on thirst feelings, but thirst (or the lack of thirst) can also be overridden by conscious control. It is important to note, however, that thirst is a poor indicator of fluid requirements or the degree of dehydration. In general, the sensation of feeling thirsty is not perceived until a person has lost at least 2% of body mass. As already mentioned, even this mild degree of dehydration is sufficient to impair exercise performance. It has also been shown that athletes tend to drink too little even when sufficient fluid is available.

Effects of dehydration

As the body becomes progressively dehydrated, a reduction in skin blood flow and sweat rate may occur. A high humidity may limit evaporative sweat loss, which will lead to further rises in core temperature, resulting in fatigue and possible heat injury to body tissues. The latter is potentially fatal.

Effect of dehydration on exercise performance

Several studies have shown that mild dehydration, equivalent to the loss of only 2% body weight, is sufficient to impair exercise performance significantly. In addition, it is often reported that losses of 4–5% of body weight or more can decrease the capacity for work by 20–30% (Figure 18.4). Even very low-intensity exercise (i.e. walking) is affected by dehydration. The capacity to perform high-intensity exercise which results in exhaustion within only a few minutes has been shown to be reduced by as much as 45% by prior dehydration (2.5% of body weight). Although there is little opportunity for sweat loss during such short-duration, high-intensity events, athletes who travel to compete in hot climates are likely to experience acute dehydration, which can persist for several days and can be of sufficient magnitude to have a detrimental effect on performance in competition. Although dehydration has detrimental effects, especially on performance in hot conditions, such effects can also be observed in cool conditions. Both decreases in maximal aerobic power ($V_{O_2 max}$) and decreases in endurance capacity have been reported with dehydration in temperate conditions.

There are several reasons why dehydration results in decreased exercise performance. First of all, a fall in plasma volume, decreased blood volume, increased blood viscosity and a lower central venous pressure can result in a reduced stroke volume and maximal cardiac output. In addition, during exercise in the heat, the dilatation of the skin blood vessels reduces the proportion of the cardiac output that is devoted to perfusion of the working muscles. Dehydration also impairs the ability of the body to lose heat. Both sweat rate and skin blood flow are lower at the same core temperature for the dehydrated compared with the euhydrated state. This means that body temperature rises more rapidly during exercise when the body is dehydrated. Finally, the larger rise in core temperature during exercise in the dehydrated state is associated with an increased rate of muscle glycogen breakdown. Depletion of these stores could also result in premature fatigue during prolonged exercise. In addition to the effects of dehydration on endurance, there are reported negative effects on coordination and cognitive functioning. This is likely to impact on all sports where skill and decision making are involved.

Heat illness

Dehydration poses a serious health risk in that it increases the risk of cramps, heat exhaustion and life-threatening heat stroke. Early symptoms of heat injury are excessive sweating, headache, nausea, dizziness, and reduced consciousness and mental function. When the core temperature rises to over 40°C, heat stroke may develop, characterized by hot, dry skin, confusion and loss of consciousness. There are several anecdotal reports of athletes and army recruits dying because of heat stroke. Most of these deaths have been explained by exercise in hot conditions, often with insufficient fluid intake. These problems affect not only highly trained athletes, but also less well-trained people participating in sport. Although well-trained individuals will generally exercise at higher intensities and therefore produce more heat, less well-trained individuals have less effective thermoregulation during exercise and work less economically. Overweight, unacclimated and ill individuals are especially likely to develop heat stroke.

Box 18.6 provides some drinking strategies for exercise in hot environments.

Box 18.6 Drinking strategies for exercise in hot environments

- In hot environments, be aware of factors that can affect heat accumulation during training or competition: time of day, length of play, conditions in indoor venues, and suitability of uniforms or protective gear.
- Players must begin each match properly hydrated. Fluid losses from previous matches or training need to be restored. It is also useful to drink immediately before a game. Players can learn to tolerate up to 5 ml/kg during the warm-up.
- Fluids should be consumed every 10–15 min. If rules of the sport prevent this practice, athletes may be able to find ways that work within the regulations.
- Players drink more of pleasant-tasting sports drinks than plain water. Sports drinks have the extra advantage of providing energy in situations where liver and muscle glycogen stores are likely to be depleted.
- Postmatch rehydration is an important part of recovery. Use drinks containing substantial amounts of carbohydrate and salts. Avoid excessive intake of alcohol.
- Athletes should practice the strategies in training so that they can implement them successfully in competition.

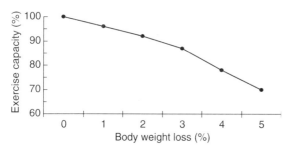

Figure 18.4 Effect of dehydration on exercise capacity.

Hyponatremia

Sweat loss results not only in the loss of water but also in a loss of electrolytes. Sodium is the most important ion lost in sweat. Replacement of electrolyte losses is necessary to maintain fluid balance, but may be more important after exercise than during exercise. A possible exception to this occurs in very prolonged exercise, where sweat losses are high and fluid intake is correspondingly high: in this situation, there may be a requirement for sodium replacement during exercise. An electrolyte imbalance, commonly referred to as 'water intoxication', which results from hyponatremia (low plasma sodium) due to excessive water consumption, has occasionally been reported in endurance athletes. This appears to be most common among slow runners in marathon and ultramarathon races, and probably arises through a loss of sodium in sweat coupled with very high intakes (8–10 liters) of water. The symptoms of hyponatremia are similar to those associated with dehydration, and include mental confusion, weakness and fainting. This means that there can be a danger of misdiagnosis of this condition when it occurs in individuals participating in endurance races. The usual treatment for dehydration is administration of fluid intravenously and orally. If this treatment were to be given to a hyponatremic individual, the consequences could be fatal.

Fluid intake strategies

Fluid intake during exercise can help to maintain plasma volume and prevent the adverse effects of dehydration on muscle strength, endurance and coordination. Elevating blood volume just before exercise by various hyperhydration (greater than normal body water content) strategies has also been suggested to be effective in enhancing exercise performance. When there is only little time in between two exercise bouts, rapid rehydration is crucial and drinking regimens need to be employed to optimize fluid delivery. Strategies for fluid replacement before, during and after exercise will be discussed in the following sections.

Pre-exercise hyperhydration

Since even mild dehydration has been shown to result in reduced exercise capacity, it has been hypothesized that hyperhydration could improve heat dissipation and exercise performance in the heat by expanding blood volume and reducing plasma osmolarity. Although some studies have reported higher sweating rates, lower core temperatures and lower heart rates during exercise after hyperhydration, some have also reported improvements in exercise performance. These results must be interpreted with caution. Some of these studies used a dehydrated state as a control condition and therefore it is impossible to conclude from these studies that hyperhydration improves thermoregulation and performance. However, the findings generally support the notion that hyperhydration reduces the thermal and cardiovascular strain of exercise.

The majority of studies have induced temporary hyperhydration by having subjects drink large volumes of water or water–electrolyte solutions for 1–3 h before exercise. However, much of the fluid overload is rapidly excreted and so expansions of the body water and blood volume are only transient. Greater fluid retention can be achieved if glycerol is added to fluids consumed before exercise. This will be discussed in the nutrition supplements section.

Fluid intake during exercise

To avoid dehydration during prolonged exercise fluids must be consumed to match the sweat losses. By regularly measuring body weight before and after a training session it is possible to obtain a good indication of fluid loss. Ideally, the weight loss is compensated by an equal amount of fluid intake. However, it may not always be possible to prevent dehydration completely.

Sweat rates during strenuous exercise in the heat can amount up to 2–3 l/h. Such large volumes of fluid are difficult if not impossible to ingest and even 1 liter may feel quite uncomfortable in the stomach. Therefore, it is often not practically possible to achieve fluid intakes that match sweat losses during exercise. Another factor that can make the ingestion of large amounts of fluid difficult is the fact that in some sports or disciplines the rules or practicalities of the specific sport may limit the opportunities for drinking during exercise.

Fluid intake may be useful during exercise longer than 30–60 min, but there is no advantage during strenuous exercise of less than 30 min in duration. During such high-intensity exercise gastric emptying is inhibited and the drink may cause gastrointestinal distress with no performance benefit.

Practice drinking during training

Although it is often difficult to tolerate the volumes of fluid needed to prevent dehydration, the volume of

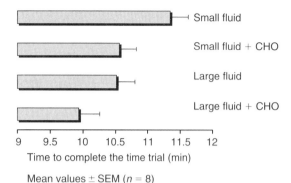

Mean values ± SEM ($n = 8$)

Figure 18.5 The effect of carbohydrate (CHO) and fluid intake during exercise is additive. Subjects performed steady-state exercise followed by a performance measurement (time trial). The shorter the time to complete the time trial, the better the performance. They ingested a small amount of fluid (no carbohydrate), a small amount of fluid plus carbohydrate, a large amount of fluid with no carbohydrate, or a large amount of fluid with carbohydrate. (Adapted from Below *et al.*, 1995.)

fluid that is tolerable is trainable and can be increased with frequent drinking in training. Often this is neglected during training. Training to drink will accustom athletes to the feeling of exercising with fluid in the stomach. It also gives the opportunity to experiment with different volumes and flavorings to determine how much fluid intake they can tolerate and which formulations suit them best.

Composition of sports drinks

Numerous studies have shown that regular water intake during prolonged exercise is effective in improving performance. Fluid intake during prolonged exercise also offers the opportunity to provide some fuel (carbohydrate). The addition of some carbohydrate to drinks consumed during exercise has been shown to have an additive independent effect in improving exercise performance (Figure 18.5). The ideal drink for fluid and energy replacement during exercise is one that tastes good to the athlete, does not causes gastrointestinal discomfort when consumed in large volumes, is rapidly emptied from the stomach and absorbed in the intestine, and provides energy in the form of carbohydrate.

Sports drinks typically have three main ingredients: water, carbohydrate and sodium. The water and carbohydrate provide fluid and energy, respectively, while sodium is included to aid water absorption and retention.

Although carbohydrate is important, a too concentrated carbohydrate solution may provide more fuel for the working muscles but will decrease the amount of water that can be absorbed owing to a slowing of gastric emptying. Water is absorbed into the body primarily through the small intestine, but the absorption of water is decreased if the concentration of dissolved carbohydrate (or other substances) in the drink is too high. In this situation, water will be drawn out of the interstitial fluid and plasma into the lumen of the small intestine by osmosis. So long as the fluid remains hypotonic with respect to plasma, the uptake of water from the small intestine is not adversely affected. The presence of small amounts of glucose and sodium tend to increase slightly the rate of water absorption compared with pure water. It must be emphasized here that the addition of sodium and other electrolytes to sports drinks is to increase palatability, maintain thirst (and therefore promote drinking), prevent hyponatremia and increase the rate of water uptake, rather than to replace the electrolyte losses through sweating. Replacement of the electrolytes lost in sweat can normally wait until the postexercise recovery period.

Rehydration after exercise

When there is little time for recovery in between exercise bouts, the replacement of fluid and electrolytes in the postexercise recovery period is of crucial importance. In the limited time available the athlete should strive to maximize rehydration. The main factors influencing the effectiveness of postexercise dehydration are the volume and composition of the fluid consumed. Plain water is not the ideal postexercise rehydration beverage when rapid and complete restoration of body fluid balance is necessary and where all intake is in liquid form. Ingestion of water alone in the postexercise period results in a rapid fall in the plasma sodium concentration and the plasma osmolarity. These changes have the effect of reducing the stimulation to drink (thirst) and increasing the urine output, both of which will delay the rehydration process. Plasma volume is more rapidly and completely restored in the postexercise period if sodium chloride (77 mmol/l or 450 mg/l) is added to the water consumed. This sodium concentration is similar to the upper limit of the sodium concentration found in sweat, but is considerably higher than that of many commercially available sports drinks, which usually contain 10–25 mmol/l (60–150 mg/l).

Ingesting a beverage containing sodium not only promotes rapid fluid absorption in the small intestine, but also allows the plasma sodium concentration to remain elevated during the rehydration period and helps to maintain thirst while delaying stimulation of urine production. The inclusion of potassium in

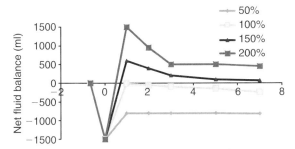

Figure 18.6 Net fluid balance after exercise with the ingestion of different volumes of a drink. Ingestion of 150% or more of weight loss is required to achieve normal hydration within 6 h after exercise. (Reproduced from Shirreffs et al., 1996 with permission of Lippincott Williams & Wilkins.)

the beverage consumed after exercise would be expected to enhance the replacement of intracellular water and thus promote rehydration, but currently there is little experimental evidence to support this. The rehydration drink should also contain carbohydrate (glucose or glucose polymers) because the presence of glucose will also stimulate fluid absorption in the gut and improve beverage taste. Following exercise, the uptake of glucose into the muscle for glycogen resynthesis should also promote intracellular rehydration.

It has become clear that to restore fluid balance after exercise much more than the fluid lost as sweat has to be consumed. This is because some of the ingested fluid will be excreted in urine. Recent studies indicate that ingestion of 150% or more of weight loss is required to achieve normal hydration within 6 h after exercise (Figure 18.6). Current American College of Sports Medicine (ACSM) guidelines on fluid ingestion before, during and after exercise, formulated and published in 1996, are shown in Table 18.2.

Table 18.2 Summary of the American College of Sports Medicine Position Stand on Exercise and Fluid Replacement (1996). Reproduced with permission.

It is the position of the American College of Sports Medicine that adequate fluid replacement helps maintain hydration and, therefore, promotes the health and safety and optimal physical performance of individuals participating in regular physical activity. This position statement is based on a comprehensive review and interpretation of scientific literature concerning the influence of fluid replacement on exercise performance and the risk of thermal injury associate with dehydration and hyperthermia. Based on available evidence, the American College of Sports Medicine makes the following general recommendations on the amount and composition of fluid that should be ingested in preparation for, during and after exercise of athletic competition.

1. It is recommended that individuals consume a nutritionally balanced diet and drink adequate fluids during the 24 h period before an event, especially during the period that includes the meal before exercise, to promote proper hydration before exercise or competition.
2. It is recommended that individuals drink about 500 ml of fluid about 2 h before exercise to promote adequate hydration and allow time for excretion of excess ingested water.
3. During exercise, athletes should start drinking early and at regular intervals in an attempt to consume fluids at a rate sufficient to replace all the water lost through sweating (i.e. body weight loss), or to consume the maximal amount that can be tolerated.
4. It is recommended that ingested fluids be cooler than ambient temperature (between 15 and 22°C) and flavored to enhance palatability and promote fluid replacement. Fluids should be readily available and served in containers that allow adequate volumes to be ingested with ease and with minimal interruption of exercise.
5. Addition of proper amounts of carbohydrates and/or electrolytes to a fluid replacement solution is recommended for exercise events of duration greater than 1 h since it does not significantly impair water delivery to the body and may enhance performance. During exercise lasting for 1 h there is little evidence of physiological or physical performance differences between consuming a carbohydrate–electrolyte drink and plain water.
6. During intense exercise lasting for longer than 1 h, it is recommended that carbohydrates be ingested at a rate of 30–60 g/h to maintain oxidation of carbohydrates and delay fatigue. This rate of carbohydrate intake can be achieved without compromising fluid delivery by drinking 600–1200 ml/h of solutions containing 4–8% carbohydrates (g/100 ml). The carbohydrates can be sugars (glucose or sucrose) or starch (e.g. maltodextrin).
7. Inclusion of sodium (0.5–0.7 g/l of water) in the rehydration solution ingested during exercise lasting longer than 1 h is recommended since it many be advantageous in enhancing palatability, promoting fluid retention and possibly preventing hyponatremia in certain individuals who drink excessive quantities of fluid. There is little physiological basis for the presence of sodium in an oral rehydration solution for enhancing intestinal water absorption as long as sodium is sufficiently available from the previous meal.

18.10 Nutritional ergogenics

The dietary supplement industry has grown enormously and annual sales were estimated to be US$ 12 billion in 1998. Up to US$ 800 million was spent on 'sports supplements'. Studies of the dietary practices of athletes report that nutritional supplements are used by 40–100% of all athletes in one form or another. There is also evidence that athletes use combinations of nutrition supplements and sometimes they ingest very high doses. The claims and the experimental evidence for a selection of common supplements will be reviewed here. Since there are now over 600 nutrition supplements on the market it is impossible to review them all, but here the focus is on the most common ones. The most important supplements will be discussed below in alphabetical order.

Caffeine

Caffeine is probably one of the most common drugs used by humans. It is an interesting and controversial substance because on the one hand most people drink coffee or tea, but on the other hand it is a banned substance for athletes. It has been claimed that caffeine improves performance and the International Olympic Committee (IOC) allows a certain (arbitrary) limit of 12 mg/l in urine.

Caffeine originates naturally in 63 species of plants. The main sources for these substances are coffee beans, tea leaves, cacao beans and cola nuts. Caffeine and caffeine-like substances can be found in a variety of foods and drinks, but the majority (about 75%) of all caffeine consumption is through coffee.

Caffeine and exercise performance

Studies in the 1970s demonstrated that caffeine ingested 1 h before exercise increased plasma fatty acid concentrations and improved subsequent exercise performance. Although not all studies have demonstrated effects of caffeine on endurance performance, the majority of studies have shown improved endurance capacity after ingesting caffeine. At exercise intensities around 80–85% $V_{O_2 max}$ improvements of 10–20% are typically found in time to exhaustion. Caffeine also seems to improve exercise performance of very high intensity (around 100% $V_{O_2 max}$) lasting for approximately 5 min, but sprint performance seems to be unaffected by caffeine.

Initially, the observed improvements in performance were explained by the increased availability of fatty acids, which would lead to a suppression of carbohydrate metabolism and consequently to a decreased glycogen utilization. However, there are alternative explanations such as effects on neuromuscular pathways, facilitating recruitment of muscle fibers or increasing the number of fibers recruited, direct effects of caffeine on muscle ion handling, enhanced anaerobic energy production or an effect on the brain, resulting in decreased sensations of effort. The central effects of caffeine are the most likely explanation for the relatively large improvements in performance and lowered rating of perceived exertion.

In conclusion, the vast majority of the studies reported an ergogenic effect of 3–9 mg caffeine/kg body weight in endurance exercise (1–2 h). Some studies did not find an effect, but this may be due to differences in the experimental protocol or day-to-day variation in the performance measurement. The mechanisms are still largely unknown.

Cognitive functioning

Caffeine also has an effect on cognitive functioning, which is likely to be important in many sports. In one study, caffeine was added to a carbohydrate–electrolyte solution, which was consumed before and during exercise. Cognitive functioning (attention, psychomotor skills and memory) was measured immediately after a time trial (approximately 1 h all-out exercise). Caffeine improved all measures of cognitive functioning and these effects were evident for the ingestion of 2 and 3 mg caffeine/kg body weight.

Dosage

Few studies have investigated the effects of different doses of caffeine on exercise performance (or endurance capacity). In one study, subjects received three different doses of caffeine or placebo 1 h before a ride to exhaustion at 75% of peak power output. The doses were 0, 5, 9 and 13 mg caffeine/kg body weight. Already with the lowest dose (5 mg/kg body weight) endurance capacity was improved by 20%, but a further increase in dosage had no further effect on performance (Figure 18.7). In runners it was shown that ingestion of 3 mg caffeine/kg body weight and 6 mg/kg body weight had positive effects, whereas the improvement in time to exhaustion with 9 mg/kg body weight did not reach statistical significance.

More recently the effect of adding relatively small amounts of caffeine (2, 3 or 4.5 g/kg body weight) to

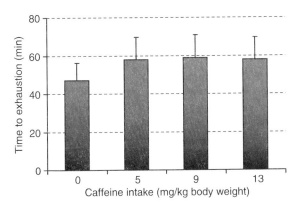

Figure 18.7 Effect of different dosages of caffeine or placebo 1 h before a ride on time to exhaustion at 75% of peak power output. With the lowest dose (5 mg/kg body weight) endurance capacity was improved by 20%, but a further increase in dosage had no further effect on performance. (Reproduced with permission from Pasman *et al.*, 1995.)

a carbohydrate–electrolyte solution was studied. Time trial performance was improved with the lowest dosage of 2 g/kg body weight, was further improved with 3 g/kg, but the highest dose did not further affect performance. Taken together, the most recent studies show that caffeine has a positive effect on exercise performance on doses that are lower than previously used (i.e. ~3 mg/kg body weight). Most importantly, it appears that caffeine does not have a dose response; that is, that larger doses do not appear to produce a greater effect on performance.

Side-effects

Caffeine has several side-effects, especially at high dosages. These include gastrointestinal distress, headaches, tachycardia, restlessness, irritability, tremor, elevated blood pressure, psychomotor agitations and premature left ventricular contractions. This is all caused by the effect of caffeine on the central nervous system. Caffeine is also a diuretic and is therefore not advisable to consume it in the hours before exercise when hydration is required. During exercise, however, the diuretic effect of caffeine is counteracted by catecholamines and urine production is minimized. Intake of very high doses of caffeine has been associated with peptic ulcer, seizures, coma, and even death.

Carnitine

L-Carnitine is a natural substance, present in relatively high quantities in meat. Oral carnitine supplementation in humans for periods of 2–3 weeks does not increase the carnitine concentration in muscle and does not have an effect on muscle metabolism at rest or during exercise. In contrast to the claims made for carnitine supplements, there is no evidence that carnitine supplementation reduces body-fat mass, increases fat oxidation or reduces glycogen breakdown during prolonged exercise. In addition, carnitine supplementation does not increase $V_{O_2\,max}$ and does not reduce lactate accumulation during maximal and supramaximal exercise.

Chromium

Chromium is a trace element that is present in foods such as brewer's yeast, mushrooms, and wheat-germ, and is considered an essential nutrient. Supplemental forms of chromium have become very popular in recent years, with claims that they increase muscle bulk and reduce body-fat levels. It has been reported that chromium increases insulin action, and insulin stimulates glucose and amino acid uptake by cells. It is thought that by stimulating amino acid uptake, there will be an increase in protein synthesis and muscle mass gain. Although there is some evidence that chromium supplements increase muscle mass and growth in animals, the effect on muscle mass in humans is less clear.

The vast majority of studies have not found effects of chromium on changes in body composition (percentage body fat, lean body mass). In a recent well-controlled study, the effect of 8 weeks of chromium supplementation, or a placebo, in untrained men who started a resistance-training program was examined. Although chromium supplements increased urinary chromium excretion they had no effect on body composition. It must therefore be concluded that the vast majority of the studies demonstrate that chromium supplements are not effective in increasing lean body mass.

Coenzyme Q10

Coenzyme Q10 (CoQ10) or ubiquinone is an integral part of the electron transport chain of the mitochondria and therefore plays an important role in oxidative phosphorylation. CoQ10 is especially present in heart muscle and has been used therapeutically to treat cardiovascular disease and post cardiac surgery. In these patients, CoQ10 supplementation improves oxidative metabolism and exercise capacity . Manufacturers have extrapolated the results of improved $V_{O_2\,max}$ in cardiac patients to healthy and trained athletes. It is claimed that coenzyme Q10 increases $V_{O_2\,max}$ and increases 'stamina' and 'energy'.

Few studies have investigated the effects of CoQ10 supplementation in athletes. Although most of these studies report elevated plasma CoQ10 levels, no changes were observed in $V_{O_2 max}$, performance, or lactate at submaximal workloads. CoQ10 is also marketed as an antioxidant.

Recently it was reported that ingestion of 120 mg CoQ10/day for 20 days resulted in marked increases in plasma CoQ10 concentrations, but the muscle CoQ10 concentration was unaltered. This observation leads us to conclude that most claims are unfounded. There may even be some negative effects of CoQ10. It has been reported that during high exercise intensity when there is an abundance of hydrogen ions in the cells, CoQ10 can even augment free radical production. Paradoxically, this is the opposite effect of what CoQ10 is claimed to do.

Creatine

Creatine became a popular supplement in the early 1990s after several successful athletes supposedly used creatine supplements. By the time of the next Olympic Games in Atlanta in 1996, approximately 80% of all athletes were reported to use creatine. The creatine consumption by athletes all over the world is now estimated to be around 3.0 million kg/year.

What is creatine?

Creatine is a naturally occurring compound mostly present in meat and fish. It is not an essential nutrient because it can be synthesized in the liver and kidney. In normal healthy individuals diet and oral ingestion together provide approximately 2 g of creatine/day. At the same time and at approximately the same rate (2 g/day), creatine is broken down to creatinine and excreted in the urine. Strict vegetarians and vegans will have negligible creatine intake because plants contain only trace amounts of creatine. They are therefore dependent on endogenous synthesis of creatine. Oral ingestion of creatine suppresses the biosynthesis. In a 70 kg man, the total body creatine pool is approximately 120 mg, most (95%) of which is found in muscle, with small amounts in the liver, brain, kidney and testes.

Functions of phosphocreatine

The role of creatine and phosphocreatine (PCr) was discussed at the beginning of this chapter. In brief, the transfer of the phosphate group from creatine phosphate to ADP results in the regeneration of ATP:

$$PCr + ADP + H^+ \rightarrow Creatine + ATP$$

Phosphocreatine is present in resting muscle in a concentration that is three to four times that of ATP, and anaerobic degradation of phosphocreatine and glycogen is responsible for a significant rate of ATP resynthesis during the first seconds of high-intensity exercise. However, the phosphocreatine store in muscle is small and could be depleted within 4–5s of supramaximal exercise. Elevated stores could potentially provide more energy. High phosphocreatine stores may also reduce the need for anaerobic glycolysis and lactic acid formation during intense exercise, and this might be another potential benefit of phosphocreatine. A third important function of creatine is its potential buffering capacity for hydrogen ions as these ions are used during ATP regeneration (see metabolic reaction above). The roles of creatine listed above suggest that elevating muscle creatine and phosphocreatine stores would benefit high-intensity exercise performance.

Effects of creatine supplementation

In 1992 Harris and colleagues were the first to describe that ingesting creatine monohydrate could increase muscle total creatine stores (creatine and phosphocreatine). In that study ingesting 5 g of creatine four to six times per day for several days increased the total creatine concentration by an average of 20–25 mmol/kg dry weight. This increase corresponded to about 20% of the basal muscle total creatine concentration of about 125 mmol/kg dry weight. About one-third of the increase in total creatine content was in the form of phosphocreatine. The authors suggested that this could improve exercise performance, but did not measure this in this study. In a subsequent study, ingestion of 20 g of creatine/day for 5 days improved performance by about 6% during repeated bouts of maximal knee extensor exercise. This initial study was followed by a large number of studies in which different modes of exercise were investigated. About two-thirds of all studies report positive effects of creatine supplementation, with the most favorable scenario being intermittent bouts of very high-intensity exercise with relatively short recovery periods (e.g. interval training, resistance training, team sports). Typically, performance improvements are found not in the first few sprints but after several repeated sprints. No studies have reported a benefit of creatine supplementation on endurance performance. Long-term creatine supplementation in combination with strength training appears to be more effective than strength training only. Creatine supplementation may allow more repetitions and thus a better quality of training, and it has been suggested that creatine may also have anabolic effects. There are some indications that creatine may have an anabolic effect.

Further studies have found that creatine loading can be achieved through a 'slower' loading protocol, with a daily dose of 3 g/day. In addition, creatine uptake and muscle total creatine can be increased more when creatine is ingested in combination with carbohydrate. In this manner, the total creatine concentration of muscle can be increased in most subjects to levels approaching the upper limit (i.e. ~160 mmol/kg dry weight of muscle). It is thought that carbohydrate ingestion stimulates muscle creatine uptake via an insulin-dependent mechanism.

Not everyone may benefit from creatine

It is important to note that not everyone may benefit from creatine supplementation. This may be related to the fact that there is considerable variation between subjects in the initial muscle total creatine concentration. The largest increase in muscle creatine concentration is observed in individuals with the lowest initial concentration, while individuals with an already high creatine concentration benefit only marginally (Figure 18.8). A concentration of 160 mmol/kg dry matter

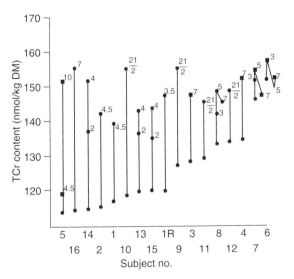

Figure 18.8 Effect of creatine loading on muscle total creatine (TCr) content. Individuals with low initial creatine concentrations seem to benefit more from supplementation than those with already high concentrations. There also seems to be an upper limit for total creatine concent of about 160 mmol/kg day weight. (Reproduced from Hultman *et al.*, 1996.)

appears to be the maximal creatine concentration achievable as a result of creatine supplementation. The reasons for these individual differences are largely unknown, but may at least partly be related to the habitual diet.

Studies have shown that individuals who display the largest increases in muscle total creatine concentration also exhibit the largest performance benefit. It has been suggested that a change in muscle creatine content of about 20 mmol/kg dry weight should be present before significant changes in performance can be observed. About 30% of all individuals will not display such large increases in muscle creatine and therefore will not benefit. These people are often referred to as non-responders.

Side-effects

Creatine supplementation is generally accompanied by increases in body weight of approximately 1 kg, although some individuals may gain minimal weight and others as much as 3.5 kg. This increase in body weight results from increases in intracellular water. The increase in body weight may be beneficial or have no effect in some disciplines, but can be detrimental to performance in weight-bearing activities (such as running or gymnastics). There are numerous anecdotal reports that creatine supplementation caused gastrointestinal, cardiovascular and muscular problems, as well as nausea, vomiting and diarrhea, but there are no scientific studies to confirm this. There is also no evidence of alterations in renal or liver function, the occurrence of muscle cramps or elevated blood pressure. However, as pointed out in a round-table discussion by the ACSM: 'The evidence is not definitive and/or it is incomplete to indict the practice of creatine supplementation as a health risk; at the same time, our lack of information cannot be taken as an assurance that creatine supplementation is free from health risks. Ignorance provides little comfort of untoward effects yet to be discovered'.

Conclusion

Oral creatine supplementation of 20 g/day for 5–6 days increases the muscle total creatine content in men by about 20% (30–40% of the increase is phosphocreatine). A subsequent daily dose of 2 g is enough for maintenance of this increased concentration. Coingestion with carbohydrate accelerates creatine loading. Creatine loading increases the amount of work performed during single and repeated bouts of short-lasting, high-intensity exercise. No studies have shown an ergogenic effect on endurance performance. Besides weight gain, creatine does not seem to have major side-effects. However, the long-term effects of creatine ingestion are unknown and therefore caution must be exercised.

Fish oil

It has been suggested that by increasing the fraction of polyunsaturated fatty acids in the phospholipids of erythrocyte membranes, membrane fluidity would be improved and red blood cell deformability increased, resulting in improved peripheral oxygen supply. Such changes in red blood cell deformability and a change in the fatty acid composition of membranes toward, a higher percentage of unsaturated fatty acids are also seen after exercise training. This could at least theoretically be accomplished by consuming a diet high in fish oil or by taking fish oil capsules.

Controlled studies supplemented trained cyclists for 3 weeks with placebo or fish oil (6 g/day). Fish oil did not alter red blood cell characteristics in this study and had no effect on V_{O_2} max, maximal power output or time trial performance. It can be concluded that fish oil could potentially have some long-term positive effects, but at present scientific evidence is lacking to support claims that fish oil improves maximal oxygen uptake and performance.

Glycerol

Glycerol has been studied as an ergogenic aid for two reasons. First, it was believed to be a substrate for gluconeogenesis and as such could provide a fuel during exercise. However, more important is probably the role of glycerol as a way to hyperhydrate before exercise in hot environmental conditions. Glycerol is a small molecule which, when ingested with a large amount of water (1–2 liters), has been found to improve water absorption and water retention in the extracellular space, especially the plasma. Hyperhydration with glycerol before exercise has been shown to decrease overall heat stress during exercise, as indicated by lower heart rate and body temperature. A recent study demonstrated that glycerol, ingested with a bolus of water 2 h before exercise, resulted in fluid retention, reduced cardiovascular strain and enhanced thermoregulation. Furthermore, this practice increased exercise performance in the heat. There are, however, quite a few studies in which no effect of glycerol was found on thermoregulation. It has been suggested that in these studies the volume of water consumed (500 ml) may have been too small.

In general, however, the ingestion of 1 g of glycerol/kg body weight with 1–2 liters of water seems to protect against heat stress and may thus have some health benefits when exercising in extreme conditions.

Side-effects of glycerol

When considering glycerol as an ergogenic aid it must be kept in mind that it can have quite a few unwanted side-effects. The most reported side-effects are nausea, heartache, blurred vision, headaches, gastrointestinal problems, dizziness and light-headedness. The large volume of fluid that needs to be consumed with the glycerol can cause some problems, and many subjects report a bloated feeling.

Conclusions

Glycerol seems to reduce cardiovascular stress and improve thermoregulation, which in some studies may have caused the observed improvements in exercise performance. However, glycerol has quite a few side-effects, including gastrointestinal discomfort arising from the coingestion of very large amounts of fluid.

18.11 Dietary supplements and failed drug tests

Dietary supplements may cause a failed doping test. There have been several recent cases in which failed doping tests were ascribed to dietary supplement use. Most of the recent attention has been on nandrolone, but other banned substances have also been found in these supplements. There are many cases in which athletes tested positive for ephedrine or caffeine after using herbal products. More recently, traces of steroids or prohormones have been detected in a variety of nutrition supplements; in fact, in one study conducted by an IOC accredited laboratory, 15% of supplements contained a banned substance (prohormone or testosterone) that was not declared on the product label. When such supplements are given to volunteers and urine samples are collected the results often indicate a positive doping test. The regulations for nutrition supplements are less strict than those for medical products and therefore it is difficult to control the quality of a product. Even dietary supplements that are labeled as being safe for use by athletes may be contaminated.

At present there is little an athlete can do to ensure that the products used are safe. Reputable brands of common supplements produced by major food and drug companies that are normally manufactured with the highest standards are likely to be safer than products from small manufacturers. The athlete will have to make a decision as to whether the supposed effect of the supplement is worth the risk of a positive drug test.

18.12 Practical issues in nutrition for athletes

Despite the sports nutrition knowledge available to modern athletes and coaches, sports nutritionists report that athletes do not always achieve the practices of optimal sports nutrition. A number of factors may be involved:

- poor understanding of sports nutrition principles; reliance on myths and misconceptions
- failure to recognize the specific nutritional requirements of different sports and individuals within these sports
- apparent conflict of nutrition goals (e.g. how can an athlete achieve increased requirements for nutrients such as carbohydrate and iron while limiting energy intake to achieve loss of body fat?)
- lack of practical nutrition knowledge and skills (e.g. knowledge of food composition, domestic skills such as food purchasing, preparation and cooking)
- overcommitted lifestyle; inadequate time and opportunities to obtain or consume appropriate foods owing to heavy workload of sport, work, school, etc.
- inadequate finances
- the challenge of frequent travel.

Given the specific nutritional requirements of sports and individuals, according to age and gender, it is impossible to prepare a single set of nutrition guidelines for athletes. Nevertheless, education tools that address key issues of nutrition for athletes are an important resource for coaches, athletes and sports nutritionists. Education strategies that focus on practical areas of food choice and preparation, and guidelines that can address a number of key nutrition issues simultaneously are most valuable. In situations where nutritional goals can be achieved by modest changes

> **Box 18.7** Strategies for eating well while traveling
>
> - Investigate the food resources at the trip destination, before leaving. People who have traveled previously to that country, competition or accommodation facility may be able to warn about likely problems, and allow the preparation of a suitable plan in advance.
> - Organize special menus and meals in restaurants, airplanes or hotels in advance.
> - Find out about food hygiene and water safety in new countries. It may be necessary to restrict fluid intake to bottled or boiled drinks, and to avoid foods that are high risk for contamination (e.g. unpeeled fruits and vegetables).
> - Take some foods supplies on the trip if important foods are likely to be unavailable or expensive. Foods that are portable and low in perishability include breakfast cereals, milk powder, tinned and dehydrated foods, and special sports supplements.
> - Be aware of special nutritional requirements in the new location. Be prepared to meet increased requirements for fluid, carbohydrate and other nutrients.

to typical population eating patterns, it may be sufficient to provide a set of behavioral strategies to guide athletes to achieve such changes. However, in situations where the athlete has extreme nutrient requirements, where nutritional goals appear to conflict or where medical problems are present, the athlete should be directed to seek individualized and expert counseling from a sports nutritionist or dietitian.

It should be appreciated that many of the practical challenges to achieving sports nutrition goals arise directly because of exercise or the environment in which it is undertaken. Goals of nutrition before, during and after a workout or training must often be compromised or modified because of the effects of exercise on gastrointestinal function and comfort. Access to foods and drinks is often restricted in the busy day of the athlete, or in the exercise environment. The frequent travel schdeules of the athlete must also be negotiated in dietary advice. In many cases the expertise of the sports dietitian is required to provide creative ways to meet sports nutrition goals. Strategies for the traveling athlete are summarized in Box 18.7.

18.13 Perpectives on the future

A significant proportion of the future reserach in the area of sports nutrition will be focussed on recovery. New strategies to improve glycogen and protein synthesis or to reduce protein breakdown will be explored.

Thus far, the work in this area has been limited because the techniques to study protein metabolism are complicated and very expensive. The work in this area will be important for all sports at high level where the amount of training that can be performed is often crucial to performance. All methods to reduce recovery time can be beneficial. In addition, refinements will be made to optimize the fluid and carbohydrate delivery from sports drinks. It is also likely that more new supplements will be promoted and researched.

Further reading

Achten J, Gleeson M, Jeukendrup AE. Determination of the exercise intensity that elicits maximal fat oxidation. Med Sci Sports Exerc. 2002; 34: 92–9.

American College of Sports Medicine. Position stand: exercise and fluid replacement. Med Sci Sports Exerc 1996; 28: i–viii.

American College of Sports Medicine. Weight loss in wrestlers. Med Sci Sports Exerc 1996; 28: ix–xii.

American College of Sports Medicine. Roundtable: The physiological and health effects of oral creatine supplementation. Med Sci Sports Exerc 2000; 32: 706–717.

American College of Sports Medicine, American Dietetic Association, Dietitians of Canada. Nutrition and athletic performance. Med Sci Sports Exerc 2000; 32: 2130–2145.

Below PR, Mora-Rodriguez R, Gonzáles Alonso J, Coyle EF. Fluid and carbohydrate ingestion independently improve performance during 1 h of intense exercise. Med Sci Sports Exerc 1995; 27(2): 200–210

Brownell KD, Rodin J. Prevalence of eating disorders in athletes. In: Eating Body Weight and Performance in Athletes: Disorders of Modern Society (KD Brownell, J Rodin, JH Wilmore, eds), pp. 128–145. Philadelphia, PA: Lea & Febiger, 2000.

Burke L, Deakin V, eds. Clinical Sports Nutrition, 2nd edn. Sydney: McGraw Hill, 2000.

Costill DL, Bowers R, Branam G, Sparks K. Muscle glycogen utilization during prolonged exercise on successive days. J Appl Physiol 1971; 31: 834-838

Hultman E, Soderlund K, Timmons A Cederblad G, Greenhaff PL. Muscle creatine loading in men. J Appl Physiol 1996; 81(l): 232–237

Jeukendrup AE, Saris WHM, Wagenmakers AJM. Fat metabolism during exercise: a review. Part III: Effects of nutritional interventions. Int J Sports Med 1998; 19(5): 371–379

Maughan RJ, ed. IOC Encyclopedia of Sports Medicine: Nutrition in Sport. Oxford: Blackwell Science, 2000.

Pasman WJ, van Baak MA, Jeukendrup AE, deHaan A. The effect of varied dosages of caffeine on endurance performance time. Int J Sports Med 1995; 16(4): 225–230

Romijn JA, Coyle EF, Sidossis LS et al. Regulation of endogenous fat and carbohydrate metabolism in relation to exercise intensity. Am J Physiol 1993; 265: E380–E391.

Shirreffs SM, Taylor AJ, Leiper JB, Maughan RJ. Post-exercise rehydration in man: effects of volume consumed and drink sodium content. Med Sci Sports Exerc 1996; 28(10): 1260–1271.

Index

Note: page numbers in *italics* refer to illustrations and boxes, those in **bold** refer to tables